**"For the
Welfare of
Mankind"**

"For the Welfare of Mankind"

The Commonwealth Fund and American Medicine

A. McGehee Harvey, M.D.
Susan L. Abrams

The Johns Hopkins University Press ■ Baltimore and London

© 1986 The Johns Hopkins University Press
All rights reserved
Printed in the United States of America

The Johns Hopkins University Press
701 West 40th Street
Baltimore, Maryland 21211
The Johns Hopkins Press Ltd, London

The paper in this book is acid-free and meets the guidelines for permanence and durability of the Committee on Production Guidelines for Book Longevity of the Council on Library Resources.

Library of Congress Cataloging-in-Publication Data

Harvey, A. McGehee (Abner McGehee), 1911–
   For the welfare of mankind.

  Bibliography: p.
  Includes index.
   1. Commonwealth Fund—History. 2. Medical education—United States—Endowments—History. 3. Medical care—United States—Endowments—History. I. Abrams, Susan.
II. Title.
R745.H38   1986   362.1'0425   85-19752
ISBN 0-8018-3199-7 (alk. paper)

*This book is dedicated
with admiration to Lester J. Evans and
with gratitude to our spouses*

The past is not dead history; it is living material out of which man makes himself and builds the future.

—René Dubos

Contents

List of Illustrations xi

Acknowledgments xiii

Introduction 1

Part I. The Early Years
1. The Harkness Family and the Genesis of the Commonwealth Fund 9
2. The Fund Searches for a Focus
   The First General Director: Max Farrand 19

Part II. The Fund Finds Its Targets
3. The Program in Psychiatry and Mental Health
   The Second General Director: Barry Conger Smith 29
4. The Program in Public Health
   The Second General Director: Barry Conger Smith 84
5. Early Programs in Medical Education and Medical Research
   The Second General Director: Barry Conger Smith 145

Part III. Expanding Interest in Medical Education
6. Support of Comprehensive Medicine
   The Third General Director: Donal Sheehan 203
7. Programs in Medical Education and Community Service
   The Second President: Malcolm Pratt Aldrich 211

        8. The University and the Community
           The Third President: James Quigg Newton, Jr.   338
        9. Integrating Medical Education into the University
           The Fourth President: Carleton Burke Chapman   461

Part IV.   The 1980s
       10. Programs for the 1980s
          The Fifth President: Margaret Ellerbe Mahoney   517

Part V.   Educating the Public and the Physician
       11. The Book Program   525

Epilogue   535

Appendixes

A Recipients of Psychiatric Fellowships   561
B Advanced Medical Fellows, 1938–1956   566
C Recipients of Fellowships in Support of Creative Scholarship, 1956–1966   571
D Grants for Medical Research, 1919–1984   587
E Grants to Medical Schools for Programs in Comprehensive Care   597
F Planning New Schools and Reorganizing Existing Schools of Medicine   598
G Capital Grants to Medical Schools   601
H Selected Grants Awarded during the Presidency of J. Quigg Newton, Jr.: The Transition   605
I Selected Grants Awarded during the Presidency of J. Quigg Newton, Jr.: The Vice-Presidency of Colin M. MacLeod   607
J Selected Grants Awarded during the Presidency of J. Quigg Newton, Jr.: The Vice-Presidency of Robert J. Glaser   610
K Selected Grants Awarded during the Presidency of J. Quigg Newton, Jr.: The Vice-Presidency of Carleton B. Chapman   613
L Institutions Receiving $1 Million or More for Medical Education, 1949–1977   616
M Commonwealth Fund Grants, 1919–1984   618

Notes and References   625

Index of Names   675

Index of Subjects   683

List of Illustrations

1. Edward Stephen Harkness   12
2. Mrs. Stephen V. Harkness   14
3. The first board of directors   20
4. Barry Conger Smith   30
5. Barbara Story Quin   31
6. Mildred C. Scoville   31
7. Hermann M. Biggs   32
8. Adolf Meyer   32
9. Thomas W. Salmon   37
10. Fellows at the Colorado Psychopathic Hospital, Denver, Colorado, 1938   58
11. Child health demonstration headquarters, Fargo, North Dakota   97
12. Lester J. Evans   98
13. Child health demonstration, Athens, Georgia   101
14. "Honor Roll" parade, Salem, Oregon   103
15. Health Center in Laurel, Mississippi   111
16. Rutherford Hospital, Murfreesboro, Tennessee   118
17. The health officer sees a case of pellagra   121
18. Alfred H. Washburn   184
19. George N. Papanicolaou   187
20. Wade Hampton Frost   189

21. Lowell J. Reed 192
22. Donal Sheehan 204
23. Malcolm P. Aldrich 212
24. Geddes Smith 213
25. Harkness House, One East 75th Street, New York, New York 213
26. James Quigg Newton, Jr. 339
27. Colin Munro MacLeod 366
28. Offshoots of the Yale Trauma Program 394
29. Robert Joy Glaser 404
30. Carleton Burke Chapman 462
31. Comparison of the traditional structure of college and medical school education with Interface Programs at the universities of Rochester and Chicago 465
32. Margaret Ellerbe Mahoney 518

Acknowledgments

We are indebted to all those individuals who were generous with their time and their help, consenting to be interviewed or providing detailed written recollections. Our special thanks go to Lester J. Evans, Barbara G. Rosenkrantz, Gert H. Brieger, Jerome J. Bylebyl, John L. Dusseau, Robert H. Ebert, Robert J. Glaser, John C. Hume, Thomas H. Hunter, John Romano, Walter Donway and Terrance Keenan for their review of all or portions of the manuscript.

Introduction

Because it deals with the vital interests of both individuals and societies—with life and death—and with so much that matters in between—Medicine has long had an unusually complex and intimate relationship to social and cultural developments at large. . . . In other words, medical history involves social and economic as well as biologic content and presents one of the central themes in human experience. After all, what is more basic in the life of any people than life itself?
—*Richard Harrison Shryock*

Established October 17, 1918, by Mrs. Stephen V. Harkness under the broad mandate "to do something for the welfare of mankind," the Commonwealth Fund has existed for over sixty-five years as a private philanthropic foundation. Throughout its history, the Fund has directed its resources primarily to developing ideas, talents, institutions, and arrangements intended to strengthen the quality of medical care in American society.

The general-purpose foundation in the United States is slightly more than three-quarters of a century old. Since several private foundations were already in operation when the Commonwealth Fund was created, the Fund had as its antecedents both the specific experiences of early philanthropists and the historical underpinnings of foundations. In the short span of thirty-five years between the end of the Civil War and the beginning of the twentieth century, the United States became the mightiest industrial power in the world. Wealthy businessmen began to use their fortunes for social benefit, creating institutions such as the Rockefeller Institute for Medical Research (established in 1901), the Carnegie Institution of Washington (1902), the General Education Board (1903), the Carnegie Foundation for the Advancement of Teaching (1905), the Carnegie Corporation (1911), the Rockefeller Foundation (1913), and the Julius Rosenwald Fund (1917). Large foundations in the early part of the twentieth century were intended to be broad and flexible, objectives exemplified by the Rockefeller Foundation's ambitious intention "to promote the well-being of mankind throughout the world."

Their charges presented a compelling challenge to foundation trustees and officers, whose responsibility extended beyond simple compliance with the donor's specific plans. Foundations were called to account: "Here is a great source of financial power, and there are the needs of the world. What do you propose to do?" The responses rested on the tacit assumption that the most fruitful means of achieving the "well-being of mankind" was to enhance what is commonly referred to as "academic research." This emphasis was a reaction to the rise of modern science, the appearance in this country of the research university based on the German model, and—even in the early twentieth century—the accelerating growth of technology. By 1918 philanthropists had begun to recognize that distributing gifts to the needy was not a practical solution: Charity had given way to scientifically disciplined giving intended to generate knowledge that would lead to improved societal conditions. The Sisyphean difficulty of trying to eliminate each individual manifestation of social distress—poverty, ignorance, and disease—led foundations to apply their resources to a search for the underlying causes of social dysfunction. The Commonwealth Fund was to be no exception.

The medical and educational foundations of the early twentieth century shared another, unusual, characteristic: the presence of strong administrators whose intuition directed the donor's intentions. Noteworthy alliances were those of Andrew Carnegie and Henry S. Pritchett, John D. Rockefeller and Frederick T. Gates (and later, Rockefeller and Abraham Flexner), and, in the case of the Commonwealth Fund, Edward S. Harkness and Barry C. Smith. These administrators limited the scope of their organizations' endeavors, delineating their own areas of interest. The Rockefeller Sanitary Commission first turned its attention to the conquest of hookworm, and the Rockefeller Foundation to improving teaching and research in medical schools around the world. The Milbank Memorial Fund, chartered in 1905, concentrated on public health. The John and Mary Markle Foundation began in 1927 by making grants for social research, but in 1935 shifted its emphasis to support of biomedical research. A principal effort of the Josiah Macy, Jr., Foundation was the Macy Conferences, the first of which was held in 1931 to encourage communication among scientists. When the Robert Wood Johnson Foundation was incorporated in 1936, it devoted most of its modest resources to programs in New Brunswick, New Jersey, and surrounding areas; at its benefactor's death in 1968, his vast fortune was turned into a major national philanthropy that now concentrates on improving the nation's resources in primary and ambulatory health care.

The vision of philanthropy shared by the founders of the Commonwealth Fund was elucidated first by Andrew Carnegie and later by John D. Rockefeller. It was Carnegie's idea that great family fortunes should be vested in charitable corporations governed objectively by distinguished, independent boards of trustees and served by officers especially trained to study opportunities for service. This view of philanthropy represented a new, mature relationship between donor and organization: Our social and economic system makes possible the accumulation of a great fortune. The person who amasses that fortune makes reasonable provision for his heirs but turns the rest of the money to the benefit of society, where the opportunities exist to make personal fortunes possible. Competent, experienced administrators apply the money to understanding the basic problems of society and to improving and enriching the lives of all men.[1]

The years since the establishment of the Commonwealth Fund have been spectacular ones for medicine: Medical education has come of age in the United States, and medical research has undergone extraordinary expansion. With an ever-increasing body of knowledge and greater understanding of the processes basic to health and disease, remarkable advances in health care have become possible. This progress in biomedical discovery and its organized application has encouraged the development of health care as a dynamic value in American society. Scientific and technological advancement has generated a second industrial revolution, accelerating the transition of the nation's population from rural to urban life, and providing a powerful economic base that has sustained an expanding population and nourished rising standards of living and levels of expectation.

The Commonwealth Fund's history is one of continuous assistance to this progress, through grants first for child guidance and child health and later for the mental health movement, rural public health services, community hospitals, professional education, and scientific research. Early in the Fund's history, the decision was made to concentrate its activities in the field of health—a field that encompasses many disciplines and organizations, some distinct and independent, some interrelated and overlapping. Certain fundamental questions, however, are common to "health" in the broadest sense: What is the real nature of illness? What are the most pressing health and medical needs of present-day society? What kinds of professional personnel are required to understand and deal with these needs? How can such people best be prepared for the responsibilities they must assume? What measures will improve the institutional and community resources through which these professionals function?

As medicine and society have changed over the years, the Fund's answers have changed as well. When medical services for children, the mentally ill, and rural populations became established features of the country's expanding commitment to better health, the Fund shifted its support to two areas that since the 1940s have become predominant, closely interwoven national concerns: the training of better physicians, biomedical scientists, and medical school teachers; and the development of improved systems for providing medical services to individuals, families, and communities. Medical education is still being challenged to prepare physicians who will be lifelong students of the best that is known and practiced in medicine, as well as leaders in extending the nation's health resources throughout the whole society. The nation's system of medical care faces like challenges—and has over time. The Fund's responses to these challenges in the past few decades have reflected a shifting relationship between medicine and society, part of a larger—and unprecedented—process of change within the American social system. The emphases have changed from decade to decade, but the fundamental goal of benefiting mankind through advancing the health and well-being of Americans has remained.

To comprehend a foundation's policies and actions requires more than just a knowledge of the programs receiving support. One must understand the reciprocal relationships of fundamental factors: the foundation's bureaucratic organization, the role of the directors, the character and responsibilities of the staff, and the interactions with potential recipients. This chronicle of the Commonwealth Fund's contributions since its founding in 1918 is as much the story of the men and women who shaped the Fund's programs as a description of the programs themselves. Each of its eight leaders brought a personal outlook and style to its work, yet transcending their individual differences were what one of them called "the subtle traditions of the Fund," a thread of continuity running through the successive programs as they were instigated and implemented. This thread can be seen in the influence of the early community programs on the Fund's later relationships with universities and their medical schools; in the persistent emphasis on preventive medicine, a theme inaugurated by the Fund's first president, Edward S. Harkness, and reemphasized by the current president, Margaret E. Mahoney; and in the importance accorded the dissemination as well as the acquisition of new knowledge.

Over the years, the Fund has benefited from the presence of talented writers and editors on its staff. The results of their efforts are reflected in the monographs sponsored by the Fund's Division of Publications; in the incisive reports of the president and staff to the board of directors; and in the annual reports. These last two series in particular provide a window on the problems of American medicine and public health over the last three-quarters of a century. Describing the basis for the directors' decisions about individual grants, they reflect the decision-making process, and they have been used extensively in preparing this book.

Another valuable source of information was the Commonwealth Fund's archives, which contain the original grant applications, notes on site visits, progress reports, and correspondence.

Finally, the inner history of the Fund emerged from extensive interviews with past and present staff members, board members, and grant recipients. Lester J. Evans was especially helpful, providing many memories of his thirty-six years on the Fund's staff along with documentary material not otherwise available and reviewing the manuscript's factual accuracy.

The steps in the Commonwealth Fund's programmatic development are documented in the chronological chapters devoted to the general directors and presidents. In addition, vignettes based on both archival material and recent interviews with grant recipients describe the Fund's important programs in detail, illustrating the nature and outcome of some specific awards. By exploring the dynamics of decision-making in a medium-sized philanthropic foundation, this chronicle attempts to reveal the methods that the Fund has used over the past sixty-five years "to do something for the welfare of mankind."[2]

**Part I:
The Early
Years**

1

The Harkness Family and the Genesis of the Commonwealth Fund

The founder of the Harkness family in the United States was William Harkness, who emigrated from Scotland to Massachusetts in 1710.[1] One branch consisted of four brothers, three of whom were physicians: Born between 1781 and 1801, William, Daniel, David, and Lamon were the great-grandsons of the original William Harkness. In the early 1800s, they moved to the Finger Lakes Region of Seneca County, New York. Stephen Vanderberg Harkness, born on November 18, 1818, was the first son (and second child) of Dr. David Harkness and his wife, Martha Cook Harkness. At the age of fifteen, when formal schooling customarily ended, Stephen was apprenticed to a local harness maker. It was an ironic choice of trade, as Stephen was later to participate in the development of the oil industry, which hastened the obsolescence of harness making as an occupation.

In 1840 Stephen V. Harkness moved farther west, settling in Bellevue, Ohio. He was a shrewd judge of values, and his vision and imagination were coupled with enterprise and determination. As his business judgment matured, he gradually abandoned his trade for more commercial ventures. In February 1854, his first wife having died, he married Anna M. Richardson, with whom he had four children. The youngest was Edward Stephen Harkness, born on January 22, 1874, in Cleveland, Ohio. By then Stephen V. Harkness had become a prominent local businessman, and his means had grown substantially from the profits of his livestock, distillery, and private banking businesses.

Investment in Oil

A few years before Edward's birth, Stephen V. Harkness had renewed a business association with Henry M. Flagler, who was married to Stephen's cousin Mary Harkness. Flagler's business was grain brokerage; he and John D. Rockefeller, then a young man buying grain for a Cleveland Commission house, shared an office in a building overlooking the Cuyahoga River, on the banks of which Rockefeller and his partner Samuel Andrews operated an oil refinery. In 1867 Rockefeller, Andrews, and Flagler formed a partnership to expand this prospering business by obtaining the new capital needed to construct additional plants. Flagler supplied an undetermined portion of this capital; the balance, estimated to be between $60,000 and $90,000, was provided by Stephen V. Harkness, a silent partner whose interest was solely that of an investor. By the end of 1869, the business was growing rapidly and required still larger infusions of new capital. It also needed a more flexible organization than was possible under the original partnership arrangement. As a result, on January 10, 1870, the four men formed a joint stock corporation, the Standard Oil Company.

It is difficult in today's world, in which petroleum is such an indispensable part of almost every aspect of our daily lives, to imagine that in those days its major need was for oil and kerosene in lamps. In 1869 no one was yet aware of the great riches that lay beneath the soil of Texas, the adjoining Gulf Coast states, California, and the Rocky Mountain area. The first oil well had been drilled just a few years before, at Titusville, Pennsylvania, to a depth of only a few hundred feet (the accompanying natural gas being discarded), and even Rockefeller himself did not foresee the enormous potential of the newly formed company. From the very beginning, however, Stephen V. Harkness placed his entire trust in this embryonic industry, whose credit was so poor that it was forced to pay ten percent interest on the money it needed to borrow. The Standard Oil Company started business with a capital of $1 million, consisting of 10,000 shares with a par value of $100 each. Of the 9,000 shares issued to the four partners, Stephen Harkness received 1,334.

The Harkness Fortune

Edward S. Harkness was only fourteen years of age when his father died in 1888. As Stephen V. Harkness left no will, the distribution of the estate followed the inheritance laws of Ohio, which gave two-sixths to the widow and one-sixth to each of the four surviving children. The oldest son, Charles, was appointed administrator of the estate.

Charles Harkness had graduated from Yale University in 1883 and later studied law at Columbia University. He was only twenty-seven years old at his appointment and faced this heavy responsibility with little experience. The estate's chief asset was the stock of the Standard Oil Company, which was then part of a chaotic industry. The most prudent course might have been to liquidate the bulk of the holdings of Standard Oil stock, replacing it with mortgages and high-grade bonds. The principal of the estate would probably not have increased beyond its current size, but at least the family would have had a steady and substantial income with a minimum of risk. Yet Charles, like his father, believed strongly in the Standard Oil Company. He knew that his father had taken a great chance in backing Rockefeller and Flagler, and he knew of his father's additional large investments in the company's stock as it became available over a period of years. Charles's decision to retain the Standard Oil Company stock led to the full development of the Harkness fortune. By itself, this enormous accumulation of wealth had no social connotation: The real test of its justification remained the determination of how it was to be used.

If the Harkness wealth was to be used effectively, its management needed "a man who had the desire to help mankind, the ability to perceive how such help could be made most effective, and the character and self-discipline to carry out specific projects."[2] Edward, the youngest son (fig. 1), possessed the qualities that made it possible for him to give social significance to the efforts of his brother and father: sensitivity, responsibility, self-restraint, and orderly patterns of thought.

After five years of preparatory education at St. Paul's School in Concord, New Hampshire, Edward S. Harkness entered Yale University in the fall of 1893. His undergraduate years at Yale were not only important for him at the time; they influenced his actions throughout the rest of his life. Always a man of strong loyalties, he continued to identify with Yale through the passage of the years.

When Edward S. Harkness was graduated from Yale University in 1897, both his mother and his brother were living in New York City. After a trip around the world with two of his classmates, Edward joined Charles in administering the family's investments. Most of the family's holdings remained concentrated in the Standard Oil Company and after the dissolution of the parent company in 1911, in the securities of its affiliates and subsidiaries. The balance lay in a variety of assets, chiefly railroad bonds and stocks.

During the first two decades of the twentieth century, the Standard Oil companies prospered along with the country as a whole, but they benefited particularly from the rapid development of the automobile. There was no federal income tax during most of this period, and Mrs. Harkness was not interested in compounding her wealth through reinvesting her surplus income in additional securities. She found herself with an increasing financial ability to accomplish good works. In the beginning

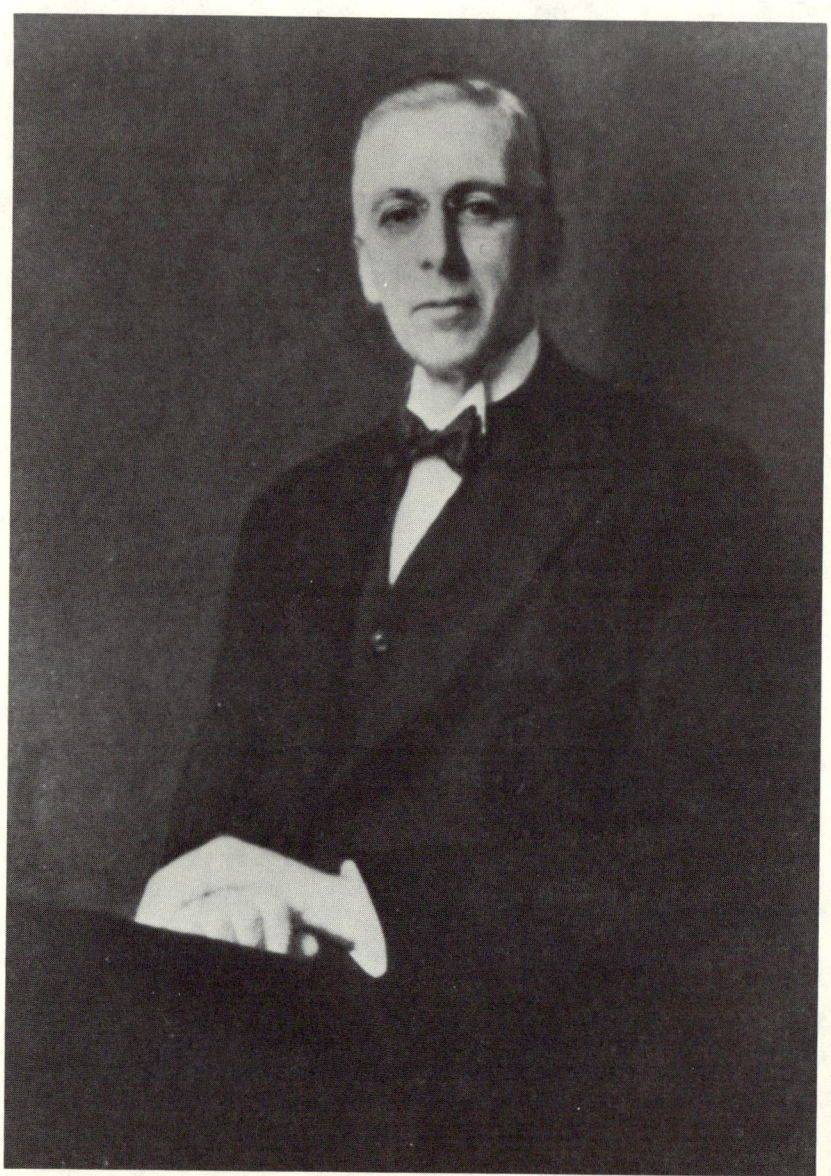

Figure 1. Edward Stephen Harkness
Reprinted from *The Commonwealth Fund: A Historical Sketch, 1918–1962*. New York: Commonwealth Fund, 1963.

she gave chiefly, though not exclusively, to religious and welfare organizations. Yale University was an early and continuing recipient of Mrs. Harkness's gifts: She financed the building of the Memorial Quadrangle, and the quadrangle's gothic tower was given in memory of Charles, who died in 1916; in 1920 she gave $3 million to increase faculty salaries.

The Birth of the Commonwealth Fund

In common with any other organized human activity, the art of effective giving can be developed only through practice, by trial and error. Edward S. Harkness had the opportunity to observe philanthropic efforts from childhood: Generosity was an integral part of his family's life. His father was characterized as "always giving," and after her husband's death in 1888, Anna R. Harkness shared this trait, on an increasing scale as her accumulating fortune permitted (fig. 2).

As time passed, Mrs. Harkness turned increasingly to her son Edward for guidance about specific projects and problems. A public-spirited woman, Mrs. Harkness contributed much to her adopted city of New York. She soon found herself overwhelmed with appeals for assistance, so that even with her son's help, it was difficult for her to decide which requests were the most deserving. After many discussions with Edward, Mrs. Harkness decided to establish a charitable foundation: a tangible framework for giving whose continuity, balance, and direction would multiply the effectiveness of her gifts.

The result of these deliberations emerged in October 1918, when the Commonwealth Fund was incorporated under the laws of the state of New York as a nonprofit institution whose purpose was "to do something for the welfare of mankind." It was an instrument with broad powers, as the first section of its papers of incorporation attests:

> The particular objects for which the corporation is formed are the application to charitable purposes of the income or the principal of such property as from time to time the corporation shall possess; including the giving of income or of principal to any other charitable corporation or corporations, and the application of the income or the principal of any property acquired by bequest, devise or gift to such charitable purposes as the testator or donor shall have prescribed by will or instrument of gift.

Edward S. Harkness became the first president of the new foundation.

The death of Charles Harkness in 1916 left Edward as the only surviving child, depriving him of the counsel that had helped to guide him for twenty years. Upon his shoulders was placed increased responsibility for the administration of the family's financial resources and philanthropic interests. For a while he carried this burden alone, but with the passage

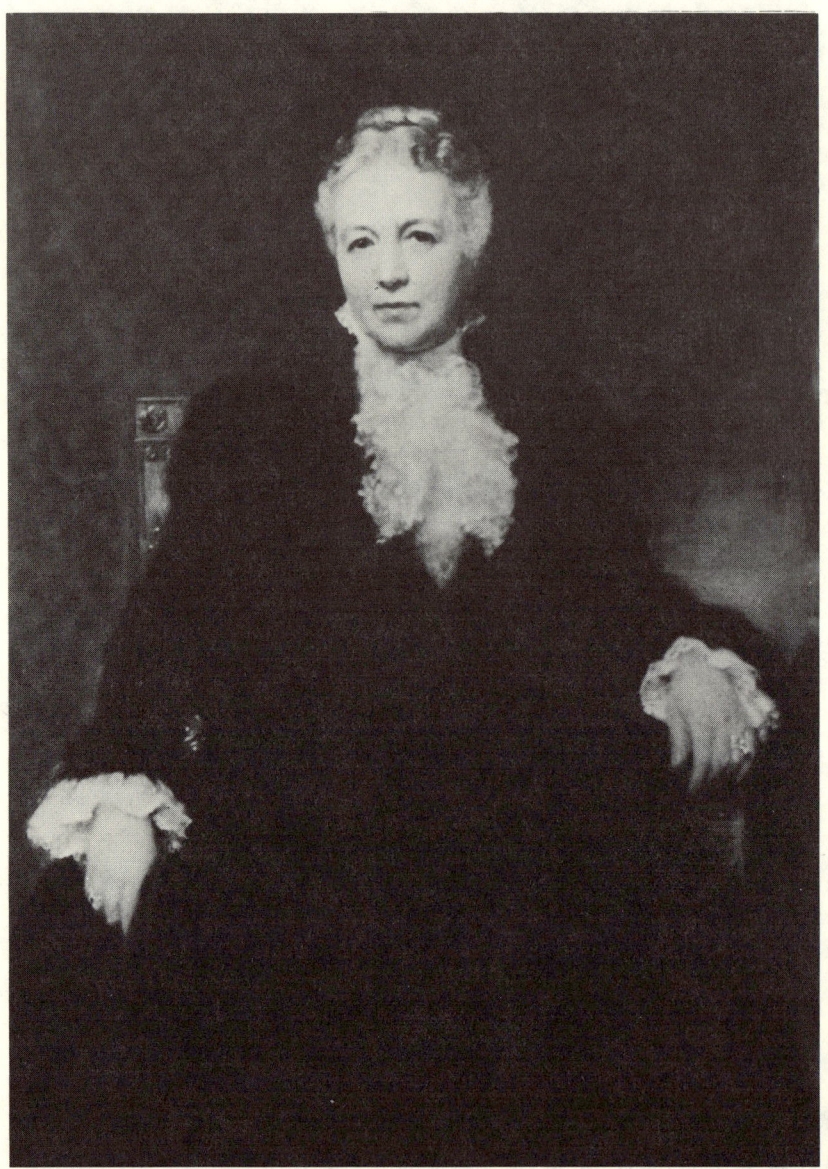

Figure 2. Mrs. Stephen V. Harkness
Reprinted from *The Commonwealth Fund: A Historical Sketch, 1918–1962*. New York: Commonwealth Fund, 1963.

of time, he felt the need for an associate—someone with whom he could discuss business and philanthropic questions and who could relieve him of many details of administering his varied interests. The man he chose was Samuel H. Fisher, a practicing lawyer in New Haven, Connecticut, and a Yale alumnus of the class of 1889. A graduate also of the Yale Law School, Fisher had served as judge advocate general on the staff of Connecticut's governor, and was for fifteen years a member of the Yale Corporation.[3] Fisher and Harkness's mutual interest in Yale and their joint service on the board of directors of the New Haven Young Men's Christian Association had brought them together; with his legal training and conservative background, Fisher was well equipped to help fill the void left by Charles's death. In June 1918 he moved to New York as personal counsel to Edward S. Harkness and his mother.

Five years later Harkness added another member to his personal office staff: Malcolm P. Aldrich, who had graduated from Yale the previous summer after an undergraduate career marked by unusual scholastic, athletic, and extracurricular attainments. Over the years the two men developed a bond of mutual respect. Aldrich was twenty-six years younger than Edward S. Harkness, with the youthful enthusiasm and drive to supplement Harkness's own planning. When Fisher approached retirement age, Aldrich was ideally qualified to take over as Harkness's representative and confidant.

Edward S. Harkness's Interest in Medicine

As founder, donor, and foundation officer, Edward S. Harkness was able to advance his own concept of philanthropy in shaping the Fund's early programs. Although the original thoughts and wording may be that of a staff member or consultant, Harkness's letter in 1910 to Robert W. deForest, chairman of the building committee of the Presbyterian Hospital, documents his well-defined philosophy of philanthropy in medicine:

> It has recently come to my attention that a basis of alliance has been suggested between The Presbyterian Hospital and the College of Physicians and Surgeons, the medical school of Columbia University, by prominent members of both institutions, subject to the settlement of details and to the approval of governing boards of these institutions. This alliance is singularly in line with my own conception of the proper relations between hospital and medical school, and I should be glad to further it.
> I have long been interested in that form of charity which has to do with the treatment of human ills, and latterly have become more and more impressed with the extent of the work that a hospital must do on the broadest scientific and practical lines if it at all adequately uses its resources.
> The scientific development of medicine has especially interested me recently,

and I have become convinced that its real underlying province and mission to humanity lies more particularly in preventing disease than in merely curing it. All this has increased a growing desire I have had to contribute something which will materially increase the usefulness of a great hospital.

I am convinced that this scientific development can best be accomplished in the hospital and the medical school, and that the two are interdependent, the one on the other. The medical school constantly supplies the physicians and surgeons of the future who in their early training must have every facility for practical experience and application which they can only obtain at a hospital where they are taught by the practicing physicians and scientific men. The hospital supplies a vast amount of material for study and research, and should realize that besides caring for the sick, it has a great obligation towards humanity to use this material both in the training of the younger men and in furthering discoveries in preventive medicine.

I believe that the visiting staff of a hospital does better work for its patients, and that its members are kept more up to date, if they include teaching in conjunction with their duties than otherwise; that the hospital and patients directly benefit thereby, the former through attracting a better class of internes and attendings because of the teaching facilities, the latter through receiving more careful attention and the latest methods of treatment. . . .

It . . . gives me pleasure to offer to the Hospital, on behalf of a donor whose name I am not now at liberty to mention, money and securities which I estimate to be of the value of $1,300,000, in trust for endowment, the principal to be kept separate from other funds and the income to be used exclusively towards the support of the scientific and educational work connected with the Hospital and referred to in this letter. As I withhold the name of the donor, I guarantee the payment or transfer of this endowment Fund to the Hospital . . . .

Both of the offers above contained are made on the following understanding and conditions:

1. That the Hospital shall admit to the wards students of the medical school to the extent and in the manner permitted by the most approved practice.
2. That the educational institution concerned may make nominations to all positions on the Hospital staff, medical, surgical and special.
3. That the persons occupying for the time being the ranking or foremost professorships in medicine and surgery in the educational institution concerned shall always be nominated to hold appropriate positions on the staff of the Hospital and that so long as they hold such offices in the Hospital they shall have no official connection with any other hospital, to the intent that under this agreement the Hospital will secure in the treatment of its patients the greatest degree of medical and surgical skill which can be furnished by the school.
4. That the physicians and surgeons of various ranks and their assistants shall have as full privileges as reasonably possible, consistent always with the welfare of patients, of instructing their students in the public wards and the various laboratories of the Hospital.

5. That the departments of pathology and bacteriology may give teaching to students in the Hospital.
6. That there shall be a Director of the surgical research laboratory who shall teach in the Hospital and who shall always be on the active teaching staff of the school.
7. That the surgical department at the Hospital shall publish an annual report of the scientific and clinical work of the year.
8. That the College of Physicians and Surgeons, the medical department of Columbia University, be the medical school with which the Hospital makes this arrangement, so long as it is in a position to carry out its share of these conditions and complies therewith. Should it not be in such a position, or fail to comply therewith, another medical school of the first rank may be selected by the Hospital . . . .

Harkness's proposed arrangements closely resembled those in effect at Johns Hopkins, the first such joint venture in the United States, where the generous endowment of a medical school and a university hospital allowed them to maintain the highest possible standards of practice and education for the day and "to give the world men who can not only sail by the old charts but can make new and better ones for the use of others."[4] Harkness's letter outlined the ground rules that must prevail in a cooperative agreement between hospital and medical school: Maintaining high standards of medical education, research, and practice requires the academic staff of the school of medicine to be responsible for key decisions.

In 1922 Edward S. Harkness and his mother together donated to Columbia University's new medical center a tract of twenty-two acres of land in upper Manhattan. The original construction plans specified two main buildings: a home for the Presbyterian Hospital and a School of Physicians and Surgeons. Ground was broken at ceremonies held in January 1925; three and one-half years later, the Columbia University Medical Center—according to one description, "the largest and most modern in the world"—was formally dedicated.[5] "From a day in the early 1920s when Edward Harkness and his friend Dean Sage sat on a wooden fence around the ball park of the New York Highlanders at Broadway and 165th Street and dreamed of a center of medical care, research, and teaching that might arise there, until that dream became a reality, and from then on throughout his life, the Medical Center was one of Edward Harkness's most vital interests."[6]

Boundaries between personal and Commonwealth Fund giving, as in support for Columbia University, were sometimes blurred. Harkness used his personal resources for projects that he considered unsuitable for the Fund, but he did rely on the Fund's staff to provide him with background information about such appeals.

Edward S. Harkness increased his donations as his resources were increased by his brother's and mother's estates. He kept track only of gifts of $5,000 or more to charitable, educational, and philanthropic institutions, and even this list was incomplete: At his death, it contained 1,332 separate entries totaling more than $129 million. It is impossible to estimate with any exactitude either the number or the total amount of the "smaller" gifts made by Edward S. Harkness during his lifetime.

2

The Fund Searches for a Focus

The perpetual enemies of the human race, apart from man's own nature, are ignorance and disease.
—Alan Gregg, 1941

The First General Director: Max Farrand (1919–1921)

The first official meeting of the Fund took place on October 23, 1918, less than a week after the papers of incorporation were signed. Five directors were appointed: Otto T. Bannard, Max Farrand, Samuel H. Fisher, Edward S. Harkness and George W. Murray (fig. 3). (Harkness remained as president of the board of directors and chief executive officer until his death in 1940.) On the day of the meeting, the Fund's accounts were opened with securities whose market value was $9,956,112. Less than a year later, Anna R. Harkness gave the Fund an additional $6,379,929 in stocks.[1] Farrand resigned as a director of the corporation in February 1919, to be elected general director of the Fund. As chief of staff, the general director was responsible for making recommendations about program development to Edward S. Harkness.

Farrand was a historian by profession. Born on March 29, 1869, he graduated from Princeton University in 1892 and spent the next four years at the Universities of Leipzig and Heidelberg. Between 1896 and 1925, he taught history at Wesleyan, Stanford, and Yale universities, serving as head of the history department at Stanford from 1901 to 1908.[2] His obligations at Yale prevented him from assuming the duties of his new office until September 1, 1919, and when he arrived, he found the work of the Fund well under way. By October 1919, 155 appeals had been considered by the Fund. Ninety-four of these projects had been formally presented to the board of directors, and twelve appropriations

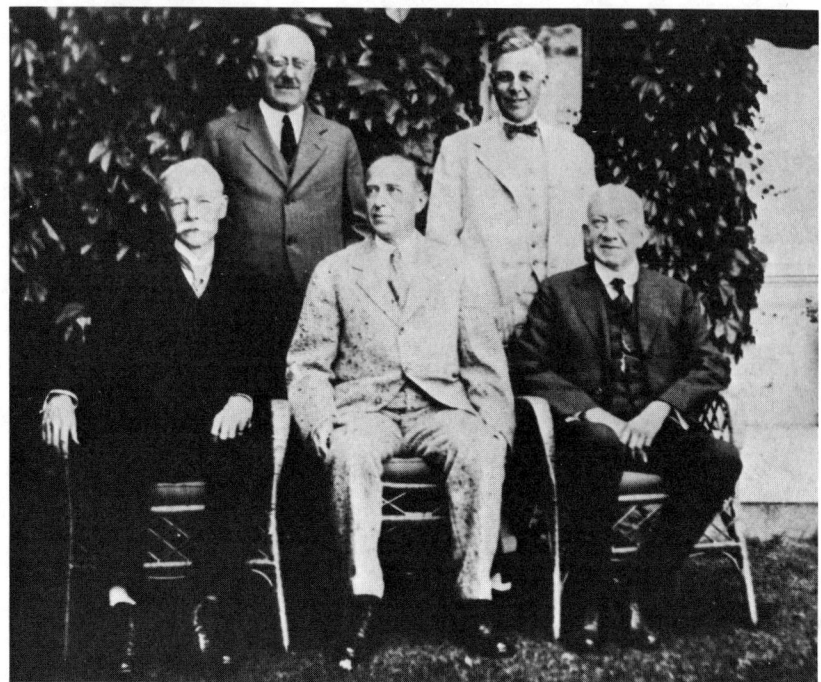

Figure 3. The first board of directors. *Left to right:* George Welwood Murray, Samuel H. Fisher, Max Farrand, Edward S. Harkness, Otto T. Bannard. Reprinted from *The Commonwealth Fund: A Historical Sketch, 1918–1962*. New York: Commonwealth Fund, 1963.

had been made, nine of which were supported in the Fund's first fiscal year at a cost of $144,000 (table 1). Two-thirds of the money expended reflected an immediate response to unusual, pressing problems of the time; the United War Work Campaign and the American Committee on Armenian and Syrian Relief, for example, each received a contribution of $50,000.

Farrand's approval of the Fund's donations was muted. Referring to himself in the third person, he revealed the frustrations that confronted him at the beginning of his directorship, particularly his growing perception of the political climate in which the Fund would have to operate:[3]

> In his innocence, he had supposed that the Commonwealth Fund would be free to undertake any worthy object that commended itself to the Directors. He found, however, that the work of the Fund is liable to be hampered by the criticisms and opposition to which it was certain to be subjected. Practically all foundations that are in any way similar to this are being attacked because

Table 1 Expenditures during the Commonwealth Fund's First Year, 1918–1919

Recipient	Amount
United War Work Campaign	$ 50,000
American Committee on Armenian and Syrian Relief	50,000
The Johns Hopkins Medical School	15,000
National Research Council	10,000
National Committee on Mental Hygiene	10,000
New York Committee on After-Care of Infantile Paralysis Cases	6,000
Babies' Welfare Association	1,500
Charity Organization Society (Bureau of Advice and Information)	1,000
Hampton Normal and Agricultural Institute	500
Total	**144,000**

Source: Treasurer's Report, Annual Report, the Commonwealth Fund, 1919.

of the conviction that they are attempts to avoid taxation and because of the belief that they are carrying out capitalistic propaganda. . . .

The Fund had the misfortune of beginning its work in an especially difficult time for foundations, a time when they were "a favorite target of official frustration and popular anxiety."[4] In the years before World War I, they were "a focus of bitter controversy between the forces of reckless capital and radical labor."[5] Again in the depression years, in the McCarthy period, and during the turmoil of the 1960s, foundations were assailed by persons of all political persuasions. Before the Fund's founding, a typical polemic came from Basil Manly, research director of the United States Commission on Industrial Relations:[6]

> The domination by the men in whose hands the final control of a large part of American industry rests is not limited to their employees, but is being rapidly extended to control the education and social survival of the Nation.
> This control is being extended largely through the creation of enormous privately managed funds for indefinite purposes, hereafter designated "foundations," by the endowment of colleges and universities, by the creation of funds for the pensioning of teachers, by contributions to private charities, as well as through controlling or influencing the public press. . . .
> As regards the "foundations" created for unlimited general purposes and endowed with enormous resources, their ultimate possibilities are so grave a menace, not only as regards their own activities and influence but also the benumbing effect which they have on private citizens and public bodies, that if they could be clearly differentiated from other forms of voluntary altruistic effort, it would be desirable to recommend their abolition.

Compounding Farrand's dismay was his unfamiliarity with the process of grant giving:[7]

> Everyone who has had experience . . . advises going very slowly—to be sure of the field of work before it is undertaken. This appeals very much to the General Director, because of his inexperience. . . . It is partly with the conscious or unconscious purpose of avoiding criticism that many urge medical and relief work or international objects or projects in foreign lands. This is by way of warning the directors that it will probably take a considerable time to mature plans and to formulate policy. . . . In undertaking his duties with all the enthusiasm that comes from approaching a new and big field of work, the General Director quickly found himself in an almost hopeless state, and in hopeless confusion of mind, for there were put to him over 50 applications for the support of projects of which he knew nothing.

Farrand sought advice from trusted friends, experts in varied fields, and other foundation executives—a course of action that directors of the Fund were to follow as a matter of policy in the years ahead. In this case, some of the last group's recommendations were contradictory. Henry S. Pritchett of the Carnegie Foundation advised Farrand not to give money to any institution without a personal visit. Abraham Flexner, on the other hand, told him that a visit was unnecessary, since the General Education Board's pool of information was always available to the Commonwealth Fund.

The charities that most interested Farrand were all concerned with medicine or public health. Some twenty appeals were shown to five men in New York, including William Darrach and Walter B. James (both associated with Columbia University and the Presbyterian Hospital). Farrand found that "the mere consideration of these concrete cases helped materially in developing lines of procedure." He concluded: "The General Director is prepared to recommend as a matter of general policy that the income of the Fund should be directed rather to the encouraging and assisting of preventive measures than in the support of what is commonly called relief work."[8] As Farrand expressed the Fund's early philosophy,[9]

> Whatever is undertaken will be certain to arouse criticism from some quarter. . . . Justification of such foundations [as the Commonwealth Fund] lies in their ability to accomplish certain things which the individual (or the government) or the community cannot do. . . . It would obviously follow that philanthropic foundations should not undertake projects which should be carried out by individuals or the community, although situations are continually arising where a foundation may act until the community is aroused to the point where it appreciates the conditions and should, therefore, be ready to act. . . . Private funds may be used to investigate, experiment, and demonstrate, but they cannot eventuate on a large scale. . . . Public funds on the other hand, are not fitted for purposes of experiment, investigation or demonstration but they can carry out the larger projects.

Here is the first elucidation of the Commonwealth Fund's abiding interest in research—an interest that led to some of the Fund's most innovative and enduring projects and one that continues to the present day. Farrand's enthusiasm was echoed by Edward S. Harkness, who believed that prevention and research should be the Fund's highest priorities. Harkness's copies of the general director's reports are generously salted with forthright marginal notes advocating support of research and in general guiding the Fund's course. When the American Society for the Control of Cancer characterized its request as primarily for the dissemination of knowledge about symptoms, his marginal note was brief: "Do not think much of this. Hope lies in research."[10] In response to an elaborate proposal to build a National Education Laboratory for the blind, he wrote: "The subject of blindness is an important one and probably worthy of our help. A much broader field, however, is search for the reasons for defective eyesight and means of prevention."[11] A request from the Presbyterian Board to support a missionary hospital led him to conclude (referring to his personal funds in the third person): "Perhaps better for ESH as it is a denominational matter."[12] A proposal to enact a law for compulsory health insurance elicited this terse comment: "Keep out of legislation."[13] Later, when the subject of the report was child delinquency, Harkness wrote: "1) Must deal with individual cases; 2) therefore, must be better trained people to care for children; 3) must not remove normal conditions by removing children from their homes."[14] Of the medical appeals received, Harkness himself favored grants to the National Committee for Mental Hygiene, the American Social Hygiene Association, the American Society for the Control of Cancer, the Johns Hopkins University School of Medicine, the Neurological Institute, the Mission to Lepers, and the Child Hygiene Association.

Urgent appeals to elevate the quality of service in hospitals also generated much discussion in the Fund's early years. Farrand said somewhat disinterestedly in a Special Report to the Fund's directors at the end of 1919: "There are some who think that public health is the present philanthropic fad, but the larger number of people who are entitled to an opinion believe that the building of the body is to be the great work of the immediate future, and that accordingly, public health is the most important field to be entered."[15] But Farrand was not yet persuaded that the Commonwealth Fund should exist at all. He believed that until the board of directors had developed a clearly defined policy upon which to stake the foundation's existence, the Fund should not be an operating concern. The opinion of the "larger number of people" notwithstanding, Farrand thought that the Fund should not commit itself to long-range plans in medicine and public health, as these fields were already receiving ample support from other sources.

Farrand restricted the Fund to making appropriations to existing organizations and encouraging the formation of new ones. He saw a double advantage in this procedure: it removed immediate supervisory responsibility from the Fund and it freed the recipient organization from much of the suspicion then attached to close ties with foundations. In Farrand's view the Fund should not confine itself to any single line of activity but should be able to turn in one direction or another to explore different interests, to change its operations or emphasis from time to time. The work of the Fund during Farrand's tenure was consequently limited to the efforts of a central staff that investigated appeals and advised the board about acceptance or rejection of support but did not administer programs directly. Should the Fund survive, Farrand believed that new directors or staff members should come from fields pertinent to the Fund's future plans. He also advised adding some younger trainees to the staff, so that they could be educated in the policy-making process and carry on the Fund's work.

Farrand left room to support special short-term appeals, such as the request from the Johns Hopkins University's Department of Medicine for funds to expand its full-time staff of clinical scientists. In the process of making this decision, the Fund consulted Abraham Flexner, who commented:[16]

> The General Education Board has in the last few years appropriated $2 million to the school, the income of which is devoted to the development and improvement of teaching and research opportunities, particularly in the fields of medicine, surgery, pediatrics and obstetrics. It happens that with the close of the war a new professor of medicine has been appointed in the person of Dr. William S. Thayer. An extension of the work of this department is now feasible beyond anything that has been possible in the past. The university now appropriates the large sum of $50,000 a year as the budget of this single department. A recent budget, which will become available within a year, will enable the university to develop the department even more liberally. In the meantime, the organization which Dr. Thayer can procure and should in the interest of medical education and science be procured involves the outlay of something like $15,000 for one year to bridge over the gap. . . . I am informed that a local appeal in the City of Baltimore is not feasible, because the citizens of Baltimore are now contributing nominally toward the fund needed to make up the general university deficit. Dr. Thayer is therefore making the effort to procure outside assistance to the extent I have indicated: While I would not wish in any way to influence the action of the Trustees of the Commonwealth Fund, I have no hesitation in bearing witness to the merit of the case.

Despite the Fund's early foray into medicine, Farrand believed that the field offering the best opportunity was research directed to improving educational conditions and the quality of teaching. The Fund assembled a group of leaders in education to recommend a plan of operation.[17] This group chose as the main subjects for study the problem of school revenues and the analysis of school subjects and systems of public education.[18] They also advised appointing a committee to supervise and evaluate any projects undertaken. Farrand became chairman ex officio of the resulting Educational Research Committee and Samuel P. Capen was made secretary. (In a similar manner the subject of legal research was taken up by the Fund and a distinguished Legal Research Committee appointed.)[19]

Porter R. Lee, director of the New York School of Social Work, was enthusiastic about the Fund's plans: "I want to go on record as believing that in your plan of a committee of selected experts to head up a study of educational work you have hit upon a device which, quite apart from your study of education, has tremendous implications."[20] A cooperative study of school finances was an immediate practical success, but Edward S. Harkness thought that improving educational conditions was too big a problem for the Commonwealth Fund alone. He wanted a central government agency to supervise the whole of American education, keeping private organizations advised of changes: "Its works would have great influence. If this is so then these men [members of the Fund's Educational Research Committee] should concentrate efforts upon getting the administration to organize a Department of Education while they themselves should work on improved methods of education and when found should get them introduced through the government Department of Education."[21]

Although the Fund's Educational Research Program lasted only until 1927, it marked the beginning of the Fund's continuing concern with the processes of teaching and learning.[22]

The Decision for Child Welfare

Farrand's third area of interest was the field of social work. One of the most important phases of public health was child welfare, he believed, and one of the greatest needs of the day was a better knowledge of the problem of delinquency and crime. And—a key point—at the time no other foundation was supporting work in this area.[23] In his first report as general director, Farrand recommended grants to the National Committee for Mental Hygiene, the New York Nursery and Child's Hospital, the Tuberculosis Preventorium for Children, the National Child Labor Committee, the New York Child Labor Committee, and the New York Committee on Aftercare of Infantile Paralysis Cases—all of whose projects dealt with problems of childhood.[24]

In 1920 Farrand was authorized to investigate the broad subject of child welfare as a possible field of activity. The resulting survey[25] identified this area as one requiring local effort and suggested the use of demonstrations to awaken communities: The Fund postulated that once a community realized the program's value, it would itself take over the work. This novel approach had worked in Framingham, Massachusetts, where the National Tuberculosis Association had organized a community health demonstration.[26] After two years the town had become quick to meet its obligations and had seized the opportunity to improve its public health facilities. The tactic was also advocated by the Fund's expert consultants. Homer Folks suggested that the Fund establish a unit similar to that of the Child Health Council, and C. C. Carstens envisioned a demonstration that would include welfare services for infants and, through the public schools, older children. Carstens, who was executive secretary of the Child Welfare League of America, devised a plan that included care for mentally, physically, and socially handicapped children—an idea that was later carried out in the Fund's child health demonstration units.

The best plan appeared to be that of Thomas W. Salmon, president of the National Committee for Mental Hygiene, who recommended establishing a Division of Juvenile Delinquency within his organization. Until this time little thought had been given to applying truly preventive measures to potential criminals or delinquents, although William Healy's preliminary work had recently attempted to categorize the personalities of potential delinquents and reveal the causes of their actions. Salmon believed that studies of juvenile delinquency should be removed from the entanglements of prison reform, criminal law, and general relief work; instead, he would undertake scientific research in social hygiene, through a division composed of a criminologist, a psychologist, a psychiatrist, an educator, a sociologist, a justice of the juvenile court, an expert in criminal law, and a child welfare worker. He also advised creating a bureau connected with the New York School of Social Work, for the treatment of maladjusted children.

The Fund's directors explored the prevention of delinquency further at a conference in Lakewood, New Jersey, in 1921.[27] There the Fund and the National Committee agreed on the shape of a joint five-year program, to be administered by the National Committee and supported by the Fund.

With the completion of the first phase of the work in education and the expiration of his leave of absence from Yale, Max Farrand resigned on July 1, 1921 as general director of the Fund. He continued his association with the Fund as an advisor and director of its Department of Education. Uncomfortable as an administrator, Farrand found this new role more congenial, as it allowed him to limit his contributions to programs in his particular field of interest.[28]

The report of the Lakewood Conference was on the desk of the Fund's second general director, Barry C. Smith, when he assumed that position on July 1, 1921.

**Part II:
The Fund Finds Its
Targets**

3

The Program in Psychiatry and Mental Health

Men who are occupied in the restoration of health to other men, by joint exertion of skill and humanity are above all the great of the earth. They even partake of the Divinity, since to preserve and renew is almost as noble as to create.

—*Voltaire*

The Second General Director: Barry Conger Smith (1921–1947)

Barry C. Smith (fig. 4) was said to be an excellent administrator, well liked by his staff—"a strong-minded person, but fair, who had definite thoughts as to how things should be done. He saw to it that the things he wanted done, were done."[1] He also had his schoolmasterish side, a sometimes unreasonable passion for detail. He insisted, for example, on keeping track of all aspects of the Fund's activities (despite adequate staff assistance)—even approving personally each expense-account item, no matter how small. Smith was the chief architect of the Fund's early programs, the general director who implemented them for twenty-six years, and the administrator who led the Fund into the broad area of medical education and research that it supports to this day.

Smith was born in Pittsburgh, Pennsylvania, in 1877, and died in New York City at the age of seventy-four.[2] His interest in education emerged early in his professional career: After graduating from Yale University, he taught at a private school for a few years, and during this time wrote a Latin grammar. A year of study at the New York School of Social Work was followed by positions in nonprofit organizations in New York City. In 1918 Smith organized the National Information Bureau, which was supported by eight of the leading "war chests" to investigate war charities and provide information for the suppression of fraudulent charitable enterprises. The Fund's staff first consulted the bureau in 1919 about relief

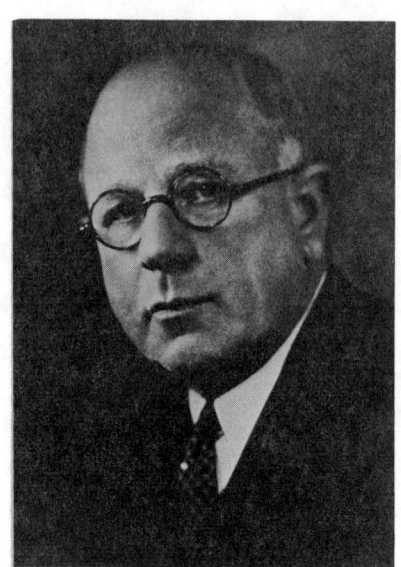

Figure 4. Barry Conger Smith
Reprinted from the Annual Report of
the Commonwealth Fund, 1947.

work in Europe. Over the next two years, they made increasing use of Smith's organization, which was growing rapidly under his leadership. In July 1921 Smith left the bureau to become general director of the Commonwealth Fund.

Barry C. Smith brought to his new post administrative experience in social welfare and knowledge of the field but none in either medicine or public health. Two of the first staff members he appointed, Barbara S. Quin (fig. 5) and Mildred C. Scoville (fig. 6), shared his professional background. Quin was a Smith College graduate with a master's degree in social work. Her professional career paralleled Smith's, as they had worked together in several of the same organizations.[3] Scoville was also a professional social worker, a staff member of the Red Cross in Minneapolis and of the National Committee for Mental Hygiene.[4]

Assisting the staff were leaders in both mental health and public health. Among the many advances in the natural sciences during the early twentieth century was the increase in recognition of the human being as a proper subject for scientific study. Innovations in mental health and public health rested on this recognition, and the Commonwealth Fund relied on experts in both fields to shape its contributions. The publications of Hermann M. Biggs (practicing physician and New York City's commissioner of health) (fig. 7), C.-E. A. Winslow (professor of public health at Yale University), and Adolf Meyer (professor of psychiatry at Johns

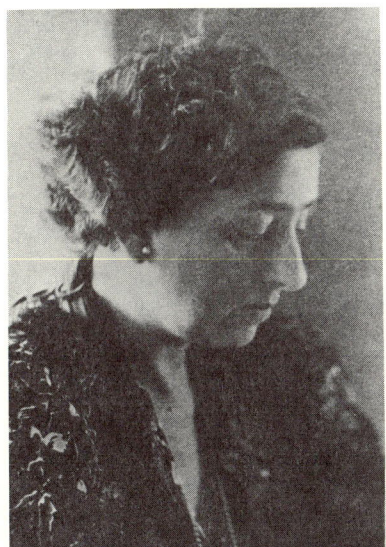

Figure 5. Barbara Story Quin Reprinted from the Annual Report of the Commonwealth Fund, 1945.

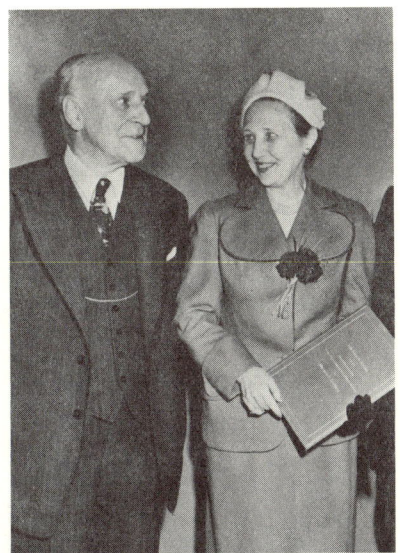

Figure 6. Mildred C. Scoville receiving Lasker Award in 1949 Reprinted by permission from the *New York Times*, November 18, 1949.

Hopkins University) (fig. 8) led Smith to seek these leaders' advice. Their concerns, endorsed by the Fund's other consultants, helped to provide the guidelines for the Fund's programs of the 1920s and 1930s, which included the child guidance clinics, the Child Health Demonstration Program, the construction of rural hospitals, and the training of psychiatrists. No less an influence on Barry C. Smith in the 1920s was the favorable temper of the times, a culmination of two decades of progress in public health and mental hygiene.

Although Smith and his staff were well equipped to enlarge the Fund's programs in educational research, legal research and child welfare, Smith was eager to acquire more information about preventive medicine and hygiene, areas already important to the Fund. He confided that he knew so little about his forthcoming responsibilities as general director that he was desperate to enlarge the scope of his knowledge.[5] As one approach, Smith read from cover to cover Milton J. Rosenau's textbook, *Preventive Medicine and Hygiene.*[6] He was particularly impressed by the chapter on mental hygiene by Thomas W. Salmon (already a consultant to the Fund's child welfare program). Salmon pointed out that the federal census in 1910 had located 187,454 persons in "institutions for the insane" in the United States—a figure that exceeded the number of students in all colleges and universities and the number of officers and enlisted men in

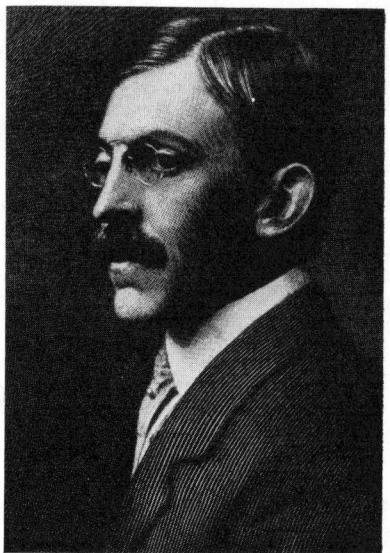
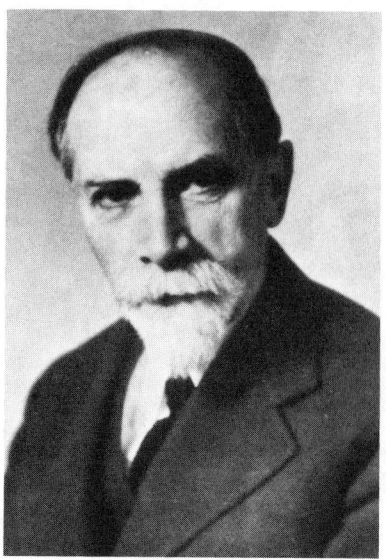

Figure 7. Hermann M. Biggs
Reprinted by permission from Winslow, C.-E. A.: *The Life of Hermann M. Biggs, M.D., D.Sc., LL.D.* Philadelphia: Lea and Febiger, 1929.

Figure 8. Adolf Meyer
Photograph courtesy of the Alan Mason Chesney Medical Archives, the Johns Hopkins Medical Institutions.

the Army, Navy, and Marine Corps. Salmon also noted the recent surge of interest in the mental life of childhood and the recognition that mental health can be endangered at a much earlier period than had been previously thought. Education, in his view, had to be fundamentally altered to fit the needs of subnormal children and those with special adaptational difficulties. More effort should be given to determining the individual requirements of school children, and the best educators should dedicate their attention to meeting these requirements. Salmon emphasized that because children and their families were rarely able to understand their situations or to take necessary corrective steps without the help of others, those who gave such help must possess psychiatric knowledge.[7]

The Background

A bodily disease, which we look upon as whole and entire within itself, may after all be but a symptom of some ailment in the spiritual past.

—*Nathaniel Hawthorne*

Psychiatry is a medical specialty, but it is also a basic element in *all* medicine and in what are known as the "helping professions." A foundation usually focuses on the specialty itself—its growth through research and graduate training—or on the application of psychiatric knowledge for the reorientation and enrichment of other professions. The Commonwealth Fund's mental health program, the legacy of Barry C. Smith and Mildred C. Scoville, pioneered in both directions. It augmented the number of specialists through training fellowships, a wise investment in view of the needs starkly brought to light by the experiences of the two world wars. At the same time, it attempted to relate modern psychiatric knowledge to the practice of pediatricians, general physicians, and public health workers.

The Fund's varied projects in mental health are too numerous to allow detailed description—or even mention—of each one. Only a few illustrative examples can be included:

I. The Program for the Prevention of Juvenile Delinquency
   A. The Child Guidance Clinics
   B. The Institute for Child Guidance

II. Education for professionals in psychiatry
   A. Fellowships
      1. The Henry Phipps Psychiatric Clinic in Baltimore
      2. The Boston Psychopathic Hospital
      3. The Colorado Psychopathic Hospital
   B. Sponsorship of the development of standards for board certification in neuropsychiatry

III. Programs linking psychiatry with pediatrics, medicine, and public health. Liaison programs between psychiatry and medicine included support for:
   A. John Romano's programs in psychosomatic medicine at Harvard University and the University of Cincinnati
   B. Developing departments of psychiatry, such as the one at the University of Rochester
   C. The Division of Mental Hygiene and the University Health Service at Yale
   D. The Pilot Clinic for a Broader Medical Service at Cornell University Medical College
   E. A program dealing with psychiatric disability in the Armed Forces
   F. A series of courses and conferences concerned with the relationship between psychiatry and medicine, and
   G. Professional psychiatric organizations, such as the Group for the Advancement of Psychiatry.

The Commonwealth Fund's contributions received lavish praise from Adolf Meyer, a leader in the development of modern psychiatry:[8]

The Commonwealth Fund and its director, Mr. Barry C. Smith, and the National Committee for Mental Hygiene and its first medical director, the late Dr. Thomas Salmon, have to their names and records the credit of having done the leading pioneer work in creating Child Guidance Clinics closer to local medical practice than to state hospitals and in supporting the extension of the necessary medical training. . . .[9] Through training fellowships, through conferences on basic organization and psychiatric education, and through the study of the status of medical education with special attention to the conditions we call mental problems and diseases, they supplemented the support given by other foundations to special research.

The turn of the century saw a major change in attitude toward the mentally ill, reflected in the more humanitarian care of the "insane."[10] The growth of psychiatric knowledge and the education of well-trained professionals led to better instruction in mental disorders—a relatively new phase of medical education, since in the latter days of the nineteenth century, "psychiatry" had little in common with its practice today.

The psychiatry of the later 1800s dealt with the "insane" as if they were a homogeneous group. Teaching and institutional psychiatry concentrated on the classification of mental diseases; no organized nosology existed until the publication of Kraepelin's *Lehrbuch* in 1883. Kraepelin, who served as the Linnaeus of psychiatry, classified mental disorders by recording individual phenomena according to essential similarities and dissimilarities. He described symptomatic clusters as entities that affected a patient much as did scarlet fever or pneumonia. Although Kraepelin stressed the disease rather than the individual, his nosology was essential for progress in psychiatry. Yet his ideas were still inadequate by modern standards: They were essentially descriptive, characterizing clinical patterns as diseases that could be clarified by biological methods without recourse to the patient's entire life history.

Two schools existed side by side in the late nineteenth century: traditional passive, descriptive psychiatric thought, limited to "insanity" and "asylums"; and the basically prognostic, "newer" psychiatry of Kraepelin, emphasizing classification rather than therapy. These two were soon displaced by a biologically oriented dynamic psychiatry, which included the whole of human nature and stressed research and teaching through daily work with patients. The mid-1890s saw a transition to child study and education and an interest in the nature of illness, rather than in just the symptomatology and incidence of disease. After 1900 the interaction of psychiatrists with teachers, schools, and the environment amplified the content of the patient's history, and a few years later, social work for patient and family was introduced into the hospital setting. An important tool was added in 1905: Binet and Simon's measuring scale for intelligence, an objective means of identifying the "feeble-minded" in the community as well as the many perplexing borderline cases. The identification of mentally deficient individuals was followed by an appreciation of their social importance.

During these same years, Adolf Meyer, later a consultant to the Fund and a recipient of Fund grants, was developing the psychobiological approach to mental illness. Meyer had worked in comparative and clinical neurology at Kankakee Hospital in Illinois and Worcester Hospital in Massachusetts. Shortly after he became director of the Pathological Institute of the New York State Hospitals in 1902, the Institute was moved to Ward's Island in direct association with a hospital for mental disease. There Meyer organized a clinical department and established training courses for staff physicians in state hospitals. It was also at Ward's Island that his important contribution to American psychiatry, the psychobiological approach, began to take shape. He contravened the custom of the time, which was to end the examination of a newly admitted patient with a single term describing his disease. By emphasizing complete case records, including information about all phases of the patient's life history, he liberated psychiatry from both its dependence upon pathology and the prevailing emphasis upon classification. From his work evolved much of the present-day content of psychiatry—the study of the normal (psychobiology), the study of the basic principles underlying abnormal behavior (psychopathology), and the more personal study and treatment of the mentally ill patient.

Paralleling the growth of the psychobiological approach was the development of the psychoanalytic school: The work of Freud, Jung, Adler, Prince, and Hall at the turn of the century enhanced understanding of the mechanisms underlying "normal" behavior and psychopathology.

A new emphasis on "mental hygiene" began somewhat later than the psychoanalytic movement, but quickly rose alongside it. In the fall of 1907, Clifford W. Beers appeared at Meyer's door with the page proofs of his book, *A Mind That Found Itself*: the vivid description of his memories and feelings as an inmate in a mental hospital. After his discharge from the institution in 1903, Beers devoted his life to abolishing the terrible abuses stemming from society's attitude toward mental disease. Included in the book were plans for improving the institutional framework of mental health work, through legislative committees and, particularly, by arousing public sentiment. The tandem efforts of Meyer and Beers joined professional psychiatry and public sentiment in a common mission. Beers offered the enthusiasm of the determined layman, dedicated to uniting physician, patient, and public; his appeal for humane treatment and compassionate understanding of the mentally ill turned out to be a powerful force for improvement. His autobiographical account was a cornerstone of the movement to promote mental hygiene and displace attempts at prejudicial legislation, freeing the insane from the strait jacket of ignorance and fear.

In 1908 Beers founded the Connecticut Society for Mental Hygiene, and the following year the National Committee for Mental Hygiene was formed. The National Committee cooperated with the inadequately supported mental hospitals to promote sound care of discharged patients and proper attention to patients even before hospitalization. It undertook studies of the personal and social factors responsible for mental illness, developing public understanding and reliable sources of psychiatric information for those in need of help. Finally, it looked outside the individual, stimulating the interest of health departments in mental health and advocating intelligent legislation.

Many entrenched attitudes had to be overcome, including the dogmatism of church, school and university faculties toward everything mental. Unwilling to recognize the emotions as part of the natural sciences, institutions held that area for their own, labeling it as the "humanities," which claimed "to know from tradition and revelation all that was worth knowing about man and his life."[11] Coupled with this protectiveness were the equally rigid ideas of medicine itself, which, in Meyer's words, had been "allowed to go the way of mechanistic materialism and elementalism, orthodox and extolled so long as it left the mind and soul and behavior to philosophy and religion." Meyer believed that an emphasis on lay development and lay organization might be a positive or negative influence toward scientific reform:[12]

> Physicians might be persuaded to lend their prestige as humanitarians to the cause of Clifford Beers, but they could not enthusiastically support practical investigation, public instruction, and research and demonstration of how to live and how to include mental health in the study of health, happiness, and a productive life. The main difficulty lay in an official agnosticism as to how to fit mind into what these medical elders had learned and thought of as science in medical school. . . . The core of the new movement—respect for and practical interest in the whole, undivided live human being—had still to be assimilated, to take the place of the traditional dualism of mind and matter, or the tripartition into mind, body, and soul, with its confusing division of interest and of labor and training.

The medical profession was so far from recognizing the relevance of mental health that at the opening of the new laboratories of the Rockefeller Institute for Medical Research in 1906, not a single reference was made to either the nervous system or mental disease—even though more hospital beds were then maintained at public cost for mentally sick patients than for all other patients combined.

Despite official neglect the national concern with mental health grew. Thomas W. Salmon (fig. 9), medical director of the National Committee for Mental Hygiene, surveyed the care of the insane and mentally deficient

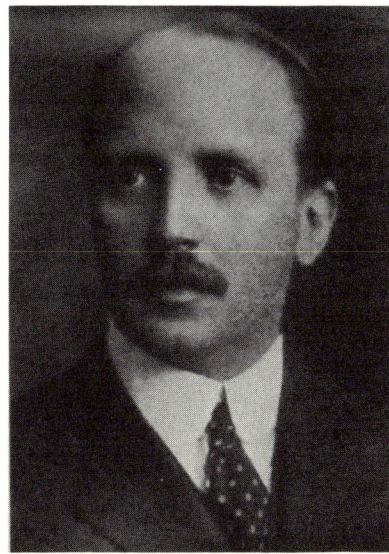

Figure 9. Thomas W. Salmon
Reprinted from Riesman, D., ed.
*History of the Interurban Clinical Club,
1905–1937.* Chicago: John C. Winston
Co., n.d.

in several states, and his efforts led the army to offer neuropsychiatric service during World War I such as no other nation provided. Psychology was also given a firm footing by the war, even though it was largely preoccupied with intelligence tests and had no clearly defined relation to modern medicine.

After World War I, through the influence of John Dewey, interest in mental hygiene shifted to the child. By the early 1920s, the mental hygiene movement was ripe for development, but it still lacked the endorsement of medical and general science. It was at this stage that the Commonwealth Fund's interest in the child began.

The Origins and Growth of Child Psychiatry

At the beginning of the twentieth century there was no body of knowledge or practice that could be regarded as "child psychiatry."[13] When good descriptions of behavior stimulated curiosity about the reasons behind behavior, Freud in Europe and Meyer in this country introduced the dynamic approach, which related the origins of the patient's present difficulties to events in his past. Biography, leading back to childhood experiences, became essential. The early textbooks had looked upon childhood psychiatry as a miniature mirror image of Kraepelinian adult psychiatry, and childhood as an "anamnestic antecedent" in the lives of adults and adolescents.

The retrospective search for early experiences as the basis of later maladjustment soon led to interest in the difficulties themselves. In 1899 Illinois and Colorado passed statutes creating juvenile courts, so that delinquent children could be handled separately from adult criminals. By 1910 children were receiving attention from several sources: the judicial system, educational psychologists, and psychiatric case workers.

The public had become aware that physical disease could be prevented, and now attention was focused on the possibility of preventing mental disease and criminal behavior. The initial step was a search for the earliest signs of misbehavior and maladjustment in childhood. What were these signs, and what remedial and prophylactic measures could be used? The psychiatrists, still sheltered in the institutions for the insane, had no ready answers. Almost nothing was known about the nature and significance of behavioral abnormalities in childhood, as no serious attempts had been made to understand needs peculiar to children.

Efforts to fill this gap resulted in one of the most significant developments in the history of modern psychiatry—the beginning of scientific efforts to comprehend and treat the emotional disorders of children. From 1910 to 1920, pioneering investigators studied the influence of intellectual and socio-economic factors on the scholastic, vocational, and communal adaptability of children. Psychometric testing was refined by Terman and others to suit the unique cultural patterns of this country, and these tests became widely used. Attention to the home situation and environmental factors resulted in the growth of social case work, as did the germinal juvenile court studies of William Healy. Healy contributed to the advance of the idea that the solution to crime lay in the study of the individual.[14] The Chicago Juvenile Psychopathic Institute, which he founded in 1909, was one of the first organizations to concentrate medical, psychological, and social study upon youthful offenders. Although Lightner Witmer's psychological clinic had been established thirteen years earlier at the University of Pennsylvania, Healy included new approaches, and his predominant interest in delinquency set his clinic apart from others whose primary service had been to education.

Mrs. W. F. Dummer, who sponsored Healy's first clinic, reminisced about the founding of the clinic and the temper of the times:[15]

> In my own case, the idea of the clinic is distinctly traceable to the thought of Mary Everest Boole and of Radot's *Life of Pasteur*, read in 1907 when, stimulated by the revelations of the Child Labor Committee, I had accepted service on the executive committee of the Juvenile Protective Association, and been shocked beyond measure at the realities of life thereby revealed to me. Brought up in an atmosphere pervaded by the Golden Rule, in which life was largely pleasure and joy, the contrast of squalor, poverty and evil offered a problem which, at one time, I feared was wrecking my mind.
>
> My reaction was,—These children are not bad. Any normal child deprived of all right opportunities would behave in the same way. There are, however,

certain exceptions: A deaf-mute boy maturing physically, but lacking education, who was corrupting various groups as he went from one neighborhood to another, and a few girls showing distinctly amoral behavior who at the time seemed far removed from normal mentality. I found myself unable to condemn that which I had always been taught abstractly was evil . . . .

Perhaps my contribution might be said to be those months of acute suffering which preceded the establishment of the Juvenile Psychopathic Institute. Emotion is said to tend toward action. I wonder if the result is in any way mathematically proportional to the keenness of the experience. The success of the clinic might so indicate in this case . . . .

I found that although progress was being made in the care of the insane, nowhere in the world was the atypical delinquent child being specially studied. My early attempts to persuade the Juvenile Protective Association that this was the most necessary step in their work in studying the causes of delinquency fell on deaf ears. I still recall the torrent of legal phraseology poured out upon me by Judge Mack, even after the establishment of the clinic, when I suggested that a wise physician, rather than a man trained in the law, would be of value in a juvenile court. However, my interest discovered others who were on the trail.

Different clinics emphasized different aspects of the problem of child guidance. The Chicago institute saw almost exclusively juvenile court cases during its early years, the Judge Baker Foundation worked with other agencies in addition to the juvenile court,[16] and the Boston Psychopathic Hospital and the Henry Phipps Psychiatric Clinic in Baltimore concentrated on problems outside the province of the juvenile courts. While in these four centers the foundations of scientific child guidance were being laid, what Adolf Meyer had called "the gradual growth and fruition of . . . a broader and more genuine comprehension of the real nature of psychiatry"[17] continued. In a few mental hospitals and medical schools, under a few leaders, physicians were being trained in the newer dynamic concepts of mental disorder. They were acquiring a broader understanding of their patients, learning to take an interest in the patients' families, schools, and communities. The original identification of insanity and delinquency as targets was commendable, but it emphasized the terminal stage, when help was needed to escape commitment to asylums and prisons. As programs progressed, professionals soon recognized that the most effective approach was to deal with "the everyday problems of the everyday child."

The increasing interest in children's health was marked by the establishment of a Division of Child Hygiene in the New York City Health Department in 1908 and in the New York State Health Department in 1914; the creation of the federal Children's Bureau in 1912; the formation of the National Child Health Council in 1920; the passage of the Sheppard–Towner Act for federal aid to local infant welfare work in 1922; and, also in that same year, the amalgamation of two voluntary organizations to form the American Child Health Association.

Now, in the early 1920s, child psychiatry was ready to offer its services to the public.

The Program for the Prevention of Juvenile Delinquency

The combination of Smith's own studies and the Fund's previous consultations and conferences prepared the way for its first long-range undertaking in the field of health, the Program for the Prevention of Juvenile Delinquency, which was announced on November 9, 1921.[18] The Fund had crystallized its interest in the welfare of children and intended to devote to this program about one-half of its income over a five-year period.[19]

The report of the Lakewood Conference on the prevention of juvenile delinquency, written by Henry W. Thurston of the New York School of Social Work, had emphasized remedial rather than preventive work, with individuals rather than groups.[20] Smith felt that the weakness of the report's proposal was its reliance upon social casework. As Thurston himself said, standards of casework in practice were far less rigorous than they should have been, largely because of the limited financial resources of social work organizations. The result was untrained, underpaid, overburdened workers. Since the caseworker did not meet the child until his social disability was already evident, any program based on casework would be ineffective in preventing neglect, destitution, or delinquency. Barry Smith had "no special enthusiasm" for Thurston's plan: "Such a program, no matter how well carried out, will not . . . produce anything like rapid results in the field."[21] Accompanying programs were needed, but at first Smith was not certain what sort of programs would be effective.

The Fund's leaders also favored a preventive approach over Thurston's remedial one, and Smith was given the freedom to set up the most effective preventive program possible, one that would treat delinquency before recourse to the juvenile court and probation systems was necessary. While children in reformatories, jails, and prisons needed attention, work with children in earlier stages seemed far more promising, both for the children served and for the country at large. Perhaps because of Rosenau's book and the board's interest, Smith came up with a detailed program that strongly emphasized prevention rather than correction. The scope of this program was even broader than its title suggested. In trying to prevent delinquency by promoting an understanding of children in general, it was really concerned with mental hygiene and child guidance and in fact was later referred to as the Program in Mental Hygiene.

Smith's Program for the Prevention of Juvenile Delinquency would develop the psychiatric study of difficult, predelinquent, and delinquent children in the schools and the juvenile courts. From this study would emerge methods of treatment and courses of training for workers in the field. The program would enhance the efforts of the visiting teacher, so that her invaluable early contacts within school systems could be used to advantage. In addition, demonstrations in widely scattered centers would show the effectiveness of psychiatric study and treatment. Finally, varied educational approaches would be used to disseminate the resulting knowledge.[22]

The Program involved the joint endeavor of four agencies:[23]

I. The New York School of Social Work. Porter R. Lee headed this institution, which trained students as psychiatric social workers, visiting teachers, or probation officers. The academic work was supplemented by field experience at the Bureau of Children's Guidance; the staff of the Bureau, directed by Bernard Glueck, studied and treated emotionally disturbed children from five public schools in New York City. The program regarded the children not as subjects for laboratory study but as individual recipients of service.

II. The National Committee for Mental Hygiene—Division on the Prevention of Delinquency. This division organized the child guidance demonstration clinics across the country. It was also responsible for two mobile demonstration teams, each of which was staffed by a psychiatrist in charge, an assistant psychiatrist, a psychologist, social workers, and clerical help.

III. The National Committee on Visiting Teachers—Public Education Association of the City of New York. A visiting teacher was placed in each of the five public schools affiliated with the Bureau of Children's Guidance to bring to the attention of the clinic those children needing its services, assist in the recommended treatment, and help in the field training of students from the New York School of Social Work. The division's second project was supervised by the National Committee on Visiting Teachers, which had been created for the purpose and was affiliated with the Public Education Association. Headed by the association's director, Howard W. Nudd, this program placed thirty visiting teachers in as many communities throughout the United States.

IV. The Joint Committee on Methods of Preventing Delinquency. This committee was organized as a coordinating agency for the entire program. It was also a publisher of educational articles and of the results of special studies, interpreting the program's work to other professionals and to the general public. The staff of the committee was organized under Arthur W. Towne as executive director; Towne was succeeded in December 1922 by Graham R. Taylor.

The Fund's four divisions were all symbiotically allied. The New York School of Social Work (Division I) provided fellowships offering "courses of training along sound lines for those qualified and desiring to work in the field."[24] Instruction in psychiatric social work was closely interwoven with field work given at the Bureau of Children's Guidance, the Fund's field center for practical training. The Fund intended to support fifteen fellowships of $1,200 each, but the program was off to a slow start: only three were given during its first year, 1921–22. By the second year, word of the program had spread, and sixty-three students applied for the fifteen places.[25]

Assisting the staff of the school were visiting teachers from the National Committee on Visiting Teachers—Public Education Association of the City of New York (Division III). Some visiting teachers were instructors in the program, but others were students: Many of the visiting teachers chosen to work in the demonstration clinics of the National Committee for Mental Hygiene—Division on the Prevention of Delinquency (Division II) were given the opportunity for special training at the school. The Fund was having a difficult time staffing these demonstration clinics. Its intensive efforts to attract visiting teachers were reflected in the proportion receiving fellowships in 1923–24: as many fellowships were given to visiting teachers as to psychiatric social workers.[26] Similarly, of the twenty-eight fellowship recipients since the start of the program, almost half had been visiting teachers.

By 1924 the Fund was starting to see results: "Graduates [of the New York School of Social Work] are increasingly to be found in important positions; and its influence in stimulating a further development of training in this field is an important factor in its usefulness."[27] The fellowships seemed to have taken hold enough to allow an increase in teaching staff at the school: thirty-one students were on fellowship (three for a second year) and twenty-seven were receiving summer scholarships. Now the Fund expanded the program to other schools as well. In 1924–25 the Fund allotted $6,000 to the Smith College School of Social Work for fellowships in psychiatric social work. The students at Smith, like those at the New York School of Social Work, were made available to the Fund's child guidance clinics for field work.

The Child Guidance Clinics

In 1922 the Commonwealth Fund's Division II began a program of demonstration child guidance clinics. A "team" of psychiatrist, psychologist, and social worker formed the nucleus of these clinics, and children's agencies were encouraged to refer children with disturbing or puzzling behavior. To psychiatric testing and study of the child was added the investigation of interpersonal relations in the home. Professionals began to correlate the behavior of the child with parental attitudes, and treatment plans took these attitudes into account.

The other divisions were working with already established institutions, but Division II had the task of providing clinical service in literally and figuratively new territory. The plan was to begin with one field clinic and add a second later, with demonstrations in not more than two cities during the first year. The demonstration service was intended to examine and treat problem children, establish methods and values, and help with the organization of the permanent clinics to follow. Once the objectives and scope of the clinical work were defined, the staff assembled, and the procedure planned, the members of the division had to find a suitable community for the first clinic, determine the length of its stay there, and help it to acquire the local backing necessary for success.

Early in 1922 announcements explaining the program's goals and the scientific basis of the work were sent to 225 juvenile courts and were published in periodicals. The Fund's choice of a community would be contingent upon local interest and promise of permanent local—preferably private—support. Replies to these announcements came from thirty-four courts; thirteen requested the service and five stated that such a service was not needed, while others suggested that the Fund help the state to deal with rural problems or to provide a traveling clinic.[28] St. Louis was selected as the site of the first child guidance demonstration in 1922, and clinics soon followed in Norfolk, Virginia; Dallas; Monmouth County, New Jersey; Minneapolis/St. Paul; Los Angeles; Cleveland; and Philadelphia.[29]

The ensuing five years for this division were ones of continuous discovery and change.[30] At first, each clinic's staff consisted of one psychiatrist, one psychologist, and one psychiatric social worker, but more staff members were often added to meet the requirements of individual clinics. Volunteer workers were sometimes available from local sources, and social work students were accepted for training.

As for the clinic's clients, many children coming into court were past the stage of prevention. Although the division had seen the juvenile court as a point of psychiatric attack on delinquency, it became apparent that other organizations, particularly children's agencies and schools, afforded a better approach to prevention. One solution was to link the clinic to these agencies so that it would be a center for clinical child guidance rather than merely a service organization for the delinquent. The predelinquent rather than the delinquent became the clinic's target, and the clinic staff began to study the prevention of other social problems such as mental disease and failure in school. Child guidance began to be at least a proximate aim in itself, and the psychiatric approach to the prevention of delinquency was no longer focused upon the courts.

These clinics also reached out to the community at large, through discussions, courses, and meetings. Lectures were given to community groups, and in Minneapolis, for example, the staff participated in courses at the University of Minnesota: a course in psychiatry at the medical school, a course in the department of education on the psychology of behavioral problems, and a seminar in the school of social work.

The program might have been considered too ambitious, and the Fund's staff considered eliminating some of its features. Both analysis and experience, however, indicated that it was unsafe to dispense with any of the parts. The importance attached to the individual objectives—study, treatment, and education—varied in different communities, but the main goal remained to establish the clinic as an integral, cooperative part of the community. Problems sometimes arose when the community was unprepared to cooperate in the casework called for by treatment plans. In St. Louis, for example, the clinic staff had to carry almost the entire burden; as a result, staff members could not live up to their standards of excellence, nor did they have time to offer educational programs in the community.

The division sought clinic staff with the best available experience, yet no one foresaw the complications that soon beset this unfamiliar project. Almost as soon as the program was established, the Fund's staff realized that there were not enough trained professionals to carry it out. In addition to studying the psychological implications of the demonstration process and community relationships in general, workers had to learn the techniques of child guidance on the job. The Fund's response was to increase its emphasis on training, and the Philadelphia clinic in particular offered a solid program for fellows in psychiatry and students of psychiatric social work.

With the completion of the Cleveland and Philadelphia demonstrations, the Commonwealth Fund's program of support for child guidance demonstration clinics came to an end. When the St. Louis demonstration was closed in 1923, its staff was transferred to Norfolk, Virginia, to establish a permanent clinic there. The bill presented to the Norfolk City Commission carried so small an appropriation, however, that this clinic was closed as well.[31] Another demonstration, in Monmouth County, New Jersey, was only partially successful. It had no permanent headquarters during its first year, and with its small staff, it received only a small appropriation from the Fund. After a year this clinic was folded into the Monmouth County Organization for Social Service.[32]

News of Division II's activities had traveled, however, and requests for assistance in planning mental hygiene work for children came from many cities in which demonstrations could not be granted. This interest was an asset to the mental hygiene movement that could not well be disregarded. To offer consultant services to interested communities, the Fund's staff decided late in 1923 to experiment with a field team consisting of a psychiatrist, a psychiatric social worker, and an office secretary. The consultant staff's contacts with these communities brought about one of the most important results of the experiment: a closer relationship between the child guidance movement and the national organizations for child and family welfare. But a consultant staff imported into a community for so short a time—usually weeks rather than months—worked under numerous disadvantages, and guiding a community's long-term programs in preparation for a clinic required broader experience. The field teams' visits were therefore discontinued, but this change in policy did not signal the end of help for cities interested in child guidance work; the division's staff continued to give short-term assistance along with its more detailed attention to the demonstration clinics and their permanent successors. Communities that had used the services of the consultant staff usually kept in touch with the division, and from time to time new communities applied for advice in organizing their mental hygiene work.

By the end of the demonstration period, visiting teachers were at work in fifty-five communities, and demonstrations had been conducted under the Fund's auspices in twenty-one of these cities. In the eight clinics permanently established through the demonstrations, the pattern of child guidance had been clarified. The focus of professional attention had shifted from delinquency and the courts to the more subtle evidences of lack of adjustment in the home and school, and much had been learned about linking the clinic with the community. The mutual responsibility of clinic and social agencies had gradually been revealed and concrete methods worked out for the agencies' use by the clinic. Many problems remained unsolved, but the strategy for dealing with them was reasonably clear.

The success of the child guidance clinics was undeniable. In the words of a contemporary psychiatrist, "The child guidance movement . . . swept the country."[33] Seven of the Fund's eight original demonstration clinics became permanent, and within the first decade after the start of the program, there were 230 locally funded clinics across the country.[34] Child guidance clinics contributed significantly to psychiatric therapy and research, psychiatric and related professional training, public education in mental health—especially education of parents—and to the concept of community responsibility for health and welfare.[35]

The clinics played a pivotal role in the origin and growth of child psychiatry. As Kanner expressed it so well, progress in child psychiatry could be represented as a series of concentric circles.[36] The outer circle symbolized the emergence early in the twentieth century of cultural trends favorable to the psychiatric study of children. The next circle included the years 1910–20, encompassing the creation of better community facilities for dealing with the problem child (for example, Healy's work in the juvenile courts, special schools and classes for retarded children, and organized foster-home care for neglected children). In the innermost circle was the effort made in the 1920s by the child guidance clinics to study family relationships and work constructively with parents on behalf of their emotionally disturbed children.

The Program in Transition

By 1926 the Fund's Mental Health Program was in transition. In April Smith presented a revision of the Program for the Prevention of Juvenile Delinquency to the Fund's board of directors. As usual, Smith had had the recommendations reviewed by prominent individuals, among them Adolf Meyer of Johns Hopkins and William A. White of St. Elizabeth's Hospital in Washington, D.C. One result of the Fund's broader interest in child guidance was a change in name for the Division on the Prevention of Delinquency, the supervisory unit for the entire program: it became the Division of Community Clinics. (The name of the program had been a liability, and all four divisions were replacing the word "delinquency" with the phrase "child guidance.") The Joint Committee on Juvenile Delinquency would be superseded by a Program in Mental Hygiene and Child Guidance; the Bureau of Children's Guidance would close on June 30, 1927, and an Institute of Child Guidance would be opened in New York City the following day. These changes reflected the revelation of the past four years that if delinquency was to be prevented, early intervention was required; once the juvenile court was involved, it was too late. Finally, the staff of the disbanded Joint Committee would become the nucleus of a Division of Publications. Publishing had been an integral part of the Fund's activities since 1921, and this new administrative unit was to plan and publish books that "explained, analyzed, or facilitated what the Fund was trying to do in all its chosen fields."[37]

Flexibility in selecting these fields was the key to success, according to Smith. It was essential, he thought, to avoid bizarre projects, to scrutinize each proposed undertaking for its theoretical soundness and practicability of operation (so far as could be determined in advance), and to consider the value of anticipated results. At the closing of the Program for the Prevention of Juvenile Delinquency, Smith formally assessed the Fund's administrative strengths and weaknesses over the five years of his general directorship.

He had used three different administrative structures to implement the Fund's projects:

1. Direct administration (as in certain phases of work in war relief);
2. Operating agencies (as in the Program for the Prevention of Juvenile Delinquency, in which administration of certain activities was entrusted to the New York School of Social Work and the National Committee for Mental Hygiene); and
3. Special administrative boards or committees.

At first, Smith had found the second structure less efficient than the other two. By 1926, however, he had come to believe that the difficulties inherent in the use of an operating agency could be overcome if the Fund retained sufficient control: "It is now thoroughly understood . . . that while the Fund has no desire to interfere in any petty way with the administration of the different activities, misrepresentation and devious policies will not be tolerated and the tonic effect is excellent."[38] The original administrative arrangement of the mental hygiene program did not allow adequate control of decision making, but this flaw had been corrected and Smith now judged all three methods equally effective.

The choice of method, Smith believed, should depend on the character of the work and the circumstances surrounding it. Certain activities required direct administration by the Fund; others required an administrative board; still others, involving a single, highly technical field, could best be carried out only by an experienced operating agency. All three structures required varying degrees of supervision by the Fund. Smith chose to enlarge his staff and involve them in the direct management of major programs. By 1926 the staff of the Fund's New York office had grown from seven to seventeen (excluding the 200 staff members of the operating agencies and special administrative boards engaged exclusively in Fund-sponsored activities). Quin as assistant director and Scoville as executive assistant continued to assist Smith in matters of general administration.

By 1927 the need for demonstration in child guidance seemed to be over. Interest in the field was widespread, and a sufficient number of stable clinics existed as examples for any community that might wish to start child guidance work. Yet in the five years of the clinics' operation, more questions had been opened up than answered. The smaller city wanted to know how to provide itself with a clinic; the city retarded in its social development wanted guidance in making progress; caseworkers felt the need for a better base of scientific knowledge and additional technical refinements. It seemed important that the National Committee for Mental Hygiene continue to guide the Fund's mental health program, and the Fund decided to retain its advisory service as a clearing-house for all child guidance clinics.

The Fund's new Division of Community Clinics offered five groups of services:

—Consultant service in established clinics, to improve clinical work and stabilize each clinic within its own community. Special services were given to all clinics receiving financial assistance from the Fund;
—Advisory service to communities planning to establish child guidance work. This type of assistance encouraged stable auspices, financing and administration, adequate personnel, and a sound relationship with the community;
—A placement service, to recommend adequately trained personnel for the child guidance clinics and to prevent the use of relatively untrained people;
—The stimulation and direction of studies of particular problems in the child guidance field and the professional exchange of information; and
—General education and informational work.

The Division of Community Clinics was a pivotal point in the Fund's mental health program. A central bureau for the entire child guidance field, it established standards for work and personnel, checked ill-considered projects, stimulated research and special studies, and evaluated clinical activities. The new division became a tool to encourage progress in organization and refinement of technique, and the soundness of its efforts and its position in the field led a steadily increasing number of clinics and communities to turn to it for advice.

The renamed division was also a logical extension of its predecessor and the term "child guidance" a more accurate label than "prevention of juvenile delinquency" for the program's activities. The purpose of the original program had also expanded during its last few years: not simply to prevent delinquency, but to establish sound methods for the well-rounded development of the child, train workers in their use, and extend their practice through demonstration and interpretation. The approach of the Commonwealth Fund to social change had shifted as well, from the narrow intent to stamp out juvenile delinquency to the nurturing of the new field of child psychiatry through the use of professional teamwork.

The Institute for Child Guidance

In reorganizing its program, the Fund used as a guiding principle the lesson that "knowledge is of little value unless there are people trained to use it."[39] The gains of the program could be lost unless special provisions were made to ensure competent and well-trained personnel for the future. And gains there were: the Fund was now certain that the psychiatric approach was the right one, and by the time the Bureau of Children's Guidance was closed, it had trained 203 students, 85 percent of whom were employed in the field.[40] Graduates of its program held positions as caseworkers in welfare organizations and psychiatric clinics, visiting teachers, psychiatric social workers with physicians in private practice, caseworkers in experimental schools, teachers, probation officers, workers in rural communities, policewomen, and institutional workers. Many went into communities where no mental hygiene work had been undertaken before. Between 1922 and 1927, more than 300 agencies had opened, serving more than forty thousand children a year; before 1922 only 170 had been in operation.[41] This nationwide enthusiasm reflected the Fund's influence, but it compounded the initial lack of qualified workers in the field. "A tide of interest throughout the country . . . bids fair to swamp the available workers," lamented the Fund's 1928 annual report.[42]

In response, the Fund's entire mental hygiene program, in all its activities, was focusing on the problems of training: "The clinic therefore needs psychiatrists, psychologists, and psychiatric social workers who are thoroughly grounded in their respective professions, thoroughly aware of the specialized character of child guidance, and thoroughly qualified, both technically and emotionally, to work as interdependent members of a staff group and as cooperating partners in a community. This is a large order, and the task of training such workers is as difficult as it is urgent."[43] As the reorganization of the Fund's mental health program continued, new purposes for fellowships came into view: Fellowships could send trained workers into direct service, but recipients, stimulated by contact with fresh ideas and new techniques, could themselves improve professional standards. To this end, traveling fellowships were given to six staff members of child guidance clinics.[44] The Fund also increased the number of fellowships at the University of Pennsylvania to eight and those at the Smith College School of Social Work to ten. The former Division III had become the third principal unit in the Fund's new program, supporting six fellows at the New York School of Social Work, four at the Graduate School of Social Service Administration at the University of Chicago, and two visiting teachers who wanted further training.

Despite the closing of the Program for the Prevention of Juvenile Delinquency and the demonstration clinics, the Fund also found a way to continue the part of its program for social workers: The Bureau of Children's Guidance was replaced with a new Institute for Child Guidance, similar but more extensive, whose purpose was "the training of psychiatrists, psychologists and psychiatric social workers in practical child guidance work."[45] Under the direction of Lawson G. Lowrey, with David

M. Levy as chief of staff, the institute represented the culmination of the Commonwealth Fund's interest in professional training during the 1920s.

Until 1916 there was but one clinic in the United States showing the characteristic child guidance structure. In 1921 there were 11; by 1926 the total had risen to 72; and by 1927 there were 102. The popularity of the movement soon threatened to outrun the capacity of the three professions involved to provide adequately trained workers. Not only were trained workers scarce, but before 1927 little research had been done to determine what kind of training was needed. Formal training in psychiatric social work during World War I had yielded increased numbers of trained workers for peacetime. Yet this training was insufficient for the child guidance clinics, which required collaboration among professionals. Though training for psychiatric social workers was improving, they also needed to learn the value and techniques of interprofessional cooperation. In pondering the advisability of setting up a training institute, Barry C. Smith solicited the advice of experts. His correspondence with Adolf Meyer reinforced his belief that the program would be valuable: "It . . . gives me greater confidence in the soundness of the plan itself to know that you believe the time is ripe for the establishment of such an Institute for Child Guidance."[46] The Fund's staff discussed the possible affiliation of the institute with one of the universities or medical schools in New York City,[47] but this link was never made, probably because none of the New York medical schools was ready to embrace such an innovative activity.[48]

The Institute for Child Guidance began its work in July 1927. No fees were charged for any type of clinical service, as the Institute was financed entirely by the Commonwealth Fund. It operated under the direction of an administrative board,[49] which included representatives of the Fund, the New York and Smith College schools of social work with which the institute was affiliated, and the fields of social work and psychiatry in general.

The institute had to provide sound clinical service, so that students could gain experience in working with clients under competent supervision, and afford some opportunity for research. By 1927 social agencies, schools, and the public were so conscious of the value of child guidance that requests for service came readily through the channels familiar to any community clinic. After some experimentation, the Institute managed to use its close relationships with a few of the large casework agencies to keep caseload and training requirements in balance, while giving occasional service to many other agencies and schools.

To integrate training and clinical functions, the institute based its organization upon a clinical team consisting of a staff psychiatrist, a staff psychologist, and two staff social workers from the group in training.

Each unit took responsibility for its own cases, which were assigned to the units approximately in rotation, and each unit functioned as a semi-independent child guidance clinic. The actual management of the case was usually in the hands of the fellows and students, with the staff workers exercising detailed supervision over study and treatment.

Primary control of both clinical work and training thus rested with the permanent staff of the units. General supervision of clinical processes and the training of psychiatrists and psychologists were vested in a psychiatrist serving as chief of staff, who was also charged with the development of research throughout the institute. A staff pediatrician and laboratory technician, serving all the clinical units, made as complete a study of each child as the case seemed to require. Suspected endocrine disorders received special attention, but the treatment of physical ailments was usually left to the family physician. To supplement the field experience of the fellows in psychiatry and psychology, two consultants, one in psychiatry and one in social work, conducted seminars during the first four years of the institute's existence. Later, this function was taken over by members of the administrative staff.

While it was expected that research activities would be part of the work of all staff members, a research unit was organized in 1930 for more intensive development of investigative projects. This unit was headed by the chief of staff (half-time) and included a psychiatrist, a psychologist (also half-time) and two or three social workers.

During its six years of existence, the Institute for Child Guidance provided training opportunities for fifty psychiatrists. Eighteen came for short periods of observation and shared only sporadically in the routine casework processes. This group included directors and staff workers from existing or projected clinics (including the clinic in London established with the help of the Commonwealth Fund), clinical directors from hospitals in New York State who were participating in a training program arranged by the Mental Hygiene Committee of the New York State Charities Aid Association, and a number of volunteers with professional connections. The other thirty-two came to the institute for structured training, normally for a full year, on fellowships either from the institute, from the National Committee for Mental Hygiene, or directly from the Commonwealth Fund. They were medical school graduates with either a general internship or at least one year of experience in psychiatry in a hospital with an active clinical service, and the Fund required that they be willing to work in an organized community clinic at the end of their training.

Of the three professions that met in the clinics, only psychiatric social work had the advantage of an established course of specialized training. When the demonstration clinics began, psychiatric social work had already been recognized as a professional specialty by the New York School of

Social Work, and psychiatry was the focus of casework at the Smith College School for Social Work.

Psychiatrists, on the other hand, often lacked the skills necessary for work with children: Many men otherwise trained had no idea how to talk to a child or how to win his confidence. Often, psychiatrists could not distinguish between diagnostic and therapeutic objectives, and between institutional practice and the complex responsibilities of community leadership. Child guidance workers generally agreed that responsibility for coordinating clinic programs and making clinic policy should remain with the medically trained psychiatrist, although large blocks of administrative functions could be delegated to an executive who was not a psychiatrist, and therapeutic tasks of considerable delicacy could be entrusted to psychologists and social workers as agents of the clinic.

Psychologists usually had limited knowledge of casework but adequate grounding in psychological theory and psychometric techniques. The training needs of the psychologists, like those of the psychiatrists, were related less to fundamental techniques than to the integration of these techniques with other approaches. Rarely before the existence of child guidance clinics had the psychologist been called upon to take a regular place in a balanced professional group. In the clinics he had to forgo some of the individual authority that the prestige of mental function tests had given him in his wartime heyday and become more sensitive to the relation between test findings and the child's whole personality.

The training offered psychiatrists at the institute was aimed directly at the requirements of the child guidance clinics, and the Fund assumed that men and women with institute experience would help to fill the vacancies in new and existing clinics. Fellows also found their way into a variety of professional connections, as this training in dynamic psychotherapy enriched the professional resources of a psychiatrist for almost any type of service. The significant later careers of the fourteen psychiatric fellows in training in the institute's fourth year reflected its wide-ranging influence.[50] The groups in training from the Smith College School of Social Work and the New York School of Social Work had thus far sent into service thirty-nine psychiatric social workers, twenty-three visiting teachers, and thirty social workers in other fields, chiefly in casework for children and families.[51]

Three fellowships were offered each year to graduate students in psychology with at least a master's degree and experience in mental testing. Seven men and eight women were trained as psychologists, and thirteen other psychologists came to the institute for shorter periods, either on special fellowships from the National Committee for Mental Hygiene (usually in preparation for specific posts in child guidance clinics) or as volunteers.

These workers were presumably already competent to carry out psychometric procedures, and some had been accustomed to using mental tests in a clinical setting. In opening its doors to psychologists, the institute intended to raise the prevailing standards in this discipline. The average community clinic was satisfied with a psychometric technician, and the field was well supplied with low-salaried workers. The Fund's demonstration clinics, however, had shown that a comprehensively trained clinical psychologist was capable of doing more for the team than simply making routine determinations of intelligence quotients.

Although the Fund increased the number of fellowships in psychiatric social work, so great was the demand for this type of training that the Institute for Child Guidance found it impossible to accept all applicants.[52] The institute's educational reach had also extended far beyond its own students: It had become a focal point for the child guidance movement. Staff workers were constantly in demand for lecture courses or single lectures in the metropolitan area and beyond; they taught at the Cornell University Medical College, the Smith College School for Social Work, the New York School of Social Work, the New School for Social Research, and the State University of New York. They also participated in courses arranged by the New York City Committee for Mental Hygiene and in institutes in New Haven, Boston, Milwaukee, and St. Louis, and contributed frequently to the regular sessions of the American Psychiatric Association, the American Orthopsychiatric Association, the American Association of Psychiatric Social Workers, and the National Conference on Social Work. Staff members took part in the International Conference on Mental Hygiene and the White House Conference on Child Health and Protection, and members of the institute's staff held office in professional associations and on committees in their fields. More than one thousand visitors from nearly every state and many foreign countries came to see it, and inquiries from all over the world about its work and its methods were answered by mail. The Commonwealth Fund itself was also supporting child guidance clinics in Great Britain.

By the early 1930s, the specialization of certain mental hygiene programs had given way to a demand for psychiatric social workers in other projects, and the Fund's training reflected the broadened field. The number entering the employ of family and children's agencies had increased: The clinics, growing less rapidly, needed fewer workers, and older agencies were increasingly hospitable to people with psychiatric training. Because visiting teachers were both requested and plentiful, in 1930 the Fund withdrew its fellowships to this profession, believing that its support of the National Committee on Visiting Teachers was no longer needed. The influence of the committee's work and its newly established standards of training had won this useful form of service a permanent place in the American educational system.

Similarly, when the Institute for Child Guidance was shut down as an economy measure in 1933, the Fund saw the closing as "less disastrous than it would have been at any previous time: the need of personnel for growing clinics was no longer urgent; training in child guidance was more generally accessible; and clinical facilities in New York had increased."[53] An editorial in the *Mental Hygiene Bulletin* concurred:[54]

> With the announced purpose of the Commonwealth Fund to discontinue its support of the Institute for Child Guidance in New York City in 1933, mental hygiene work in the United States received its first major blow from the Depression: In common with other philanthropic foundations the Fund, because of the Depression, found it necessary to decrease its commitment and after a careful study of the projects it was financing decided that the least damage would be done by retrenchment in this direction. Fortunately this withdrawal comes at a time when child guidance clinics as shown elsewhere in this *Bulletin* have reached a high point in their development and the discontinuation of this training project may perhaps least be felt since many of these clinics function as training centers which did not exist when the Institute was opened six years ago. . . . It is gratifying to note also that the economic slump has not yet seriously affected community clinic programs in the United States and that child guidance, a vital part of the mental hygiene movement, continues on its high level of progress and development. Child guidance clinics have been the heart and center of organized mental hygiene work and as the Commonwealth Fund states, they "have won their place among the accepted agencies of human betterment." To no agency do they owe more than to this Fund which has nourished and encouraged them from their inception.

The institute gave formal training to 336 persons and measurable clinic service to 2,641 children. From 1927 until its close in 1933, it educated a corps of more than 350 psychiatrists, psychologists, and psychiatric social workers.[55] The Fund could take pride in helping to train mental health professionals for the nation: A census of past students (psychiatrists, psychologists, and psychiatric social workers) in 1931 revealed that they were at work in half the states of the Union (15 in the Mountain and Pacific states, 3 in the Southwest, 28 in the Middle West, 9 in the South, and 100 in the East).[56]

The institute had always been a training center, accepting frankly the limitations of its role. As a child guidance clinic, it was atypically related to the community. By deliberate choice, it set a high standard of case work and was conservative about closing cases. It chose to offer training under specialized conditions through intensive, rather than extensive, experience.

By the mid-1930s the Fund's programs in child health and mental health had come together under the designation "child hygiene." Moralizing and punitive "correction" had been displaced by understanding and protective efforts to remove environmental disturbances. While benefiting from advances in the child hygiene movement, the Fund's programs at the same time encouraged further progress in the field. When the institute closed, many lines of inquiry were being pursued, but the structure of the institute itself created barriers to progress. The institute was firmly convinced that research in behavior and in therapy must be done in a clinical setting, yet it had to reconcile the wide gap between its desire for more accurate knowledge and the isolated bits of fact within its grasp. The child guidance clinics lacked the stimulation that would have been generated by a continuous inflow of fresh concepts, currently tested hypotheses, and new techniques developed in institutions best fitted for research into such matters. Pressed by the need to give technical service in a community setting and hurried by the pressure of the day's work, the clinics could not remedy this lack themselves. The staff of the institute concluded that significant research was impossible without more trained workers.

The quality of the Fund's service was also limited by the existing level of professional expertise. New projects were delayed; salary levels for psychiatrists were artificially inflated; and not only was there an unfortunate amount of shifting from one community to another but the Fund was finding it difficult to hold its fellowship recipients for even the length of their awards, so great was the demand for their services. The underlying difficulty was a lack of training. The expansion of preventive services of all kinds had added to the growing burden of institutional care of the mentally ill and created a serious deficiency in the number of trained men and women. Since the nature of the child guidance clinics made it necessary for even a well-grounded psychiatrist to undergo special training before he could fit smoothly into their procedures, recruiting new workers was a slow process.

Thomas W. Salmon's emphasis on the value of psychiatric knowledge was echoed by Smith's statement that "one of the greatest services a foundation can render is to assist, through scholarships and otherwise, in the training of personnel for various fields of work."[57] Many of the Fund's consultants recognized the deficiencies of the child guidance field at the time: "Despite widespread acceptance of child guidance and the popular acclaims it has received, a conscientious estimate of its validity regarding both diagnosis and treatment furnishes considerable occasion for doubt concerning its fundamental worth."[58]

The Fund attempted to compensate for these deficiencies by linking the child guidance clinics with nearby medical schools. Contacts with active practitioners of other medical specialties were also developed. Affiliation with a university usually enriched the opportunities for the clinic without robbing it of its community frontage, as might affiliation with a court, school system, or social agency. So long as the clinic was identified with the practice of psychiatry, it shared the wide range of that practice; psychiatry was already recognized as having a stake in the court, the schools, the social agencies—in everything that molded the individual. Functionally, the relationship opened the way for the clinic to influence the development of not only psychiatry but psychology, social work, and sometimes the law and the ministry as well. The physical proximity of the university hospital brought to the doors of the clinic fuller resources for study and treatment—resources that could not otherwise have been easily secured.

Educating Psychiatrists

In 1933, the American Psychiatric Association was moved to use language that from another source might have seemed exaggerated: "The dearth of competent psychiatrists is becoming a major issue in human welfare. It is no longer merely a matter of over-crowded mental hospitals in which the patients receive but momentary attention from the mental specialists. . . . We are confronted by a matter amounting to a national emergency—one not alone of producing psychiatrists enough to meet the need but one of producing, in large numbers, psychiatrists competent to handle the extremely involved problems for which their aid is more and more insistently requested."[59]

The association characterized the problem as a universal neglect of psychiatric understanding by medical educators. In the United States there existed, at that time, no established answer to the question of just what a psychiatrist was. In Great Britain the diploma in psychological medicine or the graduate degree in psychiatry was the mark of a qualified practitioner. But American medical schools had not agreed on what constituted the necessary training; clinical facilities in existence were good, bad, indifferent, or nonexistent; and there was a marked lack of cohesion in teaching objectives and methods.[60] In the opinion of the Fund's staff:[61]

> It takes many years to make a good psychiatrist—some medical educators speak of a minimum of five years after the completion of the basic medical course—as there is no great agreement at the moment as to what the form and content of this discipline should be. When the child guidance clinics were new, and most of the psychiatrists in the field had been trained primarily for such service as the state hospitals give, it was the exceptional man who was ready to step into a position where he must deal with the nascent disorders of childhood, and the clinics had to take such men as they found them. A little later, provision was made at the Institute for Child Guidance and elsewhere for specific training in the group techniques of child guidance which could be superimposed on what a psychiatrist already knew of adult psychotherapy. Then the Fund began a modest effort to encourage basic training by offering fellowships for postgraduate study at teaching centers where men might be

expected to learn a flexible and dynamic psychiatry. There is opportunity now, when emergency conditions no longer prevail among the clinics, for a fresh approach to the foundations of psychiatric training—instruction in the premedical and undergraduate medical curriculum.

In reviewing a survey made by the National Committee for Mental Hygiene's Division of Psychiatric Education, Franklin G. Ebaugh commented: "The general psychiatric teaching personnel was found to be most inadequate to meet the ordinary demands for general medical teaching. Sixteen of the 68 schools contacted, for instance, had a teaching staff of only one or two part-time men. Teachers of psychiatry, apparently, were appointed without any clearcut standards concerning qualifications of training or experience."[62]

As early as 1923, the Fund had established a fellowship of $3,500 for each of the two mobile clinics run by its Division II, to educate "young medical men trained in psychiatry who are willing to spend a year with the clinic with a view to fitting themselves to become directors of the permanent clinics."[63] The following year the Fund allotted $36,000 for five fellowships in neuropsychiatry at the University of Pennsylvania. This plan provided a course of training not even approached anywhere else in the world. Each fellowship was awarded to a graduate of a class A medical school who had had one year of internship.[64] Annual stipends ranged from $2000 to $2600, a generous sum at the time. Broad training in psychiatry was to be provided over three years, and the fellows were to be candidates for the degree of doctor of science for graduate work in neuropsychiatry.[65] Yet this program was said to have been poorly organized and the fellows taken advantage of by those responsible for the work assignments in neuropathology.[66] It nevertheless trained several men who later became directors of child guidance clinics and others who became prominent neurologists. Bernard J. Alpers, a distinguished neurologist in Philadelphia, was a Commonwealth Fund fellow, and G. H. J. Pearson, Paul E. Kubitschek, and Forrest N. Anderson headed child guidance clinics in Philadelphia, St. Louis, and Los Angeles, respectively.

The Fund also established fellowships for the general preparation of psychiatrists, at the University of Pennsylvania Hospital, Bloomingdale Hospital in New York, and Sheppard and Enoch Pratt Hospital in Baltimore. These fellows were assigned chiefly to older clinics—the Institute of Juvenile Research, the Judge Baker Foundation, and the Fund's child guidance demonstration clinics. Several community clinics, especially the one in Philadelphia, also served as training centers, providing experience for the majority of psychiatrists who later held executive positions in child guidance clinics.[67]

In 1928 Barry C. Smith and Mildred C. Scoville decided to withdraw most of their support from activities in the field and apply them to the promotion of training in psychiatry. The Fund invested $117,000, more than half the total for mental health activities that year, in ten three-year fellowships for graduates of a psychiatric internship (five at the Henry Phipps Psychiatric Clinic in Baltimore and five at the Boston Psychopathic Hospital),[68] and six two-year fellowships at the Colorado Psychopathic Hospital (fig. 10) for medical graduates intending to specialize in psychiatry[69] (see app. A).

The Henry Phipps Psychiatric Clinic

The fellowship program for training in psychiatry was initiated primarily by Adolf Meyer, psychiatrist-in-chief at The Johns Hopkins Hospital in

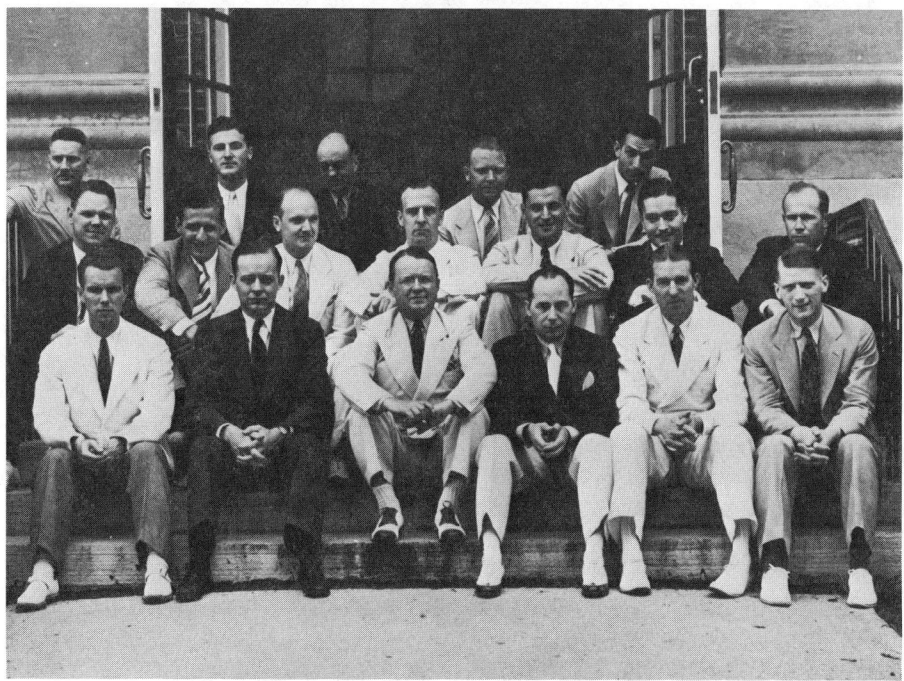

Figure 10. Fellows at the Colorado Psychopathic Hospital, Denver, Colorado, 1938. *Top row, left to right:* Unidentified (U.S.P.H.S. fellow); unidentified student; Marion Durfee (Commonwealth Fund fellow); Martin Towler (fellow from Galveston, Texas); Jack Ewalt (Commonwealth Fund fellow). *Middle row, left to right:* Unidentified (U.S.P.H.S. fellow); unidentified (U.S.P.H.S. fellow); Terrell Davis (U.S.P.H.S. fellow); Philip Franklin (Commonwealth Fund fellow); John Romano (Commonwealth Fund fellow); Edgar Findlay (U.S.P.H.S. fellow); unidentified (U.S.P.H.S. fellow). *Bottom row, left to right:* John Evans (Commonwealth Fund fellow); Herbert Parry (Commonwealth Fund fellow); Franklin G. Ebaugh (professor and chairman); Edward G. Billings (medical psychiatric liaison service); Charles A. Rymer (associate professor); John Benjamin (special fellow).
Photo courtesy of John Romano.

Baltimore. Most of the trainees at Phipps were on the threshold of specialized work in psychiatry, although some already had experience in state hospitals. The course of study provided for one year's clinical experience in the wards, the dispensaries, and the laboratories, and a second year of contacts outside the clinic—with emphasis on state hospital experience, hygiene work in a public school, and participation in a juvenile court service; third-year fellows were given special responsibilities for patients.

One of the most striking results of Meyer's program was the demand by other institutions for his young men. Even during the depression, when almost all the normal avenues of academic and hospital appointment were closed in other branches of medicine, the more advanced fellows were taken away before completing their fellowships, and the more junior fellows were able to secure important opportunities without difficulty. Mildred C. Scoville commented after a site visit on the excellence of the psychiatric staff; she singled out as the most stimulating parts of the training program Meyer's daily case conferences, his seminars on psychobiology, the wards for convalescent and neurotic patients, and his private psychiatric service.[70]

The program at Phipps continued past Meyer's retirement in 1941; funds were still made available to his successor, John C. Whitehorn, until the establishment of the National Institute of Mental Health after World War II. (After the war, Fund support was given mainly to supplement the GI Bill of Rights for individuals returning to the clinic.) During Whitehorn's tenure as professor of psychiatry and director of the Phipps clinic, the program was improved through more intimate supervision by the director and more emphasis upon the individual fellow's responsibility for therapy.

The Boston Psychopathic Hospital

A parallel fellowship program was established at the Boston Psychopathic Hospital under Charles Macfie Campbell, one of Meyer's protégés. Born and educated in Edinburgh, Campbell began his postgraduate training in 1902 under Pierre Marie in Paris; he also studied with Nissl and Kraepelin. Research with Alexander Bruce was followed by work at Meyer's Pathological Institute on Ward's Island in New York. In 1913 Campbell was appointed associate professor in Meyer's clinic at Johns Hopkins. Seven years later, he moved to Boston to become medical director of the Boston Psychopathic Hospital and professor of psychiatry at the Harvard Medical School. Fellowship recipients at the Boston Psychopathic Hospital were sufficiently experienced in psychiatry to be ready for individual research; the aim was to discover their special needs and capacities and provide them with the opportunity to round out their preparation for academic or clinical posts. Little or no clinical service was required of this group.

The Colorado Psychopathic Hospital

At the Colorado Psychopathic Hospital an effort was made to encourage psychiatric training at an earlier stage: twelve two-year fellowships in psychiatry were offered to promising medical graduates who had completed only a general internship. This fellowship program, under the guidance of Franklin Gessford Ebaugh, trained forty-four individuals. Ebaugh received his M.D. degree from Johns Hopkins and served an internship under Adolf Meyer; he then became assistant psychiatrist at the New Jersey State Hospital and in 1921 director of the neuropsychiatric department of the Philadelphia General Hospital. Three years later he assumed his position as head of psychiatry at the Colorado Psychopathic Hospital and professor of psychiatry at the University of Colorado School of Medicine. There were many applicants for the fellowships at the Colorado Psychopathic Hospital, and it was possible to select men of real promise. Candidates were admitted directly from medical internships and were subjected to a carefully organized course of instruction and clinical experience. Included were exposure to the psychiatric literature, supervised practice on the wards, in the outpatient department (especially in a child guidance clinic), and in extramural clinics; and some opportunity for clinical research on a modest scale.[71]

The recipients of these fellowships became some of the most productive men and women in their fields, taking key positions on the frontier between psychiatry and pediatrics, in psychiatric teaching posts, and in administrative and clinical positions in state and psychopathic hospitals and child guidance agencies. In 1941, on the occasion of his retirement, Adolf Meyer reviewed the history of the seventy-nine men and women who (in addition to the fifteen then at work) had held fellowships at Phipps. "Some . . . have become well known. Others are of more modest garb and grade. Taking it all in all, a noteworthy number has had the advantage of all the resources of the apprenticeship type and dispensary and community work and the theoretical training, with a widespread influence and effect."[72]

In addition to these three sets of fellowships, the Fund held five fellowships for its own staff to award in special cases. The Fund also offered annually, through the National Committee for Mental Hygiene, a group of fellowships for advanced training in child psychiatry. Eight fellowships open to psychiatrists who wished to work solely with children had been established at child guidance clinics in Philadelphia, Boston, St. Paul,

Cleveland, and Louisville. Fellowships were also available at the Payne Whitney Psychiatric Clinic of the New York Hospital and at the Child Psychiatry Clinic of Stanford University's hospital.

Board Certification in Neuropsychiatry

In 1933 the profession defined the minimal acceptable educational and professional standards for psychiatrists. The American Psychiatric Association created an Examining Board, which was instructed to "1) establish standards of fitness for the practice of psychiatry; 2) obtain information and prepare lists of universities, hospitals, and preceptors recognized as competent to give part or all of the training requisite for the practice of psychiatry; 3) arrange control and conduct examinations to determine the qualifications of those who desire to practice psychiatry; 4) issue a diploma or other evidence of special knowledge in the field of psychiatry to those who become voluntary candidates therefor and who meet the established standards; and 5) serve hospitals and medical schools by preparing lists of practitioners who shall have been certified by the Board."[73] The American Psychiatric Association established a program for board certification, and in June 1934 the first examinations in neuropsychiatry were held. Planning for these endeavors received financial support from the Commonwealth Fund.[74]

By the early 1930s, Barry C. Smith and Mildred C. Scoville had made the wise decision not to offer a larger number of fellowships for advanced work, because the number of candidates with adequate preparation in psychiatry was sharply limited. The Fund was beginning to doubt the wisdom of long-continued dependence upon the incentive of fellowships in recruiting for a medical specialty.[75] The Fund's staff recognized that their approach had only a temporary influence on the overall problem. Now the solution appeared to be in the curriculum of the medical schools. "Child guidance, like psychiatry in general, will be hard put to it for workers until the undergraduate teaching of medicine is such as to arouse an early interest in psychiatry on the part of superior students, and until the opportunities for postgraduate training and research are comparable to those offered by other branches of medicine."[76] Medical students did not benefit from the contributions of child guidance clinics, because education for the psychiatric aspects of general practice was not yet well organized in the medical schools themselves. While the clinics provided experience for residents in psychiatry, medical students were not considered sufficiently grounded in the fundamental concepts of behavior to take an active part in child guidance centers' clinical activities.

The early experiences of the child guidance clinics had also revealed the lack of close understanding between psychiatry and pediatrics. The work of the child guidance clinic should have started where the pediatrician left off, but this logical division was not possible when the pediatrician took charge of the clinic himself. Pediatricians often found themselves insecure in confronting the parental problems that played so large a part in the total service of the clinic. Those pediatricians without a general psychiatric background who nevertheless thought of themselves as qualified to practice "child psychiatry" were the most seriously handicapped, since the psychiatric problems of children usually could not be separated from those of the surrounding adults. The psychiatric staff of many clinics was left to handle cases that might be more appropriately treated by the pediatrician, largely because no one else in the community was ready to give the service these children needed. It soon became obvious to the Fund's staff that many pediatricians could benefit from programs providing psychiatric training: "Not less important than the training of psychiatric specialists is the development of some technic by which the essentials of a psychiatric point of view can be incorporated into the thinking and practice of the pediatrician, the internist, and the general practitioner. . . . There is growing recognition of the fact that what is commonly called the art of medicine may well be fortified by what we begin to know scientifically about human behavior."[77]

Liaison Programs

Psychiatry and Pediatrics

The Fund's interest in the welfare of children led it naturally to concentrate its initial efforts on linking psychiatry with pediatrics. Experience in the child guidance clinics had shown that physicians in practice, who dealt with many more children than the clinic attempted to see, were no less concerned with behavior than the specialized clinic itself. Although the interpenetration of psychiatry and social work had progressed, general medicine still had much to learn from the psychiatrist.

Spurred by Adolf Meyer's interest in integrating psychiatric approaches to the child with psychiatric practice, the Commonwealth Fund created a new element in its mental hygiene program. In 1934 it supported two experiments at medical centers of the first rank: a pediatric-psychiatric clinic at the Babies' Hospital (associated with the Columbia-Presbyterian Medical Center in New York) and a "psychological, social, and educational unit" at the Children's Hospital of Boston, the pediatric teaching hospital of the Harvard Medical School. Despite the clinics' shared purpose, their methods differed. At the Babies' Hospital, the principal clinician, W. S. Langford, had superimposed psychiatric training on training in pediatrics. In the program at the Children's Hospital, under Bronson Crothers, pediatricians were assisted by specially qualified psychologists and a consultant psychiatrist. Both units employed psychiatric social workers. The projects aimed to extract from current psychiatric and psychological thinking the most useful concepts and techniques for the pediatrician, and to find a way to add these to the equipment of physicians in training.

A similar, but smaller, program linking pediatrics and psychiatry was also underway with the Fund's help at the New York Hospital–Cornell Medical Center. By 1940 the Fund had supported this type of activity in five important teaching centers: in addition to the Babies' Hospital, the Children's Hospital and the New York Hospital, programs had been established at the University of Minnesota Hospital and the hospital affiliated with the Stanford University School of Medicine. After receiving assistance from the Fund for five years, the Babies' Hospital assumed financial support of its special unit in 1939, according to plan.

The unit at the Children's Hospital was the least typical of the group, as the psychological and educational implications of organic disorders were emphasized in a special ward. The other units worked primarily with hospital outpatient services, although there was increasing emphasis on ward service at the New York Hospital, the Babies' Hospital, and the University of Minnesota Hospital. Special intern assignments were in effect at the Babies' Hospital and the Children's Hospital; and at the University of Minnesota Hospital, graduate fellowships in pediatrics became available. Case conferences and seminars provided more formal teaching in the New York, Minnesota, and Stanford programs; formal consultations received considerable emphasis in all centers; and informal consultations were used extensively.

The Fund's staff was pleased with all five units. They varied considerably in organization, staff and procedure, but all were clarifying the psychiatric knowledge needed by pediatricians, developing the most effective ways of transmitting the information, and helping the field of pediatrics to determine the boundaries of its responsibility for mental health.

The Fund expanded its efforts when in 1937 it established three fellowships allowing pediatricians in teaching posts (or preparing to hold teaching posts) to spend two years in the study of psychiatry. The training of these men was carefully planned to enable them to teach "something which, though still undeniably pediatric, is shot through with psychiatric understanding. Perhaps such men can blend for themselves and for their students two sets of concepts which have too long been artificially separated."[78] In addition, five one-year fellowships were offered for psychiatrists wishing to prepare for clinic posts. Recipients were selected by the Division of Community Clinics of the National Committee for Mental Hygiene, and the fellowships covered a year of training at the Judge Baker Guidance Center in Boston; the child guidance clinics in Cleveland and Los Angeles; the mental hygiene clinic in Louisville; or the Philadelphia Child Guidance Clinic. Men and women who had completed this work already held appointments in the Winnetka, Illinois, public school system; in a newly organized child guidance clinic in Buffalo, New York; in state and local mental hygiene services in Nebraska, Indiana, and Ontario; and in Pittsburgh's juvenile court.

Some chiefs of pediatrics had also requested fellowships for junior men who showed an interest in psychiatric principles. By 1938 of the four awards already made, three had gone to young men holding pediatric appointments: the director of the pediatric outpatient service at the Vanderbilt University School of Medicine, a full-time staff man at the Children's Clinic of the New York Hospital, and the senior resident in pediatrics at the University of California Hospital—and the fourth to a man slated for appointment at the end of his training period. While each had some experience in the care of inpatients, their training stressed the practice of psychiatry as applied to the care of children not frankly neurotic or psychotic. To broaden their experience, the men were assigned to child guidance clinics. There was no thought of making psychiatrists out of them; that would have defeated the purpose of the fellowships. "If they become familiar with psychiatric thinking and skilled in those psychiatric techniques which are useful in the care of children the pediatrician ordinarily sees, and take this knowledge back into their teaching of pediatrics, the plan will be successful."[79]

The Fund was not hesitant to discuss the gap between the program's intentions and its execution:[80]

> The Fund is offering . . . fellowships to strengthen pediatric departments on the psychiatric side, but here it must feel its way cautiously, for the problem is not so well defined and the opportunities for suitable training are more limited . . . However strong the interpenetration [of psychiatry with pediatrics] is needed, it is not wholly clear how best to bring it about. Should the department of psychiatry plant a missionary outpost in pediatrics? Should the department of pediatrics lift itself by its own boot-straps? Should pediatrics go to psychiatry for what it needs? Where does full-blown pediatrics stop and child psychiatry begin? Should the child handicapped by an emotional stress be treated in pediatrics or in psychiatry or shuttled back and forth between them? Who takes care of the troublesome parent?

Caution slowed the integration program further in 1940. No new appointments to pediatric fellowships in psychiatry were awarded that year, as the Fund believed that "if progress is to be genuine the initiative for further experiment must come from the pediatric side of the fence."[81]

Despite these caveats, the efforts to link psychiatry with pediatrics continued. In 1942, during an extensive reorganization of the University of California School of Medicine, the Fund shared the expense of developing a unit designed for intensive service to children. Both undergraduates and graduates were taught under the direction of Karl M. Bowman, professor of psychiatry. Coupled with the interest already developed in the Department of Pediatrics around the work of a member of the teaching staff who held a fellowship in psychiatry from the Fund, this unit established a new level of care for children treated at the medical school.

These special units appeared to be useful in incorporating psychiatric concepts into pediatric thinking and practice. Histories taken by pediatricians and medical students showed increasing awareness of social and emotional factors, better selection of patients for consultation, and a tendency to retain such cases under pediatric supervision. Pediatricians were learning what to look for and how to understand the relation between physical and mental reactions. The staff at the Babies' Hospital in New York was "alert to educational possibilities and has shown discernment in the methods of approach and tact in relating this new service to established pediatric routines and procedures. Dr. [Rustin] McIntosh, Director of Pediatric Service, is well pleased and states that this clinic has been able to accomplish far more in five months than service from the Psychiatric Institute was able to accomplish in the Babies' Hospital over a period of four to five years."[82] At the Children's Hospital in Boston, "the effort is to bring psychiatric, psychological, educational, and social work techniques to bear upon the study and treatment of the problems presented, and so to make the interns, students, and student nurses, all assigned to this ward in rotation, aware of the value of such procedures in the care of sick children generally. Dr. Kenneth Blackfan, chief of pediatrics, reports that as a result of this work, 'It is becoming clear that psychological and educational observation has a real place in a hospital, whose main function is, and must be, the care of sick children'."[83]

Psychiatry and Medicine

Although these pediatric units were effective, the Fund's staff believed that departments of psychiatry in medical schools were the best place to reach undergraduate medical students. To further the link between psychiatric teaching and other undergraduate studies, in 1937 the Fund awarded a grant to the Department of Psychiatry (headed by S. Spafford Ackerly) at the University of Louisville School of Medicine. Most of this school's graduates became general practitioners in more-or-less rural districts in the surrounding area, and the program benefited the entire state.[84] The Department of Psychiatry had geared its teaching to the needs of the general practitioner: Medical students were exposed to theories regarding mental health and human behavior in all four years of the medical curriculum, and they could put this theory into practice by working with patients under the close supervision of the psychiatric staff. The curriculum did not offer a separate course in psychiatry; instruction took place while students and house staff were fulfilling their basic clinical responsibilities in medicine. Patients were usually selected for teaching purposes from the general medical and surgical wards in order to emphasize the relation between physical and mental factors. The program stressed psychosomatic relationships and the effect of lack of emotional balance on disease.

JOHN ROMANO'S PROGRAMS IN PSYCHOSOMATIC MEDICINE

In 1941 a grant to the Harvard Medical School strengthened the psychiatric component in medical teaching at the Peter Bent Brigham Hospital, where teaching services were being reshaped under the direction of Soma Weiss.

John Romano, a member of the full-time staff of the department of medicine at the Brigham for the previous two years, was responsible for clinical teaching and research in psychiatry. Assigned to him were a full-time research fellow and a psychiatric social worker. Romano wanted to make students aware of the emotional factors present in all illness, and his position in the Department of Medicine gave him more influence than a psychiatrist serving as a consultant or liaison officer. The neurological side of the medical service at the Brigham had recently been fortified by the return of Roy L. Swank from a two-year Commonwealth Fund fellowship for advanced study in London and Montreal. A report by John Romano summarized the Brigham's program:[85]

> In the first four years we have organized and conducted a psychiatric and neurologic teaching, clinical, and research service on the wards of a general hospital. The psychiatrist has not existed as a foreign body consultant nor as a liaison officer. He has been an integral part of the medical service, having both school and hospital appointments in medicine. Teaching has been directed toward nurses, students, and house officers. Methods of teaching have included lectures, conferences, clinics, and bedside instruction. The psychiatrist sees about 40% of the patients admitted to the medical wards. These problems are both neurologic and psychiatric. The principal problems are those of anxiety with or without physical disease, differentiation of the significance of the emotional factors in such people, delirium, and organic brain disease. Research has been directed along four principal channels which include 1) emotional reactions of patients to ward rounds; (2) delirium; 3) teaching methods; 4) individual case studies and neurophysiologic problems.

Romano accepted the chairmanship of the Department of Psychiatry at the University of Cincinnati in November 1941, and he remained there during most of World War II. Assisting him was George L. Engel, who had asked Romano for training while they were in Boston. The two began a liaison service in Cincinnati, receiving a Commonwealth Fund grant for fellowships and Engel's salary. One of their innovations was a teaching exercise: A resident from the Department of Psychiatry would answer a consultation request by the Department of Medicine and work the patient up thoroughly. The medical resident would then summarize his material, and either Romano, Engel, Milton Rosenbaum (of the Department of Psychiatry) or Eugene B. Ferris (head of the Department of Medicine) would interview the patient. The case would then be opened for discussion.[86] This "psychosomatic conference" put clinical clerks in psychiatry and medicine in closer touch with the psychiatric aspects of disease.

Romano left for the University of Rochester in 1946, taking Engel with him. What remained in Cincinnati was a full-time department of psychiatry that had become used to effective full-time academic leadership but now found itself in a vacuum. Maurice Levine proved to be an excellent choice as Romano's successor, encouraging a stimulating collaboration between medicine, psychiatry, neurology, and biochemistry in an atmosphere of excitement about the psychosomatic approach. When he was chosen to head the Department of Psychiatry, Levine was in full-time psychoanalytic practice in Cincinnati. His training had included time spent with Adolf Meyer in a Commonwealth Fund fellowship; and as part of his long-term interest in linking psychiatry with internal medicine, Levine had given a private seminar in his home for internists who wished to understand the role of psychotherapy in their field.

Mildred C. Scoville was particularly supportive of this department's efforts, and the Fund met the administrative costs of the program and the salaries of two fellows, one each from internal medicine and psychiatry. The first two fellows were Morton F. Reiser, who later became chairman of the Department of Psychiatry at the Yale University School of Medicine, and Robert H. Crede, who was to become head of the community medicine program and dean of the University of California at San Francisco. From this beginning grew the idea of the psychosomatic ward in Cincinnati—a ward that would not have existed without the Fund's support.

The twelve-bed psychosomatic ward was opened in 1949, with Reiser as its director. It was intended to be the one ward in the hospital that would practice holistic medicine and admit "problem" patients, such as those with bleeding and penetrating duodenal ulcers; uncontrolled diabetes; malignant hypertension and hypertensive encephalopathy; and a variety of other diagnostic entities. The service was staffed by the senior medical and psychiatric residents and specially trained psychiatric and medical nurses, and medical students were assigned to the ward as well. A patient would be kept on the ward for as long as necessary, until a thorough life history had been taken and a psychodynamic formulation and complete medical work-up performed by the appropriate subspecialists. During this time rounds would be made every day by the medical and psychiatric chief residents, and a conference about each patient's condition would be held each week. A combined treatment program devised for each patient would address his medical disorder and the underlying abnormal physiology; psychotherapeutic support would reinforce the patient's strengths rather than attacking his defenses frontally.

The isolation of patients with severe psychosomatic disorders proved to be unwise, however, since the ward took on too high a coloration of psychiatric problems and the patients tended to stay a long time. The ward also encouraged the staff to isolate the emotional components of illness: The perception was that since any patient with psychological problems relating to his illness would be sent to the psychosomatic ward, no other patient in the hospital had such problems. The assistant residents in medicine who passed through the ward for two-month tours of duty had little sense of being on a medical service and little opportunity to see more than a narrow range of psychosomatic problems, and this experience reinforced their tendency to think of psychosomatic disease as something quite apart from the ordinary run of medicine. The idea of a psychosomatic ward was therefore abandoned in 1951, and most of the beds were filled with unselected patients, assigned in rotation from the receiving ward of the hospital.

The psychosomatic ward nevertheless persisted in modified form, surviving until the early 1970s when its pavilion in the Cincinnati General Hospital was demolished. Only a few beds were still held for special referrals from the Department of Medicine, but the new mix of patients still provided an excellent opportunity for intensive study into the physical, emotional, and social aspects of their problems. Marion A. Blankenhorn, the professor of medicine, reported that "the ward now accepts in fact the responsibility for the total care of its patients."[87] The Fund felt that demonstrating "total care" in a teaching hospital was a very useful and then-uncommon service.

A second focus for teaching was the psychosomatic clinic, which met twice weekly, staffed by junior residents in medicine under the supervision of teaching fellows. The two teaching fellows worked on the psychosomatic ward and the clinic, as well as on the medical wards. During their ten-week clerkships, senior students were required to study at least one patient completely from the psychosomatic point of view. Informal weekly seminars providing detailed discussions between a group of half a dozen senior students, and an internist and psychiatrist became a popular part of the teaching program.

The year 1951 marked the Commonwealth Fund's final grant to the

University of Cincinnati's program in medical-psychiatric teaching. Blankenhorn believed that this program "succeeded in modifying considerably the teaching and practice attitudes in the department of medicine and [was] here to stay."[88] Although the program was still in need of support, it would soon be financed by the University of Cincinnati's College of Medicine and Hospital.

Reiser felt that on balance the Fund-sponsored liaison programs in Boston and Cincinnati had made an important contribution to American medicine. Students and house officers had been exposed to modern scientific psychiatry, which was in its early stage of development; they had gained a better appreciation of psychiatry throughout the rest of their medical careers. The program had also generated the beginnings of research psychiatry through partnerships with sophisticated, capable clinical investigators.[89]

THE DEPARTMENT OF PSYCHIATRY AT THE UNIVERSITY OF ROCHESTER

The University of Rochester was one of the recipients of the Commonwealth Fund's support for developing departments of psychiatry. In the late 1940s, the University of Rochester School of Medicine, always a strongly "scientific" school, had been affected by three recent developments: the Fund-supported Rochester Regional Hospital plan, a program of research in atomic energy, and the reorganization of the Department of Psychiatry under John Romano. During his first three years in Rochester, from 1946 to 1949, Romano impressed upon his colleagues a sense of the vital contribution that psychiatry could make in the teaching and practice of medicine. He had gained the support of professors of medicine and pediatrics, and he was influencing the basic policies of the school. Upon his suggestion, for example, the school began to offer a two-year general internship; this program provided six months of psychiatric training to prepare the intern for a kind of balanced general practice previously of little interest to the school. Much to the surprise of some members of the faculty, the best men in the class were asking for this type of training. Romano also presided over the completion of a new psychiatric unit in the Strong Memorial Hospital, which yielded additional bed facilities for the study of psychiatric patients.

The department was reaching out for community contacts. In undergraduate teaching, department members began to work with the freshman class, carrying these students step by step through a new four-year curriculum. The men who had come up through these courses were soon giving fresh color to the clinical work on the wards. Graduate training in psychiatry was well underway and was beginning to assume a reproducible pattern. The department was training people from medicine and pediatrics for collaborative teaching and clinical service, and other services were looking to it for help. All these changes boded well for the future of the department, for psychiatry in general, and for the specialty's contribution to medical care. In 1949 the Fund gave the Department of Psychiatry a three-year grant of $38,000 to be used at its discretion.[90]

THE YALE UNIVERSITY STUDENT HEALTH SERVICE

Another facet of the Commonwealth Fund's mental health program was the student health service at Yale University, begun in 1925 with a grant from the Fund.[91] "It is gratifying to be able to report on a prospective development in psychiatry," wrote the dean of the Yale University School of Medicine that year. "The need for such a department has been repeatedly emphasized and further evidence of the urgency of the need has been forthcoming during the year on account of the lack of available specialists to meet the requirement in this field."[92] Along with the founding of the Department of Psychiatry at Yale (also supported by the Commonwealth Fund), the student mental health service constituted an integral part of the school's development. The service was of fundamental importance because of the direction it was to give attitudes about psychiatry at Yale for at least the next twenty years.

The title given to the medical school's department—"The Department of Mental Hygiene and Psychiatry"—was of special interest. The medical school saw an enlarged purview for psychiatry: it would deal with a spectrum of emotional problems ranging from those of everyday life to those of pathological intensity requiring the patient's removal from the community. The dean's report of 1925–26 made this clear: The interests of the school of medicine have been in preventive psychiatry, rather than in outspoken mental disease . . . ; that mental hygiene and preventive psychiatry as conceived by the faculty of the school of medicine are subjects that merge with each other and cannot be arbitrarily separated; that the university administration as well as its department of student health has recognized that mental hygiene is one of the most pressing needs for the student body."[93]

Several colleges besides Yale had shown an interest in establishing a mental hygiene service for their students, but none had a program extensive enough to permit a thorough study of the problem. Answers would come only from the experience gained in actually running such a service. Mildred C. Scoville saw this project as an excellent opportunity for the Fund, and in 1925 the Fund appropriated $50,000 each year for five years to Yale's Division of College Psychiatry and Mental Hygiene. Arthur H. Ruggles was appointed head of the new service, consultant to the Department of University Health, and lecturer in psychiatry in the school of medicine.

The new division was closely affiliated with the Department of University Health and with the school of medicine. Somatic and emotional factors affecting academic performance were among the first problems to be studied intensively by members of the division's staff. At first emphasizing the emotional elements related to a student's effectiveness in his work, the staff soon recognized the importance of related questions: study and reading habits; physical difficulties affecting the learning process; reliability of the information on precollege emotional and academic development given by family, schools or physicians; and the effectiveness of remedial reading.

Yale psychologists Walter R. and Catherine C. Miles, Arnold L. Gesell, John Dollard, Neal E. Miller, and Albert B. Crawford were beginning their significant work on learning theory, and they were greatly concerned with the question of what makes for success in college. Sharing interests with the faculty meant sharing not only intellectual and professional ideas but joint participation in an area of primary concern at Yale. What questions were relevant to psychiatric knowledge? What emotional factors played a part in psychological and academic research? Through the investigation of these queries, the members of the Department of Mental Hygiene and Psychiatry found stimulating ideas and an invaluable access to key people in the Yale community. The Division of College Psychiatry and Mental Hygiene also received a stream of visitors seeking advice and technical assistance. Many psychiatrists were eager to glimpse the offerings of this new area: Some wished to gain experience in the new field as a stage in their professional formation, and others came for short periods of service, bringing fresh ideas into the department.

At the beginning of the Fund's grant, the plans for administration included an advisory committee,[94] a full-time staff of four psychiatrists in residence, a psychiatric assistant, and a group of visiting psychiatrists as lecturers and consultants. The advisory committee was confronted with the work of selecting adequate personnel and determining a broad policy for the division and its relation to the university as a whole. Four resident psychiatrists, two of whom gave full-time service to students, were appointed for the academic year 1926–27: Stewart Paton, Harry Kerns, Lloyd J. Thompson, and Clements C. Fry. Much of their time was devoted to developing ways of running the student service efficiently; they also conducted a study of the university and its life, so that they would, in addition to knowing the university community, be known by it. Their work in the first year was supplemented by a series of twenty-two public lectures given by leading psychiatrists.

Head of the advisory committee and chairman of the new division, Arthur H. Ruggles was a conspicuous figure on the American psychiatric scene. A leader in the effort to win greater understanding and acceptance of psychiatry, he promoted awareness of the widespread incidence of emotional difficulty in everyday life. He believed that psychiatrists should enlarge their understanding of these difficulties, and of "normal" growth and development, as well as widening their knowledge of the social environment. Ruggles was an excellent choice as a link between the college and the medical school, between the lay academic community and the professional one, even though he was fully available to the university only during the division's first year (when he was on leave of absence from his position as head of Butler Hospital in Providence, Rhode Island).

Although Ruggles retained only an advisory role after his first six months of full-time service, his view of the nature of the service, his ebullience, and the personal and professional gifts that made him a national leader in the field set the tone of the Yale student service. Lloyd J. Thompson, the first psychiatrist appointed after Ruggles began the enterprise, was especially interested in problems of youth and grasped the opportunity offered by a college setting to view the process of late adolescence. He, too, was eager to establish as many lines of communication as possible between the service, the rest of the Yale community, and other institutions.

During the important developmental period under the Fund's grant, Ruggles was supported by two distinguished advisors, Edward A. Strecker and Frankwood E. Williams—well known to their colleagues as enterprising, thoughtful men of wide-ranging curiosity. They were held in high regard for many years as leaders in the effort to bring psychiatry fully into the community, interested not only in the substance of the new service at Yale and its potential contributions to psychiatric knowledge, but in its "political significance" for psychiatry at large.

Full-time employment of social workers was an innovative part of the program. In line with the prevailing concept of their role, social workers brought to the therapeutic process information about sources other than the patient—from the administrative and medical services of the university as well as from school and family. Home visits and conferences with members of students' families were all part of the routine work of the clinic.

In 1932 the Fund's grant came to an end, forcing the division to reappraise its work and staff priorities. Until the end of that year, the division had first five and then four psychiatrists on its staff. Usually only two men gave full-time service to student work.[95] Assisting the psychiatrists until 1932 were four psychiatric social workers. With the end of the grant, the university budget took over responsibility for the continuing work. The staff was reduced to one full-time psychiatrist, responsible primarily for treating students and enlarging the community's knowledge of Yale's mental health program. Under the Fund's grant, routine mental hygiene examinations were a regular part of the department's work, but these were discontinued in 1932, partly because of reduction in staff and partly because of their failure as an important source of patient referrals.[96] Yale's report to the Fund for 1931–32 nevertheless expressed satisfaction that of the 261 patients seen in that academic year, 35 percent came voluntarily and 32 percent came through the contact made in the routine health examination.[97]

By the middle 1930s the clinical reach of the division had extended. Clements C. Fry became the division's head in 1931, and for the first three years of his chairmanship, the number of patients remained more or less constant at around 130 a year. In the late 1940s, a grant from the Old Dominion Foundation permitted the enlargement of the clinical service and of the training and research aspects of the program.

The Commonwealth Fund's grant had spurred the work of the psychiatric service for students. The Fund's support ended as the depression gathered momentum. Many people trained in psychiatry, in psychology, and in social work had been exposed to the psychological world of students and faculty, just as the academic world itself had confronted some of the emotional and psychological aspects of its own necessarily brought to the surface by this novel group in their midst. A residue of 3,000 files provided evidence of the five-year experience, ranging from accounts of single interviews in the routine mental health examinations to fuller histories of extended therapeutic encounters.[98] Fry's vision of the expanded service owed a significant debt to the experience made possible by the Commonwealth Fund.[99] Under the leadership of Ruggles and his equally distinguished successors, Yale's student mental health service has flourished to this day.

CORNELL UNIVERSITY'S PILOT CLINIC

Perhaps the Fund's most concentrated project in bringing psychiatrists into a teaching partnership with departments of medicine and pediatrics was the Pilot Clinic for a Broader Medical Service in the Department of Medicine at Cornell University Medical College, which received an appropriation from the Fund of $133,200 for the academic year 1947–48. Six advanced fellows in medicine were to receive continuous training for either two or three years in the care and study of patients whose physical symptoms were associated with emotional difficulties. Direction of the clinic was nicely balanced, as Harold G. Wolff, its director, held appointments in the departments of both medicine and psychiatry. His principal assistant, who ran the program on a day-to-day basis, was Stewart G. Wolf, Jr., a well-qualified internist. Although the fellows were being prepared for teaching posts, presumably in medicine, many of them became full-time psychiatrists. Their experience was intended to provide some mastery of the patient-physician relationship and its techniques, and to acquaint them with research methods in the then-emerging field of psychosomatic medicine. In practical terms, the fellows studied blood pressure, bronchial asthma, rheumatoid arthritis, and other illnesses, in relation to what Wolff called the "life situation."

Stewart G. Wolf, Jr., put the history and outcome of this program in perspective:[100]

> Immediately on my return from World War II, in October 1945, Dr. David Barr, the chief of medicine at Cornell, offered me the opportunity to organize a program that was being supported by the Commonwealth Fund. Dr. Barr was a director of the Fund at that time. He explained that one of the Fund's interests was in populating the schools around the country with internists who were accomplished in dealing with the psychological aspects of medicine. I agreed to direct the program, which was the responsibility of Harold Wolff's subdepartment of neurology. Our special clinic was known as Medicine A.
>
> The first step was to acquire a psychiatrist as part of this program. Herbert Ripley of the department of psychiatry had served with us in the Cornell-affiliated general hospital in World War II. Before that he had been assigned as a consultant to the departments of medicine and surgery and held that post all through my house staff training at Cornell. He was an extraordinarily shrewd diagnostician, a very fine teacher, and he really became one of us. When he would serve as a consultant, he would always seek one of us out to discuss the case. Ripley would tell us things that he had picked up in the history that we had not discovered. When he was able to point up relationships between symptoms and events in the patient's life, we were embarrassed at first, fascinated next, and then motivated to make sure that our work-ups of the patient did not leave anything that Ripley could discover. We never were quite successful at that, but, as you can imagine, we developed a very strong personal relationship with him.
>
> The next problem, now that we had the psychiatrist on board, was: What should the program be? To what should it devote itself? I felt very strongly that if we were going to train people to go out into academic posts in medical schools, it was important not only that they know how to talk to patients, but that they have a background in research. I insisted that the fellow's experience be half in research and half in clinical experiences; since in the course of their research, fellows would be studying, to a large extent, the patients that they saw clinically, these two activities were not really entirely separate from each other. The people at the Fund were cool to this idea, as their parallel programs elsewhere emphasized formal training in psychiatry and related psychological disciplines. However, we stuck to our plan.
>
> Dr. Barr wanted me or someone else from our group to be responsible for the whole outpatient department. I was unwilling to do this, as I thought that it would spread our activities out too broadly. Barr then selected George Reader as his outpatient director. Reader had had both his residency and fellowship training at Cornell, the latter with Paul Reznikoff, chief hematologist. He had also had a keen interest in comprehensive medicine and in the work that we were doing. His work with the outpatient department was then

supported by a new Commonwealth Fund grant. For a time, the units operated in parallel and there was a good deal of communication between the two. Nevertheless, Reader's Comprehensive Medical Care Program was not in any way an offshoot of Medicine A. Instead, it represented another of David Barr's objectives, one that I think he originally felt would be accomplished by Medicine A, but which ultimately required a separate program, separately funded.

The program trained a total of twenty-one fellows, along with five others who were not formally appointed as fellows. Nineteen of these had already begun careers in academic medicine. Of the twenty-six, all but three went right into academic posts in twelve states and Canada, Australia, and Great Britain. Two became chairmen of departments of medicine; two, chairmen of departments of psychiatry; and three, chairmen of departments of preventive medicine. The first fellow, Theodore Treuting, had been recommended by the chairman of the Department of Medicine at Tulane University in New Orleans, John H. Musser. By the time Treuting finished, Musser had died; but his successor, George E. Burch, accepted Treuting on the faculty and warmly supported his efforts. Other fellows, on completing their years of training, filled positions around the country in medicine, obstetrics and gynecology, preventive medicine, and pediatrics.

After Wolf left Cornell in 1952, a former fellow, William J. Grace, succeeded him as director of Medicine A. Another former fellow, Lawrence E. Hinkle, took over from Grace and ran the Medicine A clinic until its closing in 1955.

Psychiatric Disability in the Armed Forces

Men discharged from the armed forces after World War II (or rejected by the draft) because of psychiatric disabilities were so numerous as to constitute a national emergency. To cope with the return of discharged military personnel to civilian life, the Fund supported several projects, which further linked psychiatry and medicine. The first was a study by the New York City Committee on Mental Hygiene. The significant findings of this study were that more than 100,000 such men in New York needed psychiatric help, that only a little more than one-quarter of them were aware of that need or were willing to accept treatment, and that not more than one-quarter of the men who needed help were getting it.[101] This experience with mental illness in soldiers and veterans emphasized the need for psychiatrists to teach the concepts and techniques that all physicians require to handle psychiatric problems in daily practice.

An experimental rehabilitation clinic with a volunteer psychiatric staff opened at the New York Hospital in August 1943. The clinic, partly supported by the Fund, investigated the value and practicability of relatively brief psychiatric treatment for veterans discharged with neuroses or graver psychiatric handicaps. So much in demand were its services that the clinic was turning away more men than it was treating. It had a considerable measure of success with individual cases (especially men showing "combat fatigue"), clarified treatment procedures, and set a pattern for the twenty-five similar clinics in other cities.

The Division of Rehabilitation of the National Committee for Mental Hygiene was established in January 1944, to develop services for neurotic veterans, just as the Fund's Division on Community Clinics had been set up years ago in the field of child guidance. The new division was particularly useful as a source of printed matter and of special articles for the medical press, issuing the *Directory of Psychiatric Clinics and Related Facilities* (for the use of medical officers when discharging men from the services), the *Plan for the Organization of Psychiatric Rehabilitation Clinics*, and an excellent pamphlet of advice for veterans' wives, mothers and friends. It also coordinated the work of federal, state, and voluntary agencies, all through the efforts of a part-time director and one field worker. As partial demobilization brought the problem home to the public with fresh force, the division needed reinforcement, and a supplementary grant from the Fund provided for additional personnel.

The next year, the Fund supported a conference in Hershey, Pennsylvania, for civilian and military psychiatrists and medical educators. The recommendations of this three-day meeting were reported in a pamphlet entitled "Medicine and the Neuroses," circulated by the conference's sponsor, the National Committee for Mental Hygiene.[102] The main finding was that the rank and file of American physicians responsible for the immediate care of many thousands of individuals with neurotic reactions were for the most part unready for the task. Participants expressed the hope that many more medical officers in the Army and Navy could be trained in the essentials of psychiatry, so that upon their separation from the military they could become a leavening influence in civilian medicine, but this hope was frustrated by the unexpected speed with which demobilization occurred. Restudy of the policies and services of the Veterans Administration was also recommended, since the alliance of local Veterans Administration hospital units with medical schools offered promise for greater contributions from both. Those attending the conference also suggested that the National Committee for Mental Hygiene "intensify its efforts to arouse and inform the public and in particular the church, the schools, industrial management and labor, as to the needs and care of veterans with psychoneurotic reactions."[103] This recommendation was put into effect by the expansion, at Commonwealth Fund expense, of the committee's Division on Rehabilitation.[104] Finally, the conference participants proposed a pilot course in which a carefully picked teaching group would determine what could be taught quickly and briefly to men in practice and how best to teach it. The resulting course was also organized and supported by the Commonwealth Fund.

The sum of all these activities no doubt added something to the country's resources for meeting the immediate needs of hundreds of thousands of men whose contact with the draft or with armed service had revealed or multiplied their emotional difficulties. Over the long term, however, this was the smaller part of what needed to be done.[105]

Other Fund-Supported Courses and Conferences

The course recommended by the Hershey conference was given at the University of Minnesota in April 1946.[106] This conference incorporated three types of assistance: the presentation in simple terms of a few basic concepts, clinical practice under supervision, and abundant discussion of a very informal kind. The lectures dealt with the development of personality disorders, the interplay of the emotions and physical functions, the physician–patient relationship, and the elements of psychotherapy.

John Romano, who was one of the participants in the Minnesota experiment, recalled:[107]

> The experiment in Minneapolis broke new ground. The teaching of psychotherapeutic medicine was its objective and the conference was attended by twenty-five general practitioners from the Midwest with a wide age range. We met with them every morning; the faculty, composed of Walter Bauer, Tom Rennie, Moe Kaufman, John Murray, Henry Brosin, Douglas D. Bond, Donald W. Hastings, Harold G. Wolff, and others, were very enthusiastic and all did their best to make it a successful experience. Geddes Smith, Mildred Scoville, and Lester Evans attended from the Commonwealth Fund.
>
> This was a most interesting experiment in which we, for two weeks, lived in situ with the students in a dormitory. We ate with them and were with them all day long. In addition, we had discussions in small groups after dinner. In the mornings, we had a clinical lecture, particularly on interviewing or history taking, the psychological aspects of the physical examination, or various aspects of symptom formation such as anxiety. All of this, of course, is detailed in the monograph of the proceedings of the conference which was published by the Commonwealth Fund. In the afternoon, we saw patients more or less at random picked for us by George Aagaard, who later became dean of the University of Oregon School of Medicine. The basic idea of the conference was insisted on by the Commonwealth Fund—the notion being to bring these physicians in and, instead of lecturing them, have them participate with the instructors in the moment-by-moment examination of the patient, interviewing and so forth. It was all and all a high grade performance and everyone who

participated in it felt as though he were involved in an original and very important experiment.

For clinical teaching, the University Hospital in Minneapolis provided from its medical clinics patients with vague, often long-standing, physical complaints. Discussion was encouraged by small teaching groups and was warmed by the friendly association of instructors and students, who lived together in the Center for Continuation Study, generously made available by the University of Minnesota. Questionnaires were sent six months later to all students, and ten students were visited in their homes and offices by one of the instructors and an observer from the Fund. At this time, twenty-one of the twenty-five physicians expressed their feeling that the principles taught were "of real and practical value in dealing with patients."[108]

The general pattern of their experience was surprisingly uniform. After the course most of them went through a period of hesitant experimentation to see if what they were taught would work in their own offices. Except for a few young veterans just establishing new practices, participants found it hard to arrange time enough for the leisurely interviewing that the patient needs to ventilate his anxieties. When they did make time, the results of thoughtful and unhurried study were rewarding. No one in the group, of course, had become a really skilled psychotherapist; they all worked near the surface of the patient's problems. Yet most of the men were clearly happier after taking the Minnesota course. They were helping some patients who had previously baffled them and thinking more clearly about those whom they could not help. They had stopped blaming patients for neurotic behavior and themselves for failing after due effort to find organic causes for the patient's symptoms. The increment of freedom in their relationship with their patients was enough in itself to make them better physicians. If this is the irreducible minimum of what psychiatry has to teach the average medical practitioner, it is still a precious gain.

By 1947 many schools had had some experience in liaison arrangements between psychiatry and medicine or pediatrics. The time seemed right for a meeting to discuss their common problems. The Commonwealth Fund again organized a conference of pediatricians and psychiatrists at Hershey, Pennsylvania, in March 1947, to discuss several timely questions: What has been learned about emotional growth and development? What can the pediatrician do in the field of mental health? What are the next steps in pediatric teaching and training toward a better understanding of the emotional life of the child? What research should and can be done in this area? The answers were inconclusive, but many of the participants found the discussion stimulating and were moved to make better use of the mental health facilities they already had at hand.[109]

The Group for the Advancement of Psychiatry

Although a foundation can clarify needs in a field and indicate ways of meeting them, lasting progress can come only from those who work in the field. The Fund was particularly interested in a development within the American Psychiatric Association (APA) in 1946, one that offered leadership for the further development of psychiatry.[110] Psychiatrists serving in the armed forces had become aware as never before of the urgent demands upon psychiatry, but the structure of the APA did not allow for immediate action. Fired with enthusiasm by their successful participation in war medicine and impatient with what they considered the conservatism and lethargy of their parent organization, a small group of psychiatrists tried to bring together widely scattered information from many sources, to study the needs of comprehensive health care, and to formulate plans for meeting these needs.

The Group for the Advancement of Psychiatry (GAP) began with about 65 members, but planned to limit its membership to 150. Members had to pass rigid scrutiny of their intent and professional soundness. Most of them had military and teaching experience. The nucleus of the group contained those men who met at the Hershey conference and those who served on the faculty of the Minnesota pilot course. Brigadier General William C. Menninger was elected chairman; Henry W. Brosin, professor of psychiatry at the University of Chicago, secretary-treasurer. The group functioned entirely through working committees for medical education, psychiatric hospitals, psychiatric therapy, public education, preventive psychiatry, and social work.

Concentrating at first on medical education, the group hoped to establish standards for undergraduate and graduate psychiatric teaching, to expand and improve psychiatric training centers, and to develop better psychiatric treatment for both inpatient and outpatient care. Members expected to visit medical schools, state mental hospitals, and federal agencies; to consult with experts from other related fields; and to publish the group's recommendations. The GAP, whose sole financial assets were the few hundred dollars obtained by "passing the hat" among the members, requested the Fund's assistance for group conferences, expert counsel for committees, advisory visits, and stenographic assistance.

The spontaneous effort by the best younger psychiatrists in this country excited Mildred C. Scoville's interest: the GAP furnished a medium through which several of the interests of the Fund could be furthered, and, more important, through which psychiatry could exert vigorous and forward-looking leadership.

This aggressive and hard-working group was soon able to begin reform of the parent group, the American Psychiatric Association. By 1948 Menninger had become president of the APA and members of the GAP were a dominant minority in the larger group. Five important reports had been published and widely distributed to selected recipients: These dealt with public psychiatric hospitals, commitment procedures, shock therapy, medical education, and psychiatric social work. In each case the published committee report represented the most helpful data then available. Governmental and other agencies turned to the GAP for assistance, the Veterans Administration adopting the report on shock therapy as a basis for its own regulations. The GAP's recommendations regarding psychiatric considerations in universal military training were included in official plans. The survey of current research activities, although incomplete, was used by the Mental Health Council of the United States Public Health Service. The medical education committee, at Army request, enlisted psychiatric teams to teach in six institutes of two weeks' duration. These were patterned on the Minnesota pilot course for general physicians given by the Fund and were offered in various sections of the country for all medical officers in the army.

In 1948 the Fund responded to a request from the APA to support two new activities: Mental Hospital Institute service, a program of education for APA members; and a committee-workshop plan, closely patterned after that adopted by the GAP, to reinforce the work of the association's administrative staff. Through awards for these projects, the resources of psychiatry, then limited in both quantity and quality, would be used more effectively to prevent and treat mental disorders.[111]

The Group for the Advancement of Psychiatry spearheaded much that the Fund was attempting to do in this field. In the mid-1940s the GAP's influence was only beginning to be felt and it obviously had much unfinished business. By 1948 the GAP was well-entrenched and the Fund thought that to reach its maximum effectiveness it should continue for a few more years with an increased budget. Its achievements had been made possible through the Fund's financial assistance, and through the zeal and devotion of individual members almost unprecedented in any organization. The thoughtful position papers of the GAP, based on pooled judgments from extensive experience, were an important contribution toward establishing standards in many areas of psychiatry. Mildred C. Scoville's continued interest in the GAP and its leaders provided a ready source of expert advice for the Fund's program in mental health and psychiatric education.

Psychiatry and Public Heath

To enable public health to use knowledge from pediatrics and psychiatry in the care of the child, the Fund supported a program at the University of Louisville that mobilized teaching devices. This community was just the right place for such an experiment, as it had one particularly favorable characteristic: Nearly everyone worked well with everyone else. This harmony came about, at least in part, because of statutory limitations on the salaries paid to public officials. To recruit and hold good people the health department had to team up with the university so that salaries could be pooled. Thus the health officer of Louisville and of Jefferson County was also the professor of preventive medicine and public health in the medical school, an assistant professor of pediatrics gave half time to the State Department of Health on medical relationships, and the state director of Maternal and Child Health Services was also a member of the university's Department of Pediatrics.

Further collaboration occurred between the university and the City-County Child Health Clinics: A dozen pediatrics residents took turns in staffing twenty of the sixty-five clinics for one month each, and two of these clinics were also used for senior medical student clerkships. Fund support eventually led to the creation of a division of mental health in the City-County Health Department.[112]

The relation between mental health and public health was also explored in a two-week institute sponsored by the Fund in the summer of 1948, under the auspices of the California State Department of Health.[113] The twenty-seven students at this institute were health officers and assistant health officers of California counties and cities, or bureau chiefs in the state health department, and one representative came from each of the public health services of Tennessee, Mississippi, and Oklahoma. Eight psychiatrists, three pediatricians with psychiatric training, and five public health leaders took the responsibility for focusing the discussion.[114] The institute featured good teaching but did not really offer a course in mental health. Instead, the program was an essay in interpersonal relationships, a forum at which free discussion between two groups accustomed to working with people in different ways led to a community of feeling. The participants concluded that the best way to advance mental health in the health department might not be a "program"—as commonly understood—but an awareness of shared concern and purpose. At the end of two weeks everyone was talking "public health language." Public health had been set in a new perspective for both groups.

The Legacy of the Program in Mental Hygiene

The Commonwealth Fund recognized early in its course that if medicine is to relieve mental ill health, there must be more, better-trained psychiatrists and stronger bridges between psychiatrists and other physicians. It is fortunate that there probably will never be enough psychiatrists to treat all the neuroses that burden the American public, for the internist and general physician cannot afford to exclude the treatment of neurotic reactions from everyday medical practice. He must take into account what is referred to as the "psychiatric aspects of medicine" or leave a large part of his work undone. The key people who can meet this need are psychiatrists able to teach internists, pediatricians, surgeons, and physicians generally that core of understanding and technique that any doctor needs if he is to be fully helpful to a sick individual. This is the point at which the Fund focused its efforts to serve the cause of mental health. It offered fellowships to these men, shared in the task of planning their training, helped to organize situations in which they could be influential, and subsidized teaching clinics in which these aims were realized.

The pioneering work of the Commonwealth Fund in the field of mental hygiene was followed by interest from other foundations. In 1934 the Rockefeller Foundation expanded its financing of programs in psychiatry and mental health, and the Carnegie Corporation acknowledged the Fund's leadership in the field: "Most American foundations, our own included, were slow to recognize the opportunities open to them in the field of mental health. Today the situation is reversed and it is already evident that a problem of first importance for each trust will be one of selection, of finding that part of the general field in which it can be most useful.[115] Not only other foundations but other professional groups in education, medicine, public health, and social work became aware of the need to incorporate psychiatric work into their own activities.

With the help of Mildred C. Scoville, Barry C. Smith had conducted a program in mental health costing 6.3 million dollars, one-sixth of which supported more than 400 fellowships for psychiatric training and more than 500 fellowships for psychiatric social workers. When Scoville retired in 1954, the Fund's activities related to mental health included biological research, research in child development, clinical research, and programs offering prevention and treatment of mental illness. Her retirement coincided with the advent of expanded support for mental health projects by government, the pharmaceutical industry, and other foundations. By the mid-1950s sufficient money appeared to be available from other sources for training in psychiatry—in 1956 the National Institute of Mental Health had allocated 12 million dollars and the Ford Foundation, 3.7 million dollars for the training of investigators.

The Commonwealth Fund's Program for the Prevention of Juvenile Delinquency, which began as a bold effort to effect social change, had been transformed into the "institutionalization of professional outpatient psychiatry."[116] This change reflected the Fund's struggle in its early years to define through its philanthropic work an appropriate approach to social intervention. Unlike other major foundations, which supported community-based services, the Fund also developed an expert élite in scientific research and professional education.[117] Yet as experimental projects were organized, the lack of qualified personnel became even more acute. Although the Fund (along with the Rockefeller Foundation) had for years made available a limited number of fellowships in basic psychiatry, child psychiatry, and social work, these grants were simply insufficient. In attempting to integrate psychiatry and internal medicine, the Fund's mental health program eventually dissolved into its programs in medical education and medical research.

4

The Program in Public Health

The highest aim of scientific medicine is the eradication of disease.
—William H. Welch

The Second General Director: Barry Conger Smith (1921–1947)

The Commonwealth Fund's promotion of public health in the early 1920s, tentative though it may seem when compared with its later programs, was a bold, unconventional undertaking for the time. Government hostility to foundations coupled with the public's view of public health work as a "fad" required the Fund to proceed cautiously in choosing projects for support. In his first report to the Fund's board of directors, Barry C. Smith presented a request from William H. Park for support of his work in diphtheria immunization. Despite Park's belief that the danger of side effects was negligible, Smith pointed out that if one of the inoculated children should die, foundations would be accused of using children for experimental purposes.

Only a few years later, though, a program in public health seemed a natural outgrowth of the Fund's interest in the welfare of the child. A study had reinforced Smith's belief that a plan making a variety of public health facilities available to every child would accomplish more than the most thoroughgoing effort targeted at special classes of children:[1] 35% of the young men drafted into the armed forces in World War I had been found unfit to serve, and a high percentage of their defects were traceable to neglect in childhood. Nor was the machinery in place to improve the health of the nation's children: In the early 1920s public health units were usually run part-time, by untrained individuals. The field was ripe for a broad preventive program that would encompass such public health measures as immunization against communicable disease, provision of a potable water supply and a milk supply free of contamination, dental care, and attention to the nutritional well-being and general health of the children of each community.

The Background

The character of a health department—its basic organization, its goals and responsibilities, and the scope and limitations of its powers—depends upon the government within which it functions. The policies of government in turn reflect "existing social philosophy, which is itself the outcome of tradition, history, race, aspirations—the mores of the people."[2] In the United States, two distinct operational patterns for local, state, and national health agencies emerged from the two English "companies" formed to colonize America in the early seventeenth century.

The London Company had colonization rights from the Atlantic to the Pacific oceans, from north latitudes 34° to 38°. The immigrants to this region left England not to protest political or church affairs, but to better themselves. The land they settled invited agriculture on a large scale. These two considerations led to a form of government similar to that of their native England—with the county as the administrative political unit.

In contrast, the colonization privileges of the Plymouth Company extended from north latitudes 41° to 45°. The immigrants to this area were dissenters, having left the Church of England. Distrusting both civil and church organization, they chose government by individual congregation. The character of the land they settled, the threat of Indian attacks, and their desire to be close to their church did not encourage large-scale agriculture. As a result, their government was based on the township; county government developed later and never had more than limited authority.

As these two sets of pioneers moved westward, they took their approaches to government with them. The northern part of the United States thus tends to local government on a township basis; the southern, on a county basis; the middle zone, on a mixture of the two. Variations in state health departments and local health services also reflect the different forms of state and local government: Some states have strongly centralized state health departments with undeveloped local departments, while others have central departments functioning almost entirely through well-organized local services. The unit for local administration might be the town or the county, or a combination of both.[3]

The modern rural health unit or county health department is composed of one or more physicians, one or more public health nurses, one or more inspectors, and several clerks and other employees. But until about 1925, public health administrators and the public were both satisfied wiith merely the nucleus of health service. Public officials and the medical profession were accustomed to thinking of health-related activities as temporary; without an epidemic, there was little for a public health officer to do. Similarly, the public health problems of districts were not considered important enough politically to occupy full-time workers.

The change in the nation's attitude toward public health was powered by advances in bacteriology and the zeal of public health practitioners to extend the benefits of public health to all. Public health was seen as the science and art of preventing disease, prolonging life, and promoting physical well-being and efficiency through organized community efforts for the sanitation of the environment, the control of community infections, the education of the individual in principles of personal hygiene, the organization of medical and nursing services for the early diagnosis and preventive treatment of disease, and the development of the social machinery that would ensure to every individual in the community a standard of living adequate for the maintenance of health.[4]

Success in the first phase of the public health movement, sanitation of the physical environment, occurred through the efforts of W. T. Sedgwick of the Massachusetts Institute of Technology, who was largely responsible for developing public sanitation in the United States. From 1890 to 1910, a major public health problem was the mortality rate from typhoid fever, and sanitation was soon recognized as the most effective public health measure available for its control. A serious typhoid epidemic in 1911 brought L. L. Lumsden of the United States Public Health Service to Yakima County, Washington, to carry out an extensive campaign correcting the prevailing unsanitary conditions. Morbidity and mortality rates promptly dropped; to capitalize on these results through continuous public health service, Lumsden recommended the establishment of a county health department, one of the first in the United States.

Several cities in the United States—including New York, Chicago, Philadelphia, Boston, San Francisco, and Baltimore—have a long history of local health service provided by full-time, medically trained health officers. (The five boroughs that constitute New York City have been served since 1898 by a full-time commissioner of health, who administers the municipal health department.) But no county in the United States had a full-time health officer until 1908, when Jefferson County, Kentucky (containing the city of Louisville), not only acquired one, but provided him with a staff of sanitary inspectors. In 1911 the City of Greensboro in Guilford County, North Carolina, combined its health department with the county's, placed the health officer on full-time duty, and set up a county-wide service. In the same year, Yakima, Washington, appointed its city health officer as health officer of the surrounding county. Each of these three county health departments was organized in a locale containing a sizable city, and in each the needs of the urban population played a large part in forcing a solution to a public health problem. In 1912 the first county health department came into being in an area not influenced by the proximity of a large city: Robeson County, South Carolina, with a population of 52,500 and without any incorporated area of more than 2,500 persons, appointed a trained physician as full-time county health officer.[5] Between 1908 and 1934, 811 counties (more than one-fourth of the total number in the United States) appointed full-time local health officers, and by the end of this period the service was still operative in 541–two-thirds–of the counties.[6]

Another boost for county health service was a program supported by John D. Rockefeller to study and control hookworm in the South. In 1910 the Rockefeller Sanitary Commission, under the direction of Wickliffe Rose, organized and administered the five-year program, which depended on the collaboration of state health departments. The first half of the campaign was devoted to educating the medical profession and the public about the importance, prevention, distribution, diagnosis, and treatment of hookworm disease. Later, financial aid was provided for sanitation and the establishment of county health departments. The program's influence spread: These departments grew rapidly when it became clear that only the ones headed by a full-time director could adequately provide health services and meet the individual needs of rural areas. In 1918 there were 30 health units in the United States operating on a full-time basis; in 1935, there were 762; and in 1940, 1,577.[7]

The second phase of the public health movement in the United States, the application of bacteriology to the control of contact-borne infections, was almost entirely the work of Hermann M. Biggs. Health departments established in the nineteenth century were concerned primarily with the control of communicable diseases through environmental sanitation. Their programs identified cases, detected conditions likely to result in outbreaks of disease, and applied engineering skills to prevent or eliminate these conditions. Chiefly responsible for disease prevention were physicians, sanitary engineers, and chemists. Health professionals in the United States, although contributing relatively little to the growth of background knowledge, were more alert than their European colleagues to the practical applications of the new information in bacteriology and immunology that had become available in the late 1800s.

It was in New York City, in fact, that the new bacteriology was first used for the prevention and control of disease. In 1892 at Biggs's instigation, a small diagnostic laboratory was set up in response to the threat of a cholera epidemic. The next year this laboratory was expanded by Biggs's associate, William H. Park, into what could be called an institute of applied microbiology, where a wide variety of infectious diseases were studied, including diphtheria, tuberculosis, dysentery, pneumonia, and typhoid fever. Within a few years, almost all states and large cities in the United States had established diagnostic bacteriological laboratories.

So influential were these laboratories in diagnosing communicable diseases and providing biological products for their treatment that by 1889 the American Public Health Association (APHA) had established a Section on Bacteriology and Chemistry. Knowledge contributing to the prevention of disease and the promotion of health led to further recognition of the value of preventive medicine: In 1907 the APHA established a Section on Municipal Health Officers and a Vital Statistics section, followed by Sociological and Sanitary Engineering sections in 1911, a Section on Industrial Hygiene in 1949, and a Section on Food and Drugs in 1917. Four important new sections were launched in the 1920s: Child Hygiene (1921), Health Education and Publicity (1922), Public Health Nursing (1923), and Epidemiology (1929). Throughout the 1920s and 1930s, the Commonwealth Fund participated in the programs of the APHA, backing it financially and enlisting its collaboration to evaluate the Fund's public health programs.[8]

Advisors to the Fund, including Biggs and his colleagues Homer Folks, Livingston Farrand, and C.-E. A. Winslow, were among the leaders of the third phase of the public health movement—popular health education in the principles of personal hygiene. The campaign for public health featured an elaborate array of health bulletins, health news services, health lecture bureaus, health exhibits, and cinemas. All these educational devices were intended to secure popular support for health programs and to help health clinics reach out to the community. The mainstay of these clinics was the public health nurse, whom William H. Welch designated one of America's unique contributions to the cause of public health.[9] Public health nurses were ideal carriers of the message as well as the service. District (or visiting) nurses were introduced into America in 1877 by the Woman's Board of the New York City Mission, and the first group of nurses organized especially for this purpose, the Industrial District Nursing Association, was established in Boston in 1886. From then on, the teaching of hygiene became one of the standard duties of the district nurse, and in 1902 school nursing was introduced into America by Lillian Wald of New York.

Biggs also took the lead in organizing the fourth aspect of the public health movement, medical service for the prevention and early detection of disease. By the early twentieth century the physician had become an effective force in preventive medicine, as technological advances allowed effective medical examination of well persons and those in the first stages of disease. The tuberculosis dispensary and the infant welfare station did more than express the educational emphasis of the time—they implied an entirely new relationship between the physician and the patient. Even then it was recognized that before medicine could become truly preventive, a radical alteration had to occur in the basis of payment for medical service. Winslow and many of his colleagues knew that without compelling symptoms of disease, the average individual is unlikely to resort to the care of his physician if he will be incurring an immediate financial obligation.[10]

The new relation between physician and patient led to the growth of a systematic plan for the medical supervision of school children. Sweden appointed what was probably the first school physician in 1868. The idea soon spread: The first effective use of the school physician in the United States occurred in Boston in 1894, during an epidemic of diphtheria. The main duty of the physician was to detect communicable disease—to protect one child from another. At that time a proposal to establish school clinics for detection and treatment of noncontagious physical defects would have been labeled a dangerous form of paternalism. The medical inspection of school children during the first fifteen years of this century led to the recognition of malnutrition as a factor in lowered vitality, the development of nutrition clinics, and the program of popular health education inaugurated by the Child Health Organization in 1918.

The two main forces in public health—education and medical service—were complementary and inseparable, dominating the health programs of the era. The United States pioneered in the campaign against venereal disease and, through Biggs's work, tuberculosis.[11] As early as 1901 Biggs had claimed cancer and disease of the heart, arteries, and lungs as among the preventable maladies that would be targets for the health programs of the future.[12] Control of these diseases required educating the public not only in the generalities of personal hygiene but in the particular kind of personal hygiene that took into account an individual's specific limitations and environment. This aspect of public health practice therefore depended on a preliminary medical diagnosis and the use of the physician in a preventive role, rather than as a repairman after the damage was done.

Biggs became aware of the serious deficiencies in rural health service during the poliomyelitis epidemic of 1916 and the influenza epidemic of 1918—deficiencies corroborated by the results of a survey he ordered in 1919. He proposed the creation of local health centers, which would include hospitals, dispensaries, laboratories, district health services, and public health nursing services. In 1919, at Biggs's request, the Public Health Council of New York prepared a memorandum on these health centers,[13] and the following year, at the start of his second term as New York State's commissioner of health, Biggs saw that a bill providing for these centers was introduced in the New York legislature. Biggs's program was intended to develop school medical service, public health nursing, and public health education throughout the state; to coordinate all existing public health activity within specified rural or semi-rural areas; "to encourage and provide facilities for an annual medical examination to detect physical defects and disease; to assist the local practitioner of medicine by bacteriological and chemical laboratory diagnosis, x-ray facilities and expert clinical consultation service; and to provide for the residents of rural districts, for industrial workers and all others in need of such service, scientific, medical and surgical treatment, hospital and dispensary facilities, and nursing care at a cost within their means, or, if necessary, free."[14]

The plan was a bold attempt to solve at one blow a problem growing out of these conditions, one that had to be neutralized if medical knowledge was to work preventively for all classes in the community and for all geographic areas. But the bill was defeated: Many members of the medical profession still feared any steps taken by public authorities that seemed to threaten the individualistic practice of medicine. Although the plan was far ahead of public opinion—particularly medical opinion—in 1920, it captured the interest of Barry Smith and through him the directors of the Commonwealth Fund.[15]

The health center bill was defeated again in 1922, but Biggs's ideas continued to spread. That year Biggs delivered an address on the problem of health in the rural districts before the New York State League of Women Voters,[16] and it was probably this lecture that impelled Barry C. Smith to approach him.[17]

When the bitterness of the controversial health center bill had died down, Biggs made another attempt to provide medical service in rural districts. Alfred E. Smith was once more governor, and the state health department could count on his support. Bills were passed that adopted the principle of state aid to rural counties for "the construction, establishment or maintenance by such county of a county, community, or other public hospital, clinic, dispensary or similar institution, or for the purpose of defraying the expenses of such county in any public enterprise or activity for the improvement of the public health. . . ."[18] The practical translation of this idea was support for public health work in states and counties and the financing of county laboratories.

The far-reaching vision of men like Biggs expanded the field of public health until it encompassed the entire range of physical disability. Their efforts led to the establishment of special groups such as the American Society for the Control of Cancer (1913) and the Association for the Prevention and Relief of Heart Disease (1915), both of which were later supported by the Commonwealth Fund.

The nation's burgeoning interest in public health was matched and encouraged by the Commonwealth Fund's four major programs in the field. Child health demonstrations gave way to formal liaisons with state and county health departments, implementing the construction of rural hospitals and the transformation of existing hospitals into regional ones. As the scope of public health was enlarged, its approach to service changed as well: The physical aspects of the community became less important than the health and welfare of the people in the community. Through its own programs, the Fund adapted to this shift, adding experimental projects to governmentally supported activities. The Fund's unique contributions were supplemented by assistance from voluntary groups, which were able to use varied strategies not available to public institutions.[19]

The Child Health Program

Every child knows that prevention is not only better than cure, but also cheaper.
—Henry E. Sigerist

The Child Health Program was adopted by the Fund's Board of Directors on June 7, 1922, and the Child Health Demonstration Committee was formed to supervise the work. Two trends opened the way for the program: the mobilization of community resources and the application of increasing scientific knowledge to personal health.[20] Yet when the program was initiated, neither the recent national reduction in infant mortality nor the public's heightened interest in prevention of disease had made any substantial progress in influencing the child health practices actually in effect in the average American small town. In a survey of eighty-three large cities in 1920 and 1921, the Committee on Municipal Health Department Practice found that "infant hygiene is one of the more recent divisions of municipal health departments and few are yet prepared to carry the entire responsibility for infant care . . . . Only a small proportion of the cities has given very much consideration to the child of preschool age."[21] In few cities was there any unified concept of child health service. Approaches to the problems of maternal hygiene, infant welfare, preschool health, school health supervision, and school health teaching had been made from many different sources. Although information on the extent of health service in rural areas is mostly inferential, efforts to promote health education and protective services for children appear to have been much more sporadic than in the larger cities. When the American Child Health Association studied health work in American cities with populations between 40,000 and 70,000, the cities' average rating in maternal hygiene was 39 percent of a reasonable standard, in infant hygiene 58 percent, in preschool hygiene 32 percent, and in school hygiene 44 percent.[22] In 1921 a rural health survey sponsored by the local tuberculosis organization in Tippecanoe County, Indiana, gave equal space to two items: the collection and disposal of refuse, and school hygiene.[23] It was assumed that work in public health should concentrate on communicable disease control; further service, with its inevitable concomitant of larger budgets, was suggested only hesitantly. The Fund recognized the difficulty of persuading the public to support public health efforts:[24]

> The progress of public health handicaps its friends. If yellow fever threatened an American city money would be poured out for protection. But when a generally healthy group of people has set up a decent minimum of safeguards against disease, and few gross dangers seem to threaten the average household, it becomes harder and harder to prove to the taxpayer that he will get his money's worth out of larger payments for public health service . . . . The health staff which cramps its work because of bad judgment, limited imagination, or inadequate personnel is an expensive luxury just as truly as one which is overgrown . . . . It is certainly possible for one part of the health department program to absorb so much of the funds and time available that a lopsided piece of work is done, essential fields are neglected, and thoughtful citizens lose confidence in the health officer's leadership. Most rural health departments are now so sadly understaffed that the practical problem is to build them up. But there was never a time when it was more important to plan shrewdly for maximum output with a limited staff, in order to hold the ground already gained and clear a path for future advances.

The Commonwealth Fund's Child Health Program was not so much an innovation in public health thought as a novelty in public health experience. It was based on four fundamental assumptions:[25]

> That child health service formed an essential part of a well-rounded health department; that it could not be soundly planned except as a part of such a program; and that it represented a useful point of departure for interesting a community in public health.
> That the community, in meeting its responsibility for child health, must be concerned with the whole child throughout childhood.
> That the interest of private citizens in public health work was too valuable to be wasted in the support of unrelated enterprises, but could be developed into a powerful force for health education if it was intelligently related to a unified public program.
> That if the value of health work was shown convincingly, there would be no need to set arbitrary limits to possible appropriations for its support; but that small cities and rural communities could and would meet the cost of a well-balanced health program, including reasonably adequate work for children of all ages.

None of these assumptions was original with the Fund. "Child health specialists agree," wrote Barry C. Smith, "that they possess the knowledge of what to do and how to do it; that the public is keenly receptive in its attitude towards the whole problem of child health and alive to its importance. Nowhere, however, has a complete program been carried out."[26] Smith's purpose in spreading the idea of "keeping well" rather than "getting well" was to show that a sound, well-balanced public health program could take place outside the larger cities and could be incorporated permanently into the range of accepted, tax-supported public services. The techniques of providing service were established; decidedly untried, however, were the ways by which a vague concern with child health could be converted into intelligent participation in public health service.

For one year beginning October 1, 1922, the Fund appropriated $232,750 for child health demonstration programs in three communities chosen on the basis of infant mortality rates. One or more visiting teachers would be placed in each community, and the Fund's traveling psychiatric clinic would be at their disposal. The program was submitted to fifteen individuals for their comments,[27] and, as was customary in the Fund's early programs, an affiliated committee was set up to carry out the project.[28]

Responsible by contract for the administration, statistics, and publicity for these demonstrations was the American Child Health Association, a newly created amalgamation of the Child Health Organization of America and the American Child Hygiene Association. Herbert C. Hoover had accepted the presidency of the new joint association; he was elected partly because of his prestige and partly because he had made it clear that general financial support would be forthcoming from the American Relief Organization (ARO).[29] As the American Child Health Association's president, Hoover sought to control its policies and place staff of the ARO in strategic positions, making things difficult for the general director, Courtenay Dinwiddie. When it came time for Hoover's reelection, he first declined the nomination but then made it clear that if he were allowed to withdraw the ARO would terminate its support. Hoover was summarily reelected and set about revamping the organization. Dinwiddie, in turn, refused to continue as executive director, even though the association's board of directors was unanimous in its approval of his stewardship. Barry C. Smith's temporary solution was accepted:[30] Dinwiddie would resign from the association, with the official explanation that the Commonwealth Fund and the association had recognized the Child Health Program's need for a full-time director. One of Hoover's plans was to fold the association into the ARO (an idea that Smith related to Hoover's attraction to publicity), and Smith saw in the distance Hoover's wish to remove the administration of the Child Health Program from the association. It was wise, Smith felt, to prepare the Fund's staff by giving the Child Health Committee a separate office and staff—a plan that would avoid direct administration by the Fund yet assure the committee's continuation of control. It was through Smith's skill as an administrator that the entire situation was handled without any open disturbance, to either public health workers or the public at large.

Courtenay Dinwiddie was an administrator with considerable experience in both governmental and private organizations concerned with public health.[31] Smith believed that if the health benefits in these demonstration communities could be supported by statistical evidence, the national reaction would be favorable and his belief that, in Hermann M. Biggs's words, "public health is purchasable," would be vindicated. Planning this research component of the Child Health Program was George T. Palmer, director of research for the Child Health Association.

Since the program's central purpose was to demonstrate the possibility of establishing and maintaining maternal and child health services as part of a balanced public health program in the ordinary small community, the Child Health Committee was determined to select typical centers for its work. A successful demonstration was seen as an experiment in partnership and an episode in community self-education. The committee placed the initiative squarely on the local community, issuing a general invitation to communities in specified areas to make their needs and resources known if they wished to be considered. Communities had to meet three general requirements, whose fulfillment would ensure the validity of the "experiment":

1. The community should evince no striking departure from average conditions that would make its health problems atypical.
2. It should have important, unmet health needs.
3. Its officials and citizens should furnish evidence of their interest in a well-proportioned health program and of their intention to carry on, through local support, any work that proved its value.

The pool of applicants was therefore confined to places with an appetite for progress sufficient to enable local groups to present a united front when the community asked for their participation.

The first meeting of the Child Health Committee took place on June 15, 1922. By the end of September, thirty-three cities had applied for the first demonstration; Dinwiddie and William J. French left on December 1 to inspect the more promising ones.

The Commonwealth Fund did not insist that Dinwiddie and the committee employ any fixed procedure for selecting the demonstration sites, as adaptability to local conditions was regarded as a prerequisite for success. Because general community health included environmental conditions and other matters not directly related to problems of children, the Fund wanted the demonstration sites to be well reinforced by routine public health services subject to epidemiological study. The quality of state health work under the public authorities was thus an important factor in selecting the demonstration cities. The decision was to put the first demonstration in a city with a population of fifteen to twenty-five thousand, in a state in the general region of the upper Mississippi Valley. Three months later, the choice had been narrowed to Hutchison, Kansas; Fargo, North Dakota; Salinas, Kansas; Jefferson City, Missouri; and Winona, Minnesota. Hutchison and Fargo presented nearly equal opportunities, but since a somewhat similar health demonstration was being conducted in Mansfield, Ohio, a manufacturing town, the Committee was inclined to Fargo, an agricultural trading center. This city was finally chosen as the site of the first child health demonstration program, and other demonstrations followed in Athens (Clarke County), Georgia; Rutherford, Tennessee; and Marion County, Oregon.[32]

The term "child health" was used somewhat loosely in connection with the more rural of the demonstrations. Child health activities in the Fund's urban demonstrations supplemented the work of local health departments. But in Rutherford County, a health department had to be built and a local organization set up to perform all the functions of a county department of health. This department's large budget set it apart from most other rural health units, and it was able to engage at once in diverse and intensive activities.[33] The success of the entire program depended upon varied means of support, so that child health services could take their natural place in relation to basic activities for communicable disease control, such as sanitation and the recording and interpretation of vital statistics. In Fargo the need for full-time health department service was met by city appropriation. In Rutherford and Marion counties, the staff of the demonstration was accepted as the health department by the county and city authorities; this function of the demonstration gradually gave way to a locally supported health department as public funds became available. An early advantage for these departments was regular appraisal by the American Public Health Association, which tended to keep their programs on an even keel.

Although the pattern of service introduced in the four demonstration communities was standardized, variations in community needs and resources demanded flexibility in applying this pattern, and by the end of the five-year demonstration, no two of the areas had precisely the same program. In general, however, the idea was to discover whether a uniform plan, shaped as nearly as possible to conform with the best current public health practices, might be practicable for small cities and rural counties.

The Administration of the Child Health Demonstrations

The Child Health Demonstration Committee turned for advice to the American Child Health Association, the American Public Health Association, and the National Association for Public Health Nursing; and pediatrician Henry F. Helmholz of the Mayo Clinic served as a consultant. Cordial relationships were established with the United States Public Health Service, and Surgeon General Hugh S. Cumming arranged to give his chief assistant a leave of absence to visit the demonstrations and advise the Fund about the technical aspects of public health work. The committee's efforts were intended to be nationally significant: The relation of child health to general community health was considered to be of paramount importance, as the demonstrations involved health concerns, environmental conditions, and other matters not directly related to the problems of children.

Smith's new administrative policy eliminated many of the problems that had beset the Fund's previous efforts. The Program for the Prevention of Juvenile Delinquency had been run by at least three independent executives, leaving the Fund without direct control. The Fund's staff had also experienced administrative difficulties in coordinating the work of the training clinic under Bernard Glueck with that of other clinics and in the use of visiting teachers. Glueck was a genius of highly temperamental personality, and it was difficult to obtain his cooperation in general administrative tasks, such as supplying material needed by the supervising committee and keeping the necessary records. These difficulties did not hamper the program's ultimate success, but the Fund's staff was forced to devote excessive time to the nuts and bolts of the program as a whole.

To avoid a repetition of this problem, the Fund centered executive responsibility for the Child Health Program in a small committee headed by Barry C. Smith. The decision was presaged by Porter R. Lee's resignation in 1923 as chairman of the Joint Committee on Prevention of Juvenile Delinquency because he believed that the position should rest with the Fund's director. Before the conflict with Hoover, Dinwiddie himself thought that although the staff of the Child Health Association should supervise the demonstrations, a committee within the Commonwealth Fund—with Barry C. Smith as chairman—should retain full power regarding general policies. Smith agreed that "where operating agencies are employed in carrying out any program of the Fund the reservation of final administrative authority of the Fund, through the Director, is essential. . . . Given the authority to issue orders, no orders are necessary; without such authority there is a tendency on the part of individuals of a certain type to do exactly as they please. The conclusion would seem to be correct that in the adoption of future programs and in the revision of the Delinquency Program, which is likely to occur two years from now, it is of the utmost importance whenever operating agencies are employed to reserve definite final authority to the Fund."[34]

The four demonstration units themselves used an organizational procedure based on the Fund's work in child guidance. A small staff gave

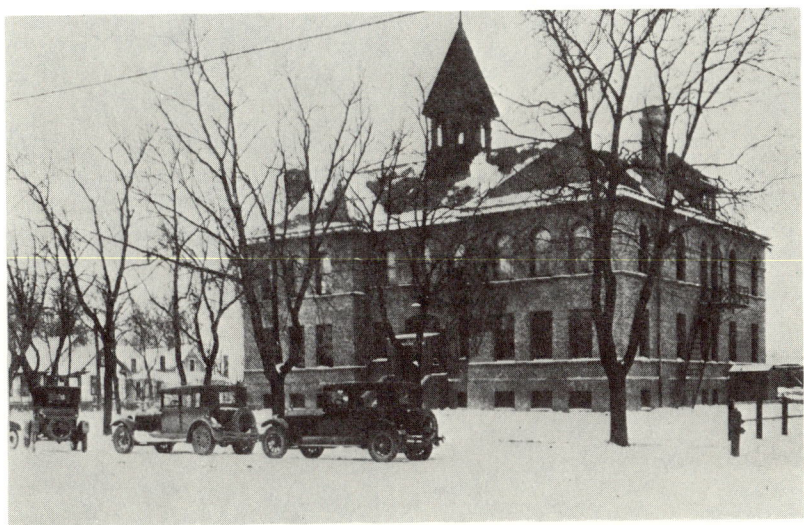

Figure 11. Child health demonstration headquarters, Fargo, North Dakota Reprinted from the Annual Report of the Commonwealth Fund, 1925.

educational service and nursing care from the prenatal period through school age and conducted health education programs in the schools. The success that these pilot operations achieved is best indicated by the spread of comparable health units to neighboring communities and the accompanying demand for the support of public health activities on both county and state levels.

Staff organization followed the same general lines in all of the demonstrations. A director was responsible for coordinating services and maintaining good working relations with the community. At first the director also served as health officer in the two rural counties, but as the demonstrations progressed, administrative leadership was gradually shifted to the permanent health officer. Medical service was entrusted to a pediatrician employed full-time. Each nursing staff had its own director, and this section of the program was fortified by integrating existing services and adding new personnel until nursing districts covered an average population of four to five thousand.[35] A full-time director of health education was provided for the schools of each community. Recording and measurement in each demonstration were assigned to a full-time statistician, who was aided by a clerical staff, and sanitary inspectors were provided in the rural counties where the demonstrations functioned as health departments.[36]

Lester J. Evans and the First Child Health Demonstration

In 1923 when the demonstration began, Fargo, North Dakota, had a population of about twenty-five thousand (fig. 11), and the town contained

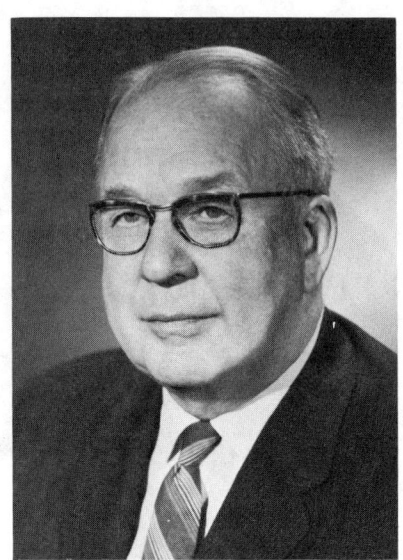

Figure 12. Lester J. Evans

four elementary schools and one high school. Its chief assets for health were an excellent water supply, the beginning of control of the milk supply, a limited nursing service, good hospital facilities—and more important for the future than any of these—an intelligent public sentiment toward health and a cooperative and able group of physicians.

The success of the demonstration in Fargo was due largely to the efforts of Lester J. Evans (fig. 12), the program's medical director, who was so well accepted by the local physicians that he was elected secretary of the local medical society. It was this demonstration unit that brought Evans into contact with the Commonwealth Fund. Evans was born and educated in Kansas, moving to the Washington University School of Medicine in St. Louis for his medical school years and residency training. Early in his medical school career he had decided to specialize in pediatrics. A year at the Boston Floating Hospital showed him the difference between midwestern medicine and eastern medicine, and he returned to St. Louis to join the faculty at Washington University. In 1923 he was approached by a representative of the Fund's Child Health Demonstration Committee, who was looking for a young pediatrician to run the newly formed child health demonstration in Fargo. Evans had never heard of the Commonwealth Fund and knew little about any foundation. (He had, however, examined the possibility of entering the field of public health with the Rockefeller Foundation but concluded that his limited laboratory training did not justify further inquiry.) Although his interests throughout medical school and during his residency were primarily clinical, he had become thoroughly familiar with the philosophy of scientific search and proof. Evans saw the job in Fargo as an opportunity for him to use his full knowledge of pediatric medicine, particularly its preventive aspects.

He nevertheless recognized the disparity between his experience and the task he was considering. For one thing, he was moving from the care of sick children to the care of well ones. For another, he was inexperienced in community relationships; all he knew about hospital service to the public and about staff organization was what he had acquired in his six years of training in St. Louis. Evans's only immediately useful preparation was his voluntary work at Washington University's first Well-Baby Clinic (an effort his fellow house officers considered foolish. Their attitude, which was probably general at the time, was "Why take care of well babies?")

Yet Evans's early years in the midwest would help him to adjust quickly to life in Fargo. He knew well the educational, ethnic, and occupational characteristics of the population. Most of all, he was looking forward to seeing, for the first time, medicine practiced in the raw—never before had he dealt directly with community physicians, nor with local hospitals, nor even with what then passed for public health activity.

The work in Fargo started with the organization of a general citizen's committee, from which an eleven-member executive committee was elected. This group advised the staff throughout the duration of the demonstration. The staff itself consisted of a director, who was responsible for general administration; a medical director; a director of public health nursing; six public health nurses; a statistician; a health educator; a newly appointed health officer whose only staff was one sanitarian; and, in the later years of the program, a staff dentist. Many of the residents of Fargo were of Scandinavian background, and, among the doctors, Evans found several well-trained graduates of Scandinavian medical schools. In addition to conducting infant and preschool clinics and making regular health examinations in the elementary schools and the high schools, Evans consulted with the doctors of the community, attended the staff meetings of the hospitals, and arranged for visiting pediatric teachers.

Fargo's two hospitals, one Lutheran and one Catholic, each had a separate staff. Evans described his efforts to circumvent the hospitals' rivalry:[37]

> In Fargo I had my first taste of what a hospital looks like from the outside. The staffs of the two hospitals in Fargo did not speak to each other except when necessary. They certainly did not attend staff meetings and when I organized the first teaching clinic there, asking McKim Marriott [Evans's mentor at Washington University] to conduct a two-day session on infant

> nutrition, I could not hold those clinics in either of the hospitals because the staff doctors of the other hospital would not attend. So I arranged the necessary facilities in commercial club rooms downtown. I selected about 20 patients (with their mothers) to come in so Marriott could question and examine them. There was little discussion or question by the doctors but the exercise convinced them that there was something to "preventive medicine" although that term was never used.

Evans's work with the hospital staffs represented the first postgraduate medical activity financed by the Fund. He also spoke frequently to lay audiences about preventive medicine; dealt with the local board of health; met with the City Commission on Public Health Planning; and involved the leaders of the Rotary, Kiwanis, and other service clubs, all of whom had volunteered to help with the development of the demonstration. For the first time, too, the administrative staff of the Fund—Barry C. Smith, Barbara S. Quin, and Mildred C. Scoville—looked at health and medicine in a community setting as they visited Fargo to see how the program was progressing.

When the program reached its end in 1927, the city chose to adopt as its own all the essentials of the demonstration. The community's final takeover of public health activities proceeded smoothly. Before the demonstration Fargo was a typical prosperous, small community unburdened by any unusual health deficiencies, unawakened to the value of systematic public health. At that time the functions of a health department were divided among a part-time health officer, a sanitary inspector, a state employee in a branch of the state university laboratory (located in Fargo), a school nurse, and a Red Cross nurse. Health work was scattered and uncoordinated, and the city was rated by the APHA's Committee on Administrative Practice at 320 points out of a possible 1000. The community budget for public health, including the maintenance of an isolation hospital, was not low as compared with prevailing small-city standards—eighty-eight cents per capita—but sixty cents supported the hospitalization of persons with communicable diseases and only twenty-eight cents was devoted to preventive work and health promotion.

The direct effect of the demonstration was the city's hiring of a full-time health officer, at a time when less than 40 percent of all American cities with a population of ten thousand or more had taken this primary step. Around the health officer the demonstration then built a carefully coordinated structure of health services. The Board of Education, the Red Cross, and later the Tuberculosis Association shared in the cost, and the city gradually increased its financial stake in the program.

By 1928 Fargo's full-time health officer, sanitary and food inspector, part-time school physician, six public health nurses, director of school health education, and two clerical workers were all carried on the public payroll. Only the school dentist was supported from private funds. The budget for public health activities rose to $1.51 per capita; and while the appropriation for the isolation hospital fell to 38 cents per capita, $1.13 was devoted to the general purposes of the health department and of health education in the public schools. The volume and standard of public health services increased so rapidly that in 1926 the American Public Health Association appraised Fargo's performance at 814 points out of a possible 1000.

Other Demonstration Units

The second demonstration unit, opened in 1924, was situated in Athens, Georgia, a city characterized as "progressive," with an unusual interest in health and societal activities (fig. 13).[38] The encouraging factors in the selection of the city and surrounding Clarke County were the assured cooperation of the state departments and officials, including the governor, the state board of health, the superintendent of education and the state council of social agencies. On the other hand, very little maternal and child health work had been done (in 1925 the infant mortality rate for blacks in Athens was over 100 for every 1000 live births),[39] and the town had a serious tuberculosis problem. One specific benefit of the child health demonstration was improvement in dental hygiene: According to the

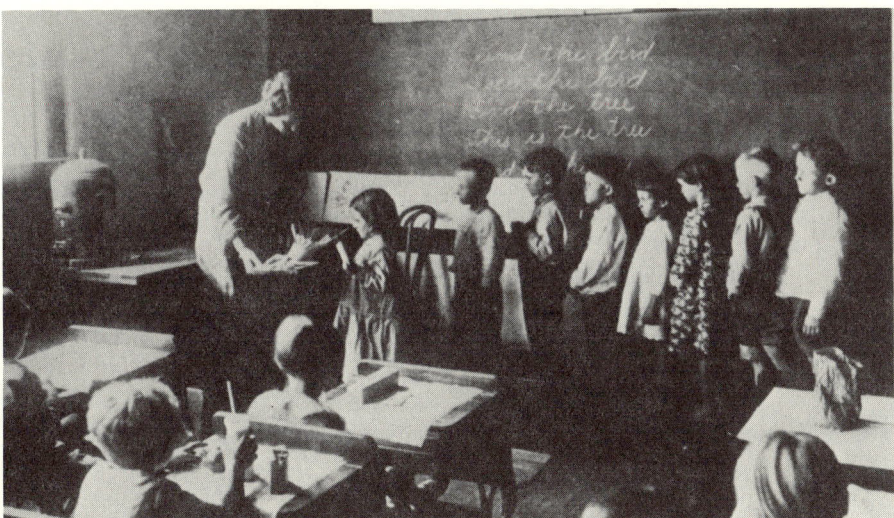

Figure 13. Child health demonstration, Athens, Georgia. "In all schools, milk is served with a cracker and a straw at the mid-morning recess."
Reprinted from the Annual Report of the Commonwealth Fund, 1926.

records of local dentists, most dental defects were corrected in the five elementary schools serving white children. The school board contributed to the success of the dental program: Although the board was already carrying most of the salary of the director of school health education, it made room in its budget for an oral hygienist.

Also begun in 1924 was a third demonstration unit, in Rutherford County, Tennessee. Here quite different arrangements had been made. This county of 33,000 inhabitants had practically no health department, and many of the rural inhabitants were unfamiliar with modern health safeguards. Little in the way of constructive results could be expected unless the director of the demonstration had complete authority over fundamental matters of public health. The county and state health authorities therefore arranged to have the demonstration's director appointed county health officer, and state and county funds were placed at his disposal. With careful boundaries established between official and unofficial duties, the two projects, demonstration and county health work, became, for practical purposes, one. A department of sanitary control was also established to deal with communicable diseases, abatement of nuisances menacing to health, milk and water supply, and sanitary conditions. The demonstration also set up a bacteriological laboratory—an essential, although previously non-existent, part of the county's public health armamentarium.[40] Immunization against communicable diseases in the county reached a new high, and sanitary activities were greatly strengthened by the addition of a deputy health officer and a second sanitary inspector. The excellent results achieved in Rutherford County were reflected in the vote of the county court in 1928 to support the health unit by replacing the three-cent levy fixed in 1926 with a tax of five cents per $100 of valuation.

The demonstration in Rutherford County also inaugurated health education in the schools, an aspect of the program that could not be controlled by the health officer or the medical society. Attached to the demonstration was an experienced teacher who offered her assistance to the county superintendent of education. Her most valuable work was as a liaison between education and medicine. After the demonstration ended, she participated in a comprehensive study of the state's health curriculum. This project was conducted by the University of Tennessee College of Education, which arranged a group of courses for the training of health teachers, and helped the state commissioners of health and education to set up a program of health education in the state's elementary schools.

The Fund decided to extend the duration of the Child Health Program from five to seven years, in order to consolidate the public health positions already staked out and facilitate the task of gathering, comparing and interpreting the results of the experimental efforts. This extension also allowed the final demonstration to achieve results of its own. In the fourth demonstration unit, in Marion County, Oregon, interest in school health had taken a long stride under the special stimulus of an "honor roll" campaign (fig. 14). In the first eight months of 1927 a county-wide educational effort led to the administration of 3112 diphtheria inoculations, compared with 31 in all of 1926. The raising, gathering, and shipping of fruits, hops, and flax in the area raised new questions in industrial health, and personnel of a local hop yard supervised the health of hop workers and their families.

Results of the Child Health Demonstrations

The success of the child health demonstration in Rutherford County showed that the rural public would react favorably to intensive service

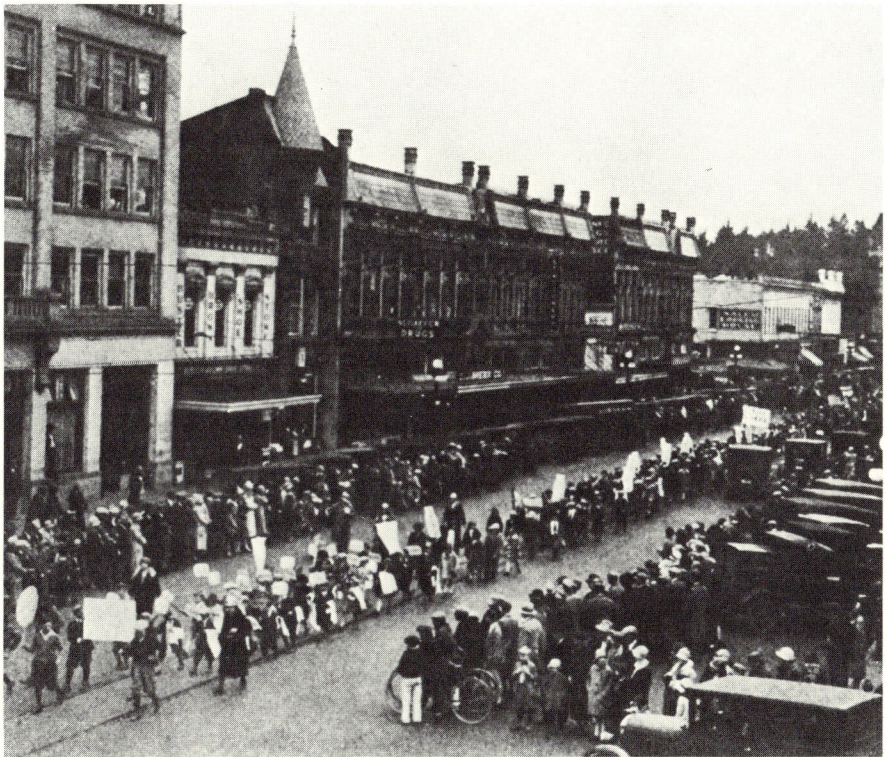

Figure 14. "Honor Roll" parade, Salem, Oregon. "Twenty-two percent of all children in Marion County elementary schools qualified for this distinction on the basis of health, behavior, and scholarship, and 2200 of them marched in the parade."
Reprinted from the Annual Report of the Commonwealth Fund, 1927.

and that material gains were possible with a modest budget. Many problems that had at first appeared almost insurmountable had been solved. Measured by the APHA's Rural Appraisal Form, a health service scoring 110 points out of a possible 1,000 in 1923 had grown to one scoring 814 in 1928. Friendly relations had been established with the medical profession at an early stage of the work, and the policies of the demonstration had gained the physicians' cordial support. The schools had accepted health education, in practice as well as in theory, as a part of their routine function, and the community's interest in health had crystallized into strong local health committees and parent-teacher associations. A local health department was strongly supported as a community necessity, and a balanced program was operating smoothly. The transfer of well infants to private physicians for health supervision was becoming a reality, and protective inoculations, sanitation, and other control measures for communicable diseases were seen as essential.[41]

At the end of the Rutherford County demonstration, the county court saw fit to perpetuate the program with state aid at a cost of approximately $1 per capita, and a community health program with a budget of more than $31,000 was established. The health department carried on with a slightly reduced staff but an essentially unchanged program. The county voted a ten-cent tax for the program's support each year until 1932, when the depression cut the rate to eight cents. In 1934 the ten-cent levy was restored by overwhelming vote of the county court. During this period the maternal mortality rate was decreased almost one-third, from 6.3 to 4.4 per 100,000 population; the stillbirth rate more than one-fifth, from 50.4 to 38.7; the infant death rate about one-fifth, from 66.5 to 53.4; the death rate from diarrhea and enteritis in children under two years of age almost two-thirds, from 45.5 to 17.3.

The Child Health Demonstration Committee secured a complete appraisal of public health performance in all four communities by the APHA's staff. The Committee also began a publishing program that placed informal reports of the demonstration in the hands of approximately twelve thousand community leaders. The results of the intensive demonstration of child health services fell into roughly three groups. The most immediate, and the easiest to measure, was the emergence of a structured public health program, incorporating services to mothers and children, staffed by suitable personnel, and receiving sufficient public funds. Each demonstration represented an informal contact between the Commonwealth Fund and the community, the Fund providing good public health services for children at its own expense, and the city or county supporting the program's continuation.

A second group of results, more difficult to measure but of underlying importance, related to the health status of the group directly served. Vital statistics were important, but only when a long period of time showed genuine trends as distinct from temporary fluctuations; figures could be trusted only when the body of cases on which rates were computed was large enough to outweigh the effect of accidental variations. In a five-year period in a community of fifty thousand or less, only slight progress could be visualized from the vital statistics readily available.

A third group of results was to be found in community attitudes that followed the educational work of the demonstrations. The outlook toward public health service and private health progress, and the general political opinion about the results, showed that the demonstrations were proving their case, not only with officials but with the sound business sense of the community.

The comments of Tennessee's commissioner of health, Dr. E. L. Bishop, about the program in Rutherford County were equally applicable to the other Fund-sponsored demonstrations:[42]

> If public health work be a responsibility of government, then the assumption of this responsibility carries the obligation for an approach in a spirit of critical analysis not only of technical activities but of administrative methods. Study of administrative practice has lagged far behind abstract research in other fields, and this is not as it should be, for in administrative practice is found the application of technical knowledge. If technical knowledge is to be of practical value, the science of its application must be developed. It must be confessed, however, that until recent years the public health program in Tennessee, in common with most states, was lacking in exact definition as to objectives and as to methods of approach in the attainment of objectives. Realizing this weakness, there has been a conscious and sustained attempt on the part of the state Department of Health to study its problems, to define objectives, to test methods, and to develop policies and procedures that will most effectively service the public health interests of the state.
>
> With this in mind, the state Department of Health welcomed the establishment of the Child Health Demonstration in Rutherford County in 1924, as constituting an initial step toward a critical and objective approach to our public health situation. This method of approach, which was consistently followed by the demonstration throughout its history, is perhaps the most valuable contribution it has made to public health work in the state, for the influence has extended far beyond the limits of local activity. It was recognized by those in charge of the demonstration that certain fairly well-defined principles had already been developed in rural health work, and with these as a foundation, its program was projected to include the study of current administrative practice, the exploration of new fields of activity, and the development of sound technique. It was this philosophy which enabled the demonstration to contribute so largely to the public health practice of Tennessee. For example, there has gradually developed a broader conception of the relation of preventive practice to the general medical field, our ideas of the loosely used term "adequate health service" have been revised; and we have come to a new

understanding of methods by which health education may be integrated with the work of education organizations and into the community as a whole.

That success has in large measure been attained by the demonstration is proved by its influence on the public health program of the state as a whole, by its stimulus to similar methods of approach in the fields of both technical and administration methods, and by the fact that it has been continued as the county health department of the local community with adequate financing, the last being an evidence of successful achievement as measured by that most sensitive index—the public pocketbook.

After four years on the staff of the Fargo demonstration project, Evans was asked to come to New York to assist the staff of the Child Health Demonstration Committee in evaluating the data from the four demonstrations. "In retrospect," he recalled, "I realize that I could not have had better preparation than the experience with the child health demonstrations for the variety of situations and activities I was to encounter throughout my life with the Fund—dealing with people and evaluating programs. I had learned something of medicine and health in the social setting, how community medicine could be viewed critically, and how cooperative action could be developed between professionals, organized as hospital staff or in some other capacity, and lay leaders of the community."[43]

The success of the child health demonstrations rested on principles emerging from public health work during the preceding decade: The rural public health program had to be generalized and balanced, local official status secured, and a public health undertaking accepted as a community responsibility, the community providing the greater part of its financial support. From the last of these fundamentals came an inevitable corollary: Community financial support must rest upon public health education. These general principles, apparently so simple now, were arrived at by trial and error. Official status and local support were not initially seen as essential to success. Only gradually was it understood that although the initial approach might concentrate on a disease (e.g., tuberculosis or typhoid fever) or a particular age group (e.g., infants), the degree of success of the program depended upon its success in solving the community's public health problems as a whole.

The Fund's experience with the child health demonstration units led it to assist medical schools in developing training facilities for their students in public health and preventive medicine. The need for these facilities emerged from conversations with older physicians, particularly those practicing in the smaller centers, who had never had the opportunity to become familiar with the important contributions of public health.[44] The Fund had always enjoyed a high degree of cooperation from the practicing medical profession, partly because the staff recognized the importance of the private practitioner's viewpoint. In this case, the private physician felt that the public health worker was subjecting him to unreasonable expectations. Medical schools were just beginning to teach preventive medicine, and the Fund encouraged them to assume the responsibility for training future physicians in the principles and practical techniques of public health and to delineate the private physician's specific role in securing the health of the community.

From 1922 to their end in 1929, the Fund's four demonstrations of child health services broadened current concepts of public health, helped improve public health records, drew the Fund's attention to the utility of postgraduate education for practicing physicians, and set a pattern for a few good local health departments.[45] The skillfully promoted participation of community organizations made the resulting progress in public health the object of local effort and a matter for local pride. On the whole, though, the demonstrations were disappointing as instruments for the complete development of public health services. Once again the Fund perceived the need to broaden its services to accomplish its goals.

The Fund Expands Its Program in Public Health

The Fund's Child Health Program ended formally on December 31, 1929, when the demonstration in Marion County, Oregon, was closed and the Child Health Demonstration Committee disbanded. Even before the program's official end, however, Barry C. Smith was expanding the Fund's ventures in public health. Between 1928 and 1932, he created three new administrative units, the divisions of Public Health, Rural Hospitals, and Health Studies; he took in several new staff members to run the units; and to accommodate the Fund's growth, he arranged for it to move from adapted offices in the Vanderbilt mansion to larger offices in the Fuller Building around the corner, at 41 East 57th Street.

Smith characterized 1930 in particular as a year of transition, one in which the Fund's staff developed old and new enterprises intensively and reevaluated underlying principles.[46] To Lester J. Evans, these years of expansion did not seem significant at the time, but he later realized that it was in the early 1930s that the patterns of the Fund's future had been set. The additions to the staff increased the Fund's composite experience in fields of increasing concern. Evans described the general feeling within the staff: They had come through a fruitful infancy and adolescence in preparation for mature roles in the Fund's chosen field of action. Staff energy, imagination, and optimism were high.

Evans himself was invited to become an associate in the Fund's new Division of Rural Hospitals in 1928—the first physician to be employed as a staff member. He also helped with projects in medical education in the Division of Public Health, which was headed by William J. French, a physician experienced in public health work who had directed the Fargo demonstration in its early years. French proved unable to work with the communities effectively and was succeeded in May 1931 by Clarence L. Scamman, deputy commissioner of health of Massachusetts, under whose direction the work of the division progressed rapidly.[47] Scamman's background was useful in programs derived from the child health demonstrations, and he was especially adept at promoting collaboration between state and county health departments.

Harry E. Handley, a pediatrician and a graduate of the Johns Hopkins University School of Medicine, became Scamman's able partner in administration and education.[48] Formerly with the Tennessee State Health Department, Handley was especially concerned with scholarships for medical students, fellowships for practicing doctors, extension programs for physicians, and all aspects of public health nursing. His particular interest in nursing led to the Fund to increase its support of education programs in this field.

The Division of Health Studies was directed by W. Frank Walker, one of the leading authorities in the country on the evaluation of health activities.[49] Walker had degrees in both engineering and public health. Before joining the Fund, he was a research associate of the American Child Health Association, surveying health work in 86 American cities, and field director of the APHA's Committee on Administrative Practice. "With the backing of the experienced personnel of this Committee and with his own admirable approach and keen insight, he created a new state of mind in public health workers. He did not 'inspect' their departments but, with rare tact, made them inspect themselves."[50]

Carolina R. Randolph, a statistician, was Walker's assistant and a member of the division from 1933 to 1955.[51] She had worked at the Virginia Department of Health, the Tennessee State Health Department, and the health department of Rutherford County, Tennessee, in projects supported by the Commonwealth Fund.

Aside from general administrative know-how, the staff possessed skills in psychology, education, medicine, social work, nursing, public health, epidemiologic research, and writing and reporting. They also hoarded their time, concentrating on their work at the Fund. Although individual staff members participated in their respective national associations and were frequently called to hearings as consultants, they did not become active in the many commissions then in vogue. The staff was well aware that the studies of these commissions tended to be sterile, and it was an unwritten Fund policy that staff time needed for the Fund's ongoing activities was not spent on the activities of national committees. The Fund's plans for its future rested on hard-won practical experience in the field, not on hypothetical formulations by social planners. On this practical experience was based the Fund's own continuing critical evaluation of its programs.

George E. Vincent, president of the Rockefeller Foundation, commented on the rapidly expanding scope of public health work in 1927: "It now includes much more than sanitation, quarantine and vaccination. The idea of prevention is no longer merely negative; it seeks to promote positive and vigorous health. Emphasis shifts from water supplies, sewers and immunization to hygiene; and this in turn takes many forms—infant, maternity, school, industrial, social and mental."[52] To help with the Fund's growing program, Smith empaneled a Committee on Public Health. The membership of the committee changed often, but it included individuals well known to the Fund's staff in medical education, public health, public health nursing, preventive medicine, the practice of medicine, the federal government, and psychiatry. The committee was strictly advisory, never taking any action of its own;[53] the Fund's staff always made the final decision, a wise policy that kept the staff from commitment to any committee decision representing only the least common denominator of opinion.[54] In 1939 the advisory group became the Committee on Health Activities, and its membership was augmented.[55] This gave the Fund access to an even larger panel of experts in varied fields who could serve as a sounding board for discussion of any areas in which the Commonwealth Fund had a developing interest. It was an excellent way to maintain a cadre of knowledgeable advisors without committing the Fund to the group's specific recommendations. Changing with the years, the committee always reflected the primary interests of the Fund. When it was disbanded in 1946 its membership was heavily weighted toward medical education and research.[56]

The Division of Public Health

The Fund had advanced beyond the current state of the art in its child health demonstration units. Without neglecting the protective side of public health—for example, sanitary control and prevention of communicable disease—it had emphasized other services such as health education, public health (home) nursing, children's health centers, and the practice of preventive medicine by private physicians. Now an entirely different approach to public health seemed necessary. Although the term "public health" encompassed the Child Health Program, the Division of Rural Hospitals, and a number of miscellaneous smaller projects, the Fund's staff believed that rural communities needed aggressive development of general medical services. The Fund's study of rural health indicated the need for a broader approach to public health and preventive medicine.

In its Rural Hospital Program the Fund was endeavoring to develop the hospital as a health center and a remedial institution, stimulating new activities and raising the standards of medical practice. But subtleties and constraints of rural health planning were also becoming evident: The Fund recognized that in many rural communities a hospital was impracticable and in some instances even unnecessary.

The Division of Public Health did not actually administer programs; its duties were advisory and investigative, and its main role was to keep the Fund's staff in close touch with the state and local administrators of Fund-supported activities—a degree of control that Barry C. Smith saw as essential to successful programming. First-hand contact with workers in the field was also intended to keep projects adaptable to changing conditions. The Fund's staff had recognized the importance of securing the cooperation of local participants, particularly members of the medical profession, and because demonstration programs had been conducted only through agreement with local medical societies, physicians did not feel that the Fund was trying to interfere with their practices. Friendly relations with the American Medical Association were another asset that could not be taken for granted: Lester J. Evans recalled his summons by the association to defend the free administration of typhoid vaccine in the Fargo child health demonstration unit. The approval of the American Public Health Association was equally important; it had made regular surveys of the Fund's child health demonstration units, and the Fund reciprocally appropriated money for the APHA's study of methods for appraising rural health work.[57]

The division was a response to the lesson taught by the Fund's experience in child health: the need for an integrated approach. It intended to better the full range of local—particularly rural—health service through formal cooperation with state health departments. In Rutherford County, Tennessee, one of the four child health demonstration areas, the Fund began an experiment with model health units at the county level. Working not only where the need appeared greatest, but where the county government was especially suitable, the Fund set up similar demonstration units in three counties in Tennessee,[58] in three counties in Mississippi (fig. 15), and in two counties in Oklahoma.[59] Later, modified units were established in Alabama, Louisiana, Kentucky, and Florida.

The Development of Local Health Units

The prevailing pattern for public health, particularly in the South, had been established by the Rockefeller Foundation's intensive work with endemic public health problems. It was based on a county health department staffed by a physician, a sanitarian, and one public health nurse.

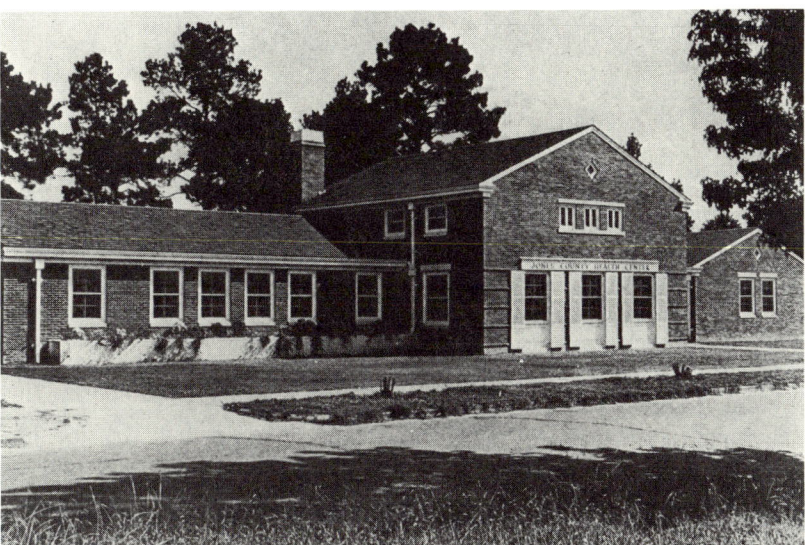

Figure 15. Health Center in Laurel, Mississippi (Jones County)
Reprinted from the Annual Report of the Commonwealth Fund, 1943.

The Fund's program set up another source of support for county health departments—the field unit.

In Tennessee the Fund's Division of Public Health provided field consultant service to one of the former child health demonstration communities and helped other communities and institutions with new activities. It also established necessary cooperative relationships, made continuing arrangements for the gathering of educational material and the study of results, and furnished technical and investigative services. In all these endeavors, the Fund's staff hoped that this program would serve as a model for other states. Health authorities in Tennessee and Mississippi actively supported the plan, and an exceptionally able staff in Massachusetts disseminated information about the program to other professionals.[60]

Running these units required intensive supervision at both state and local levels. Statistical services, training for record clerks and laboratory technicians, and field training centers were occasionally supported with small honoraria and salary stipends to assure the employment of competent personnel, particularly health officers. Commitments were almost always made through a take-over plan so that after several years, the cost would be carried by state or local funds, and the Fund would be released from its obligation.

The field unit proved to be one of the most effective tools for strengthening plan and performance in public health.[61] An innovation in rural health organization, it fortified local programs through technical advice. The core team included a physician trained in public health, a nurse, a sanitarian, and a clerk, all of whom acted as intermediaries between the state health officer and the local health department. Additional specialists in fields such as epidemiology, venereal disease, dental hygiene, and nutrition were sometimes attached to a group. The unit maintained close ties between the state and county health departments and through advisory visits improved the health services given by each local unit to the community. Dr. E. L. Bishop, state health commissioner for Tennessee, believed that "no service we have ever developed in this department has a more profound influence in the development of both better quality and better quantity of public health activity."[62]

Experience with the field units led the Fund to conclude that the best machinery available to improve the standards of rural health work had two aspects: a mobile unit teaching good medical practice as it shuttled back and forth among the local health departments, and work in a specimen county in which better than average standards could be demonstrated. The field unit helped to build the demonstration; the demonstration in turn gave the field unit teaching material—fresher and more interesting material than could perhaps have been drawn from long-established services.

Study of the topography, population, economy, culture, and vital statistics of the communities indicated that no single formula could be applied to the solution of their health problems or to the measurement of their accomplishments. Before the organization of the field unit, the staff of the state health department in Mississippi ordinarily visited a community only when it was necessary to save a budget by intensive effort, to adjust differences of opinion, to cope with an epidemic, or to stiffen a drive for elementary sanitation. Now the staff of one unit traveled to every one of the twenty-eight organized counties in the state to establish working relations with the local staff and made complete factual studies—the first ever attempted—of twenty-four. The unit also helped local personnel to think objectively about their work. In one county where the health officer, interpreting his local situation too casually, was complacent about conditions relating to diphtheria, the field unit cut through to the facts of the case; as a result, 3,056 immunizing treatments were given in four months, as compared with 272 for the preceding ten years.

The administrative situation in Massachusetts differed sharply from that in the three southern states. Public health responsibility was diffused among a great number of separately incorporated cities and towns; and the state health department wielded only so much authority as it could earn for itself by persuasion and manifest technical leadership. Distances were not as great as in the southern states, and the staff of the state health department was more readily on call. The field unit in Massachusetts, therefore, played a less important role than its counterpart in Mississippi or Tennessee.[63]

The experience in Tennessee showed how striking advances in the status of public health could be brought about in a relatively short period. In 1924, when Bishop was appointed commissioner of health, the state was appropriating for its health department $77,320 a year, or 3.1 cents per capita, and ranked forty-seventh among the forty-eight states in this respect. State services were weak: There was, for example, no official state program for the control of tuberculosis. Ten years later, although appropriations in general had fallen below pre-depression levels, Tennessee ranked in the upper third of states in appropriations for public health, providing the equivalent of 9.9 cents per capita. This sum was considerably augmented by funds from outside the state. Fifty percent of the rural population had full-time health service, in contrast to 15 percent a decade earlier, and every full-time county health officer had received at least a minimum of postgraduate training. By 1935, with one exception, all six Fund-supported counties scored more than 825 points out of a possible 1000 on the Appraisal Form of the American Public Health Association.

The state health department contributed to this progress by offering supervision and advice but placing the primary responsibility for service on the local community. The department also subsidized county units on a continuing—not a temporary or diminishing—basis. Finally, it insisted that local service be given by trained workers, and eventually the public became convinced that only the service of such workers was worth paying for. In executing these policies, the state welcomed help from outside agencies—the United States Public Health Service, the United States Children's Bureau, the Rockefeller Foundation, the Rosenwald Fund, and the Commonwealth Fund. Staff members of the Fund's Division of Public Health also helped to develop ancillary local services—for example, they prepared the first edition of the *Manual for the Conduct of County Health Departments.*

The lessons learned in Rutherford County—the specimen county and the site of one of the original child health demonstration units—were shared with the state through the mobile unit and the movement of staff workers to other training facilities. A field technical service implemented the supervisory functions of the state health department and raised the quality of full-time county service. The special subsidies given jointly by the state and the Fund to Gibson and Sullivan counties in Tennessee also made possible a marked advance in local health work and pointed the way for the more aggressive promotion of rural services. Harry S. Mustard characterized these programs as the "turning point" in American public health.[64] The gains of ten years were unmistakable.

The Division of Health Studies

This statistical support system for the Division of Public Health was inaugurated in April 1931 to encourage local public health activities through practical methods of recording and periodic analyses of service rendered. "Unless health service is analyzed objectively and measured where measurement is possible, the health officer can hardly do a job which satisfies either his own professional standards or the skepticism of the taxpayer."[65] The division also surveyed the Fund's rural hospitals and mental health activities, measuring results in the Fund's separate areas of health work and examining evidence of progressive integration. Its influence extended beyond the Fund's immediate programs, as it strengthened the Fund's already excellent relations with the United States Public Health Service and other leading organizations in the field. Out of W. Frank Walker's analysis of accumulated data and experience came such books as *Recording of Local Health Work* (1935), *School Health Studies* (1941) (both in collaboration with Carolina R. Randolph), *Influence of a Rural Health Program*, and *Ten Years of Rural Health Work*. Walker's death in 1941 was a severe blow to the division, and when his successor, F. L. Moore, resigned three years later, the remaining staff and activities of the division were merged into the Division of Public Health.

Just as the child health demonstrations had shown the way to better organization and promotion of rural health, the creation of the divisions of Public Health and Health Studies, midway through a transitional time, had moved the Fund from a demonstration period to a more broadly based program.

The Rural Hospital Program

The emergence of the hospital as a health center has been occasioned by the success of medical science. The doctor has seen himself changed from an intuitive, independent artist far removed from the hospital as a House of Despair to a scientific social worker heavily dependent on what is now a House of Hope, with its centralization of specialists and expensive machinery.

—*John H. Knowles, 1965*

In the twenty-two years after its formation in 1926, the Fund's Division of Rural Hospitals built and supported rural hospitals in fifteen towns.

Edward S. Harkness had a particular interest in hospitals: "Purposes: 1) Better hospitals in the U.S.; or 2) Establishing hospitals in needy parts of the world on conditions that they be supported by the communities. Fundamental principle to be remembered is prevention rather than mere relief."[66] More specifically, "Might it not be that the Commonwealth Fund could better confine itself to giving money to help build new hospitals when and where needed, imposing certain conditions with each gift such as . . . that each patient pay what he is able to; an adequate sum should be charged to endow a bed; a social service and follow-up system should be maintained; a certain amount of endowment should be secured to start with; a dispensary and outpatient department should be maintained."[67] The Fund's staff had also realized that "the pressing importance of two related phases must not be overlooked; namely, the apparent inadequacy of our rural hospital facilities and the negro hospital problem which appear to be intimately connected, the rural situation being more acute in states where negroes predominate."[68] "Inadequacy" covered both the paucity of hospitals and the defective state of existing ones, which were not only poorly built but deficient in administrative organization and record-keeping.[69]

The Fund's first programs in child welfare consumed its resources in the early 1920s. Yet exposure to Hermann M. Biggs's plan for rural health centers convinced Barry Smith that the Commonwealth Fund could do no greater service than to meet the need for hospitals for rural communities and for areas in which the black population predominated.[70] Smith was impressed with Biggs's figures for New York state alone: 250 incorporated villages were without the services of a physician, and no fewer than eleven counties were without a hospital.

Biggs's death in 1923 was a setback to the hospital program, but Smith acquired other excellent advisors: S. S. Goldwater of the Mount Sinai Hospital in New York; John G. Bowman, a director of the American College of Surgeons; Winford H. Smith of the Johns Hopkins Hospital (whose report was strongly endorsed by William H. Welch); A. R. Warner, a secretary of the American Hospital Association; and Edwin R. Embree of the Rockefeller Foundation. The proposals now reaching the Fund concerned establishing new hospitals in various communities (most were outside the United States); hospitals for blacks in the South; and improvements in hospital management and equipment.

By June 1925 Smith had developed an extensive memorandum for the board of directors: The Fund should secure a consultant to select a suitable community, make a preliminary study and report with recommendations for the building of a hospital.[71] Choice of location would be a formidable problem: Of the 3,027 counties in the United States, more than 50 percent lacked hospital facilities. This first hospital would be a pilot endeavor; if it succeeded, Smith proposed to establish a Division of Rural Hospitals, which would erect one or two fifty-bed hospitals a year in strategic locations and provide a consultant service to help with their operation. The board received the memorandum enthusiastically, and Henry C. Wright was appointed to survey the situation and select the community for the first rural hospital. Wright's report, presented eighteen months later, supported all Barry C. Smith's recommendations, suggesting in addition that the Fund provide an advisory service for communities erecting small hospitals at their own expense and give small scholarships for further study to physicians in the chosen communities. He also advised against delaying the formation of the Division of Rural Hospitals: A new administrative unit of the Fund should be responsible for hospital construction from the very beginning.[72]

The implications of these recommendations touched both the Fund's administrative structure and its program arrangements. In fact, the Rural Hospital Program marked a turning point in the administrative structure of the Commonwealth Fund. The program offered the Fund its greatest experimental opportunity to date. Unlike the child health demonstrations, this program would be operated solely by the Fund's staff, and in the process of improving health in rural communities, the staff would acquire valuable field experience. The educational aspects, which brought the staff into contact with university schools of medicine, were the basis of the Fund's later contributions to medical education and research.

Henry J. Southmayd, who had served as hospital consultant on the staff of the Cleveland Welfare Federation, was engaged as director of the new division, and the architectural firm of Edward S. Harkness's Yale classmate James Gamble Rogers was hired to draw up the hospital plans.

In announcing the new program, the Fund emphasized the great disparity of health services between rural and urban areas. The staff hoped that the rural hospital would combine public health and medical services by creating modern hospital facilities (provided the local community could meet operating costs and a one-third share of capital cost), by improving standards of local medical practice through attracting young physicians to the community, and by giving good physicians an incentive to remain. Developing community public health activities around the hospital would influence surrounding communities to improve their own hospital facilities. Although a fifty-bed hospital offered a narrower range of teaching material than a large-city institution, the smaller hospital had an advantage in stimulating local health services and sustaining the morale of local physicians. If properly located, it also could operate on a sound financial basis.

Although many communities applied for help, the Fund could choose only those combining a need for hospital facilities with sufficient local resources and interest to ensure successful maintenance of the hospital once the Fund's support had ended. The Fund defined a likely district as a circle with a thirty-five mile radius containing no town with a population of more than twelve thousand. Once such a district was identified the applicant town's financial, civic, and medical assets and liabilities were surveyed. An essential consideration was always the willingness and ability of a local group to maintain community services that could eventually be self-supporting and to conduct the hospital in accordance with the standards set by the American College of Surgeons and the American Medical Association. Finally, the district had to fit into the Fund's plan for distributing these rural hospitals across the country.

These hospitals were to be community organizations, controlled by the public and not by the medical profession. The Fund's staff believed that its program could be fully successful only if the community rose to its opportunity and used the hospital freely and imaginatively. They told aspiring communities:[73]

> We will give approximately two-thirds the cost of building and equipping a well-designed hospital of fifty beds if you will undertake to run it in accordance with accepted standards and will underwrite the deficit which it will quite properly and inevitably incur. We will also help in such ways and to such a degree as seems desirable in the development of as good a public health organization as you and your state health officer think you can permanently support. We will help your physicians to better practice by paying the cost of several months of post-graduate study for an average of five of them each year, and by making it possible for the hospital staff to hold medical and nursing institutes.
>
> In return we look to you to recognize the hospital as a community asset— not merely a workshop for your physicians, and as a community servant— not merely a luxury for the well-to-do. We expect that as soon as practicable you will offer out-patient service to the indigent sick, as well as admitting them to hospital beds with full and conscientious care when they need it. We expect you to encourage your health officer to use the hospital whenever that makes for public health progress and to cooperate with him in well-considered plans for sanitation, the control of communicable diseases, and preventive services. We expect your physicians to consider themselves working partners of the hospital in preventing disease and promoting the general health, and to put the health interests of the community and the hospital before their individual interests as private practitioners.

From a large number of communities that had applied for participation in the Rural Hospital Program, the first six locations chosen were: Farmville, Virginia; Murfreesboro, Tennessee (fig. 16); Glasgow, Kentucky; Farmington, Maine; Beloit, Kansas; and Wauseon, Ohio.

The First Six Rural Hospitals

The first hospital in the Fund's Rural Hospital Program opened in November 1927. Farmville was a growing community: Its population had increased from 1500 to 4000 in the previous six years. It served an area thirty-

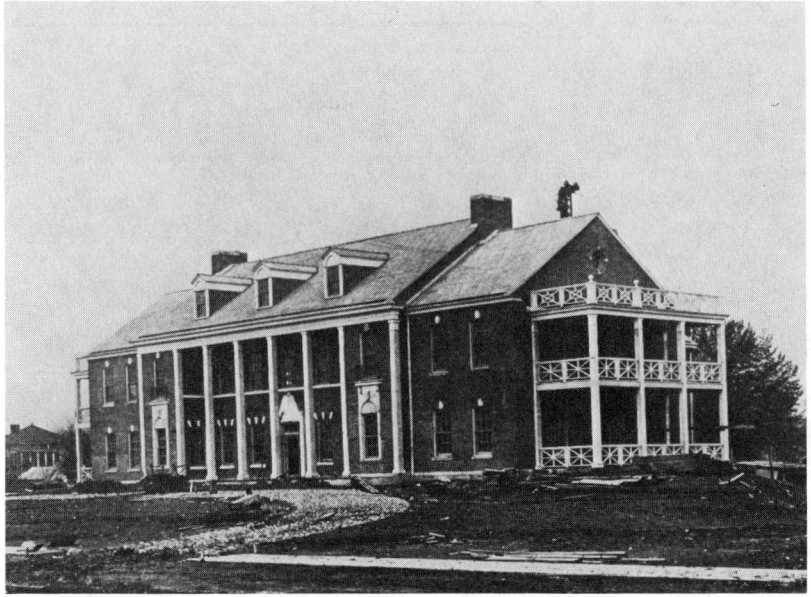

Figure 16. Rutherford Hospital, Murfreesboro, Tennessee
Reprinted from the Annual Report of the Commonwealth Fund, 1926.

five miles in radius, including all of Prince Edward County and parts of eight adjoining counties; the area's total population was sixty thousand, of whom twenty-seven thousand were black. The nearest hospital facilities were in Lynchburg, fifty-nine miles to the west, and Petersburg, seventy-five miles to the east. Local health services had been provided by a part-time health officer and a sanitary engineer, who worked with a single public health nurse employed by a private organization.

The community responded eagerly to the prospect of a hospital by raising local funds to meet the cost of the site and one-third of the anticipated cost of construction and equipment. The Fund, on a contractual basis, paid for the building plans and specifications and for the remaining building and equipment costs. A lay hospital board was organized and incorporated under the state laws for charitable purposes; it retained full property rights and full responsibilities for the construction and operation of the hospital. Along with the usual clinical services, the hospital was to provide x-ray and laboratory facilities. The local health department would be housed in the hospital, and a system for keeping medical records would be devised for inpatient, outpatient and public health services. The Fund planned to build on the experience of the child health demonstration communities, where the "family health records" were supervised by the public health nurses.[74] (This type of inclusive medical record was a predecessor of the "problem-oriented" record system.)

A second hospital was established in Murfreesboro, Tennessee (Rutherford County), as an extension of that location's child health clinic. The Rutherford Hospital was operated by a five-member, incorporated, self-perpetuating board of directors, composed entirely of laymen. The hospital performed both medical and surgical work and was accredited by the American College of Surgeons. Staff members had to be medical school graduates licensed in Tennessee and of good ethical and personal standing in the community. Appointees were designated as either visiting or associate staff members able or not able to use the hospital's facilities for major surgical procedures.

The Rutherford Hospital had twenty-one beds available at need for free care—ten for black and eleven for white patients. In addition to the major operating room, the hospital included a delivery room; an operating room for eye, ear, nose, and throat cases; an operating room for patients with infections; and an emergency room. A laboratory was maintained which, in addition to performing the routine work of the hospital, furnished information for the health department and received in return $50 a month. All classes of cases except certain of the communicable diseases were accepted; typhoid fever and influenza cases could be admitted but patients with diphtheria and tuberculosis could not.

The deficit in hospital operation was met by a county appropriation of $2,000 per year, supplemented by Murfreesboro's commitment of up to $14,000 per year.

When four additional hospitals were established in different states between 1926 and 1930, the Fund's six rural hospitals were serving about 410,000 people. The six communities differed greatly. Glasgow, Kentucky, the county seat, was a town of 4,000 people and served as a trading center for a wide area to the east. Highways focused on Glasgow, and a regional population of 113,000 was for the most part evenly distributed over good farm land. The community had only limited private hospital facilities, and little public health work had been attempted. Farmington, Maine, was known as "the cleanest town in Maine," and lay at the transportation center of Franklin County. The nearest hospital facilities, forty miles away, were inaccessible half the year because of heavy snows and spring thaws. Beloit, Kansas, was the county seat in the center of an area with a population of about 78,000, a district devoted chiefly to wheat farming. Public health work was limited, but a recent epidemic had awakened the public to the need for preventive service. Wauseon, Ohio, was a prosperous town of 3,100.

All the hospitals were directed by representative lay boards; all had medical staffs open to any reputable physician; all gave care without considering race, color, creed, or economic status. Not all of them, however, really encompassed the full spirit of the community hospital. Many staff doctors were complacent and remained competitive, and too few influential citizens grasped the difference between a community institution and a business.[75] Yet both doctors and board members slowly grew in competence, and patients, who had been unaccustomed to hospitals because of their low income, began to fill the waiting beds.

The Fund sponsored many diverse projects to improve a hospital's efficiency and strengthen its staff. Accounting procedures and rules and regulations were worked over in detail. The fixed, or inclusive, rate schedule was introduced at most of the hospitals to better both patient care and public relations. Direct educational programs were instituted along with indirect educational influences such as diagnostic laboratory and x-ray facilities, outside consultant services, discussion of cases at staff meetings, and accurate record-keeping. Once a year in each hospital, a medical institute was conducted by eminent physicians and surgeons. Lectures, clinics, and a nursing institute with leading nurse instructors were also offered. The visiting lecturers at Farmville in 1928, for example, were Joseph C. Bloodgood, associate professor of surgery at the Johns Hopkins University, and Stewart B. Roberts, professor of clinical medicine at Emory University. At the Rutherford Hospital, the speakers included W. S. Leathers, dean and professor of preventive medicine at Vanderbilt University; Barney Brooks, chairman of the Department of Surgery at Vanderbilt University; Willis Campbell, a noted orthopedic surgeon at the University of Tennessee; and K. S. Howlett of the Tennessee State Medical Association.

The resident physician in particular held a strategic place, and to help him, the Fund developed *The Resident Physician's Handbook,* one of several publications prepared for use in the rural hospitals. Its principal author, William L. Noe, Jr., had served on the resident house staff of the Philadelphia General Hospital and was a resident physician in the Fund's Farmington hospital. This volume, the forerunner of today's popular house-staff manuals, was intended to encourage the development of high-quality routine procedures within the hospital. It also suggested standards for technical procedures, an important endeavor in an institution treating a wide variety of clinical conditions, and served as a foundation for the development of additional routines as hospital service was augmented. Beyond these general efforts to improve the competence of the medical staff, the Fund used the device that had served it so well in its child welfare programs—the fellowship.

Outpatient care was developed in some hospitals under the guidance of specially trained nurses; at their best, these clinics illustrated the benefits of collaboration between hospitals and health departments (fig. 17). This was a new endeavor for the Fund. It confessed: "Here one is on quite uncharted ground, and it is not easy to trace the lines along which definite cooperative service can be developed. The out-patient department is obviously a promising field for such development, and the

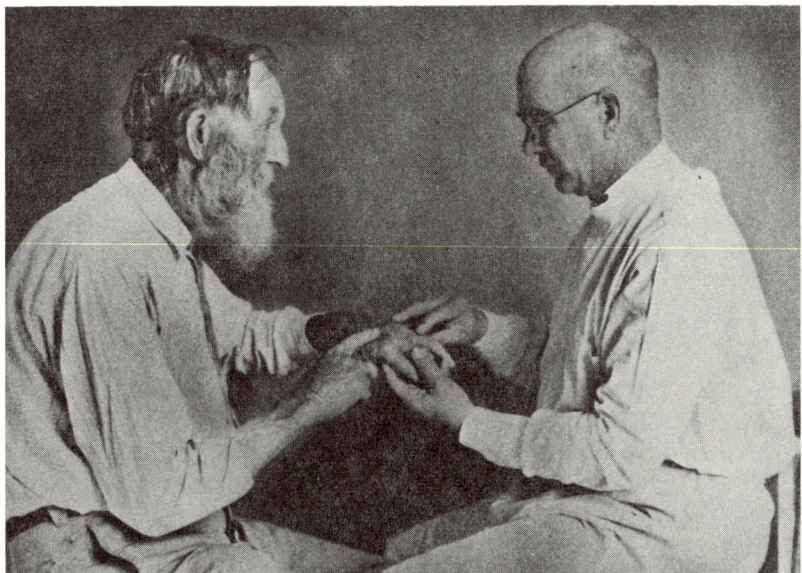

Figure 17. The health officer sees a case of pellagra. "The medical staff of the rural hospital and the rural health officer can cooperate effectively in outpatient services."
Reprinted from the Annual Report of the Commonwealth Fund, 1931.

physical resources of the hospital—the laboratory and x-ray apparatus, for instance, can without great difficulty be put at the service of the health officer. But the extent to which the hospital, both as a physical plant and as a focus of public thinking, can become a health center for the community is not likely to be determined without a long process of trial and error. The elements are in the melting-pot, but there is no crystallization yet."[76]

Progress in the Rural Hospital Program

By 1930 the Fund could assess the preliminary results:[77]

> While local conditions vary so widely that no generalizations are wholly true for the group, these hospitals have shown somewhat similar tendencies in their initial stages. The first reaction on the part of the public is one of pride and satisfaction in the visible evidence of community progress which the new building offers. The financial requirements are taken lightly; the community rests on its oars after raising the money necessary to meet the offer of the Fund and to get the building finished. The riper physicians and a few far-seeing laymen recognize the opportunities for public service which the hospital offers and quietly assume responsibility for realizing them. Other physicians,

contemplating with pleasure the fresh and ample equipment of the hospital, think of it chiefly as an asset for their private practice, and watch its early developments closely to make sure that no competitor reaps undue advantage from it. Patients are received, necessary regulations are enforced; bills are presented. Free cases come; operating deficits make their appearance; trustees become nervous; the more conservative physicians hesitate to accept the substitution of free hospital service for private charity work, fearing the loss of some vague lien on the patient's future; strains creep into the relations between staff and superintendent and board. Medical factions jockey for positions at the hospital. Meanwhile, the care of patients goes on more or less steadily—well below the capacity of the hospital, in most instances, but gradually increasing. Malcontents criticize the hospital administration, but the majority of patients, recognizing advantages that before the opening of the hospital would have been entirely or relatively unattainable, begin to spread favorable comment. Gradually the community becomes acquainted with this hospital; there is a friendliness under the surface that can be counted on in an emergency; the hospital gathers momentum as a going concern. More of the physicians, exposed to a variety of educational influences through the hospital, catch a glimpse of its possibilities as a center for disinterested medical service and professional progress; the less imaginative begin to feel the tide of public favor which swings toward the hospital, and shape their own course accordingly. Eventually the growing understanding of what the whole enterprise is worth to the community finds expression in a stable financial policy and generous interest in its development to maximal usefulness.

It would be unfair to imply that all the unfavorable items in this chronicle have been true of all the hospitals, and misleading to suggest that the favorable ones have yet been completely attained. Not all the hospitals have reached the happy state of equilibrium which is marked by assured support for a broad-gauge policy of hospital service. But the developments of the past year have shown encouraging progress in that direction. Certainly, there is, in all six communities, a growing sense of community proprietorship which is a foundation for real achievement.

The rural hospitals' educational aspects in particular attracted wide attention. In a letter to Barry C. Smith, Dr. Edward Hume, chief executive of the Postgraduate Hospital and Medical School, said:[78]

> Two weeks ago it was my privilege to attend the Institute held at the Southside Community Hospital in Farmville, Virginia. . . . I am convinced that the activities at Farmville represent one of the most important developments in graduate medical education that has been attempted. . . .
>
> 1. The doctors of the area are definitely learning how to use a hospital.
> 2. Even more important is the educational value of the hospitals in training them to analyze their cases rather than merely to give them medicine.

3. The presence of a resident physician will make it possible for the physicians to add laboratory facilities to their diagnostic procedure.
4. The doctors are being stimulated to keep better records.
5. The Institute itself was a genuine educational value . . . because the doctors of the community recognized their need of education and came to be taught.
6. The very enthusiasm of the doctors of the community for the opportunity offered to go away for study was significant. That they should apply for scholarships in the way they do indicates the educational value of the hospital movement.
7. The community itself . . . is learning that it must shoulder certain responsibilities in connection with the prevention and treatment of disease and . . . it is learning to expect and demand better medical practice.

I congratulate the Commonwealth Fund that it has launched upon this program for rural hospitals and congratulate you on the way in which a community such as Farmville has learned to think of you as a counsellor and friend.

After the first six hospitals had been built, financial conditions worsened and further building ceased. For the next five years, the Fund concentrated on strengthening the existing hospitals. The six hospitals shared with similar institutions in the United States the severe handicaps caused by reduction in the general income level. As fewer patients were able to pay the usual rates for hospital service, the demand for free or part-pay service was increased. The average occupancy in these six hospitals, which was rising until 1931, declined in 1932, and the local boards were forced to cut expenses. Yet not one of these six hospitals closed its doors or suspended service for one day.[79]

All the hospitals weathered the depression and by 1934 it was possible to resume building. The first unit of this new group of hospitals was located in Kingsport, Tennessee, and some of its successors were built in more densely populated communities. A more concentrated population facilitated the introduction of hospital insurance, since it brought the hospital into contact with large groups of industrial workers.

Lester J. Evans described the selection of additional sites:[80]

I was the first staff person to be involved in the selection of Tupelo, Mississippi, and Provo, Utah. In our new selections, we wished to widen the geographic distribution of our hospitals. Our experience in selecting the first six hospital sites and evaluating the hospital performance provided a baseline for what we wanted to look at in new communities. . . . We were able to get a sense of the background of the doctors in the area by noting their schools of graduation. We knew what hospital facilities already existed locally in the form of proprietary institutions. In Tupelo the doctors came from southern schools, essentially from Tennessee and Mississippi. In Provo the situation was quite different, since Utah had only a two-year medical school. The doctors in that area had, as medical students, come East to complete their training in places such as Harvard, Washington University, and Northwestern. It was possible to judge the relative competency of the doctors in the two areas by comparing them with what we had seen in the earlier communities. As to public opinion and expression of need for hospital facilities, we had the usual Chamber of Commerce information and other expressions of special interest along with the usual vital statistics. Only rarely had the local medical society or county medical society gotten together information that might be convincing as to the need for a hospital. We looked for the inadequacies in practice and potentialities for improvement if adequate bed and laboratory facilities were made available.

In Mississippi the selection had to be made between two communities. In one it was obvious from the first hour of the visit that the public officials were simply looking for someone to make a contribution to the area. . . . In the second community, Tupelo, it was evident from the beginning that they had problems which they thought a hospital would help solve, and that the public expression was not so much a matter of civic pride but rather an expression of needed community service. . . . I recommended Tupelo wholeheartedly. Interestingly, it started with a bed capacity of only 49 and 10 bassinets. It now has a bed capacity of between 350 and 400 and is the principal medical center for northeast Mississippi, with strong consultant relationships with Birmingham, Alabama, and Memphis, Tennessee. . . .

Provo has become much the same type of medical center for its section of Utah even though it is not more than thirty-five or forty miles from Salt Lake City. This has been due to the industrial expansion in the area and also, I believe, to the backing of the Mormon church in that region.

Seven other awards were made in rapid succession for new buildings, bringing the total number of hospitals built by the Fund to fifteen (table 2).[81]

The Legacy of the Rural Hospital Program

A hospital built in an accessible town would not work automatically, and the introduction of these hospitals into virgin soil presented a community with many unfamiliar problems. A technically appropriate and economically feasible plant had to be designed, the medical staff had to grasp the opportunity the hospital offered for professional progress, the public had to understand the ways in which the hospitals could serve a growing clientele, a reasonable course of public health development had to be tailored to the community, and the board and staff had to adopt sound standards of performance. These requirements called for a genuinely experimental attitude, and none could be solved by any rigid adherence to preconceived ideas. In each community the Fund stimulated local administrative authorities first to want the technical knowledge and grow-

Table 2 Rural Hospitals Built by the Commonwealth Fund

Southside Community Hospital, Farmville, Virginia
Opened November 9, 1927, with 38 beds and 8 bassinets; enlarged in 1942 to 55 beds and 16 bassinets.

T. J. Samson Hospital, Glasgow, Kentucky
Opened September 3, 1929, with 51 beds and 9 bassinets.

Franklin County Memorial Hospital, Farmington, Maine
Opened June 26, 1929, with 49 beds and 9 bassinets.

Community Hospital, Beloit, Kansas
Opened December 11, 1929, with 49 beds and 6 bassinets.

De Ette Harrison Detwiler Memorial Hospital, Wauseon, Ohio
Opened January 8, 1930, with 46 beds and 7 bassinets.

Holston Valley Community Hospital, Kingsport, Tennessee
Opened August 9, 1935, with 53 beds and 9 bassinets; enlarged in 1941 and 1942 to 92 beds and 17 bassinets.

North Mississippi Community Hospital, Tupelo, Mississippi
Opened October 3, 1937, with 49 beds and 10 bassinets.

Valley View Hospital, Ada, Oklahoma
Opened July 24, 1938, with 50 beds and 10 bassinets.

Utah Valley Hospital, Provo, Utah
Opened September 10, 1939, with 51 beds and 13 bassinets.

Marion Sims Memorial Hospital, Lancaster, South Carolina
Opened June 8, 1940, with 52 beds and 11 bassinets.

Illini Community Hospital, Pittsfield, Illinois
Opened January 25, 1942, with 40 beds and 9 bassinets.

Central Michigan Community Hospital, Mt. Pleasant, Michigan
Opened April 2, 1943, with 50 beds and 12 bassinets.

Missouri Delta Community Hospital, Sikeston, Missouri
Opened December 1, 1948, with 45 beds, 4 cribs, and 13 bassinets.

Rutherford Hospital, Murfreesboro, Tennessee
This hospital, built by the Fund without local participation in construction costs, was opened May 2, 1927, with 40 beds and 8 bassinets.

Kings Mountain Memorial Hospital, Bristol, Virginia
This established institution was reorganized and remodeled with Fund assistance between 1938 and 1940. Its capacity was increased to 50 beds and 7 bassinets.

ing experience of a trained staff and then to capitalize on the advantages of staff assistance.[82]

Barry C. Smith spoke of the Rural Hospital Program in glowing terms: "The number of delicate problems involved in securing the establishment of a successful hospital, with accompanying rise in standards of medical service in a community absolutely without experiences in modern methods is very great. . . . No project undertaken by the Fund has aroused more interest and favorable comment, none has presented greater difficulties, and none has shown more marked results in a period of equal length."[83]

The Fund's Division of Rural Hospitals took the best that hospital experience had to offer and adapted it to the rural community and the small town rather than experimenting with new instruments of health service that might be designed specifically for rural needs.

Postgraduate Education for Rural Physicians

Rural practice was suffering not only from a shortage of hospitals but from deficiencies in medical knowledge and technique. As in its Child Guidance Program, the Fund's staff quickly found a severe shortage of competent personnel. Again, the Fund used the device that had served it so well in its earlier program—fellowships for several categories of professionals involved in medical care and public health work, including physicians, nurses, and technicians.[84] Some fellowships served a general purpose (for example, brush-up courses for general practitioners) and some were more specifically intended to meet particular community needs. Henry C. Wright's report had foreseen the lack of competent physicians in particular, anticipating the need to help doctors in rural hospital communities with "small scholarships" for brief postgraduate courses or observational trips.[85] Of all the needed personnel, the physician had the least professional incentive either to establish himself or to remain in the small towns. In some rural communities the number of physicians was actually declining—Rutherford County, Tennessee, for example, which had thirty-four physicians in 1915, a decade later had only twenty-seven.

The Fund's staff recognized that[86]

> one of the chief handicaps to the practice of medicine in the country is the sense of isolation which the rural physician is likely to feel. If he is alone in his village, he has no one to whom he can turn easily for helpful discussion of a knotty case. If he is one of two or three doctors, he hesitates to lay his problems before a competitor. Good general hospitals are few. It is not easy to make the break and get away for study. One plods along. Before the motor-car and good roads made it easy to get about, this isolation was accepted as part of the job; indeed, it is doubtful whether the average man was even conscious of it. Now that it is no great trouble to drive to a district medical meeting now and then, the doctor is likely to catch a glimpse of progress outside his own range of experience which makes him a little dissatisfied. The man in that frame of mind is ripe for postgraduate study.

For those who might still be "green," the Fund was ready to encourage the maturing process: "Staff education in a hospital begins when two or three men swap case stories in the corridor; it can go a long way before the resources of local clinical material are exhausted. But it gets nowhere unless there is the appetite for knowledge, the habit of reflection. In most rural groups, these must be stimulated. Sometimes giving a physician a chance to study away from home for a few months provides such stimulation."[87]

Beginning in 1927 the Fund's Division of Rural Hospitals awarded an average of five fellowships a year in each hospital area for postgraduate study by members of the hospital staff.[88] Each fellowship lasted no longer than four months, and consisted of a grant of $400 per month with transportation.[89] Recipients studied at the New York Postgraduate School; Harvard, Vanderbilt, and Tulane universities; and other schools of similar rank. The purpose of these fellowships was not to encourage specialization, but to afford local physicians an opportunity to observe the best current practices. Programs of study conformed to the standards of the Council of Medical Education of the American Medical Association, and the first group of recipients—eleven physicians from Murfreesboro and Farmville—undertook three- to four-month postgraduate courses. In selecting recipients and planning the educational program for each, the Fund worked closely with the local medical group.[90] The Fund was also careful to equalize the geographical distribution: Men from larger towns were included as well as those from outlying rural districts. The program soon expanded to include training for dentists, and a few appointees to executive positions in Fund-supported rural hospitals were given special courses in preparation for dealing with what the Fund termed "the somewhat unusual professional problems" that these hospitals presented.[91]

The Division of Public Health also provided fifteen postgraduate scholarships annually, five in each of the targeted counties and five in the state at large. Recipients were encouraged to concentrate on fields of general interest—general medicine or obstetrics, for example—and to avoid training in relatively limited areas such as the surgical specialties. While the Division of Rural Hospitals allowed its recipients to choose their own institutions and, with advice from the Fund, to plan their own courses of study, the recipients in the Division of Public Health theoretically fitted into structured courses of study at selected universities. In fact, even as early as 1930, the individualized programs of study tended increasingly toward generalized instruction. Recipients were exposed to training in "the work that a man needs in a smaller place . . . majoring in medicine and pediatrics and diagnosis."[92]

The Fund also established four-year undergraduate scholarships, five each year, for first-year medical students who agreed to enter practice at the end of their basic training in towns with populations of less than five thousand. If the student disregarded the terms of the stipend and went into urban practice, he would be required to treat the stipend as a loan. The scholarships were offered in three medical schools in the Fund's three target states (Vanderbilt University[93] for students in Tennessee, Tulane University for those in Mississippi, and Tufts University for students in Massachusetts), and between forty and fifty students applied for the program in its first year. The Fund's staff was divided about the wisdom of giving scholarships to entering medical students in return for their agreement to enter into a particular kind of practice. Lester J. Evans argued that the premise of the scholarships was unwise: Not knowing what the practice of medicine really entails, most first-year medical students are not ready to make a decision about the rest of their professional lives. His intuition proved correct: Later studies by the Fund showed that very few of these scholarship students stayed in rural practice.

Participating schools received substantial grants for instruction in public health and preventive medicine. New York University received a five-year grant to develop a department of preventive medicine;[94] at Tulane and Tufts universities, new professorships of preventive medicine were created; and an award was given to Vanderbilt University, whose medical school dean, a former state health officer, already occupied a chair of preventive medicine.[95]

The Fund altered all the segments of its fellowship program as it increased its knowledge of the rural setting and of the needs and wishes of its recipients.[96] As early as 1931, the Division of Rural Hospital's postgraduate program did seem to be successful: Grateful letters arrived from fellowship recipients, and the Fund concluded that the men who were most ready for professional growth were receiving an opportunity that few could carve out for themselves. But most hospital staff members qualified to benefit had already received fellowships. Several physicians studied under a second, briefer grant, but few could afford to be absent from their practices. Accordingly, the Fund reduced the number of fellowships available in this category. With the depression, the Fund had seen diminishing interest in all of its postgraduate fellowships, in both Rural Hospital and Public Health programs: "Times are hard. . . . As the lists of eligible physicians in an area dwindles, and older men complete the initial period of study, demand for fellowships decreases. Younger men, better able perhaps to adjust themselves to the complicated environment of the modern medical school, will continue to welcome interludes of study, and some of the older men will want second courses, but other means must be found to stimulate the majority."[97]

The Division of Public Health was baffled by the particularly small demand for fellowships in Massachusetts, far less than in the other participating states. Perhaps, the staff speculated, rural physicians in Massachusetts were not as isolated as in the southern states; or physicians in Massachusetts might have special, unrecognized needs. A study of the situation by a group at Harvard University led the Massachusetts Medical Society to organize, without expense to the Fund, a program of extension teaching for Massachusetts physicians that the society hoped would also stimulate interest in the Fund's fellowships.[98] The Fund's direct solution was to break the four-month fellowship into segments of one or two months. The appeal of a shorter absence from practice was carried over into the general brush-up courses offered in the southern states. To meet the preferences of these recipients, the Fund split the four-month courses at Vanderbilt University into four units of one month each, to be taken separately at the physician's convenience. A similar choice was offered at Harvard University for physicians in Massachusetts.

The decline in the fellowships' appeal was but one of the problems confronting the Fund. The older physician had been a legitimate target of attention: "One need only recall the great gulf between medical education before and after the Flexner Report in 1910 to appreciate the handicaps under which many men who graduated 30 years or more ago are now working."[99] But the psychological difficulties inherent in this return of older men to medical school militated against the program's success:[100]

> For some men of this sort, a blend of defensiveness and bewilderment tends to block the most earnest efforts to understand what they hear. For others, long experience in managing the ills of their neighbors and friends has created a degree of self-sufficiency which makes them impatient of the wisdom of younger men. For some, the question of professional prestige is involved; one physician who was glad to accept a scholarship gave it out in his home town that he had been invited to teach a postgraduate course at the university to which he was sent! Some men must be tactfully made aware of their deficiencies; others must be weaned away from their timidity. This is a job for skillful teaching. Postgraduate teaching for men long out of school . . . must have two objectives; first, to bring their basic knowledge and their point of view about medicine to a level where they are capable of grasping new techniques, and second, to show them when and how to use these techniques.
>
> At Vanderbilt, where postgraduate education had hardly been begun before the Commonwealth Fund began its scholarship program, it was possible to face this twofold problem frankly and to shape a curriculum to meet it. It was agreed between the school and the Commonwealth Fund that a four month course should be set up and that, generally speaking, men on postgraduate scholarships should be required to take the full course. . . .
>
> Certain problems are common to all . . . institutions and indeed are characteristic of postgraduate teaching. At most teaching hospitals clinical facilities are set up definitely for the instruction of undergraduates working under staff supervision. The clinical clerk has a recognized place; the limits of his authority are well established and ward and clinic patients are accustomed to his attentive ministrations. The older man who had carried a large degree of individual responsibility for the life and death of his patients for many years and who yet fails to measure up to the standards which prevail currently in a teaching hospital is something of an anomaly. He cannot be given full responsibility nor can he, without occasional heartburning, be treated as a mere medical student. Moreover, there is not always material enough to serve the needs of both postgraduate and undergraduate students without fatiguing the patients.

In this dilemma some instructors feel themselves thrown back on a purely didactic teaching method. Cases are discussed and principles of diagnosis and therapy are explained in informal lectures to groups of ten or a dozen students. . . .

There are then a number of unanswered questions in postgraduate education. How far can postgraduate refresher courses be planned and prescribed in a systematic way? How far can the men who take them be given actual clinical experience? How large a group can be handled effectively at one time? How far can didactic instruction be relied on to meet the students' needs? Should an age limit be set in awarding scholarships for such study, and if so, at what level? The Fund believes that these questions are important, and that only careful experimentation, systematic observation, and a judicious weighing of results can reveal the answers.

By 1936, 379 postgraduate fellowships had been awarded through the programs of the Fund's two divisions.[101] But a few years later, during World War II, one doctor was doing the work of two or three in both the medical school and in the village, and the postgraduate training of physicians in practice was inopportune.[102] At Vanderbilt University, for example, the medical faculty was simply too busy to offer training during the war. The war years consequently saw a sharp reduction in the number of fellowships awarded to physicians in both public health and rural hospital programs.[103]

Shorter fellowships were one solution, and in 1945 the Division of Public Health planned a new award, intended to place well-qualified young physicians for a preliminary three months in a health department where they could try the field and be tried out themselves. If both results were favorable, the candidate would be given a year's training at a school of public health. The exigencies of World War II made it impossible to put this plan into operation right away, but neither did the return of soldiers to civilian life flood rural communities with health professionals. Men who were health officers before the war hesitated to return to the narrow salary scales of the prewar years. As a result, the Fund could find only five satisfactory candidates to fill its eight fellowships for health officers, and all recipients had been previously committed to a public health career.[104]

By 1949 federal funds were replacing foundation grants for technical study in the field of public health. The Fund's Division of Public Health was therefore discontinued as a separate unit, and public health programs were phased out. Fellowships in the Division of Rural Hospitals, too, were absorbed by the Fund's other programs.

Coming at the beginning of postgraduate medical education in the United States, the fellowships offered through the Public Health and Rural Hospitals programs were particularly valuable to the Fund's staff, who developed extensive contacts with other organizations, including the American Medical Association, the extension divisions of a few state universities, and several professional societies. As for the fellowships' recipients, it was difficult by and large to judge the value of these short periods of postgraduate training. The Fund did not believe that rural medicine would be "revolutionized" by offering postgraduate fellowships to country physicians, but that those who faced forward would benefit. Although only a limited number of men could be reached through postgraduate fellowships, they probably shared their gains with their colleagues:[105]

> Each of them has had three or four months at a good school, with the opportunity to brush up against an infinite variety of new experiences. Many men pick up a wealth of new information which they are able to put to work promptly in their everyday practice. Four months is a short time in which to fall in step with the amazing progress of medicine in the last decade or two, but even when the physicians' capacity for grasping new technic is limited by his age and previous isolation, he is likely to be so stirred by his adventure that his whole professional outlook is fresher. This may be revealed in very homely ways: sometimes the most noticeable change is that a man goes home and spruces up his office, or buys a microscope. Sometimes a group of men who compete closely for patients have gotten together and worked out a set of record forms which they have printed at their joint expense.

The Fund concluded that perhaps half of the men receiving postgraduate fellowships really increased their professional stature. A Fund-supported study of rural health in Tennessee showed that while younger and middle-aged men learned the most, the older men had made the greatest relative improvement. A thorough follow-up study in 1934 of thirty men who had completed the course showed that twenty-six had demonstrated sufficient improvement to justify the investment in their postgraduate training. When these men purchased equipment and improved their offices, the effect on their competitors was obvious. When they took part in medical meetings, they were heard with respect. When they made thorough examinations, they set a standard that patients were quick to appreciate. One concrete piece of evidence was a demonstrably greater use of hospital facilities in communities where physicians had undertaken such training; the Fund believed that this increase reflected the public's growing confidence in the physicians staffing the hospitals.

The Fund's staff felt that medical schools were not making the necessary special effort to reorient general practitioners long out of school: "While we believed that the general results of the postgraduate effort with doctors were worthwhile, we were faced with the fact that adequate methods of postgraduate teaching had not been generally accepted by educational institutions."[106] Here was the seed of the Fund's later interest in direct assistance to medical schools to cover the complete spectrum of health education.

The entire weight of progress in education could not be placed on the medical school, however; the ultimate responsibility rested with the individual. The Fund's staff believed that its influence could extend only to setting the stage for competent service within a hospital. The men at work must form the habit of evaluating their own output and must carry within them the wish for self-education. As this fellowship program wound down, the Fund concluded that "something can be done to modernize the work of men trained before the turn of the century and isolated most of the time since. More can be done for men in their prime. Most can be accomplished by getting good youngsters into the medical schools, giving them sound training for general practice with due attention to preventive service, and offering them a chance to find real satisfactions in rural practice. . . . As . . . educational opportunities are spread more widely, the problems of rural medicine, as such, will tend to disappear in the larger issues of medical progress."[107]

Regional Hospitals

In 1942, with its last award to a rural hospital, the Commonwealth Fund turned to the next phase of its program, the regional organization of hospitals and related services. Basil C. MacLean, president of the American Hospital Association and director of the Strong Memorial Hospital in Rochester, New York, discussed the future of community hospitals at the Fund-supported annual meeting of the American College of Hospital Administrators. He predicted important changes in hospital and medical care during the war years and in the postwar period. The hospital could find itself in an increasingly strategic position as an instrument of public health—in many communities the center of public health activities. The entire field of public health, he believed, was poised for rapid expansion.

One type of expansion involved "regional organization," which in the Fund's conception would coordinate hospital services around a population center containing a full complement of medical personnel and hospital institutions. The dimensions of a region would vary considerably, depending upon population density and size, character, number, and distribution of outlying population centers. The radius of a region could extend between 75 and 100 or more miles, but in densely populated areas or urban states, regions would be considerably smaller. A regional organization would distribute hospital facilities throughout the outlying parts of the region; promulgate standards in all hospital departments; offer joint services that might be considered desirable locally (including joint purchasing); provide regional consultation in clinical and laboratory medicine and in institutional administration; and offer continuing educational programs for physicians and other hospital personnel in a more organized fashion than was possible in the single rural hospital.

Henry J. Southmayd's confidential memorandum to the Fund's staff in September 1943 reinforced the staff's repeated observation: Rural hospitals closely linked to hospitals and consultants in larger centers offered a higher standard of service than those without such ties.[108] Southmayd believed that a plan to promote better standards should allow the rural hospitals surrounding a large center to have easy access to consultation services in pathology and x-ray and in clinical specialties such as pediatrics, obstetrics, and orthopedics. A regional association would also make it easier for local community hospitals to obtain competent hospital administrators, nurse executives, dietitians, and other hospital personnel who could profit from close relationships with their counterparts in the larger center. Some of the more fortunately situated hospitals had been able to work out collaborations with their neighboring centers; but in other areas, distance and cost, local indifference, and some open opposition to the presence of consultants were practical barriers that a single hospital could not easily surmount.

After much staff discussion, the idea of supporting a regional organization was approved by the Fund, and a public announcement was made. There is no record of the number of inquiries that followed this announcement, but two were of particular interest to the Fund: Rochester, New York, and Richmond, Virginia. Southmayd favored Rochester, but Evans preferred Richmond.[109] In Southmayd's view a regional organization existed primarily to promote better administrative standards in hospitals; education and patient-care services were secondary considerations. Evans argued that the quality of patient care was most important and although hospital administrative standards needed to be raised, the Fund should select a region whose professionals could benefit from improved educational programs. Evans believed that the level of sophistication in the Rochester area mitigated the need for the Fund's educational efforts; a program in the several counties involved would improve only hospital administration. Through the Rural Hospital Program, Evans was in frequent contact with the Medical College of Virginia in Richmond and the University of Virginia in Charlottesville. Richmond, Evans thought, offered a fluid situation in which improvements in medical education, patient care, and hospital administration could be demonstrated more quickly.

The Fund's board of directors shared Southmayd's point of view, and the decision was made to proceed with an intensive investigation of the Rochester area—an investigation encompassing the attitude of the medical school faculty toward regional development and their willingness to participate as well as the strength of the services of the Strong Memorial Hospital, the Monroe County Hospital, and the larger private hospitals in Rochester, some of which were not then affiliated with the University of Rochester's medical school. Evans spent a week visiting every hospital in the nine counties that the Fund originally intended to include. These hospitals were not unlike the Fund's own rural hospitals in size, but they had no programs for staff education and no formal relationships with other hospitals in Rochester or with the medical school. In general administration, organization, and functioning, the small hospitals were inferior to many of the hospitals that the Fund had assisted. The Fund's assessment was that the region's programs were weak in ways that a regional organization could remedy, while community enthusiasm and the presence of the university gave the area the potential for leadership. The final decision of the Fund was for Rochester.[110]

The Rochester Regional Hospital Plan

At the end of 1945, the Fund set up its initial experiment in the seven counties surrounding the city of Rochester. The Rochester region covered 4,715 square miles, and the combined population of the seven counties was 713,862 (with fewer than half the inhabitants living in the city itself).

The program in Rochester was an experiment in methodology, an effort to show how the existing resources of rural medicine—good, bad, or indifferent—could be effectively supplemented by those of a regional center, and the Rochester Regional Hospital Plan turned out to be the prototype for local and regional hospital associations.[111] Yet the idea of regional organization of community efforts was not new. In 1920 the Lord Dawson Report[112] in Great Britain adapted this concept to health services and recommended the development of a network of hospital facilities within which hospitals and medical services could be integrated. In the United States, the first significant experiment in the regional organization of health services was initiated in 1931 in Maine, by the Bingham Associates Fund, to overcome the isolation of practitioners by establishing an intimate working relationship between community hospitals and physicians in Maine and the New England Medical Center in Boston. After World War II, several regional programs had been inaugurated by university-affiliated medical schools, but the programs in Maine and Rochester remained those with the broadest scope.

The assets of the Rochester area included an outstanding medical school; an active hospital council consisting of six voluntary hospitals; relatively adequate regional hospital facilities; and a generally favorable level of economic and social development.[113] Three areas of action seemed promising: joint planning of hospital building and expansion; joint operation of certain institutional services that could be performed more efficiently by the group than by individual institutions; and pooling of clinical, administrative, and technical skills.

Basil C. MacLean proposed that the Rochester Hospital Council assume responsibility for getting the program underway. After a series of conferences with representatives of the Commonwealth Fund, a new organization, the Council of Rochester Regional Hospitals, was incorporated on February 18, 1946, and a five-year agreement with the Fund defining the responsibilities of the two organizations was signed eight days later.[114] The Fund's support would allow the Council to provide financial aid and planning for distribution of hospital facilities throughout the region; promulgate approved procedures for hospital organization and operation; develop consultation services in clinical and laboratory medicine and in institutional administration; organize and administer an educational program for physicians, dentists, and hospital personnel (emphasizing postgraduate study); and offer other health services mutually agreed upon by the contracting parties.

The program's staff consisted of a part-time executive director (Albert D. Kaiser, health officer of Rochester), a physician as full-time associate director, a part-time nursing associate, an administrative secretary, and a part-time business manager who was also executive secretary to the Rochester Hospital Council. This council and the Council of Rochester Regional Hospitals began as discrete agencies sharing office space and staff; in 1951 they were consolidated into one organization, the Rochester Regional Hospital Council.

The business of the corporation was managed by its board of directors; two directors from each member hospital were elected for a two-year term. The board was responsible for determining policy, financing, employment of staff, and action on applications for membership, and for ensuring effective working relations with other health agencies. Most of the detailed discussions of policy were conducted by the executive committee, which was composed of the officers of the board and five directors. Capital grants were allocated through a separate committee until 1951, when the moneys provided by the Commonwealth Fund for capital improvement (over $1 million) had been completely expended.

During its first five years of operation the Regional Council's major financial support came from the Commonwealth Fund under the terms of their basic agreement: The Fund would support general administration and education with annual contributions of up to $75,000 a year for five years. Supplementary matching funds of no more than $25,000 would be available for special projects. Furthermore, the Fund would provide $200,000 a year for construction of hospital facilities. In turn, the corporation agreed to raise $10,000 a year for operations and matching funds for supplemental grants. A complete review of the council's program was made in 1949 and 1950, and a request for continued support from the Fund was approved for a three-year period at a diminishing rate ($50,000, $40,000 and $20,000). Toward the end of the Fund's support, the Council obtained money by assessing member hospitals according to the number of beds in each.

Some of the most tangible results of the council's activities were found in the field of hospital administration and medical education. Postgraduate courses were designed to explore problems of current interest in the council program; for example, an institute on the use of blood and blood derivatives was given at the Strong Memorial Hospital in 1948, when the regional blood bank had just come into operation. In many respects the council's services were in themselves educational. It functioned as a clearing center through which administrative techniques found successful in one hospital could be transmitted to others, and meetings of administrative and advisory bodies, institutes, and seminars provided forums for discussion of organizational problems.

The council was also interested in the field of nursing education and offered advisory services, recruiting activities, institutes and conferences, fellowships for special study, in-service training, and formal education for undergraduates, graduate nurses, and practical nurses. Advisory support was also provided for other hospital personnel, including medical record librarians and accountants, and programs were aimed at the education of trustees.

The council's interest in research was subordinate to its program of education. Most of the council's studies were designed to answer specific questions related to administration of the program. A few were organized for purely administrative purposes, and many would not ordinarily be classified as research but as analyses of administrative controls.[115] The more significant studies examined changes in health behavior and health attitudes in the Rochester region resulting from the regional hospital demonstration; delineation of hospital service area; community health and medical-care statistics by hospital districts; comparisons of appendectomy rates; surveys of nursing and other hospital personnel; allotment of nursing time; and cost of nursing education. The council also developed a system of periodic reporting and analysis of professional activities, an important step toward measuring the quality of care.

Like other council proposals, the plan for regular visits by consultants at first met with reserve from the medical staff of the community hospitals; the Fund thought the staff members feared an effort by the medical school to dominate medical practice in the area. As time passed, however, the medical staffs' wariness was overcome, and the council provided consultants in varied phases of hospital operation, such as dietetics, laboratory procedures, and hospital construction. These advisory services were usually designed to meet the needs of smaller institutions lacking a variety of specialized personnel, and much time was devoted to in-service training. Over the years the council developed into a source of general information for hospital personnel throughout the region, and hospitals profited greatly from an orderly approach that allowed them to obtain information on a wide range of subjects. One particularly useful procedure was the council's briefings for hospitals before inspection by the Joint Commission on Accreditation of Hospitals.

Many of the solutions emerging from meetings of the Rochester Subregional Committee were later adapted to the rest of the region. An administrators' conference was established as a forum for hospital administrators in the region—an opportunity to consider common problems, formulate recommendations to the board, and see their hospitals' operations in the perspective of the whole region. A medical conference was also set up, as a subdivision of the council, to exchange information among member hospitals and formulate policies about medical staff organization, activities, and education. Specific areas were handled by new committees—blood banks, laboratory and diagnostic procedures, and nursing, for example. As the committees gained experience, their structures were altered to meet the member hospitals' needs. Other common problems were addressed when a field medical librarian was hired in 1949 and a central purchasing program established in 1953.

Hospital administrators in particular appreciated the opportunity to associate with others in the region. They felt free to call and visit, to discuss such problems as wage scales, personnel policies, and departmental relations within the hospital. A Committee on Records, Reports, and Statistics, established in 1947, developed standard nomenclature suitable for hospitals in the region, planned consultation services, and prepared a manual concerning medical records. Standards for hospital organization were developed, and upon their retirement, several untrained administrators were replaced with formally trained personnel.

Appraising the value of educational programs like the Rochester Regional Hospital Program is extremely difficult because so many groups and disciplines were involved. Although it is possible only to record impressions, the educational efforts of the council appeared to promote greater cohesion between the professional and nonprofessional groups. Hospital administration seemed to benefit more than professional education, although the educational programs for medical record librarians and accountants appeared to be very efficient. Continuing education of physicians, still in an experimental stage, could not be readily evaluated but was not obviously improved by the activities of the council. The formal efforts at trustee education and education incidental to the proceedings of the boards of directors and other committees did have a beneficial effect—as shown by the high degree of enthusiasm that many of the trustees displayed for the council's operations.

The efforts of the council to improve regional hospital facilities complemented those of other official and voluntary agencies. The New York State Joint Hospital Survey and Planning Commission, established in 1947, was responsible for the administration of the federal Hospital Construction Act in New York, as well as for developing a plan to coordinate hospital facilities within the state. To distribute hospital construction funds, the Joint Hospital Survey and Planning Commission appointed regional hospital planning councils in each of the state's seven regions. The executive director of the Rochester Regional Hospital Council served as the state planning council's secretary, and many members of the Regional Hospital Council's board of directors were also members of the planning council. Criteria devised jointly by the Capital Grants Committee and the Commonwealth Fund's staff led to the approval of eight projects in hospital construction, which would receive almost $1 million from the planning council—almost one-quarter of the Rochester region's $4 million expenditure for this purpose.

Widespread interest in this regional hospital program convinced the Fund that a report of the experiment should be available for those unable to visit Rochester in person. In 1954 the Institute of Administrative Medicine at Columbia University was asked to develop an objective description of the program, use the program's experience to suggest principles of organization and administration appropriate to the appraisal of regional health services, measure the effects of the program on medical facilities and professional services in the area, and formulate recommendations for the program's further development.

The resulting study unearthed ample evidence of the program's success. Through its committees and advisory bodies the Rochester Regional Hospital Council had stimulated the interest of community leaders in a broad range of fields. The willingness of participating hospitals to increase their contributions to the program's support confirmed the study's finding: The council had become a significant part of the area's hospital services. Regional organization had become a process for improving communication and establishing a pattern of cooperation among independent communities and specialized agencies in a functionally constituted area. Because it was a process, rather than a specific form of service, its ultimate potential could not be precisely defined. Once the process was established in a region, it would be adapted to meet many, often unanticipated, needs. Regional organization could be compared to a railroad system: Once the structure was built, it served to distribute a variety of products as they became available and as demand for them developed. The region offered a kind of meeting ground for the medical school, the hospital planning group, and public health and medical care agencies. Only through their coordinated efforts could the basic unity of essential preventive, therapeutic, and rehabilitative services be achieved. The multiplicity of independent organizations, each with its own objectives and policies, presented a continuing challenge to the development of regional service. This diversity was not an insurmountable obstacle, although it did impose a slower rhythm of development, one that allowed time to educate the public to identify with a larger community and to make professional groups aware of the potential benefits of enlarged objectives.

The study concluded that the Rochester region had made significant progress in the face of complex problems. The organization of the program had ensured wide dissemination of information about council activities and encouraged confidence in the regional program. The board of directors and the several advisory bodies were broadly representative of the region and reviewed issues comprehensively. The council's experimentation with a great variety of services allowed the council and the Fund to visualize the potential of this form of organization and to measure obstacles much more precisely. The council's wealth of experience also provided a valuable resource for planning by other regional programs.[116]

This program also benefited the small hospitals built or remodeled under the Fund's Rural Hospital Program, transmitting the techniques of more efficient administration emerging from the Rochester experience. Some of these scattered hospitals had already been linked with larger institutions that might serve as regional centers, and the Fund hoped that this small project might be augmented.[117] Once again the Fund's interest had turned from ameliorating the deficiencies of a strictly local situation to improving health services over a broad area.

The Rochester Regional Hospital Council Today

Robert L. Berg, professor of preventive medicine and chairman of the department at the University of Rochester, recently put into perspective the current status and overall effectiveness of the Commonwealth Fund's first major investment in the Rochester area.[118] When he arrived in Rochester in 1958, the program relied on three groups: the administrators, the physicians, and the board of trustees and its committees; and at first Berg spent a great deal of time meeting with the administrators and physicians. In 1960 he was drafted to serve as director of the Strong Memorial Hospital—a temporary job that extended over eighteen months. From this vantage point, it appeared to him that the Regional Hospital Council was not serving any constructive purpose: Its functions seemed limited to joint purchasing and joint bill collecting. Until 1977 or 1978 the program—and the overall effort to regionalize hospital services—seemed to Berg in many respects a failure.

More recently Berg concluded that the program had accumulated enough experience to "take off" and that health planning in Monroe County and the entire region had advanced faster than elsewhere. Because a large number of people were involved, more time was needed for them to begin to trust each other, to stop "wondering what everyone was up to."

Once this initial hurdle was overcome, the Regional Hospital Council was able to create an organization marked by understanding between members at different levels.

Albert D. Kaiser was the local force behind the formation of the Rochester Regional Hospital Program, but it was Marion B. Folsom, treasurer of the Eastman Kodak Company and the patron saint of health in Rochester, who took the program in hand. The presence of the Eastman Kodak Company was a special resource in Rochester, and Folsom had brought to Rochester his experience as Secretary of Health, Education and Welfare under President Eisenhower. Folsom had Kodak's support, and "what he said usually went pretty well."[119] His enthusiasm would have been far less useful, however, had he not been able to draw on the council's accumulated experience. Folsom's contributions included adroit organizational arrangements, "making things happen that otherwise would only have been talked about." When asked to serve as the chairman of a general hospital fund drive, he stipulated that he would do so only if the hospital would agree never to add new beds without first obtaining the permission of a hospital planning group. The group to which he referred was the Patient Care Planning Council; originating in 1961, it was the first organization in the United States to give "certificates of need." Folsom next persuaded the New York legislature to enact a law mandating this procedure for the state at large. His success made New York the first state in the country to enable such legislation, and this plan ultimately became the model for the federal Planning Act of 1966. Folsom was also adept at involving local people, who would know more about community situations than so-called outside experts and, most important, would be involved in implementing the decisions made. The participation of the local community was a new idea for the council, whose studies had previously relied only on these outside experts, and the result was greatly strengthened planning.

Through Folsom's efforts the University of Rochester School of Medicine also became involved in health planning. By the early 1960s the department of preventive medicine had shifted its emphasis from comprehensive medical care for the individual patient to the organization of studies related to use of hospital beds, care of the aged, and other issues requiring a team approach. The department's recruitment of faculty reflected its interest in this new direction, the organization and financing of health care.

The present name of the council is the Regional Hospital Association, and it is now fundamentally a trade group. The power that evolved from the original regional plan is no longer vested in that association, but has been shared by other groups "piggy-backing" on the entire program. One such group is the federally ordained and supported Finger Lakes Health Systems Agency, whose major function is deciding whether a hospital can add beds or new services. The Agency not only emerged from the Rochester Regional Hospital Plan but superseded it, receiving the power that would otherwise have gone to the new Regional Hospital Association.

The lessons of the Rochester Regional Council derived from its long history of enabling diverse groups to work together and its ultimate beneficial effect on the area it served. The Commonwealth Fund's important contribution was its initiative in supporting the early phases of the Rochester Regional Health Plan, a function that government agencies and even other private foundations would have found difficult. These groups were not likely to see such a program as a worthwhile investment if the positive result was to be 15 to 20 years away—even though these long-term gains may have proved to be the most substantial of all.

Ancillary Programs in Public Health

The significance of the word "demonstration" evolved over the years from 1920 to 1940. At first it meant a form of public health salesmanship aimed at persuading a particular community to take over and maintain a demonstrated program. Later, the task of "selling" a broad-gauge health program to a county was left to the state health department and was virtually complete before a demonstration began. This shift in responsibility allowed the Fund to undertake projects in public health that united its seemingly diverse activities in this broad area.

To ensure the objective evaluation of health programs, from 1937 to 1947 the Fund supported the plan of the APHA's Committee on Administrative Practice to review health services in any state, on the request of the governor or state health officer. As state health departments and the United States Public Health Service had often contributed funds to these programs, their assessments would be open to charges of bias. In contrast, the committee's surveys were not influenced by local politics or the wishes of the local personnel. The evaluations of this national body proved indispensable in promoting legislation to raise standards of public health. Conducted by a staff headed by Dr. Carl E. Buck, they were undertaken in Oklahoma, Michigan, Florida, Illinois, Washington, California, Oregon, Utah, Idaho, Colorado, Wyoming, Montana, and North Dakota. Recommendations were made to state and local health departments, and follow-up visits assisted in carrying them out. Accounts of these visits are among the most exciting portions of Buck's reports, revealing particular accomplishments in Illinois, Colorado, and Oregon. In Colorado, for example, where a state health survey was conducted in the winter of 1945–46, extraordinary local leadership was available in the person of Florence R. Sabin. Buck reported that of nine bills for the promotion of public health introduced in the 1947 legislature, only two failed to pass. The successful legislation removed the state health department from the executive branch of the state government, where it had been a division directly responsible to the governor; facilitated the establishment of full-time local health departments; improved the civil service; reorganized the board of health; defined qualifications for the position of state health officer; and established a division of health education within the state's department of health.

The Fund also supported the nation's first survey of educational units in the field of public health. Started in 1945 by the American Public Health Association, this process of evaluation and accreditation led to substantial improvements in public health education. By 1947 ten schools of public health in the United States and one in Canada were accredited.

The Fund's Accomplishments in Public Health

The Fund entered the public health field through its interest in special services for children. Although developed by pediatricians and educators, these services had won scant acceptance in public health programs outside the larger cities. This relatively specialized effort by the Fund soon gave way to its broader commitment to the cause of rural public health service. County health services were enriched and reasonably high standards of public health established, while the point of contact between the Fund and the field was shifted to the state health department. Later, the Fund began to supplement its standard programs with more experimental services, such as the assignment of staff nurses to bedside service at home deliveries. Its long-range hopes were to strengthen the services of state and local health departments, encourage state authorities to enlarge the content of their services, and keep pushing standards closer and closer to the point of maximum return on the investment of the taxpayer and the Fund—a point that itself moved forward as medical knowledge increased. Since the states learned slowly from one another and there was a wide span from the best to the worst, the Fund continued to emphasize personnel training and sound technical guidance. Federal and state subsidies were raising the median level of local health work, leaving philanthropic foundations such as the Commonwealth Fund free to explore its upper reaches by fostering new concepts of field service.[120]

The Fund's child health demonstrations and the wider program that followed established the principle that if county health work is worth doing at all it is worth doing with an ample staff. Fifteen years of activity by the Fund's Division of Public Health led to vastly improved standards of public health, through demonstration health departments in rural communities and strengthening of state health departments. County health departments broadened their work, expanded their staffs, improved their records, consolidated measures for protection against some of the communicable diseases, and generally increased their efficiency. These gains came about largely because of deliberate stimulation by a number of foundations, including the Commonwealth Fund, and partially because of the vision and energy of a few outstanding state leaders and increased interest from the United States Public Health Service. By the 1940s the committee on local health units of the American Public Health Association had completed a master plan for the expansion of a reasonably well-standardized health service that would cover the entire country.

The Fund chose to continue its efforts to improve the public health by filling gaps in the programs of better-than-average county health departments. The progressive development of state service was encouraged and the training of public health workers fostered. By 1945 federal support was so extensive that there was no further need for foundation aid in the geographical expansion of public health services.

The national success of the Commonwealth Fund's efforts in public health led to a citation of merit from the American Public Health Association in 1935, provoked newspaper editorials,[121] and influenced President Roosevelt's Committee on Economic Security, which was preparing a federal public health program. The Subcommittee on Public Health requested the help of W. Frank Walker and Ira V. Hiscock, a member of the Fund's Committee on Public Health. Their recommendations were modeled on the Fund's public health program and called for modest assistance to states and local communities in the development of local health units. Walker commented: "It is, we believe, a significant endorsement of the Commonwealth Fund's public health program that this national plan, drawn so extensively from Fund studies and experience, was the only one of the reports in this section of the Committee on Economic Security studies which was endorsed practically as written by the professional advisory group. It was furthermore favorably commented on editorially on two occasions by the Journal of the American Medical Association."[122]

The Commonwealth Fund programs in public health also provided an important example for the framers of the Hill–Burton Hospital Survey and Construction Act.[123] In 1942 the American Hospital Association and the United States Public Health Service formed the Commission of Hospital Care with financial support from several foundations, including the Commonwealth Fund. The Hospital Survey and Construction Act of 1946, which was based largely on the recommendations of this commission, gave the states money to build hospitals.[124] Smith invoked the Commonwealth Fund's experience in public health and rural hospitals to caution the federal government:[125]

> It is practically certain that the institutions so erected will be publicly owned and operated. The Fund has been exclusively interested in the voluntary

> hospital operated under private auspices. To what extent or in what ways modification of the Fund's program may be advisable cannot be foreseen until the federal program becomes a reality. However, it would appear that the Fund's emphasis on standards is likely to be as important in connection with this proposed undertaking as it was in the expansion of the public health service three years ago. Indeed this is already proving to be the case. . . . Officials of the [United States Public Health] Service and of the Children's Bureau have called at the office and requested information repeatedly as to methods and standards of building and operation employed by the Fund; Mr. Southmayd and also Dr. Walker of the Division of Health Studies have been asked to state the Fund's views before the Technical Committee in Washington. . . .
>
> The dangers of cheap and inadequate construction; of scattering hospitals in undesirable and unnecessary locations on a pork-barrel basis; of poor medical, nursing and general operating standards; and of various forms of political control are sufficiently great to warrant at least making the importance of standards widely known. This we are trying to do and it is gratifying, if not important, to have the associate director of the American College of Surgeons remark that more can be learned from the Commonwealth Fund than from any other source as to rural community hospitals and how to operate them.

Contrary to Smith's fears, this piece of legislation made possible an almost ideal working relationship between the federal and state governments. By 1965 the federal government had provided almost $2 billion to match $4 billion given by sponsors for the construction of 6700 projects, involving 285,000 hospital beds and 800 health units located in rural areas; more than half of the projects were located in areas that previously had no hospital service.[126]

In addition to its work with rural hospitals, the most important contribution of the Fund's public health program may have been its emphasis on the prevention of disease. With national health-care costs now at 10.5 percent of the gross national product,[127] public institutions have turned their attention to prevention as a cost-saving measure. Although it has been called a "blind spot in U.S. health policy,"[128] prevention has been a cornerstone of all the Commonwealth Fund's programs since its inception. Current proposals to provide the consumer with information about prevention of disease, establish preventive procedures paid for by a governmental program, and encourage prevention-oriented primary care are echoes of programs devised and supported by the Commonwealth Fund fifty years ago.

Beyond any immediate benefits to individuals, states, and the practice of medicine in general, the Fund's efforts in public health brought it into contact with many problems in health education. The benefits of this exposure emerged in the Fund's later programs in medical education, which were built on this bedrock of experience.

5

Early Programs in Medical Education and Medical Research

Every good laboratory consists of first-rate men working in great harmony to insure the progress of science; but down the hall is an unsociable, wrong-headed fellow working on unprofitable lines, and in his hands lies the hope of discovery.
—Lord Rutherford

The Second General Director: Barry Conger Smith (1921—1947)

Medical education did not assume an identity of its own at the Commonwealth Fund until 1932, when it appeared as a separate heading in the annual report. Medical research was also not mentioned separately in the annual report until 1930. Yet during the previous decade, the thread of the Fund's interest in both fields had run through its writings and its programs. The Fund's third annual report recorded two grants in support of medical research and commented: "The interest of the Fund in health work has been chiefly expressed in three ways during the year; namely, by assistance to medical and hospital work, to medical research and to organizations dealing with health conditions and engaged in educational work along health lines."[1] As in its programs in medical education, the focus of the Fund's support for medical research was at first confined to its major area of concern at the time: the welfare of children. In the early 1930s the Fund made grants for specific research projects, directing its support toward ways of preventing and curing disease and methods of understanding normal function. The Fund's staff considered these approaches just as important as the teaching and field programs that showed the way to put existing knowledge to work. Nevertheless, it was not until 1937, mid-way through Barry C. Smith's tenure as general director, that the Fund acquired the resources to develop formal, freestanding programs in medical education and medical research.

The Harkness Gift

In 1937 Edward S. Harkness added $5 million to the Fund's endowment: "Mr. Harkness stated that he would arrange to provide a sufficient increase in the endowment of the Fund to increase the annual income by 200,000 dollars, this additional income to be expended for such projects as medical research and medical education including the teaching of preventive medicine, strengthening of postgraduate teaching at medical schools, and granting of fellowships to promising medical men with the emphasis placed upon medical research."[2] This gift changed the thinking of the Commonwealth Fund's staff: it marked the moment when the Fund began to consider medical education and research as specific entities, separate from existing programs.[3]

It also allowed the full development of the "trickle-down approach" to philanthropy, a device that had particular appeal for Edward S. Harkness. Institutions of high quality would be identified, and either the institution would receive a direct grant or first-rate investigators in that institution would be chosen for support. The students and fellows in the investigators' orbits would in the course of their own careers go on to other institutions, starting a chain reaction with potentially far-reaching influence. Through this approach fellowships from the Fund produced outstanding men and women in all branches of medicine and bioscience. Research grants to distinguished scientists such as Dickinson W. Richards, Walter Bauer, Selman Waksman, and Fritz A. Lipmann provided research and clinical training to a generation of fellows who in turn became established clinicians and scientists teaching the next generation.

Medical Fellowships and Medical Research

The Fund's fellowships before 1937 reflected its long-term interest in child welfare, mental health, hospitals, and public health. In medical schools the number of full-time professorships in both basic and clinical sciences had increased, but recruitment and training of faculty members remained a pressing problem. One solution was postdoctoral medical fellowships, first offered by the Rockefeller Foundation during World War I.

Barry C. Smith wanted the Commonwealth Fund's medical fellowships to strengthen the teaching resources of medical schools at strategically important points. To supervise the Fund's Fellowship Program and its projects in medical research, Roderick E. Heffron was recruited from a Fund-supported program in Massachusetts.

Heffron was born in the midwest, but came east for his medical education, graduating from the Harvard Medical School in 1928. While waiting for his internship to begin at the Massachusetts General Hospital, he worked in neurology at the Boston City Hospital under Stanley Cobb. Jobs were scarce during the depression, and when his internship ended in 1931, Heffron considered himself fortunate to secure a position with the Massachusetts State Department of Public Health. Under the direction of George H. Bigelow, he participated in a study of the use of antipneumococcal serum in the treatment of pneumonia, a project financed by the Commonwealth Fund. This subject so absorbed his interest that when the study ended in 1935, he used the residual money from the Fund's grant to write a book on pneumonia.[4] The Fund invited him to join the staff as a medical associate in 1937, and he remained until his retirement in 1966.[5] With Heffron in charge, the fellowship and medical research programs survived the vagaries of four general directors. For almost three decades, many of the brightest men and women in American medicine passed his scrutiny as he oversaw the Fund's Advanced Fellowships in Medical Education (1938–56); their successor, the Awards in Support of Creative Scholarship (1957–66); and the grants of the Medical Research Program.

Heffron was assisted by Charles O. Warren, a medical associate of the Fund from 1946 to 1959. Warren had both the M.D. and Ph.D. degrees (the latter in biology), and his experience included years as an assistant professor of physiology and anatomy at Cornell University and as an associate in the Office of Scientific Research and Development.[6]

The Fellowship Programs

Our universities have become the research and training centers on which American defense and industry and agriculture and the professions depend. Our progress in all these fields depends upon a constant flow of high-caliber and skilled manpower, upon new ideas and the ability to apply these skills. Thus, today, the university is, in the words of Woodrow Wilson, "the root of our intellectual life as a nation."

—*John F. Kennedy*

As one of philanthropy's more productive ventures, the fellowship allowed the Commonwealth Fund to provide individuals with unique, sometimes previously nonexistent capabilities. Although the Fund's intentions have remained stable over sixty years, the interpretation and execution of its aims changed. Fellowships in the early 1920s were backed by a strong organizational structure: As in the Rural Hospital Program, recipients were chosen to fill specific slots created to support the Fund's programmatic interests. But forty years later the Fund's staff was giving fellowships to scholars at mid- or even end-career, scientists and physicians whose purposes were sometimes as vague as "to travel" or "to be exposed to new ideas." These varied fellowships reflected a judicious interpretation of Edward S. Harkness's—and the Fund's—stated mission, "service . . . rooted in sound clinical practice by trained practitioners."[7]

Hospital staff members in the Rural Hospital Program had received postgraduate medical experience to encourage professional growth and improve hospital care. Fellowships also raised the level of competence of health officers, nurses, and other public health workers in county health demonstrations and in positions of state leadership. At the same time, fellowships for the study of psychiatry, previously offered with the needs of that specialty in mind, had been made available to pediatricians and later, on similar terms, to internists who wished to carry some degree of psychiatric training back into the teaching of medicine. These groups of awards—flexible, opportunistic, and highly individualized—set the pattern for the most active years of the Fund's fellowship program.

Advanced Medical Fellowships

Smith saw the Fund's fellowships as a link between medical education and medical research, and he therefore targeted the fellowships at the basic clinical departments—internal medicine, pediatrics, and obstetrics. Edward S. Harkness's gift had also made it possible to support permanent staff members of such departments actually engaged in teaching and research and to connect fellowships with other departmental awards. The Fund's formal program for young teachers was the first concrete realization of these intentions.[8]

Small schools and large, preclinical and clinical departments—the Fund considered all evenhandedly. In offering fellowships, the Fund followed the path it had taken in child health and mental health: Programs began simply but eventually led to broader interests. At this time the Fund wanted to put its limited resources to work at points where the medical schools themselves saw a concrete need.

The tendency to make one discipline feed another was then conspicuous in medical education: Electrophysics was nourishing neurology, physiology was enriching obstetrics, biochemistry was invading physiology. In one year the Fund sent a physiologist to the Massachusetts Institute of Technology to study hydraulics. It helped a dermatologist to work in pharmacology, a physiologist to administer physical therapy, and a bacteriologist to learn public health. One of the first fellowship recipients eventually held a dual appointment in medicine and physiology. Still another defined the relationship between the practice of public health and the teaching of preventive medicine. In some cases, the school contributed by providing new laboratory facilities upon a fellow's return.

The continuing use of these fellowships enabled a university to take someone from his familiar academic environment and stretch his mind in a new and broader setting. It was obviously advantageous for a young teacher well grounded in clinical medicine to have some uninterrupted firsthand experience with investigative methods. Many of these fellows quickly displayed brilliance as investigators, their contributions to research providing an early return on the Fund's investment (see app. B).[9]

When this program began in 1938, the Fund's staff hoped that it would have nationwide importance as a model for other foundations and universities; more concretely, they wanted to give promising young investigators an opportunity to grow more rapidly than they might without such help, and to improve the faculty in good medical schools. Finally, the Fund hoped to do something more subtle by "exposing a good mind to the stimulus of a year of work outside its chosen field, so that cross-fertilization could take place."[10] As the staff said, "The appointees are mature enough to have shown the stuff there is in them, young enough to be impressionable. As they go back to their posts, they should be more competent teachers, more stimulating colleagues. Some of them may come to be leaders in teaching and research. They are good risks, and the Fund is glad to back them."[11]

A recipient had to meet four general criteria:

1. He should already be a member of a university faculty, or ready to join a faculty after his fellowship;
2. He should provide recommendations from the dean of his school and his department head;
3. His program of study could encompass either teaching or research, or both, in any department—clinical or preclinical—as long as it was related to his future departmental responsibilities;
4. Upon completion of the fellowship, he would be required to return to a post waiting for him at his own school.[12]

The program was marked by great flexibility not only in the choice of applicants, but in the selection of their parent schools. A school's financial need mattered less than the presence of "thinking brains" on the faculty.[13] Two types of schools were favored: the medical center of nationwide influence, where a particular phase of departmental activity needed rounding out; and the small, regional school that habitually turned to its own graduates for staff recruits and would welcome an opportunity to expose its teachers to a new academic environment. In schools where a full-time faculty seemed to be an unattainable luxury, the deliberate preparation of young men for faculty appointments seemed to hold promise for raising teaching standards.

The amount of the stipend was variable, as was the length of the fellowship, and the center chosen for fellowship study might be in the United States or abroad. The Fund also took a flexible approach once the award had been made: "After the Fund is once assured of the qualifications of the applicant and of the intention of the school from which he comes to use him to advantage, and after a plan has been worked out for his study, it has been the policy to let these fellowships run their course with a minimum of administrative attention."[14] The structure of the program itself reflected this policy of flexibility: Psychiatrists, nurses, medical administrators, foreign psychiatric social workers—all were eventually included.

The first set of ten awards in 1938 spanned eight different fields at nine institutions, and the amount appropriated was $29,100. By the following year the Fund had perceived—cautiously—not only the program's eventual far-ranging effects but more specific categories of problems it could address: "In one department, the need of the moment may be to stress a scientific approach to a field where clinical experience needs interpretation; in another, to reinforce clinical skills as a make-weight for prevailing emphasis on structure and mechanism. Sometimes, it is the man himself who needs reinforcing, and a year away gives him sufficient confidence to make full use of his resources. More often, a neglected area of subject matter needs cultivation."[15]

The program expanded rapidly in its first three years, but when World War II reduced the pool of applicants, the number of fellowship awards also declined. In 1944 all fellowships were awarded either to women or to men ineligible for military service, and in 1945 only three were given, the fewest in the history of the program. The war also cut off foreign study, but because war in the tropics gave tropical diseases unprecedented importance in American medicine, applicants were permitted to study these diseases in Mexico and in Central or South America. As early as 1939, fellowships had been deferred or interrupted, and the program was handicapped until the return of peace. It was also impossible after 1941 to hold strictly to the requirement that the fellowship recipient have or be assured of an academic appointment upon completion of study.[16]

Despite these difficulties, the Fund was buoyantly enthusiastic about its new program:[17]

> The current crop of advanced medical fellowships in four medical schools in the city of New York happen to illustrate clearly the range and possible usefulness of such awards.
>
> During the year Dr. John Mulholland, assistant clinical professor of surgery of the New York University College of Medicine, returned to his post after

spending a full year in a methodical and meticulous observation of surgical services and teaching in nine universities and one independent clinic. He has now been promoted to the rank of clinical professor of surgery and placed in charge of the University's surgical service at Bellevue. Few men could bring to a similar task so wide an acquaintance with the ways in which surgery is taught at representative medical schools. This fellowship may be considered a direct contribution to good teaching.

The same might be said of the fellowship awarded last year to Dr. Robert Dickes, Jr., resident in medicine at the Long Island College Hospital. In this case a young man just at the beginning of his career, who has shown a flair for teaching, was sent to a department of medicine (at Western Reserve) where in addition to participating in departmental research he has been given a share in a well-coordinated teaching program and has an opportunity to join the discussion of curriculum revision. Dr. Dickes is the third young physician destined for a part-time appointment at the Long Island College of Medicine to receive a fellowship. Such awards make it possible to enrich the experience of teachers who will at best find it difficult to live up to their academic possibilities while they are building up practices. . . .

A fellowship in another category, but also pointed directly at the improvement of teaching, was awarded last year to Dr. Kent A. Zimmerman for two years' training in pediatrics and psychiatry at Cornell University Medical College. As a house officer in pediatrics at the New York Hospital Dr. Zimmerman was strongly influenced by his contact with Dr. Milton J. E. Senn, assistant professor of clinical pediatrics (in psychiatry), who has brought to the inpatient service for children a sound psychiatric viewpoint which the Fund helped him to get through an earlier fellowship. . . .

Some of the advanced medical fellowships are given to men who have already shown a special gift for research. Dr. John S. Labate, returning to the department of obstetrics and gynecology at the New York University College of Medicine this year after two years' study (in the department of anatomy) of the uterine nerves, has received a part-time teaching appointment which leaves two days a week free for continuation of his research. Dr. Joseph C. Turner, released from teaching duties in the department of the practice of medicine at the Columbia–Presbyterian Medical Center to spend two years working with Dr. A. R. Dochez on immunological aspects of cancer, has returned to his permanent assignment. It is felt in this department that cancer must be studied in departments of medicine as well as in more specialized institutions, and Dr. Turner's experience on fellowship is correspondingly valued. Dr. Jacob Haskell Milstone, assistant in bacteriology at the New York University College of Medicine, is in the second of two years to be spent on a problem in enzyme chemistry with Dr. John H. Northrop of the Rockefeller Institute for Medical Research at Princeton. This is another case in which a fellowship is being used to enable a given department to broaden its frontage on basic and difficult problems.

By 1945 the Fund was looking to the future, making plans to use its fellowships liberally for the benefit of men newly released from the armed forces and eager to advance as they returned to academic medicine. In 1946 the appropriation for domestic Advanced Medical Fellowships more than doubled from the previous year, from $14,450 to $35,100.

The end of the war also marked a shift in the Fund's method of selecting recipients and appropriating money. Awards made individually kept the applicants waiting, sometimes for several months, while the Fund's staff and board of directors deliberated. "While this may be unimportant in the case of those who are very young, it may be a decided inconvenience for candidates who have family responsibilities and are already well started on a professional career."[18] Accordingly, in 1947 the board delegated to the staff the authority to grant awards. The Fund also decided to use the plan that had worked so well with its mental health fellowships: It appropriated a lump sum at the start of the fiscal year to be awarded for fellowships at the discretion of the staff. For 1947–48 the amount decided upon was $44,000, to cover the cost of ten fellowships with a contingency fund of $4,000 for emergency adjustments. The estimate of cost proved too low; seven fellowships representing nine fellowship-years were awarded, and the Fund expected the available money to be exhausted by October 1948. The sum allotted for the following year was therefore raised, to $48,000. During these immediate postwar years most fellowships lasted from six to twelve months, and the stipend for an unmarried recipient ranged from a low of $400 to a high of $9,800. Over two-thirds of the total appropriation from 1945 to 1948 was given to men in clinical work; those in the basic sciences received the remainder.[19] As the scope of the program expanded, the name of this set of fellowships changed accordingly: It became "Advanced Fellowships in Medicine and Allied Fields."

The Fund also changed its procedure for selecting recipients. Until 1950 fellowships had been awarded by a group of staff members in general medicine and by individual staff members in the mental health, public health, and rural hospital programs. In 1950 Heffron was made chairman of a staff committee to select the recipients. During the next four years, the committee's procedures were well standardized by its six members. Inquiries from students working in areas remote from the field of health and from those clearly unable to meet the program's special requirements were advised of their ineligibility by the committee's secretary. All borderline cases were reviewed by Heffron himself, but only interesting applicants technically eligible for awards were discussed by the entire committee. If the candidate was interviewed outside New York, he met with one committee member; the usual procedure was to invite the candidate to meet with at least two committee members in the Fund's offices. Although this method of handling fellowship applicants was time-consuming, the Fund felt that the success of the program over the years warranted meticulous attention to the selection of the recipients.[20]

Awards to United States citizens and those to noncitizens were kept separate, but awards to domestic advanced fellows were combined, by considering all candidates—including those specifically interested in psychiatry—as a common pool. Candidates interested in the social sciences were also brought into the Advanced Fellowship Program: Fellowships were opened to applicants from the medical and public health fields who wanted training in social sciences and to those from the social sciences seeking training in any medical field.[21] During the early 1950s, the Fund singled out for particular attention psychiatric fellows wanting training analyses. The result was a set of varied awards to domestic candidates. Six went to men and women identified with teaching and research in medical fields other than psychiatry. These included a professor of anatomy who wished to spend three summers expanding his knowledge of microscopic anatomy and physiology to cover a wide range of biological material, particularly invertebrate forms of life; an assistant professor of surgery preparing himself for larger responsibilities by a year's exploration of physiological research; a pediatrician who would become the first well-trained pediatric endocrinologist in Canada; two young internists anticipating special responsibilities, for endocrinology and metabolism in one instance and clinical neurology in the other, in their respective medical schools; and a recipient with already proven ability in research who was being groomed for an academic appointment. Nine awards were given to men and women for psychiatric training or for the observation of psychiatric teaching. A social scientist and an anthropologist in the Department of Social Relations at Harvard University received fellowships for psychoanalytic training designed to sharpen their skills in their individual fields of research.

Awards in Support of Creative Scholarship

In 1955, the Fund began to explore the possibility of offering a new kind of fellowship. The staff was receiving requests that current policy left them powerless to meet. Inquiries and conversations during field visits to universities demonstrated the potential usefulness of awards that would stimulate the creative contributions of mature scholars and scientists.[22] Funds for training, laboratory investigation, and other kinds of empirical research were available from many sources, and the competent and mature scholar who wished to conduct research along with his usual duties could ordinarily secure the necessary financial support. But the scholar or scientist who wished to devote an uninterrupted year or two to scientific writing, to analysis and correlation of data from previous research, or to exploring a new research area had great difficulty in securing funds. The pressure of daily routine on able, productive men was often very great and their opportunities for creative intellectual work correspondingly narrowed. The Fund's staff believed that "In the field of medical science . . . there was no dearth of new facts, but . . . creative work by individual scientific minds is a commodity in short supply. . . . It could be very helpful to provide for a few outstanding scholars the freedom from daily routine which would give them an opportunity to put some of these new facts into relationships which may reveal new truths."[23] In the mid-1950s, they had nowhere to turn for the kind of individual support involving chiefly a stipend for themselves.[24] The staff's experience with its previous fellowships led them to incorporate a similar flexibility into this new endeavor. No single form of support would be effective in all cases. To be relieved of regular duties, a recipient would probably need a stipend equal to his academic salary. In other instances he might require funds for clerical, editorial, or research assistance (with or without a stipend for the scholar himself) or support for a moderate amount of travel.

As for the characteristics of the recipients, this program was not for the promising young beginner. The staff intended to seek out mature men and women from all areas of the field of health, including some areas not currently receiving Fund support. Applicants would also be considered from the natural and behavioral sciences, as long as their primary interests were in some aspect of health or medicine. The chief determinant was not to be the focus of the candidate's interest but the candidate himself: his accomplishments to date and his qualities of originality and creativity. As a scientist, he should have done significant, widely recognized research; as a scholar, he should have been concerned with the relationship of his own work to the larger questions in his field. In addition to outstanding ability, zeal, and integrity, he should be an original thinker with creative ideas that he was eager and competent to develop. The Fund recognized that only some such men were well known and prominent; others were to be found in specialized fields and were known to only a few thoughtful and scholarly colleagues. It was this "hidden" type of scientist that the Fund would make a special effort to locate.

The staff planned not to solicit applications at first but to proceed informally, without public announcement. As in the Advanced Medical Fellowship Program, the Fund appointed a staff committee to review the qualifications of any potential recipients, using outside consultants when necessary. At this point the staff did not intend to allocate any money to the program; domestic and foreign awards in the Advanced Medical Fellowship Program had been consolidated in 1955, and these fellowships were being phased out. Funds that had been appropriated for the Advanced Medical Fellowship Program would be sufficient to carry the new project through its early stages, and the committee wanted to evaluate the

Awards in Support of Creative Scholarship after the first year before deciding whether they should be continued or terminated.

The first two grants in this program were made in 1956 to Florence Powdermaker, a psychiatrist and psychoanalyst, and Clayton Loosli, professor of preventive medicine in the University of Chicago's Department of Medicine. Loosli intended to analyze original data collected over many years on the structure of mammalian lung tissue and on the origin and development of bacterial blood infection. Powdermaker would complete research and write a monograph on a hitherto undescribed character disorder stemming from early frustration of the inquisitive "instinct" or the individual's "need to know."[25] Powdermaker's award of $15,750 covered a stipend for her as well as funds for a part-time collaborator and a secretary.

Increasing interest in the creative fellowship program was reflected in 1958 by the 10-to-1 ratio of applications to acceptances. As the proportion of creative fellowships increased, the median age of fellowship recipients rose: Ages ranged from thirty to sixty-three, with a median age of forty-four. Formerly many fellows were younger than thirty-five years of age, but in 1958 there were only three in that age group.[26] As the median age rose, so did the academic standing of recipients: by 1964 twenty of the fifty-two domestic recipients were full professors, twenty-two were department heads, and five were deans or subdeans.

There was considerable variation in the amounts of the awards, in their duration and purpose, and in the academic or institutional rank of the fellow and of the field from which he came. Most of the creative fellowships lasted for one year, but in some instances $2,000 or less was adequate for four to six weeks of travel in connection with a specific program of teaching, observation, or study of special developments in a given field; other awards called for more general support over a longer period of up to two years. One-half of the recipients required full support as well as travel or other assistance (more than half of the American recipients went abroad), and the rest needed help to supplement salaries for sabbatical leaves.

During the late 1950s, for example, Sydney S. Gellis, professor and head of the Department of Pediatrics at the Boston University School of Medicine, was given an award of $3,925, enabling him to spend four months studying clinical, pathological, and epidemiological manifestations of an obscure form of liver disease in infants. H. Stephen Weems, professor and chairman of the Department of Radiology at the Emory University School of Medicine, received $2,750 (including $1,250 for travel) to broaden his experience and strengthen his departmental program by observing and talking with colleagues during visits to leading radiological centers.

The program's continued expansion into the mid-1960s reflected the demonstrated usefulness of the awards, the increasing number of well-qualified candidates (by 1965 the Fund was receiving about three hundred fellowship applications a year), the growing volume of research in medicine and health affairs, and the widening interest in many aspects of medical education. In 1963 fellowships accounted for almost 20 percent of the Fund's total expenditures, and the Fund awarded more fellowships in 1964 than in any previous year in its history.[27]

The mid-1960s saw a redefinition of the program's purposes. Many recipients of the early Advanced Medical Fellowships, those awarded between 1938 and 1948, were now returning for further aid. Some were continuing their previous work: For one recipient, the second fellowship enabled him to expand his association with staff at the Atomic Bomb Casualty Commission in Japan, an association he had used his first fellowship to initiate. Another had taken his first fellowship when modern toxicology as a science was just becoming a reality. The outcome of that fellowship was a small textbook, *Essential of Toxicology*; the second fellowship allowed the author to acquire the "added perspectives" that enabled him to write the second edition of that book.[28] A third fellow spent his first fellowship mainly in Copenhagen, where he worked simultaneously in the Laboratory of Zoophysiology with August Krogh and at the nearby Institute for Theoretical Physics with Georg Hevesy. This work enabled him to become "among the very early workers with radio-isotopes as tracers of metabolism in this country." This recipient's fellowship in 1960 returned him to Scandinavia, where his work dealt with x-ray crystallography and microradiography of calcified tissues.

Others received second fellowships to acquire new information as advances in technology and the expansion of medical knowledge made their earlier skills obsolete. One recipient was retrained as a teacher and practitioner of internal medicine after nearly a quarter of a century in medical administration; another pursued an interest in the possibilities of noninvasive techniques in cardiac diagnosis, a field that grew steadily over the next twenty years. One wrote: "The Commonwealth Fellowship exposed me to a first-class biochemistry department for the first time in my life and got me started on an interesting new and productive line of investigation. . . . I worked in the laboratory of Ronald Whittam and learned all about sodium-potassium-ATPase at a time when it was still new. I was then able to apply this in the field of renal physiology and to get a head start in opening up a relatively unexplored area of investigation in transport physiology."

And another said: "The first, in 1947–48, made it possible for me to work with the late Fuller Albright at the Massachusetts General Hospital. This great opportunity molded my entire future. At that time I had had reasonably good training in internal medicine, and had taken a Ph.D. in endocrinology under the late Herbert McLean Evans. The experience with Albright made it possible for me to put the two together in a career of clinical investigation. . . . The second Commonwealth Fund Fellowship made it possible for me to work with Dame Honor Fell . . . in 1963 at the Strangeways Laboratory in Cambridge, England. This was fundamentally a program to learn a specific technique."

Some of the more numerous first-time recipients of Commonwealth Fund fellowships used them for retraining. One wrote: "Since 1948 I had been a part-time member of a two-man cardiac catheterization team at the Buffalo General Hospital. We studied only two or three patients per week and were aware of the shortcomings of our diagnostic studies of patients with cardiac disease. We gradually came to the realization that we needed to extend our diagnostic capabilities by adding the technic of angiocardiography. [The] fellowship permitted me to spend six months at the Karolinska Sjukhuset in Stockholm, studying all aspects of angiocardiography in the laboratory of Professor Ulf Rudhe." From another came this letter: "My academic career was threatened by elimination of the Family Medicine course and because I had no "bench research" skills. Furthermore, clinical behavioral research was very suspect. Fortunately, before my sabbatical year in '59 to '60 I had determined that I would try to gain some skills that would allow me to pursue behavioral and clinical neurophysiological studies. . . . It was with this decision to focus my attention on the behavior and neurophysiology of the newborn and infant that I went to Dr. Minkowski's research unit in Paris for my sabbatical year. Two members of this research unit were important for me: Dr. Sainte-Anne Dargassies had recently published a book on the neurology of the newborn and premature infant and Dr. Dreyfus-Brisac, numerous articles on the development of the brain electrical activity of premature and full-term newborns. There were no other people in the world with as much clinical experience in the study of the nervous system and behavior of newborn infants as these two people."

Fellowships awarded by other organizations, such as the National Institutes of Health, the American Cancer Society, and the American Heart Association, were for the most part limited to individuals whose primary aims were to carry out specific types of research in specific fields. But the flexibility of the Fund's program allowed the staff to provide assistance for diverse purposes:[29]

> Help may be given to a fellow who wishes to take a year or so to write a book in his field, summarize past research, review recent literature, or consult colleagues in various countries about medical education, teaching programs, or developments in his field. Awards may enable American medical school staff members to assist as visiting professors in strengthening the educational and research programs in medical schools of under-developed areas. A Fund

award enabled a capable scientist to study higher mathematics, which he found he needed in his work; other recipients have obtained advanced training in biochemistry or biophysics to enhance their competence.

The increased availability of fellowships from the federal government, coupled with Roderick E. Heffron's retirement, led to a reappraisal of the program in 1966. Left without adequate staff to carry out the program on the scale it had attained, the Fund's president and staff decided to reduce its size over the next few years. The proposed reduction would not invalidate the Fund's agreements with Harvard, Cornell, Columbia, Johns Hopkins, Tulane, and Stanford universities to consider an occasional request for a special fellowship for a senior, distinguished person from outside the United States, or for a younger, brilliant person with a promising future. In limiting the program, however, the Fund's staff intended to favor recipients who wished to prepare monographs. This use of the Fund's fellowships had already produced a number of important manuscripts, some of which were published under Fund sponsorship.

The planned curtailment of the program began June 1, 1966, three months before Heffron's retirement. For 1967, $350,000 was appropriated, $200,000 less than the preceding year. The number of awards also declined, from seventy-two in 1966 to twenty-eight in 1967. By the end of the program, fellowship recipients were participating in special research programs with colleagues in other institutions both within and outside the United States; securing knowledge of new fields essential to progress in their work; studying teaching methods and the curricula of medical schools in this country, Europe, and elsewhere; or serving as visiting professors abroad (see app. C). Obvious benefits accrued to the individual recipient, and foremost were the intellectual rewards. One recipient said: "The fellowship so kindly granted me was a real life-saver at the time in that I had gotten hopelessly behind in writing up research results. That year . . . made it possible to write approximately twenty papers and complete a badly stalled monograph."

Another wrote: "The sabbatical in London, at the University of London in the Department of Eugenics under the leadership of Dr. Lionel Penrose, was a rejuvenating, intellectually stimulating period. I found myself among many very talented geneticists in the Gower Street environment and freed up from the teaching and patient care responsibilties I had in New York. I had time to study, learn new techniques, and participate in ongoing investigations. I caught up with the exploding genetics-scientific revolution that was going on. I was forced to learn the methodology of biostatistics, human tissue karyotyping, drosophila and mouse genetics and had a whole new world of scientific inquiry open up to me. My 'batteries were recharged' and I returned to the world I had left fresh and eager and with a feeling of enthusiasm I believe I was losing prior to the London experience." Other benefits were more personal. A recipient said: "The financial support for continued work was of real value, but even more valuable was the psychological effect. The terminus of retirement, so sharp and definitive, was blunted. . . . Someone—in this case, the august Fund—had faith that there was still some good, some productive strength left in the individual. . . . Since my retirement and the receipt of the Fund's fellowship, I have written near to thirty papers and published about twenty-five." And another wrote: "Having spent most of my life in the middle west and mid-south, my views were circumspect, parochial, and in many cases, unfounded. I started for Nigeria pretty much an anglophobe and became, if not an anglophile, at least lacking in group prejudice. I arrived in Nigeria with a better than average knowledge of the anthropology of Black Africa and came away a year later with my attention shifted to an appreciation of the contemporary sociological problems of at least one Third World country. I came to realize that different did not necessarily mean better or worse." The recipients' medical schools often benefited directly as well: "I expended three months in travel to European centers to discover changes then taking place in the mental health delivery system particularly as they might relate to our community mental health movement. Undoubtedly the most striking observations made there were connected with the organization of the mental health services in Great Britain, Holland, and the U. S. S. R. Those experiences made it possible for me to introduce a number of differing usages of personnel in the mental health delivery systems around this medical center, provide input to our Division of Community and Social Psychiatry as well as on the national scene, and to prepare me for the tremendous difficulties which led to the social upheavals of 1968, '69 and '70."

And in the largest sense, the fellowship recipients contributed to the field of medicine: "Overall my experience in medicine during the fellowship period in Sweden greatly broadened my concepts of the practice of medicine. I left with the belief that the practice of medicine in Scandinavia was the most efficient and best delivered of any in the world and that it should provide a model for the future development of health care delivery in America. This has influenced my thinking in later years as these matters are deliberated on the American scene. With the insight obtained from this experience abroad, perhaps I can contribute to the evolution of an improved health care delivery system in this country with emphasis in the area of preventive cardiology." Another said: "My fellowship from the Commonwealth Fund was largely responsible for us developing two [original] radio labeled compounds. . . . The first compound is the radioiodine labeled chloroquine analog for the diagnosis of the ocular melanoma and for trials in the therapy of the malignant, metastatic, dermal melanoma. . . . Most recently, we have been greatly heartened by developing another chloroquine analog which shows the rather fantastic concentration of 25% dose/gram uptake in melanoma. . . ."

Several of the appointees in the program's later years helped their medical schools plan extensive curricular revisions. The Fund's staff believed that other rewards for the recipient's institution were less tangible: "In other cases, the benefit to the institution is less direct but no less real, in that anything that contributes to making a member of the faculty a better teacher or research worker thereby strengthens the institution."[30]

The success of the Commonwealth Fund's advanced fellowships derived not only from the qualities of the grant recipients, but from the ineffable contributions of the Fund's staff. As one recipient said: "The type of continued interest and advice by a wise and experienced person of Lester's ability played an enormous role in my own professional development and is an example of responsible foundation relations with grantees—a difficult but proper blend of continued involvement, yet not meddlesome." Another said: "In the 1960s, the Commonwealth Fund and Rod Heffron, in particular, gave me a period of time to exercise my intellectual and creative potential to the fullest degree possible, without any constraints. The support I received was much more than financial; the moral support was perhaps more important. The Commonwealth Fund fellowship demonstrated to me that at least some people, reasonable and responsible, believed in me and what I was trying to do; that the project I undertook, though off the beaten track, was important, and worth supporting though 'risky' and likely to fall far short of global expectations. In a word, the Fund was not afraid to support efforts which might turn out to be failures."

When the Fund discontinued its formal program of fellowships in 1967, it was supporting the largest number of awards to individuals in its history. Five ancillary fellowship projects were spreading the Fund's resources to ethnic and professional groups outside the area of American medicine dominated by white physicians. The Fund's tradition of innovation was reinforced by its contributions to the birth of programs to train physicians' assistants (including surgical assistants), nurse practitioners, child health associates, and pediatric nurse-practitioners. The strength of some of these additional programs allowed them to continue even into the 1970s and '80s, beyond the termination of the Fund's formal fellowships.

Special Awards to Individual Medical Scholars

In closing down its program of medical fellowships in 1967, the Fund stated: "...Further fellowships will not be awarded. Thus, the Fund's medical fellowships are no longer a formal part of its philanthropic program."[31] Despite the apparent finality, the word "formal" allowed the staff to keep the door open. In a sense the fellowships became a supplement to the Fund's programs for educating professionals and providing services in medicine and health: Applications were no longer invited or considered, but the staff reserved the prerogative of making a few awards each year for "individual activities of special relevance to the Fund's philanthropic program,"[32] or to medical schools of particular interest.

The less structured program offered two advantages: It avoided the necessity of disappointing the scores of candidates bound to apply for the fellowships as long as they were a formal part of the Fund's program, and it allowed the Fund to make fellowship appointments with much greater flexibility than was possible under an open program. The financial structure of the program also reflected its closer relation to the Fund's efforts in medical education: Instead of going directly to the scholars themselves, the fellowship costs were paid to and administered by the scholars' universities.

The program of special awards ended when the Tax Reform Act of 1969 was signed into law midway through the Fund's 1970 fiscal year. The act appeared to restrict individual grants to formally structured programs open to all applicants who met stated eligibility requirements. Ten awards made during 1969–70 were the final grants dispensed. In dismantling the program, the Fund canceled its appropriation for 1970 and restored the balance of $114,384 to general funds for use in other programs in fiscal year 1969–70.

In its informal fellowship program of the late 1960s, the Fund had given $885,616 to 702 scholars (145 domestic, 557 foreign).[33] During the past thirty years the Fund has spent more than $8 million, with awards going to more than 400 United States citizens and 130 noncitizens.[34]

The Program in Medical Research

Without theory, practice is but the routine born of habit. Theory alone can bring forth and develop the spirit of invention. It is to you specially that it will belong not to share the opinion of those narrow minds who disdain everything in science which has no immediate application. You know Franklin's charming saying? He was witnessing the first demonstration of a purely scientific discovery, and the people around him said: "But what is the use of it?" Franklin answered them: "What is the use of a newborn child?"

—Louis Pasteur

The advance of medical education and the results of research are separated only with difficulty, as progress in one depends so heavily on progress in the other. New knowledge flows from research efforts, serving as a continuing impetus to medical education, which must stay abreast of new research findings or gradually stagnate. Similarly, the presence of research activities acts as a continual spur to members of any medical group. Research, too, is responsible for progress in health care, and worthwhile research in a medical school or in the field imposes a degree of intellectual discipline on staff and students alike.

Private foundations in America have been influential in creating an academic research community and encouraging research itself, but no one model has predominated in the variety of patterns developed by American foundations for their programs in research. Under Heffron's leadership the Commonwealth Fund based its research grants mainly on the rankings by staff and consultants of programs' intellectual and medical significance. Fund-supported investigation between 1937 and 1958 into normal and abnormal living processes led to the study of fundamental biological problems with roots in biochemistry, physiology, and biophysics (see app. D). As knowledge in the basic sciences increased, medical research led to an even closer relationship between these sciences and medical practice.

Each foundation must find its own answer to the primary question: How much control should the foundation exert over the conduct of research? Some foundations took the road of endowment support, relieving themselves of all responsibility except the identification of the recipient institutions. (Quality control through evaluating the recipient's progress is relatively recent, albeit now universally accepted.) The major difficulty with this laissez-faire attitude is that the foundation nevertheless assumes a measure of responsibility for the results, exposing itself to political and intellectual criticism for work over which it has not had definitive control. And how much control should the staff have in formulating programs? If the trustees exert tight control, the programs are more likely to be very conservative. But if greater freedom is given to the staff, greater opportunity for adventurousness and flexibility follows. Like most American foundations, the Commonwealth Fund found a balance between the two extremes.

The First Research Period (1919–37)

The Fund awarded its first grants for medical research soon after its founding. In 1919 Columbia University's Neurological Institute received $10,000 for the investigation of epilepsy and multiple sclerosis, and its College of Physicians and Surgeons was given $4,000 for an investigation of the roles of diet and calcium in the cause and prevention of rickets.[35] J. W. Jobling, professor of pathology at Columbia University, had proposed the latter project, planning to pursue the unproven possibility that rickets was due to lack of a specific vitamin and should be considered a deficiency disease.

The Fund's interest in research increased markedly in the early 1930s, although it still had no formally organized program. Edward S. Harkness was obviously considering medical research as the object of his forthcoming gift to the Fund in 1937, for in the summer of that year Lester J. Evans was asked to survey the expenditures in the United States for research on chronic disease, poliomyelitis, and cancer (he found that only about $350,000 was being dispensed nationwide to support research in these fields each year), and Esther Everett Lape of the Fund's staff was asked to prepare a brief, confidential summary for Harkness of the results of the eighteen projects in medical research supported by the Fund over the previous five years:[36]

1. *Causes of Dental Caries. Columbia University School of Dental and Oral Surgery.* Microscopic, chemical and x-ray examination of the structure of the tooth led to a proposed explanation of the decay process. Caries was produced in experimental animals for the first time with a diet affecting the surface of the tooth; and chemical, bacteriological, and hematologic studies of caries-susceptible and caries-immune individuals were said to reveal differences between these two groups.

2. *Growth and Development. Child Research Council of Denver.* The long-term, longitudinal study of the physiological growth of normal children from birth to maturity was intended to show individual variations within the normal range and to develop more exact standards of what could be called "healthy" and "unhealthy" as an aid in the diagnosis, prevention, and cure of children's diseases (see p. 183).

3. *Effectiveness of Placental Extract. Harvard Medical School.* The original purpose of the investigation was to demonstrate the effectiveness of placental extract in the prevention of measles. Next, a search for other disease-preventive properties resulted in the chemical differentiation of several component protein parts, one of which was discovered to be effective in the treatment of hemophilia. Later, this project was aided by Edwin J. Cohn's work on the separation of serum proteins by ultracentrifugation, work also supported by the Fund.

4. *Pediatric Clinic for Cardiac and Rheumatic Cases (Research in Rheumatic Fever). New York Hospital* (see p. 179).

5. *Rheumatic Fever. House of the Good Samaritan, Boston.* The hemolytic streptococcus was thought by many to be the cause of rheumatic fever, as it was known that many patients with rheumatic fever were also infected with streptococci. This study investigated the as yet unproven relationship between the streptococcus and the pathogenesis of the disease.

Early Programs in Medical Education and Research

6. *Insulin. Johns Hopkins University School of Medicine.* John J. Abel demonstrated in this study that insulin was a protein, accounting for the essential chemical elements in the molecule. Abel succeeded in obtaining crystals of insulin, but his attempt to synthesize the active principle was not successful.

7. *Tuberculosis in Childhood. Johns Hopkins University School of Medicine.* An intensive investigation of the infant exposed to tuberculosis was a continuation of a Fund-sponsored, joint clinical and epidemiological study begun in 1921. These studies, which extended over many years, were among the first to provide an accurate and complete account of the diagnosis, treatment, pathology, and epidemiological behavior of this disease in infancy (see p. 169).

8. *Pneumonia Serum Treatment. New York University.* Later work in serum therapy of pneumonia was based on the results of this study of the use of serum in the treatment of pneumonia in children. The common types of pneumococcus causing pneumonia in children were identified, methods that shortened the time for laboratory typing of the pneumococcus were developed, new type-specific antisera were produced, and cases were successfully treated under controlled conditions.

9. *Pneumonia. Massachusetts Department of Public Health.* A five-year program in the laboratory and field covered all aspects of lobar pneumonia and its treatment with serum. Many lives were saved; for Type I pneumonia alone the fatality rate was reduced by 56 percent. The project led to similar work in five other states, served as a model for a study in Michigan, and guided other programs in combating and controlling the disease.[37]

10. *Pneumonia. Michigan State Department of Health.* Initiated in the summer of 1936, this program made excellent progress in refining antipneumococcus serum and lowering the cost of production. It is one of the ironies of medical research that completion of this work coincided with the introduction of the sulfonamides—as a result, serum therapy was placed in mothballs.

11. *Study of Normals. University of Pennsylvania School of Medicine.* Under the direction of Theodore H. Weisenburg, this project focused on speech and sensation, including vibratory, pain, and temperature sensibilities. It produced striking information about normal and abnormal speech and resulted in an important monograph on aphasia.[38]

12. *Central Brucella Station and Culture Collection. Michigan State College.* Little was known of the life history of Brucella organisms, which not only caused undulant fever in the human but posed an important economic problem in the cattle industry in the midwest. Through chemical, bacteriological, and pathologic studies, the biological characteristics of the organism were determined; the incidence and manner of transmission of infection among animals were elucidated; a method of typing the organism was developed, useful in tracing sources of infection; and a vaccine assuring temporary immunization was perfected.[39]

13. *Puerperal Mortality. New York Academy of Medicine.* One of the causes of the excessively high maternal mortality in New York City was found

to be poor obstetrical practice. The investigators discovered that patients were receiving inadequate prenatal care, poor judgment and lack of skill were displayed by many physicians in the handling of complicated situations, operative interference at delivery was either too frequent or methodologically incorrect, hospital delivery facilities were often inadequate, and even the simplest precautions to prevent infection were neglected. Two-thirds of all deaths studied could probably have been prevented had the patient been cared for properly. At least fifteen other communities used this study as a model for similar investigations.[40]

14. *Structure and Development of the Brain. Columbia University College of Physicians and Surgeons.* Headed by Frederic Tilney, a distinguished neurologist and neuropathologist, the objective was to study the relation of the brain to behavior by examining the development of normal brain structure. The investigators hoped to accumulate information that would enable them to study factors that upset or retard normal development— factors related to nutrition, endocrine function, and disease.

15. *Multiple Sclerosis. Neurological Institute, New York.* One of the initial studies of multiple sclerosis, this investigation of the pathology and pathogenesis of the disease revealed that it was not caused by bacteria; that as the disease progressed, myelin—the covering of the nerve fibers— disappeared; and that some ferment in the blood was thought to be responsible for the myelin degeneration.

16. *Trachoma. Washington University.* Trachoma was yet another example of a disease causing extensive morbidity in children.[41] Here, Louis A. Julianelle's investigations disproved Hideyo Noguchi's claim that *Bacterium granulosis* was the cause. Nutrition studies ruled out a dietary causative factor, and pannus, a phase of the disease affecting the eyesight, was shown to be secondary to the original infection. Julianelle showed the disease to be caused by a virus, which was resistant to methods of cultivation then available.

17. *Function of the Kidney. University of Pennsylvania* (see p. 171).

18. *Essential Hypertension. Johns Hopkins University.* One of the early, well-organized studies of a widespread affliction in the United States, the investigation took a long-range view of the natural history of a little-understood form of hypertension. A group of patients was brought under clinical observation and treatment; methods of physical and functional examination were developed; and parallel studies on experimental animals were started.

Edward S. Harkness's gift came at a time when basic scientific knowledge was expanding and many opportunities were available for its clinical application. The absence of federal agencies such as the Department of Health, Education and Welfare and the National Institutes of Health (and the lack of agencies to accredit professionals) gave the Fund unlimited freedom to build on its own experience. Ideas for grants were often discovered during visits to ongoing projects in the field or in universities. The Fund believed that the money at its disposal did more good if it was concentrated rather than scattered, and it tended to support research projects closely related to the objectives of its field enterprises. Grants were almost equally divided between those initiated by the Fund—grants to organizations for work related to the Fund's own programs—and those made in response to outside inquiries. Many of the latter were in areas of basic medical research, some leading to long-time support. Throughout, the Fund preferred to subsidize workers whose professional standing made them good risks for investment and whose affiliations offered the promise of suitable control and orderly administration.

The staff screened the grant requests first, deciding which were worthy of presentation to the Fund's board of directors; all final decisions were subject to the board's approval. The first consideration was that the topic of inquiry be obviously and especially important. The Fund's initial preference was for action of demonstrable value to humanity as compared with "knowledge for its own sake," and it usually chose to support investigations with direct clinical application rather than those concerned with pure science. At first the Fund tended to choose projects that looked as though they would pay off within a fairly short time. This emphasis on quick return avoided committing the Fund to long-term projects that might handicap the staff in meeting unforeseen demands and unpredictable changes. Grants usually covered a single year—rarely more than three years—and each project was restudied before its support was renewed. Later, the staff's attitude changed, and many grants extended over several, or even many, years.

Quality control was encouraged by progress reports and visits to the laboratories by staff members, but there was no attempt to exert any influence over the direction of the work once the grant was made. Projects were evaluated by the board at least every third year. Field investigations were always made before a project was presented to the board, but in the course of a grant, a visit was made at least once a year and recipients were responsible for submitting periodic reports. Measurement of progress toward the original objectives was often difficult: New leads would cause the direction of an investigation to shift. At times a study had to be terminated simply because no methods were available for its next stage. Although the results of a particular piece of research might fall short of meeting the original objectives, its findings might be important for other areas of research. The consequences of good work were unpredictable; for example, a narrow project in immunology—the use of placental extract in measles—helped to lay the foundation for the fractionation of blood, which was accomplished with an ultracentrifuge placed by the Fund in Edwin J. Cohn's laboratory at Harvard University.

A seemingly simple problem could develop into a long, involved study, as was the case with the investigation of rheumatic fever at the New York Hospital. The Fund's first grant there supported an inquiry into the therapeutic value of a streptococcal vaccine for rheumatic fever, but the results of the study were negative. Yet the material accumulated by the investigator, May G. Wilson, on the natural history of the disease was yielding such fruitful information that it seemed essential to continue collecting data; the Fund continued to support the project for the next twenty-four years. The outcome was a comprehensive description of the natural history of rheumatic fever in the child.

The Second Research Period (1937–44)

In the eight years following Edward S. Harkness's gift, the Fund supported fifty-eight research projects fostered by twenty-seven different organizations. Almost half of these awards were given to university schools of medicine,[42] and about half of the projects received aid for at least five years. The Fund's appropriations for medical research between 1937 and 1945 amounted to approximately $2,757,250. As work on a single project extending over one year represents one project-year of study, the total of the investigations covered approximately 249 project-years of research—two and one-half centuries of scientific endeavor.

About one-third of the projects were concerned with bacteria and related agents, infectious disease, and immunity, and the rest with aspects of chronic disease and general physiological problems. The physiological and biochemical aspects of chronic and degenerative diseases were assuming greater importance as an increasing proportion of the population reached older age.

By 1942 the Fund was selecting for support chiefly those projects that promised direct usefulness to war medicine, offered significant contributions to the physiological underpinnings of medicine, or rested on continued, consecutive observation that could not be interrupted without losing hard-won information. As one of the recipients of a grant said, "In general what we have in mind is to make our abilities, techniques and facilities available to the national effort wherever they can be useful, and still try to keep unbroken the thread of scientific research which we have been following."[43]

Fund-supported projects during World War II were concerned with aviation medicine, gas warfare, infectious disease, vision at low levels of illumination, the treatment of pulmonary edema and gas casualties, influenza and meningococcal meningitis, gonorrhea, shock, the metabolism of individuals stranded in life boats, steroid hormones, the epidemiology of airborne infections, respiratory infections, immunity, wound infections, and the application of the cyclotron in biological and physical research.

Much of the work done during the war was confidential, but the Fund's staff correctly predicted that war-related work would be useful in postwar civilian medicine, as well as providing a basis for continued medical research.

Progress in research, the Fund's staff believed, could be measured only with a yardstick with one end in the future. The correct description of diabetes took thirteen centuries, and another third of a century elapsed before the information could be used. The discovery of insulin in 1921 was but the final stage of investigation, and the clinical results—so brilliantly successful—were the outcome of the patient, quiet effort of many workers in many fields of science. These efforts could rightly be valued only in retrospect. It would be rash to appraise work done on the great unsolved problems of medicine in terms of immediate practical results.

This point of view led the Fund to support a broad range of investigations between 1937 and 1944. Its Medical Research Review of 1944 included:

1. *Chemical Factors Involved in Resistance to Disease. Western Reserve University School of Medicine, Institute of Pathology. E. E. Ecker, Ph.D., in charge (average annual grant $12,680; 6 years).* Four components of complement were identified and were shown to act one after another in a cascade. This work contributed much to knowledge of these important biologically active factors and resulted in the identification of properdin, the important alternate pathway of complement activity.

2. *Apparatus for Protein Studies. Harvard Medical School, Department of Physical Chemistry. Edwin J. Cohn, Ph.D., in charge (average annual grant $6,666; 3 years).* Cohn's principal contributions were made during the search for blood substitutes. Two ultracentrifuges were obtained with the Fund's grant. Proteins were sedimented at rates roughly proportional to their weight: With one ultracentrifuge, proteins could be recovered in concentrated form, and with the other, the rate at which the particles settled could be measured. The investigators combined information obtained from centrifuge studies with other data to progress significantly in isolating important proteins in pure form and characterizing many of their biochemical and biophysical features. The ultracentrifuges also advanced the department's wartime studies of the preparation of purified albumin, plasma, and other blood substitutes, and fractions of human serum.

3. *Antibacterial Substances of Natural Origin. New Jersey Agricultural Experiment Station. Selman A. Waksman, Ph.D., in charge (average annual grant $9,600; 2 years).* The possibility of developing chemical substances for the treatment of infection had attracted interest for many years, and the introduction of the sulfonamide drugs was an important step. Naturally occurring substances were also capable of killing many kinds of bacteria, and organisms representing some of the lower forms of plant life—bacteria, molds, fungi—were found to produce these agents. The most striking

was penicillin, derived from a common mold. Waksman had developed methods for the rapid assay of organisms from soil, to determine whether they produced substances antagonistic to bacteria. He isolated four antibacterial agents, the most important of which was streptomycin. Waksman later received the Nobel Prize in medicine for this work.[44]

4. *Quantitative Community Studies of Disease. Johns Hopkins University School of Hygiene and Public Health. Lowell J. Reed, Ph.D., in charge (average annual grant $15,215; 5 years).* Reed, professor of biostatistics, and Wade Hampton Frost, professor of epidemiology, studied the impact of chronic diseases on a limited community to which statistical analysis could be applied with almost microscopic intensity. These and other Fund-supported studies by Frost helped to provide the methodology for the fundamental approaches used in modern-day "clinical epidemiology." An important part of this program was the training of statistically and epidemiologically minded scientists, who were responsible for later advances in public health (see p. 188).

5. *Tuberculosis in Childhood. Johns Hopkins University School of Medicine. Miriam Brailey, M.D., and Lydia Edwards, M.D., in charge (average annual grant $4,182; 8 years).* Central questions about this disease were the reason and the mechanism behind the particular vulnerability of adolescents to the acute infection, and the relation between these adolescent breakdowns and the patient's exposure to tuberculosis in infancy and childhood. This study, begun in 1921 and aided by the Fund since 1933, laid a firm foundation for the answers to these questions, and its findings influenced local public health practice.[45] The study measured the relative hazards of exposure at various ages in white and black children and underscored the importance of separating children instantly from active cases within a household.

6. *Kidney and Vascular Physiology. New York University College of Medicine, Departments of Physiology and Medicine. Homer W. Smith, Sc.D., in charge (average annual grant $12,140; 5 years).* Whatever the nature of essential hypertension, understanding of that disease depended on study of the kidney as an important control point for the circulating blood. This study used ingenious clinical and laboratory methods to learn more about kidney function in man and its relationship to vascular disorders, particularly essential hypertension. Information was obtained in part from animal experiments, but chiefly from hundreds of normal individuals and diseased patients. By applying tests devised previously, the investigators were able to draw far-reaching inferences about the interplay of blood-flow and renal function from the rate of excretion of various substances (either naturally present in the blood or artificially introduced into it). The amount of blood passing through the kidney was found to vary significantly in health and disease. This flow of blood in persons with high blood pressure and advanced kidney disease was markedly lessened in comparison with normal individuals, decreasing progressively as the disease became more severe. The study was an example of the outstanding research supported by the Fund in the basic physiology of cardiovascular and renal function.

7. *Neurology. Columbia–Presbyterian Medical Center, Neurological Institute. Tracy J. Putnam, M.D., in charge (average annual grant $40,663; 3 years).* All the known techniques of biophysics, biochemistry, physiology, and pharmacology were applied in this study. Advances were made in all areas, especially in electrophysiological studies to diagnose and treat neurological disease; in the studies of epilepsy, including fundamental biochemical investigations of the mechanism by which impulses are transmitted by nerve cells; and in the development of new drugs for treatment. A new anti-convulsant was discovered, and the work partially revealed the mode of action of this and other preparations in modifying the chemical environment of the brain.

8. *Inherited and Other Physiological Factors in Susceptibility to Experimental Cancer. Roscoe B. Jackson Memorial Laboratory, Bar Harbor, Maine. C. C. Little, Sc.D., in charge (average annual grant $4,500; 3 years).* The Jackson Memorial Laboratory had developed a number of highly inbred strains of mice of known susceptibility to cancer. These mice were used to study genetic and nongenetic mechanisms in the transmission of susceptibility to leukemia and other cancerous processes. The Jackson Laboratory was particularly interested in a virus-like factor, which on passing from mother to offspring in mice, had been found to make the latter susceptible to transplanted mouse-leukemia. The Fund-supported work indicated that functional differences, even in the intricate interrelations of the endocrine glands, could be inherited just as well as structural differences and that these inherited physiological differences had a direct bearing upon susceptibility to cancer.

9. *Diagnostic Uses of the Vaginal Smear. Cornell University Medical College, Departments of Anatomy and Obstetrics and Gynecology. George N. Papanicolaou, M.D., in charge (average annual grant $3,750; 4 years)* (see p. 186).

10. *Endocrinology. Harvard Medical School, Department of Pediatrics. Alan Butler, M.D., in charge (average annual grant $3,858; 3 years.)* The study of endocrine function had been accelerated by the development of practical methods for measuring the amount of hormone in blood and urine. Biological procedures had recently been replaced by chemical ones that reduced the time needed for testing and added fresh momentum to this field of study, and this project emphasized the further development of these chemical tests. Diagnostic tests were developed for three chemical fractions of the total output of male sex hormones. Improved methods determined the output of male sex hormones in the urine; permitted the measured of thyroid hormone in the blood; and, in general, determined the range of hormone values encountered in health and disease.

11. *Obstetrics and Gynecology. New York University College of Medicine, Department of Obstetrics and Gynecology. W. C. Studdiford, M.D., and H. C. Taylor, Jr., M.D., in charge (average annual grant $13,312; 8 years).* Results of these studies of the toxemias of pregnancy and infections associated with delivery improved understanding of the physiology of

pregnancy and the mechanisms of endocrine function, particularly of the relationship between endocrine and kidney function.

12. *Respiratory Physiology. Columbia–Presbyterian Medical Center, Department of Medicine, and Bellevue Hospital. Dickinson W. Richards, Jr., M.D., in charge (average annual grant $10,180; 5 years)* (see p. 176).

13. *Kidney Function. University of Pennsylvania, Department of Pharmacology. A. Newton Richards, M.D., in charge (average annual grant $19,242; 7 years).* Observation of the kidneys of cold-blooded animals, using new micro-puncture techniques, had yielded much information about what actually takes place in the kidney as it separates essential elements from waste. The procedures included analysis of microscopic samples of fluid from the glomerulus and tubule of the living kidney to obtain a clear picture of the physical and chemical changes that intervene between the filtering of fluid from the bloodstream and the eventual formation of urine. The investigators planned to continue their observations on the secretory processes of the tubule and to extend their studies to the mammalian kidney.

14. *Peripheral Circulation and Shock. Western Reserve University School of Medicine, Department of Physiology. Carl J. Wiggers, M.D., in charge (average annual grant $8,380; 5 years).* This work was chiefly a laboratory study of shock in dogs, using a comprehensive battery of experimental procedures developed to quantitate the dynamics of blood circulation. A standardized procedure (repeated bleeding) evolved for creating irreversible shock experimentally yielded much-needed precision. Persistent low blood pressure was the most important basis for predicting the development of irreversible shock.[46]

15. *Treatment of Shock Due to Hemorrhage and Burns. Washington University School of Medicine, Department of Surgery. Robert Elman, M.D., in charge (average annual grant $9,156; 3 years).* The intravenous injection of amino acids was a new method of restoring the protein content of the blood in acute and chronic conditions, such as shock from hemorrhage and burns. The principal investigator had for several years been injecting protein components into the blood to relieve chronic lack of protein and to build up malnourished patients in preparation for surgery. Solutions of amino acids, while not as effective as whole blood or plasma, were shown to be an excellent therapeutic supplement.

16. *Clinical Study of Marijuana. Research Council of the Department of Hospitals, New York City ($7,500; 1 year).* In 1939 marijuana was a problem of fairly recent origin in this country, and little was known of the effects of drug addiction or the complications of its use. A preliminary study carried out by the New York Academy of Medicine had recommended two investigations: a sociological study of the people using the drug and its influence in producing anti-social acts; and a clinical study of the effects of varying doses, the cumulative effect of continued use and sudden withdrawal, the changes in behavior occasioned by its use, and the drug's

possible therapeutic effect in the "tapering off" process for narcotics addicts. The city agreed to finance the first study and the Fund, along with two other foundations, supported the second.[47]

Research in the Postwar Years (1944–51)

During the Fund's next research period (October 1944 through December 1951), awards were given for fifty-seven separate investigations at thirty institutions; almost two-thirds of the latter were university schools of medicine.[48] Twenty-eight projects were initiated, forty-four terminated, and nine others remained active. Appropriations for these studies totaled approximately $2,987,000. During any one calendar year, the amount ranged from $337,000 to $447,000, averaging $410,308. The average annual budget of a grant was slightly over $11,000, with a range of $2,000 to $50,000. The number of grants operative during any one year averaged thirty-seven and the average period of support of the projects terminated during this interval was 6.8 years. Many studies in infectious disease, chronic disease, and general physiology were discontinued or scheduled for discontinuance, and the Fund was not currently supporting any research in epidemiology and cancer.

By the end of the war, the Fund's view of medical research had become more sophisticated. It recognized that the problems that overlapped, sprawled a little, or were too big to be mapped clearly in advance were often the ones worth putting money into. Individual projects had to be judged in the perspective of the problems around which they clustered, and immediate and ultimate goals kept distinct. Current "failures" might be laying the foundation for future successes and the importance of today's successes might shrink in the light of tomorrow's new discoveries. It was clearly a mistake to hold the watch on the growth of a new concept or the maturation of a new technique. Some kinds of research obviously needed long-continued support—the longitudinal study of a chronic disease like arthritis or the tracing of the growth pattern in childhood and adolescence—and most research thrived best in an atmosphere of unhurried observation and reflection.[49]

As a result, while it reviewed its grants for research at intervals of two or three years, the Fund was careful not to disturb the pace of studies that needed a long time to mature. In choosing between one project and another the Fund found it necessary to weigh to the best of its ability the growth possibilities of ideas. By drawing a baseline for the understanding of a physiological process, devising and demonstrating new techniques for measuring physiological events, or creating a new frame of reference for the study of chronic disease, the Fund was helping those studies that were laying the groundwork for current and future medical advances.

Changes in the Fund's approach to medical research in the late 1940s and early 1950s were largely influenced by the Fund's increasing interest in "comprehensive medicine" (see p. 203), the need to develop research in relatively unexplored fields, and the availability of considerable sums of public and private money for "popular" disease-centered studies—ones for which appeals could be readily made—such as cancer, infectious disease (including poliomyelitis) and cardiovascular disorders.

The Fund's early reviews of medical research classified grants as a matter of convenience, placing those grants with common features in one of six categories. Four were essentially disease-oriented: Infectious Disease, Epidemiological Studies, Chronic Disease, and Cancer Studies. The remaining two, Endocrine Studies and Studies of a General Physiological Nature, indicated the Fund's strong interest in physiology. The Fund's Third Research Review in 1952 retained the old system, but added a new method of categorizing grants according to the staff's assessment of the Fund's major objectives in supporting research:

I. Studies Primarily Concerned with Organism-Environment Interaction
II. Studies Primarily Concerned with Integrative Processes within the Organism
III. Other Studies

The new classification system reflected the staff's intention to direct support of research in channels that would most clearly further the Fund's other programmatic interests. The inclusion of Category III, however, showed that the staff was willing to accommodate occasional meritorious projects outside the interests of its other programs.

"Comprehensive medicine" was occupying the Fund in the postwar years, underscoring the central theme of "organism-environment interaction." Directing attention to "processes" (or mechanisms) implied that research would include physiological investigations not too dissimilar from some of the studies supported in the past. There was one important difference, however: The Fund favored integrative studies of organs and of the interaction of the whole organism with its environment over studies of processes occurring in individual organs.

Category I contained only two projects: Alfred H. Washburn's at the University of Colorado and Milton J. E. Senn's at Yale University, both longitudinal studies of growth and development in children. As efforts to obtain a clearer description of the constitutional makeup of children and a richer understanding of developmental processes, these projects were "longitudinal" studies, in which a particular population ("experimental" or "control," sick or healthy) is kept under observation for protracted periods of time. The Fund had long recognized the need for longitudinal research, which is particularly valuable in studies of growth and development and of chronic disease. One study (Janet Hardy's investigation of tuberculosis in childhood) had been supported by the Fund for seventeen years.

The five programs in Category II emphasized the body's two integrative systems, neural and endocrine, and included Nathan B. Talbot's endocrine studies and Horace W. Magoun's neurological investigations.

"Other studies" (Category III) consisted of six investigations. One group included three longitudinal studies of chronic disease (Walter Bauer's of arthritis, May G. Wilson's of rheumatic fever, and Max Lurie's of tuberculosis); the other, Seymour Cohen's chemical study of virus formation, Alexander Weinstein's of genetics, and Heinrich Klüver's of porphyrins, each notable for the excellent qualifications of the senior investigator.

Since the Fund's previous Medical Research Review, substantial changes in the financing of medical research in this country had begun to affect the thinking of the Fund's board of directors and staff. Publicly supported organizations and groups sponsored by industry were receiving larger sums for research support. Each year branches of the federal government were making available more funds for research. The United States Public Health Service, in particular, was providing more money for medical research than any other single agency in the country. Commercial firms, especially the pharmaceutical companies, aided medical research directly or had large intramural research programs of their own.[50] The Fund's Medical Research Review of 1951 nevertheless concluded that increasing federal support had not diminished awards from private sources and that there was no evidence of unreasonable duplication of research support by government and private agencies. The Fund's report showed most grants to be small, but at least 50% of all projects received a minimum of three years' support, and aid had been given in a wide variety of fields. The Fund's staff approved of the diversity of funding sources, as concentration of all research funds in one agency—especially a powerful, specialized agency—could be a threat to freedom of inquiry.

Despite the proliferation of other sources of support, the Fund's staff believed that medical research was still a worthwhile beneficiary of the Fund's attention. The Fund itself profited from the program in medical research: Contact with investigators helped the staff to understand the problems of medical education, maintain productive relationships with educators, plan advanced medical fellowships, and give perspective to field programs. As for the fields of inquiry themselves, the staff was careful to choose for support neglected areas of knowledge needing assistance.

A varied group of projects was supported between 1945 and 1952, including:

1. *Mechanisms of Antibody Formation. University of Pennsylvania School of Medicine, Department of Pediatrics; Children's Hospital of Philadelphia. T. N. Harris, Ph.D. (Initiated October 1948, terminated July 1953. Annual budgets $6,300–$11,100.)*[51] The answer to the central question of just where and how antibodies are produced was far from clear. Harris's previous work pointed strongly to one type of white blood corpuscle, the lymphocyte, as the principal site of the process. The Fund's grant enabled him to check his earlier findings and fill in some of the details. He showed that, along with antibodies, the lymphocytes manufactured increased amounts of nucleic acid in the cytoplasm of the cells.

2. *Hemophilia. Harvard University Medical School, Beth Israel Hospital. Benjamin Alexander, M.D. (Initiated October 1947, terminated October 1950. Annual budget $7,000.)*[52] Alexander had kept patients in good health by repeated intravenous injections of normal blood plasma. He succeeded in obtaining concentrated preparations of antihemophilic plasma (AHP), but the preparations were still contaminated with other substances and the effort to secure AHP in pure form was unsuccessful. He did discover a new factor (prothrombin accelerator) implicated in the mechanism of blood clotting.

3. *Relation of the Endocrine Glands to Growth and Development. Johns Hopkins University, Harriet Lane Home. Lawson Wilkins, M.D. (Initiated April 1938, terminated July 1950. Annual budgets $7,300–$14,500.)*[53] Wilkins's longitudinal study followed a decade of discovery about the properties of the endocrine glands. Hormones were isolated and synthesized, but little was known about their usefulness and safety in treating problems of growth and development in children. In 1938 Wilkins set up an endocrine clinic for the threefold purpose of establishing diagnostic criteria for endocrine abnormalities, instituting proper therapy, and conducting animal experiments bearing on the clinical investigation. The initial investigation sought diagnostic procedures for distinguishing true dwarfism, due to underfunction of the thyroid, from "borderline" cases. The clinic expanded rapidly as patients with all sorts of endocrine dysfunctions were included, and a metabolism ward of ten beds was established, enabling Wilkins to conduct complete biochemical tests on patients with chronic disorders. By 1948 the clinic was one of the best diagnostic and therapeutic centers in the country for the study of endocrine factors in growth and development.[54]

4. *Cellular Metabolism. Massachusetts General Hospital. Fritz Lipmann, Ph.D. (Initiated June 1942, terminated July 1953. Annual budgets $3,200–$21,492.)*[55] At the start of the Fund's awards, the principal investigator was a German refugee whose work was little known in the United States. By the end of the decade of support, he had become professor of biochemistry at the Harvard Medical School and one of the most highly respected and influential biochemists in America. Lipmann showed that energy is stored principally in a particular chemical grouping, the "high-energy phosphate bond," which he identified in various compounds occurring in living

cells. Lipmann was the discoverer of one of these compounds, acetyl phosphate, and the delineation of its role in metabolism marked the second phase of his work. Experiments with this compound led in turn to the discovery of a new enzyme, co-enzyme A. The purification, chemical characterization, and definition of the functions of this enzyme system marked the third phase of this work and made a major contribution to the understanding of life processes. In 1953 the Nobel Prize in medicine or physiology was awarded jointly to Hans Krebs for his discovery of the citric acid cycle and to Lipmann for his discovery of co-enzyme A and its importance for intermediary metabolism.

5. *Integrated Enzyme Action. University of Wisconsin, Enzyme Institute. David E. Green, Ph.D. (Initiated June 1948, terminated June 1952. Annual budget $7,500.)*[56] The Enzyme Institute of Wisconsin was an independent unit of the university devoted to the study of the enzymatic tool chest used by living cells. For four years, the Fund subsidized the work of David E. Green, one of the institute's two directors. Green's particular purpose was to determine the natural biological unit of organization in which enzymes function. What the intact cell could do was generally known; what relatively small individual compounds, generally known as enzymes, could do when other compounds were present was also known in many instances, and long sequences of chemical transformation could be described with some accuracy. What was not known was the natural organization of aggregations of enzymes. Green and other workers made it clear that for many of the transformations known to occur inside the living cell, the necessary enzymes were found in the mitochondria.

6. *Cardio-Respiratory Physiology. Columbia University, College of Physicians and Surgeons. Dickinson W. Richards, Jr., M.D. and André Cournand, M.D. (Initiated October 1939, terminated October 1950. Annual budgets $9,700–$22,400.)*[57] Throughout its eleven-year span, this program elaborated upon increasingly refined methods of obtaining deeper physiological understanding, more accurate diagnoses, and more effective therapy of respiratory and cardiac diseases. New clinical and laboratory procedures were devised to permit more accurate assessment of pulmonary function before and after surgery and to help physicians select optimal methods of treatment. Cardiac catheterization, which permits the measurement of pressures and the sampling of blood directly from the heart and was previously employed only in isolated instances abroad, was perfected and its full potential explored.

This dramatic accomplishment did not retard the development of simpler methods of approaching other problems, such as assessing the efficiency of the lungs in the exchange of gases between inhaled air and the blood. Nor did the emphasis on methodology ever obscure the primary objective of this study, which was to secure refined physiological knowledge of function in health and disease.[58] The Bellevue Laboratory, the site of this research, became the parental training ground for a steady stream of young investigators. Few projects could compete in accomplishment with this study either in the advancement of medical knowledge and skills or in training for research. In 1956 the Nobel Prize in medicine or physiology was awarded to Cournand, Richards, and Werner Forssmann (who first discovered the feasibility of cardiac catheterization) for their development of this procedure.

7. *New Techniques in Respiratory Physiology. University of Pennsylvania Graduate School of Medicine. Julius Comroe, M.D. (Initiated December 1947, terminated December 1950. Annual budget $15,500.)*[59] The principal purpose of Comroe's study was to exploit the use of new instruments— a nitrogen gas analyzer, a flow-meter, and a carbon monoxide analyzer— in making rapid and relatively simple assessments of the efficiency of the lungs in normal individuals and in those with a variety of pulmonary diseases. The research focused particularly on demonstrating and measuring the uneven distribution, in certain diseases, of the respiratory gases within the various parts of the lungs and the consequences in terms of the impairment of pulmonary functioning. As in the studies by Richards and Cournand, Comroe measured the rapidity with which gases are exchanged between the air in the lungs and the blood, and the results of the two studies complemented each other.

8. *Physiological Studies of Children with Congenital Heart Defects. University of Alabama Medical School, Department of Medicine, transferred from Johns Hopkins University School of Medicine, Department of Surgery. Richard J. Bing, M.D. (Initiated October 1945, terminated June 1953. Annual budgets $11,500–$18,620.)*[60] Alfred Blalock and Helen Taussig's successful repair of cardiac defects in "blue babies" required better diagnostic tests to select those patients for whom the operation would be beneficial. Bing devised physiological tests, based primarily on the technique of cardiac catheterization, to aid in accurate preoperative assessment of cardiac status. After preliminary experiments on dogs, he worked out the difficult technique of placing the catheter in man, in the principal vein that drains the heart musculature. He was thus able to obtain blood samples from which he could calculate the amount of metabolic fuel utilized by the heart as well as its energy consumption.

9. *Histochemical Studies of the Nephron. Long Island College of Medicine, Department of Pathology. (In 1948, this school became a part of the University of New York, as the State University of New York College of Medicine at New York City.) Jean Oliver, Ph.D. (Initiated June 1947, terminated June 1950. Annual budgets $11,000–$7,000.)* Jean Oliver was an outstanding anatomist who brought to the study of kidney function a particular interest in how the kidney retains proteins and prevents their elimination in the urine. Another important phase of his investigations dealt with the nature of the kidney damage frequently observed in shock, which was widely assumed to result from toxic products circulating through the kidney. Oliver's work revealed that, on the contrary, the damage is due to an impaired supply of oxygen to the kidneys.[61]

10. *Emotional Development in Early Childhood. Child Study Center, Yale*

University. Milton J. E. Senn, M.D. (Initiated May 1950, terminated 1959. Annual budgets $17,820–$34,000.)[62] Senn's intensive longitudinal study of the relationship between the child and his environment focused primarily on interpersonal relationships within the family to discover significant factors that determine the course of the child's physical and emotional development. A team of psychiatrists, psychologists, pediatricians, and social workers in the Yale Child Study Center was making independent observations on the formation of family attitudes and behavior from early in the mother's pregnancy to the end of nursery school. The research methods employed were principally interviews and observations, but the thoroughness of the detailed records was unique. The investigators' thesis was that a baby's actions and feelings cannot be described adequately in language, so during interview sessions minute-by-minute drawings were correlated with simultaneous observations of the mother's behavior. The mother-child interaction was thus observed through time in great detail. The investigators made periodic predictions based on psychoanalytic theory about the probable effects of family relationships on the course of the child's development. These predictions were then checked, within the limits enforced by time, against the actual developments.[63]

11. *Control of Pituitary Function. Harvard Medical School, Department of Surgery, Peter Bent Brigham Hospital. David M. Hume, M.D. (Initiated January 1949, terminated 1961. Annual budgets $5,000–$13,433.)*[64] This research centered on the question of how the activity of the pituitary gland was itself controlled, the subject of much current interest and study. Hume was concerned particularly with the anterior pituitary lobe, which governs the activity of the adrenal cortex and acts in situations involving stress (e.g., surgical trauma). He experimented mostly on dogs, but his findings were also supported by clinical evidence in man: In stress, the pituitary-adrenal system is activated by nerve impulses arising in damaged tissues and carried to the hypothalamus before being transmitted to the pituitary gland. His evidence also suggested that this last step in the chain—the brain-pituitary link—was itself an endocrine rather than a neural mechanism: The brain tissue secretes a hormone which, carried in the bloodstream, stimulates the pituitary gland.

The Fourth Review of Medical Research (1952–58)

Only twenty-seven investigations were supported in the six years covered by the Fund's fourth review, far fewer than the fifty-seven projects supported during the previous seven years. Fifteen projects were begun, nine terminated, and seven others continued throughout the span of the report. Funds provided for these projects totaled approximately $3,892,000. Annual (calendar-year) appropriations ranged from $465,000 to $802,000, averaging $673,000. The annual project budgets ranged from $6,300 to $126,000, averaging just over $29,500. These increases reflected both the Fund's new willingness to assist larger research undertakings and the generally increased costs of operation. Of the nine grants that were terminated, the illness of the principal investigator intervened in one instance. In three other cases, support became readily available and the Fund was not asked for further help, and four awards were terminated when it seemed likely that the work could command help elsewhere. At least six of the nine studies appeared likely to be continued with assistance from other organizations, chiefly the National Institutes of Health.

By 1958, although the National Institutes of Health was supporting much of the nation's medical research, the Fund continued to provide grants for investigation, particularly when the studies were related to its interests in furthering medical knowledge and promoting good health care.[65] Characteristically, the Fund looked to its projects in medical research to train junior personnel in research attitudes and techniques. Many of the research projects supported by the Fund afforded young workers opportunities for this type of experience. Among the investigators offering such training were Homer W. Smith, whose area of interest was vascular and renal physiology; George N. Papanicolaou, cytology; Fritz Lipmann, enzyme chemistry; Dickinson W. Richards, Jr., and André Cournand, cardio-respiratory physiology; Richard J. Bing, cardiac physiology; Carl J. Wiggers, vascular physiology; Alfred H. Washburn, growth and development; Nathan B. Talbot, endocrinology; Horace W. Magoun, neurophysiology; and Walter Bauer, rheumatology.

Representative projects supported between 1952 and 1958 reflected the staff's decision to give awards to fewer projects and to channel the Fund's research interests into a smaller number of areas:

Category I. Studies Primarily Concerned with Organism-Environment Interaction.

1. *Rheumatic Fever. New York Hospital, Department of Pediatrics. May G. Wilson, M.D. (Initiated June 1929, terminated 1962. Annual budgets $25,900– $39,413.)*[66] For nearly half a century Wilson studied and cared for children with heart disorders, and for 40 years she concentrated her efforts on rheumatic fever. Her study was an extensive clinical and laboratory investigation to establish the natural history of the condition, determine the mechanisms that produce it, devise successful methods for its treatment, and ultimately develop effective means for its prevention. Through extended contact with many of her original patients, their parents, and later their children, Wilson accumulated detailed information on three generations of rheumatic and nonrheumatic individuals. Her conclusion that susceptibility to rheumatic fever is inherited from generation to generation slowly gained acceptance. With cortical hormone therapy, active carditis was brought to an abrupt halt, clinical symptoms melted away, and recovery took place without either residual heart damage in patients with initial attacks or increased residual damage in patients with recurrent attacks. In another phase of the program, clinical studies determined mortality rates for patients

with heart lesions and established criteria for the selection of suitable cases for heart surgery. Finally, a six-year study of more than 100 patients tested the effectiveness of the daily use of penicillin to prevent streptococcal infections and consequent attacks of rheumatic fever. Wilson's investigation was the research project receiving the longest support from the Fund, and it probably contributed more important information about rheumatic fever than any other single program.

2. *Arthritis. Harvard Medical School, Department of Medicine. Walter Bauer, M.D. (Initiated December 1937, terminated December 1958. Annual budgets $30,000–$40,286.)*[67] This exhaustive study of rheumatism, the most intensive and penetrating investigation of joint disease ever undertaken, received Fund support for twenty-one of its thirty years of operation. In all, well over two thousand patients with joint disorders were studied, and more than half were found to have rheumatoid arthritis. Attention was focused upon this condition because of its frequency, severity, and prolonged course—and because relatively little was known of its cause, character, or methods of treatment. While the investigation remained clinically oriented, it included physiologic, pathologic, immunologic and chemical laboratory work in conjunction with research on the influence of social and psychologic factors. In general, Bauer's research confirmed the theory that rheumatoid arthritis was a distinct type of chronic inflammatory disease, involving the body as a whole but characterized by its effect on the joints. The consensus was that multiple factors were probably involved, including microbiologic agents and stresses upon the host. A vast amount of information resulted from this research, much of which was published in nearly 200 journal articles and several books. The first publication emerged from the most comprehensive study ever made of joint fluid and the changes produced in it by joint diseases,[68] and the second offered both longitudinal and cross-sectional findings over more than twenty years in a series of nearly 300 patients with rheumatoid arthritis—the most complete scientific description and analysis of the natural history of this condition ever compiled.[69]

Category II. Studies Primarily Concerned with Integrative Factors within the Organism.

3. *Pediatric Endocrinology. Harvard Medical School, Department of Pediatrics. Nathan B. Talbot, M.D. (Initiated December 1941, terminated June 1958. Annual budgets $40,824–$49,986.)*[70] The first part of this project developed new techniques for assaying the status of endocrine organs and their hormonal products. The second carried out highly technical studies to determine the role of the neural and endocrine systems in influencing homeostasis, the body's maintenance of a stable chemical environment amidst constantly changing external conditions. Also explored were the metabolic processes by which the body deals with various food constituents, minerals, salts, and water, and the ways in which these processes are influenced by hormones from the pituitary, adrenals, pancreas, thyroid, parathyroids, and sex glands. Normal children were studied, as well as

children with growth and developmental abnormalities and children with acute or chronic disease. This research demonstrated that the endocrine system as a regulator of body equilibrium reacts to and affects almost all disease states.[71]

4. *Neural Correlates of Mental Activity. University of California School of Medicine (Los Angeles), Department of Anatomy. Horace W. Magoun, Ph.D. (Initiated August 1949, terminated June 1957. Annual budgets $15,445– $49,816.)*[72] This research started with the discovery that the reticular formation, an area deep within the brain stem, exerts a general controlling influence over the entire cortex. When the reticular formation is functioning, the whole brain is "activated"; when it ceases to function, or is damaged, the activity of the brain is depressed and the individual loses consciousness. Because of these overall influences, the reticular formation, together with its connections to other parts of the body, is called the "reticular activating system." Its functioning is essential for all forms of perception, and it also affects motor activities, notably those concerned with posture. Earlier work had shown that this system was the one suppressed by anesthetics and other drugs that alter levels of consciousness.

Much more detailed knowledge had been obtained in recent years about the intimate physiologic processes evoked by the reticular activating system. In some instances it was possible to show how it affected individual nerve cells in the brain, and from this finding came a clearer understanding of the nature of neural activity in general. Magoun and his collaborators demonstrated that the reticular system was anatomically and functionally separable into two parts: a grosser and more continuously operating component in the lower brain stem, which makes relatively general alterations in the level of brain functioning, and a more forward area in the thalamus "with greater capacities for fractionated, shifting influence upon focal regions of the brain."

5. *Neural Mechanisms in the Regulation of Pituitary Thyrotropic Hormone Secretion. Washington University School of Medicine (St. Louis), Department of Internal Medicine. Seymour Reichlin, M.D. (Initiated July 1956, terminated June 1958. Annual budgets $13,685–$17,062.)* This project involved both laboratory studies of animals and clinical investigations of patients. It was known that the pituitary gland secretes thyroid-stimulating hormone (TSH), which largely controls the thyroid's activity. It was also known that the rate of TSH secretion by the pituitary is, in turn, regulated by the amount of hormone that the thyroid gland pours into the bloodstream. This feedback phenomenon was well recognized, but its detailed operation was not fully understood. Preliminary research revealed that the hypothalamus, regarded generally as the coordinating center of the involuntary, or vegetative, nervous system, somehow directly influenced the part of the pituitary that stimulated the thyroid.

Category III. Studies in Basic Biology.

6. *Chemical Studies of Virus Formation. University of Pennsylvania School of*

Medicine, Department of Biochemistry; transferred from the Department of Pediatrics and the Children's Hospital of Philadelphia. Seymour Cohen, M.D. (Initiated October 1949, terminated 1961. Annual budgets $20,666–$30,837.)[73] These imaginative and effective studies, conducted for more than a decade, yielded a comprehensive understanding of the series of chemical events occurring when a bacterium is infected with a destructive virus (bacteriophage). The process begins with the insertion of nucleic acid from the virus into the bacterial cell, an action that interrupts and redirects the normal metabolism of the bacterium. The result is a rapid, vigorous production of particles composed largely of virus nucleic acid and virus protein. Cohen discovered the particular component of the virus nucleic acid, hydroxy-methyl-cytosine, that makes it chemically unique in nature, the component producing a virus nucleic acid resistant to enzymes present in the bacterium that would otherwise break it down. This chemical event was a crucial one in the infectious process, for it appeared to be responsible for the manufacture of virus nucleic acid by the bacterium at the expense of its own metabolism. Understanding the nature of the process of virus multiplication, at least in these organisms, was made much more complete, and Cohen's contributions won wide acclaim, including one of the annual awards of the American Association for the Advancement of Science.

The Fund's fourth review suggested deemphasis of medical research as a part of the Fund's overall program, even though the support of research continued to be consistent with the Fund's programmatic objectives. The large amount of money available from other sources had decreased the importance of the Fund's contributions; nor had support of medical research retained its value to the Fund's staff as an aid to medical education and the planning of fellowships. The review suggested that the emphasis for future grants be directed toward a few investigators with interesting but unorthodox ideas who were unable to secure other funding. From time to time, too, the staff might wish to support research projects on problems of special interest to the Fund. Yet the Fund's staff believed that its awards in this area were no longer as vital to the health field as was its support of medical education, and in 1958 the Fund's Medical Research Program was dissolved.

Three Projects in Medical Research

It is not unusual that some research projects produce wholly unanticipated results, and some projects that appear to have only a slight chance of success (but represent unique ideas that should be given a chance) succeed to an unexpected degree. In the first category fell the longitudinal study of child development conducted for many years at the University of Colorado by Alfred H. Washburn; in the second, the study of exfoliated normal and cancer cells by George N. Papanicolaou at the Cornell University Medical College. Unexpected rewards came from both of these programs and from the studies of Wade Hampton Frost and Lowell J. Reed, which established epidemiology as an important branch of clinical science.

The Child Research Council Study of Growth and Development

A pioneering effort, this longitudinal study attempted to determine the cause of abnormal processes in the adult through studies of the newborn. The investigators intended to continue their investigations as the child grew into adult life, predicating that preventing or retarding the diseases of old age requires consideration of the conditions of the middle-aged individual; the young boy or girl at maturity; the child in grade school; the preschool child; the infant; the neonate; and finally the parents—especially the mother—before, during, and after the birth of the child.

In 1929 George Worlin, president of the University of Colorado, presented a request on behalf of the Child Research Council, for a three-year appropriation of $8,000 annually to broaden the scope of the council's work. The council had been founded two years earlier as an affiliate of the university and had been supported by the Salomon Winter Foundation. W. Walter Wasson, the foundation's director of research and a practicing radiologist in Denver, had become interested in refining a rapid technique for performing radiographs of the thorax, and he was studying serial x-rays of the chest and sinuses of children to determine whether sinus disease was a cause of lung infection. All the work was carried out in his office, where he was assisted by more than twenty part-time, unpaid practicing physicians and staff members from several departments of the university's medical school.

No grant was made in 1929, but in considering the application, Lester J. Evans suggested that the council reorganize its administrative arrangements. The project obviously needed a full-time director; Wasson did not have the time to fill the post, but the next year Alfred H. Washburn (fig. 18) was appointed. The council also clarified its objectives, and the group moved into quarters in the medical school. These changes made the council a more attractive organization to the Fund, and in 1930 the Fund gave it an award of $30,000.

The next few years were marked by disagreements between Washburn and the part-time investigators and conflict among the members of the council's board of trustees. Staff and board underwent many changes in personnel, and by 1936 Washburn was free to fashion a sound program. The university's respect for the council's work was demonstrated first by Washburn's appointment to the Department of Pediatrics and later

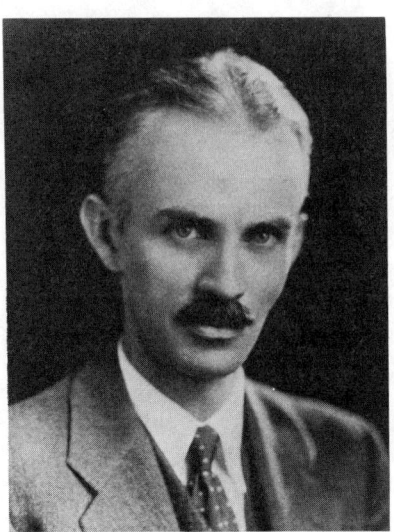

Figure 18. Alfred H. Washburn
Reprinted from the Annual Report of
the Commonwealth Fund, 1935.

by the transformation of the council into the Department of Human Growth at the university's school of medicine, with Washburn as the new department's head. The council continued, however, as an independent research institute with a separate administration and board of trustees.

The early work of the council was concerned with normal growth and development, but there was in its program manifest application to preventive medicine. Eventually, the detailed study of the child throughout life was directed toward recognizing the earliest evidence of abnormal conditions that might influence his development. The council's work might then contribute to the understanding of the origins of such conditions as hypertension, vascular disease (including coronary artery disease), allergies, and emotional problems. Although the objectives of the study remained constant, there were changes in the specific areas of development surveyed. Unfortunately, studies relating to mental health were not added until relatively late in the program.

The council's work represented the patient accumulation of innumerable observations over a long period of time. A few other studies of growth were being carried out at other centers in the country, but none was as thorough as this one: "A year ago, the four members of the Fund staff most concerned with medical research agreed to list all the research projects the Fund was supporting, ranking them in terms of what each man thought the Fund ought to be doing in research and which projects were most worthy of continuation. Independently each of them put the Child Research Council at the head of the list on both counts."[74]

The Fund hoped that this study would provide a foundation for the practice of comprehensive medicine, one of the Fund's major interests after World War II. The faculty of the University of Colorado School of Medicine—and the Fund's staff—believed that the work of the council was responsible for important changes introduced into the postwar curriculum at Colorado and for the developing appreciation of creative scholarship there. Washburn and Roderick E. Heffron both felt that the council had a reciprocal influence on the Commonwealth Fund's efforts in medical education and research.

Although the council also received grants from other foundations (including the Rockefeller, Markle, and Ford Foundations) and from the United States Public Health Service, its continuation was jeopardized when support from the National Institutes of Health was diverted to the new National Institute for Child and Maternal Health. A joint survey in 1953 by the Commonwealth Fund and the Rockefeller Foundation was very favorable, however, recommending not only continuation of the work, but supplementary staff such as a biostatistician and personnel with training in psychology.[75] The survey report recognized the unique problems involved in longitudinal studies, in contrast to the usual studies of children, which obtained information from a cross-section of the population at a moment in time.[76]

The joint survey led the Commonwealth Fund to renew Washburn's grant for three years, increasing the annual budget from $35,000 to nearly $50,000 to add a biometrician, who it was hoped would help to prepare material for publication.[77] By 1954 the program had produced 112 books and articles, including an atlas of physical growth, which was used in the University of Colorado's medical curriculum.

In 1964 the entire staff of the Child Research Council received appointments in the university's Department of Pediatrics and were housed in a separate, new division of the department. A nine-man team whose members represented all the significant areas of activity throughout the university was also created as a permanent advisory group to the council. These administrative shifts were intended to satisfy the requirements of the National Institutes of Health, which had been asked by the council for a seven-year grant of more than $3 million, that the council be part of the medical school structure. Even with these changes, the grant did not materialize.[78]

The Child Research Council's subsequent difficulties were described by Robert W. McCammon, who replaced Washburn on the council when he retired:[79]

> We were able to continue our research with support from NIH and other private foundations until the middle of 1966. With the decision at NIH, made that year, that longitudinal research is all non-productive, our grant was not renewed along with those of several other studies. We did obtain a contract for two years under which we converted all the physical and physiological

data to computer form, did cross-sectional analyses, and published a book devoted to these analyses.[80]

A tacit agreement that we would be eligible for another contract under which more meaningful longitudinal analyses would be undertaken if we fulfilled the original contract did not withstand the rapid turnover of personnel at the National Institute for Child Health and Development. By 1969, no one there had ever heard of such an agreement and our application was turned down. . . .

I found it necessary to disperse [the accumulated records] to a number of other centers whose interest in and regard for segments of the data gave some assurance of their preservation.[81]

Although the grant for completion of the work did lead to publication of the manuscript for the first of three projected volumes,[82] efforts to publish the results of these studies as a series after Washburn's death did not materialize.

The fate of the Child Research Council study illustrates the problems associated with the conduct of long-term longitudinal investigations. Changes that inevitably take place over time—in this case, shifts in the program's leadership and improvements in the methods of data storage and retrieval brought about by the advent of modern computer technology—alter such studies in unanticipated ways. The study was in many respects successful, particularly in its stimulating effect on research at the University of Colorado, but the accumulated material was never fully evaluated, and the stored files may never be fully used.

George N. Papanicolaou, Father of Exfoliative Cytology

The work of George N. Papanicolaou (fig. 19) and Herbert F. Traut at the New York Hospital–Cornell University Medical College gave the Fund a rare opportunity to support the development and application of a new technique, the microscopic examination of vaginal smears for diagnosis of cancer of the genital tract.[83]

Papanicolaou studied problems of sex differentiation with Richard Hertwig in Germany, investigations that led to a Ph.D. degree and eventually to his greatest discoveries. Learning of research opportunities in the United States, he came to New York in 1913. Thomas Hunt Morgan at Columbia University was familiar with Papanicolaou's dissertation work and arranged a technical position for him at New York Hospital in the Department of Pathology. Papanicolaou soon became a research assistant in the Department of Anatomy, under Charles Stockard.

Papanicolaou had postulated that sex was determined by the X and Y chromosomes in spermatozoa and ova, and his studies required mature ova that had not yet been extruded from follicles. To obtain them he needed the ability to predict ovulation, and since all female mammals

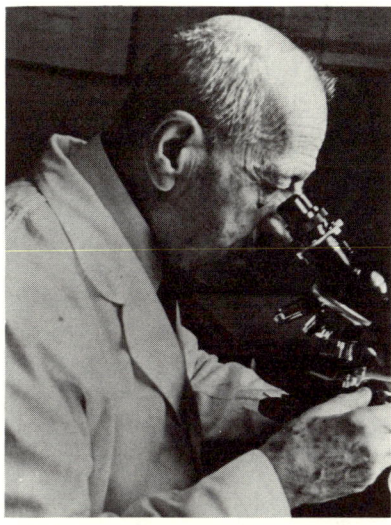

Figure 19. George N. Papanicolaou Courtesy of the Medical Archives, New York Hospital–Cornell Medical Center.

have a periodic vaginal discharge, he began to study daily vaginal smears under the microscope. He was soon able to determine the estrus cycle by correlating the observed sequence of distinctive cytologic patterns with changes in the uterus and ovary. Publication of these findings in 1917 led others to recognize that the vaginal smear was useful for studying the sex cycle in mammals other than rodents. Studies were carried out in many laboratories, and Willard Allen used the smear technique as an assay of follicular hormone, isolating the first sex hormone–estrogen.

Papanicolaou started a large-scale study of vaginal smears in women in 1923. He found cancer cells to be unmistakably different from normal cells in his preparations. Presenting his important findings at the Race Betterment Conference in Battle Creek, Michigan, that same year, he pointed out that the cells of cervical cancer were recognizable with greater ease in his preparation than in embedded sections, in which they were crowded one against the other. The diagnosis of cancer from individual cells was inconceivable to pathologists at that time, however, and they refused to use Papanicolaou's techniques. Discouraged, he turned away from cancer diagnosis, and concentrated his efforts on cytologic studies of ovulation.

It was not until 1939 that Papanicolaou returned to the use of exfoliative cytology, beginning a long collaboration with Traut, a gynecologist at the New York Hospital. Using the vaginal smears that Traut obtained from all women admitted to his service, Papanicolaou established clear proof that this technique permitted detection of otherwise asymptomatic uterine cancer and earlier diagnosis than was possible by biopsy. Finding great difficulty in obtaining money for his work, Papanicolaou turned to the Commonwealth Fund, which recognized the potential value of his research.

The story is told in a letter from Papanicolaou to Roderick E. Heffron in 1953:[84]

> At this moment as I am writing what is possibly my last report to you, my thoughts return to the time some eleven and one-half years ago when our first application for financial support was submitted to the Commonwealth Fund. That was one of the most critical periods in my scientific career as it was then that I found myself totally deprived of funds for the continuation of my research.
>
> Having decided to withdraw from the field of sex endocrinology, I had tried to obtain support for a study of one of two major problems, the first being the exfoliative cytology of uterine cancer and the other, the incidence of spontaneous tumors in the senile guinea pig and its relation to the functional state of the endocrine glands. Both projects were rejected by every one of the societies supporting cancer research to which I turned for help.
>
> It was then, at a moment when every hope had almost vanished, that the Commonwealth Fund, a society not primarily devoted to cancer research, stepped in. . . .
>
> As I write these lines my eyes are moist from the memory of those critical days. It is with a feeling of deep gratitude that I want to express my appreciation to the Commonwealth Fund for having extended to me since that time the financial and moral support which made possible the continuation of my scientific studies. . . . What appeared to be a speculative project eleven years ago is now a recognized and well founded contribution to the biological and medical sciences. This could never have been realized without the inspiration and help which came from the Commonwealth Fund and more particularly from Dr. Evans and you.

Wade Hampton Frost and the Coming of Age of Clinical Epidemiology

Support of research was a reciprocal process for the Fund. The talented individuals who were beneficiaries of grants from the Fund often provided the Fund's staff with excellent counsel. One man whose help was crucial at the beginning of the Fund's research program was Wade Hampton Frost (fig. 20), professor of epidemiology and later dean of the Johns Hopkins University School of Hygiene and Public Health. The Fund's early interest in child health led it to support studies of diseases affecting children, particularly tuberculosis, and investigations of this disease were carried out at Johns Hopkins under Frost's aegis.

Frost received the M.D. degree from the University of Virginia in 1903. A commission in the Public Health and Marine Hospital Service appealed to him more than the practice of medicine, and he spent the next seven years on epidemiological assignments around the world. In

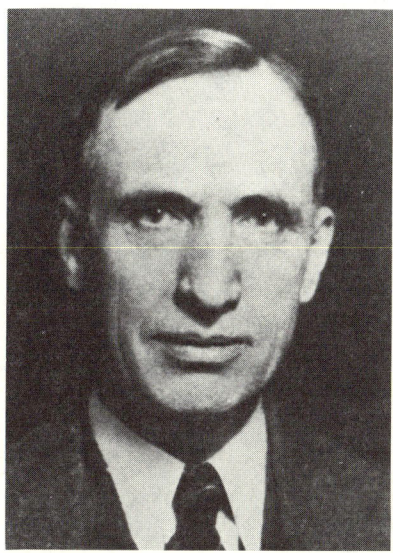

Figure 20. Wade Hampton Frost
Reprinted from the Annual Report of
the Commonwealth Fund, 1938.

1910 Frost embarked on his first field investigation of poliomyelitis epidemics. The following year he wrote a critique that was an abbreviated American forerunner of the important Peabody–Draper–Dochez monograph on poliomyelitis.[85] Frost's paper contained new data: the recorded age incidence of cases in several epidemics under different environmental conditions.

By 1913 no other investigator had obtained statistical studies on as many epidemics as Frost, nor had others been in a position to draw conclusions based on three methods: intimate clinical observation, statistical analyses, and laboratory experiments. Frost's accumulated data strongly reinforced the view that the disease was spread by personal contact.

In 1916 New York experienced one of the most devastating epidemics in the history of poliomyelitis. After analyzing the data from this epidemic, Frost reached four important conclusions: Poliomyelitis is a human infection transmitted from person to person; the infection is far more prevalent than is apparent from the incidence of clinically recognized cases; the most important agents in disseminating the infection are the mild abortive cases ordinarily escaping recognition; and an epidemic of one to three recognized cases per thousand immunizes the general population to such an extent that the epidemic declines spontaneously because of the exhaustion or thinning out of susceptible material.[86]

Two years later the great pandemic of influenza had reached America, and Frost made an epidemiologic and statistical study of that disastrous plague. Frost had by now gained experience in depth with laboratory and field investigation, studied many of the major infectious diseases, and displayed unusual skill in both research and administration. With Edgar Sydenstricker he had developed new methods of handling morbidity surveys and family studies and had formulated new statistical techniques for epidemiological research—techniques that are widely used in modern-day clinical epidemiology.[87]

Meanwhile, William Henry Welch had established the School of Hygiene and Public Health at Johns Hopkins and was looking for a physician capable of developing the scientific potential of epidemiology. He had no difficulty in singling out Frost, who was appointed resident lecturer in epidemiology in 1919. Thus began a fruitful academic period that endured for twenty years, until Frost's death. Frost rose to the position of professor of epidemiology in 1921. In the growth of the young school, he shared a close association with such men as William H. Welch, William H. Howell, Raymond Pearl, and Lowell J. Reed.

The first project of the new department of epidemiology was a study of diphtheria in Baltimore, conducted in cooperation with the Baltimore City health department and the Department of Immunology in the School of Hygiene and Public Health. This work, which began a long series of studies on the epidemiology of diphtheria, was continued in the health department's Eastern Health District. The district, which was especially equipped for teaching and investigation, had been established in 1932 by the School of Hygiene and Public Health, the city health department, and other agencies under a five-year grant from the Rockefeller Foundation.[88] The district comprised the sixth and seventh wards of the city, an area of about one square mile with a population of about sixty thousand. It was well provided with clinic service by the Johns Hopkins and Sinai hospitals, two municipal dispensaries for tuberculosis and venereal diseases, and two infant welfare clinics. It also included a large part of the territory covered by the outpatient obstetrical service of the Johns Hopkins Hospital. For many years the Eastern Health District acted as the "population laboratory" for both research and practical teaching of public health students. There Frost and his students, working with a large stable population about which they already knew a great deal, were able to undertake extensive work on diphtheria, tuberculosis, influenza, the common cold, syphilis, and rheumatic fever.

The Eastern Health District was the centerpiece for Frost's Fund-supported activities. A special census of the district was conducted in 1933 and every three years thereafter to provide a field training group for both faculty and students. These epidemiologic and administrative studies were internationally acclaimed and laid the conceptual foundation for what came to be known as a "human population laboratory." The censuses and morbidity reports also served as the basis for the development of a national health survey.

Frost recognized in the mid-1930s that the subject matter of epidemiology was changing: Acute epidemic infectious diseases were being replaced by chronic long-term diseases. Until then his work had been concentrated entirely on infections of short duration, but now he turned his attention to the special methodological problems involved in studying these chronic diseases. He collaborated with Lowell J. Reed (fig. 21), members of the staff of the School of Hygiene and Public Health, and graduate students, to elaborate the techniques and methods of approach to the epidemiology of chronic illness. Again he used the material of the Eastern Health District. By arrangement with Edwards A. Park of the Johns Hopkins Hospital's Department of Pediatrics and with a grant from the Commonwealth Fund, he began a study of tuberculosis in infancy and childhood. Miriam Brailey was placed in charge of a special tuberculosis clinic in the Harriet Lane Home, and her cooperative study was supported by the Fund for many years.[89] Frost also arranged a collaborative study of the epidemiology of acute rheumatic fever involving Park, the United States Public Health Service, and the cardiac clinic of the Harriet Lane Home.

Methodologically, Frost's studies of tuberculosis led to the development of what is now known as the "nonconcurrent prospective study" or the "historical cohort study." In Frost's own words:[90]

> Observation of the exposed group must extend over a sufficient number of years to define rates of morbidity and mortality prevailing in successive periods throughout the usual span of life. To keep a sufficiently large group of people under systematic observation, each observation for such a length of time is a difficult task which has, indeed, been undertaken in various places, but to the best of my knowledge has not been carried much beyond a decade. However, such simple facts as lie within the knowledge and memory of the average householder may be obtained by retrospective investigation, tracing familial histories backward into the past. . . . The procedure, except in collection of data, would be essentially the same in analysis of records obtained by keeping a group under planned observation.

This method is now in widespread use, especially in epidemiologic studies of occupational exposure to hazardous agents.

Wade Hampton Frost set the pace for teaching and research in epidemiology in the United States: To no one more than Frost is due the credit for establishing epidemiology as a biological and statistical science, a central discipline of public health and medical research and practice in the United States. The doctoral theses of Frost's students reveal the development of the methods used to study tuberculosis, syphilis, and rheumatic fever,[91] and many of those he trained in the Eastern Health District went on to splendid careers in epidemiology and public health.

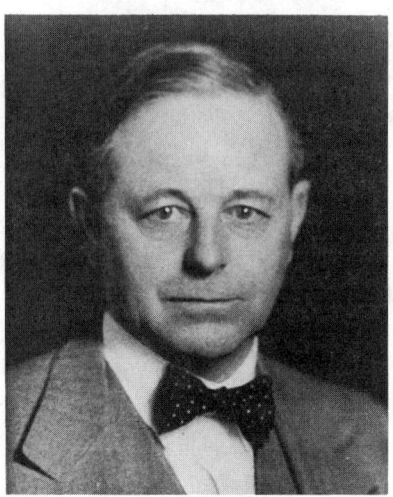

Figure 21. Lowell J. Reed
Reprinted from the Annual Report of
the Commonwealth Fund, 1940.

With Lowell J. Reed and others, Frost showed how quantitative methods could be used to discriminate between conflicting theories of disease causation, and he refined the existing methodological tools for gathering and organizing data. He made epidemiology an analytic discipline based on the accumulation of field data by intensive surveys—data from which meaning was extracted by statistical methods.[92] Through teaching, research, and consultation, he gave epidemiology a new definition: In his hands it evolved from a philosophy to a science.

Medical Research after 1960

By the mid-1960s the Fund had discontinued its formal program for medical research and its support of fellowships for research training. Constant and automatically increasing support from the National Institutes of Health (NIH) for medical research had lulled foundations and universities into believing that this type of project was an accepted, and permanent, obligation of the NIH. The Commonwealth Fund and other foundations had assumed that the important programs created with their seed money would be permanently funded by another source—usually the federal government. In the early 1970s, however, NIH training grants, direct traineeships and fellowships, and all Career Development Awards were discontinued, and in the ensuing years the money available for research support diminished. The NIH had adopted not a new policy but a strict interpretation of its concept of "buying" programs, discontinuing the "purchase" when the programs were no longer needed or no longer effective.[93] The NIH was only coping with the decision of the United

States Congress not to provide automatic increases in its funding, and foundations and universities were forced to realize that federal support to research was also temporary.

Yet the same university faculty members were both influences on governmental policy and recipients of NIH grants. Faculty members also served as advisors to the voluntary health organizations and the foundations, and members of the NIH's study sections and councils. Robert H. Ebert has pointed out that their devotion to university needs was secondary to their loyalty to their NIH responsibilities, and they frequently failed to remember that they were, in fact, the "university."[94] The competition for categorical grants created many problems, not the least of which was that research funds—particularly for basic research—were not necessarily distributed in the most effective way. What the faculties forgot was that when the NIH felt that it could no longer "buy" research programs, only the university remained with the final responsibility for their support.

By the 1980s faculties had learned their lesson and were no longer considering NIH grants as "hard money." Ebert believes that the struggle between universities and the federal government could be beneficial if university faculties were to use it as an opportunity to reexamine public policy for research and research training. Action to resolve this difficult situation could revitalize medical school faculties, leading them to accept the responsibility for making plans as a group within a university, and not as loose "federations of individual entrepreneurs."

Better coordinated faculties that considered their institution's and the nation's research needs would recognize the advantages of support for basic research to solve the major problems of disease, rather than support for task forces tackling certain categorical areas. As Lewis Thomas has pointed out, halfway technologies designed to deal with the consequences of disease or to postpone death are enormously expensive in contrast to the "high technologies"—such as immunization against poliomyelitis—which are relatively cheap. Foundations are in a position to stimulate thoughtful consideration of these and other issues of national policy on medical research.[95]

One of the untoward aspects of the federal largess of twenty years ago was the blurring of boundaries between the funding of medical education and medical research. As research funds were diverted to support education, medical education became a by-product of medical research. As federal funds have diminished, full-time staff have increasingly been torn between medical practice, medical research, and medical education. Ebert believes that foundations should consider these situations as old problems in new shapes and reconsider their overall programs accordingly: Foundations should now support pressing areas of medical research and training that are not receiving sufficient attention from the NIH.

The Commonwealth Fund has reentered the field of medical research under President Mahoney, supporting several institutions' studies of Alzheimer's disease and osteoporosis. Looking at the health problems of the elderly, the Fund's staff has selected as worthy of support disease syndromes of apparently increasing frequency.

The Commonwealth Fund's role in medical research has been catalytic, influencing the development of an academic research community, then encouraging and monitoring the concomitant work. Geddes Smith of the Fund's staff wrote eloquently of the difficulties inherent in assessing results:[96]

> It will be noticed that there is no attempt to make a clearcut separation between successes and failures and little comparison of one project with another. This is deliberate. It is impossible to say categorically that a given project has been successful or unsuccessful. The word "project" itself is an administrative artifice set up for the convenience of donors, deans and bookkeepers. There are research problems without end, and a man may spend his life at a single one of them, but the boundaries of a problem and a project rarely coincide. Occasionally, a limited problem can be so tightly defined as to fit comfortably into a neatly budgeted project; more often the problems that overlap, or sprawl a little, or are too big to compass in any predictable span of time, are most worth putting money into. . . .
>
> It is rash to appraise work done on the great unsolved problems of medicine in terms of immediate results or the lack of them; no man living may be wise enough to say what may come of it in the long run. The staff presents these reports, therefore, not as a mere balance-sheet of grants and gains, but as an exhibit of intellectually sound, technically proficient, pertinent and therefore hopeful work for the welfare of mankind through the enrichment of medical knowledge.

The success that has attended the research programs of the Commonwealth Fund attests to the wisdom of those who administered them and those who made the important decisions about expenditures. The Fund's program was highly successful not only in the specific knowledge that it generated, but in its potent multiplier effect, through support of the many young scientists trained in new projects who later made important contributions of their own.

Ancillary Projects during Barry C. Smith's Presidency

Not all the grants awarded during Barry C. Smith's directorship could be neatly categorized. Smith's perspicacity and strong will involved the Fund with projects on the fringes of child welfare, public health, medical education, and medical research—projects that sometimes appeared isolated and inconsequential but in retrospect were among the most valuable recipients of Fund support.

One example was his almost single-handed implementation of grants for the support of the American Society for the Control of Cancer (ASCC), the predecessor of the American Cancer Society.[97] Cancer research in the early 1920s was thought to be adequately funded, but no efforts had been made to educate the public about the need for early detection and treatment. A small group of physicians—James Ewing, Howard C. Taylor, Thomas S. Cullen, Frank F. Simpson, and Joseph C. Bloodgood—had drawn up plans in 1914 for a new society to "disseminate knowledge concerning the symptoms, treatment and prevention of cancer, to investigate conditions under which cancer is found, and to compile statistics in regard thereto." In 1921 Smith received a letter from Francis Carter Wood, a physician in New York, asking the Fund to support the ASCC. Smith's reply took the form of a plan that he presented to the Fund's consultants William Darrach, W. W. Palmer, and Hans Zinsser, who agreed to a five-year grant. The Fund's subsidy allowed the society to capitalize on its previous extensive educational work with health departments, medical societies, women's clubs, and nurses' organizations, and to build a strong field department and an endowment of over $1 million. As a result of the Fund's grant, attention throughout the country was focused on cancer as never before. Mrs. Robert G. Mee, chairman of the ASCC's Finance Committee, referred to the "substantial assistance which the Commonwealth Fund has given in establishing the Society on a firm financial basis during its first halting years." She continued, "We wish to give full credit to the Commonwealth Fund for its share in spreading the educational message of this society far and wide throughout the country." Typically, Smith used the ASCC's expertise for the Fund's benefit: When an appeal arrived for the investigation of x-ray therapy in the treatment of cancer, among Smith's advisors was Charles A. Powers, the society's president.[98]

Another project of especial interest to Smith was the effort to settle on a uniform nomenclature for disease. The best-known classification systems were those at the Bellevue Hospital, the Massachusetts General Hospital, the Presbyterian Hospital in New York, and Stanford University, but the army, navy, and United States Public Health Service (USPHS) had their own individual systems as well. The diversity resulted in much confusion and prevented physicians from comparing morbidity and mortality statistics. In 1928 representatives of a dozen national medical associations met to discuss the need for a uniform system. A National Conference on the Nomenclature of Disease was organized; its executive committee included chairman George Baehr, of New York's Mount Sinai Hospital, and representatives of the USPHS, the Bureau of the Census, the Metropolitan Life Insurance Company, the American Medical Association, the American College of Surgeons, and the American Hospital Association. The following year, E. H. L. Corwin appealed to the Fund for a two-year grant for the project. Smith intuitively considered this project to be very important, and the Fund's board of directors agreed on a modest award. The result of the Fund's grant was a book that Henry A. Christian recommended for use in every hospital in the country.[99] Henry Alsop Riley also praised the Fund's contribution to this project: "The Commonwealth Fund should take great satisfaction in the publication of this nomenclature. I believe this publication should have great educational value . . . and contribute to the ease with which statistics may be compiled and research carried out. . . . In all probability, no special grant ever made by the Fund has had so far-reaching an effect as those to this organization."[100]

Another project that captured Smith's interest was a proposal by the National Board of Medical Examiners "to establish a standard of examination and certification of graduates in medicine for the whole United States and its territories through which, by the cooperation of the state and territorial boards of medical examiners, its diplomates may be recognized for licensure to practice medicine."[101]

Once again, small but strategic grants helped construct the basic framework of medicine in the United States.

The War Years and Planning for the Future

During World War II, the Fund's income dropped and expenditures for all programs were reduced—partly because of a shift to projects for war relief that were costing between $100,000 and $400,000 a year. In its central office, as well as in the field, the Fund lost personnel to the armed forces. Those who remained at the Fund began to focus their attention on postwar projects. The federal government was beginning to consider support of medical research and other health activities, and in 1944 Barry C. Smith was called to testify before the Senate's Subcommittee on Wartime Health and Education. Smith reviewed the Fund's activities before the committee, and added: "In my opinion, no plan for governmental assistance to civilian medical research should be formulated until a responsible and independent group of scientific workers, clinicians and educators has been asked to report to the Congress as to the overall need for Federal financial aid in medical research and if such need is demonstrated to suggest apparatus by which it may be met."[102] Typically, Smith's comments reflected the Commonwealth Fund's fear of governmental invasion into the private sector.

Without foreseeing federal programs such as those of the National Institutes of Health; the Hill–Burton Act; or the broad scope of the future Department of Health, Education and Welfare, the Fund's staff pursued programs based on its own experience—ones that would be most likely to continue despite future governmental action. Although the programs of the previous twenty years had largely fulfilled their purposes, the Fund never considered leaving the health field. Its staff was looking instead for new programs that would be as innovative and provocative as those of the past.

One result of the search was Lester J. Evans's extensive memorandum in 1945 proposing postwar activities in medical education.[103] Evans recognized the new perception of health as a societal responsibility. He anticipated that government would move into the field and believed that the Fund should lead the way in experimentation and demonstration. Another theme of his report was that the Fund should concentrate on helping medical students understand the patient as a human being—an idea emphasized in later Fund-supported programs in medical education.

Barry C. Smith's guidance had placed the Fund in an especially favorable position: In the years to come, it could exert a profound influence on the character of the nation's health services. The Fund was leaning toward work that would reorient medicine around an understanding of man in society and not just around the techniques, instruments, specialists, and facilities that in the eyes of the public meant "medicine."

A Summary of the First Twenty-Five Years

The foundation is a device for steering a middle course between the inflexibility of fixed endowments and the inconsequentiality of random giving. Its success can be measured, in part, by the balance the foundation strikes between consistency and adaptability. The Commonwealth Fund completed its twenty-fifth year on October 17, 1943, and over its first quarter-century undoubtedly made mistakes in searching for this balance. Yet there was a thread of continuity in its giving and progress in its learning how to give.

The appropriations of the first twenty-five years amounted to about $41 million. In the Fund's first five years, it devoted nearly half its total appropriations to war service and overseas relief. At the same time, however, it was developing a pattern of giving that it would be able to follow under more normal circumstances—at first by scattered gifts to many independent agencies, later by coordinated grants that taken together formed a "program."

The Commonwealth Fund pursued four main philanthropic channels, choosing to emphasize the welfare of children. Delinquency was the first target when in 1921 the Fund launched its initial major long-range undertaking, the Program for the Prevention of Juvenile Delinquency. As the child guidance clinics progressed, training became—and remained—the core of the program. The immediate result was not only to use psychiatrists in areas outside state hospitals, where they could formulate varied approaches to the problems of daily living, but to call attention to "child psychiatry" as a specialized, more dynamic form of psychiatry. Soon psychiatrists had formed more effective liaisons with pediatricians and internists.

The Fund's second project was its Child Health Program. Turning again to the method that had been effective in the child guidance clinics, the Fund established four demonstrations of child health services to provide preventive and educational pediatric care, nursing assistance for children and mothers, and leadership for health education in the schools. When the demonstrations had accomplished their purpose, a new public health program was built around the development of county health work and parallel strengthening of state health departments. These coordinated efforts led to technical advances in local health service, which were soon diffused throughout each state. Because public health work was only one part of a broad field in which the family physician had the larger role, the program included grants for the teaching of preventive medicine and fellowships for postgraduate study by physicians in private practice.

Hospitals engaged the support of the Fund in its earliest years, but at first only as isolated projects. Gifts were made to build or enlarge institutions in missionary areas, but not until 1925 did the Fund turn to this aspect of health service in any systematic way. After a study of rural hospital facilities, a program of hospital construction and development was launched, and half a dozen small community hospitals had been built when the depression intervened. The Fund continued to study the administrative and educational problems of hospitals, however, until building operations could be resumed in 1933; this type of investigation played a large part in all the Fund's public health projects, which stressed the hospital as a tool of medical progress.

The Fund's early giving for medical education was sporadic, with emphasis again on support for missionaries, but some small gifts had already been made for postgraduate education before it became an objective of both the rural hospitals and the public health programs. Beginning in 1926 fellowships for postgraduate courses at medical schools and clinical education at the rural hospitals shared support with that for extension teaching in several southern states and intensive programs for residents at one northern school. Direct subsidies to medical school departments, beginning with the Department of Medicine at the Johns Hopkins University in 1919, were used chiefly for the development of preventive medicine and psychiatry. In 1938 this aid took a subtler form, with the offer of Advanced Medical Fellowships to instructors identified by their deans and department heads as potential leaders in the growth of a given school. Later grants permitted interschool visits by outstanding teachers as a means of freshening the stream of instruction. In medical education the Fund felt no need to confine itself to any single method of forwarding its broad purposes.

The physician, the health department, and the hospital formed a triad of health service. In support of their common and distinctive functions, the Fund appropriated nearly $16 million, or 39 percent of all its grants for the quarter-century. Gifts for medical research ranked as the largest single program of the Fund during its first twenty-five years. Grants under that heading were consistently eclectic, as neither the duration nor the amount of individual subsidies, nor the choice of problems for investigation, was held to a preconceived pattern. Although the Fund's interest was drawn repeatedly to certain broad fields of inquiry—e.g., cardiorenal physiology and disease—this focus did not interfere with the selection for subsidy of individual problems as far apart as the chemical aspects of complement and growth patterns in children. If there was a trend, it was toward a broader view of the relation of underlying physiological investigation to clinical progress.

In his summary of the Fund's first twenty-five years, Barry C. Smith said:[104]

> One of the knottiest technical problems encountered in the task of giving away a million and a half to two million dollars a year is the choice of a channel. The simplest way to translate such sums into social action is to hand them over to established agencies for the furtherance of their own programs. A large part of the Fund's giving in its earliest years took this pattern, which was useful and often necessary. But the established institution, by definition, is already able to command support from other sources, and the foundation should be backing needed work that no one else is ready to pay for. Moreover, many established agencies tend to harden around a fixed idea; the most alert find it hard to avoid the lag that creeps in between administrative routine and the changing realities of the world outside.
>
> The foundation may try to act more directly by setting up its own programs to meet what it believes to be pressing needs, entrusting their execution to existing or *ad hoc* agencies, with varying degrees of supervision through its own technical staff. This the Fund has done in several fields. Such programs differ in specificity and in duration. The short-term program set up for a limited purpose, like the Fund's first mental hygiene project, has the advantage of coming to an end before it gets out of date, and its results are relatively easy to measure. It is vulnerable, however, on other counts. Unless it is carefully considered and administered with an open mind, it may be ephemeral, or miss the real point of the situation to which it is addressed. Lasting progress is likely to come slowly. No program is as good when it is first written down as it is after people have lived with it in the field. The advantage of close connection between a foundation and a field staff is that the foundation can learn as well as lead through such contacts. The shift in the Fund's public

health activities in 1930, when the Child Health Program based on isolated demonstrations gave place to a program geared to state leadership, was the fruit of such experience.

The long-term project with fixed objectives has the advantage of allowing time for such adjustments, but sooner or later it runs the danger of becoming dated or arbitrary; there is a temptation to fit situations to the programs instead of the program to the situation. The more specific the program, the more quickly events may leave it behind: all such programs need periodic overhauling.

Selecting Barry C. Smith's Successor

The Commonwealth Fund's consideration of future directions and plans occurred just at the end of Barry C. Smith's directorship. Smith himself was active in choosing his successor. Early in 1947 Smith compiled a list of what seemed to him the most important qualifications for the next director of the Fund:[105]

1. Administrative experience, ability and skill, preferably in some field of social effort, such as philanthropic, scientific or educational work;
2. Some knowledge of the techniques of investigation and appraisal combined with good judgment of people;
3. A nice combination of flexibility and tenacity of purpose with the ability to say "no" and not make enemies, and patience in waiting for results coupled with determination in securing them;
4. A scientific attitude, good powers of observation, and the ability to learn with reasonable speed the essentials of various fields of activity;
5. A mature and constructive, but not too radical, point of view about social development.

He considered for the position the broadcaster Edward R. Murrow, who was at one time connected with a philanthropy, but Murrow expressed no interest. As time went on, Smith's views became more specific. Malcolm P. Aldrich wrote to another member of the Fund's Board: "Barry takes a strong position now against anyone who has not medical, hospital, and public health knowledge. I am afraid he has forgotten that he had none when he came to the Fund!"[106]

Barry C. Smith retired on September 1, 1947, after twenty-six years of service.

Part III: Expanding Interest in Medical Education

6

Support of Comprehensive Medicine

Medical teaching organized around the student's need to learn and the patient's need for care will prepare students to meet the responsibilities of medicine as a social institution more effectively than medical teaching organized around the preoccupation of teachers with what they as specialists think they ought to teach.

—Annual Report,
The Commonwealth Fund, 1952

The Third General Director: Donal Sheehan (1947—1948)

When Barry C. Smith retired, the directorship of the Fund passed from a social worker to a basic scientist with a medical degree. Donal Sheehan (fig. 22) was born in Carlisle, England, in 1907 and received the bachelor's and master's degrees in science and two medical degrees from the University of Manchester, England. Between 1932 and 1935 he held Dickinson and Rockefeller fellowships, studying medicine in Vienna, Breslau, and Amsterdam and at McGill and Yale universities. After two years as a lecturer in neuroanatomy at the University of Manchester, he became a resident of the United States. From 1937 until he joined the Fund on September 1, 1947, Sheehan was professor of anatomy, director of the anatomical laboratories, and acting dean of the New York University College of Medicine.[1]

Sheehan entered into his new duties with vigor, producing an elaborate Special Report on General Policy for the board of directors only six months after joining the Fund. This prescient document encompassed the thinking of all the staff members, particularly Lester J. Evans; it emphasized problems that were to concern medicine in the years to come and served as the basis for many of the Fund's future programs. Sheehan's evaluation of the Fund's experience and resources led him to one conclusion: The Commonwealth Fund should continue to concentrate on medicine and health.

Specifically, the Fund should support what Sheehan termed "compre-

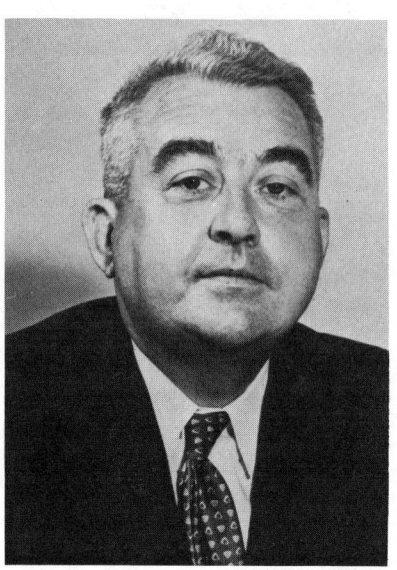

Figure 22. Donal Sheehan
Photograph courtesy of the New York
University Medical School Archives.

hensive medicine." Sheehan saw the current practice of medicine as fractionated, ignoring the patient's total personality, the interplay among physical condition, emotional makeup, and environment. Ideal medical care would consider man in health and sickness as a whole and not as an aggregate of component parts. Comprehensive medicine recognized that the patient cannot be understood in the isolation of a laboratory or hospital ward, apart from his own past and his present environment. His behavior cannot be fully interpreted without evaluation of his physical and emotional constitution and without a knowledge of the cultural pattern of his society. Medicine had always leaned heavily on the physical sciences, but dedication to comprehensive medicine involved understanding derived from the social sciences as well.

Sheehan believed that the quality of the medical schools in any country at any period in history coincided with the quality of medical service available to the people of that country twenty-five years later. The most effective method of raising the standards of medical care on a wide scale, therefore, was to effect change in the underpinning of medicine—the centers where future clinicians and investigators were being trained. Medical schools in the United States, however, had improved substantially since the turn of the century. To cope with developments in medical science, schools were providing teaching and research laboratories, organizing full-time faculties, and setting standards of qualification for medical practice. The result was to place American medicine ahead of anything else known in the world. For the first time, young physicians in search of postgraduate education had turned toward the United States. The full effect of this change on standards of medical practice was still to be realized: The public was being educated to demand high-quality medical care, but at the same time the growth of research was leading to diminished interest in the individual patient. It was time for medical training to reconcile these aspects of medical practice.

Sheehan was suggesting a reorientation of medical education around the study of the normal, whole person. When the student is trying his hand at dealing with sick people, he needs continuity of contact with his patients, so that he may become sensitive to the importance of time in physical and emotional adjustment. He needs more contact with chronic constitutional disorders of the aging, more contact with his patients' personal, social, and economic environment. He also needs experience with ambulant patients at a stage when the earliest deviations from "normal" appear. Sound training in diagnosis and therapy will always be necessary, but it is not enough to expose the future physician to the late stages of disease and the major illnesses assembled in large teaching hospitals; in this setting, attention is inevitably directed to diseased organs rather than to the patient, to diagnosis and cure rather than prevention.

The inevitable increasing complexity of medical and surgical techniques had resulted in the almost complete neglect of any organized program of training for the general physician. For day-to-day practice a new type of internist was needed—a physician skilled in diagnosis; able to deal with ordinary difficulties, whether primarily physical or emotional; and stressing the maintenance of health rather than the cure of established disease. Such a physician would be given a new dignity and importance as the future leader of preventive and comprehensive medicine in the community.[2]

Once a physician was launched in practice, either in a group or on his own, there should also be facilities for continuing education. For the physician already in practice who lacked the appropriate training, postgraduate education offered the only hope of increasing his usefulness to the present generation of patients. Here again, the Fund's emphasis on "continuing medical education" occurred before its necessity was widely recognized.

Sheehan saw the study of human biology as the foundation for integrating the components of comprehensive medicine. The best way to advance the cause of comprehensive medicine, he thought, was to give medical schools large subsidies that would allow small groups of students ample facilities for tutorial instruction, and offer staff the opportunity to engage in research and participate personally in clinical teaching.

Few organizations besides the Fund had the knowledge and experience necessary to help comprehensive medicine become firmly established.

Because the Fund's programs had already contributed to the evolution of this idea, the Fund now had a unique opportunity to capitalize on its past work.

Sheehan had been a faculty member at a medical school receiving Commonwealth Fund support. Now, as a member of the Fund's staff, he had the advantage of viewing the Fund's work from the inside as well. The topic of medical education was in the air; at a staff meeting near the end of Smith's tenure, staff members had begun to discuss the entire educational process for medical students, the ten- to twelve-year period past high school that included premedical as well as medical education.[3] Lester J. Evans felt that the Fund now stood in an especially favorable position to influence American medicine. The war was over, and the Fund's accumulated experience would allow it to accelerate the progress of medicine and to extend the kinds of activities that had contributed to its growth in the prewar years.

Evans advanced the idea of unrestricted grants to medical schools, a type of award that might encourage experimental changes in course content and teaching methods and relieve the schools' grave financial difficulties. The public did not fully appreciate that although the tuition paid by the student was high, it represented less than one-third the cost of his education. The remaining two-thirds of the budget in private institutions came principally from two sources: endowment, which in most schools was small, and the general university budget, which depended largely on revenue from endowment. There was already a shortage of teachers and investigators in the basic science departments of medical schools. Salaries were low and it was becoming increasingly difficult to attract the ablest individuals into the fundamental branches of medicine.

Some schools had already taken steps toward teaching comprehensive medicine by linking the teaching of internal medicine with that of psychiatry, setting up special courses in preventive medicine, and exposing students to their patients' home environment. To better relate the basic sciences to the rest of medical education, Evans also proposed reorganizing the first two years of medical school. A new curriculum at the University of Colorado School of Medicine allotted a generous amount of time in the first year to the teaching of human biology in terms of normal growth—a natural sequel to the long-term studies of growth in children conducted by the Child Research Council of Denver. Sheehan felt that such beginnings should be developed as rapidly as possible:[4]

> [the medical student] is starting his career, which demands a knowledge of man not only as a biological organism, but as we have already said, as an active member of a human society. Thus, it is only logical that the future doctor should come to know his future patient as he will find him—a living, growing, maturing, feeling and reacting person living in an environment. To

learn this he must have more opportunity early in his medical course to study the living person as well as the material now offered in departments such as anatomy, physiology, and biochemistry. The subject matter of these departments and others, without which the human organism cannot be understood, will become meaningful to the student if he can use it to illuminate such natural phenomena as growth, development, maturation, organism-environment interaction and total behavior as he observes them in the people he is studying.

Sheehan also wanted to extend this emphasis on comprehensive medicine to the Fund's support of medical research. Longitudinal studies of comprehensive medicine should be part of the Fund's program, he believed, along with five-year grants for research in the fundamental medical sciences. In whatever research the Fund decided to support, Sheehan felt that the quality of the investigator was more important than the attractiveness of the project.

Sheehan advanced his proposal at a propitious time: The Fund was looking for a new vector as the federal government encroached on its territory. National expenditures for scientific research and development in medicine and allied fields amounted to $110 million annually (of which private foundations contributed only $10 million).[5] The United States Public Health Service had a budget of more than $15 million annually for state and local health work, another $25 million was allotted for control of specific diseases, and the Hill–Burton Act had authorized the appropriation of $75 million a year for hospital construction. Under the National Mental Health Act, new grants of between $4 and 5 million were allocated annually for training, research, and community services in psychiatry and mental health. Once again the Fund's pioneering efforts had been taken over by the federal government, enabling the Fund to phase out its support. The Fund's staff believed that as government funding of psychiatric fellowships increased, foundations should save their grants for individuals advanced in teaching and research. They recognized, however, that the direction and intensity of federal support were subject to the caprices of governmental funding. Some programs (for example, training for workers in child guidance clinics) would have been crippled without the Fund's continuing awards. In other cases, even the large sums available from the federal government had not ended the need for private contributions—as in the field of psychiatric research.

The government grants demonstrated public approval of the objectives of the Fund's programs, but they also placed a new burden—overlapping programs—on the Fund's director and staff. A shift to comprehensive medicine would provide one answer to the problem of duplicate effort. To seize this opportunity, Sheehan wanted the Fund to use its financial resources in bold and experimental ways. He proposed taking full advantage of Edward S. Harkness's gift of 1937, whose flexible terms made it an ideal vehicle for the execution of this new plan.[6] Sheehan suggested spending not only the income but a portion of the principal as well to support the teaching of comprehensive medicine in a few medical schools. In selecting schools for support, Sheehan would consider geographical distribution, faculty interest, and potential ability to develop programs in comprehensive medicine; he would favor less well-established institutions whose graduates were nevertheless providing most of the country's medical care.

Related to the training of the general physician was the larger question of community health. Again, Sheehan proposed a bold, innovative program, a series of experiments in community health care that would integrate public health and hospital service with physician and nursing care and with strategically situated teaching centers. Experimental methods of organizing, administering, and distributing health care were also included in Sheehan's plan. Projects would take place in settings where community health care was reasonably integrated and medical care reasonably accessible to all the population. Experimentation of this sort was already underway in Rochester and Richmond: Regional hospital plans were improving medical education in the field by placing teacher-consultants in small outlying communities, where they could have a continuous influence on the local practice of medicine.[7] Specific plans would be tied to a community's needs and readiness for change—they could not be worked out at a desk but were to be tested in the field.

Sheehan saw psychiatry as a potent force in advancing the practice of comprehensive medical care: "It is a basic element in *all* medicine and in other professions that serve human beings". . . . As new patterns are being found for improving the quality of medical care—group practice clinics, complete family health programs, home care of the aged and chronically ill, rehabilitation of the physically handicapped—all these and other exploratory measures in providing health services must necessarily include psychiatric knowledge."[8] During his tenure the Fund began its program of awards to nine medical schools to improve their instruction in psychiatry and mental health: to the departments of psychiatry at the universities of Louisville,[9] California, and Long Island; to pediatric departments at Columbia, Cornell, and Stanford universities, and to those of the universities of Minnesota, California, and Cincinnati;[10] and to departments of internal medicine at Harvard University, Cornell University, and the University of Cincinnati.[11]

Recognizing the inadequacy of the supply of teachers and clinicians in psychiatry, the Fund had provided psychiatric fellowships since the start of its mental health program.[12] Under Sheehan's direction, the focus of the medical fellowship program was sharpened, aligning it with the Fund's other programs in medical education. Awards for pediatricians and internists were added as an additional bridge between psychiatry and other fields. Sheehan also continued the Fund's sponsorship of conferences concerning problems in teaching and service.

The panoply of programs encouraged by Sheehan could not have been carried to fruition without the support of the Fund's board of directors. In 1946, the first physician joined the board, which had previously been composed exclusively of educators, businessmen, lawyers, and financiers. The new board member was David Prestwick Barr, chairman of the Department of Medicine at the Cornell University Medical College.[13] He was enthusiastic about Sheehan's plans to involve the Fund in the teaching of comprehensive medicine, and he particularly liked the idea of a pilot clinic in a medical school and teaching hospital. Based on the principle of group practice, this clinic would include diagnosis, therapy, preventive care, and home care, with opportunities for instructing students, interns, and residents. With Barr's assistance a clinic was instituted at Cornell under the guidance of Harold G. Wolff (see p. 73); it served as the precursor of a more comprehensive effort directed by George G. Reader (see p. 226).[14]

To support these experimental programs, Sheehan was counting on released money: In 1948 substantial support of training in psychiatric social work by the United States Public Health Service permitted the Fund to drop its twenty-seven-year-old program of grants to social work schools, and federal and state grants for public health projects allowed the Fund to phase out its support of rural hospital budgets. The discontinued programs came from both of the Fund's administrative categories. During Sheehan's tenure, administrative functions at the Fund were divided into general administration (including administration of the Program in Mental Hygiene and of special grants for medical research, medical education, and miscellaneous purposes) and divisional administration (including administration of the field programs in the Divisions of Rural Hospitals and Public Health, and the Publications program). Current budgets called for the expenditure of 14.2 percent of total income for the first division and 11.7 percent for the second. Obviously, total administrative costs were high. With the discontinuation of programs, Sheehan hoped to reduce these costs from 25.9 percent to under 20 percent of total annual income.

Sheehan's time at the Commonwealth Fund was an interlude in a career devoted to academic medicine. Before the end of 1948, Sheehan had decided to resume the chairmanship of the Department of Anatomy at New York University. John Romano, a colleague and admirer, speculates that Sheehan's decision to return to academic medicine may have been related to the presence of Barry C. Smith, who remained in place at the Fund even after his resignation. Smith still involved himself in decision making, and as a result, Sheehan had to deal with divided loyalties and resulting administrative conflicts.[15] Health problems also played a role in Sheehan's decision to return to academic life.

Donal Sheehan left the Fund on September 1, 1948. Although Sheehan spent only one year as its general director, his imprint was deep. He was the theoretician who summarized the Fund's past and gave the Fund a direction for the future. It was left to Malcolm P. Aldrich to set up the programs that would reinforce Sheehan's early belief in the primacy of medical education for the improvement of medical service.

7

Programs in Medical Education and Community Service

A rare blending of learning and humanity, incisiveness of intellect and sensitiveness of spirit which occasionally come together in an individual who chooses the calling of medicine; and then we have the great physician.

—Hans Zinsser

The Second President: Malcolm Pratt Aldrich (1948—1963)

Malcolm P. Aldrich (fig. 23) was born October 1, 1900, in Fall River, Massachusetts. His undergraduate career at Yale University was marked by academic and extracurricular honors: He was captain of the varsity football and baseball teams, president of the undergraduate athletic association, and recipient of the Francis Gordon Brown Prize.[1] He received the bachelor's degree in 1922 and one year later joined Edward S. Harkness as a member of his personal office staff.

The Fund's attention to education was compatible with Aldrich's background and interests. When Harkness's first assistant, Samuel H. Fisher, retired in 1923, Aldrich became Harkness's representative and confidant, and a close bond developed between these two men. Without a son of his own, Harkness looked to "Mac," twenty-six years his junior, for the youthful vigor, enthusiasm, and drive to supplement his own thinking.

At Harkness's death in 1940, Aldrich became executor of his estate and trustee of the charitable trust established under his will. Edward S. Harkness had remained the first president of the Commonwealth Fund until his death. When the title passed to Aldrich on September 1, 1948, he became both general director and president—and thus chief of staff and chief executive officer of the Fund.

Aldrich assumed the leadership of a foundation with a changing administrative staff. Barbara S. Quin, administrative assistant to the general director, died in 1945; Barry C. Smith had resigned in 1947, and his

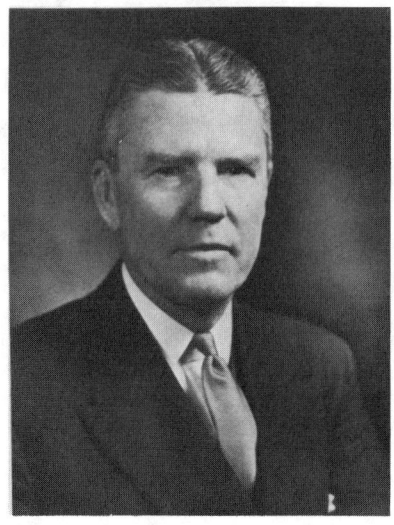

Figure 23. Malcolm P. Aldrich
Reprinted from *The Commonwealth Fund: A Historical Sketch, 1918–1962.* New York: Commonwealth Fund, 1963.

successor had stayed only one year; Henry J. Southmayd, since 1926 head of the Division of Rural Hospitals, retired in 1949. Long-time staff members Mildred C. Scoville, Geddes Smith (fig. 24), and Lester J. Evans were promoted in 1950 to executive associates, for administration, general administrative duties, and medical affairs, respectively.

Shifts in the Fund's annual appropriations between 1945 and 1952 reflected these changes. Support of mental health programs decreased. A larger amount was given to programs in medical education, especially those combining medical and psychiatric teaching, and medical fellowships. A new classification for appropriations, "Experimental Health Services," was instituted in the late 1940s.

In 1952 the Fund's offices were moved to the Harkness family's house at 1 East 75th Street (fig. 25). Staff turnover continued: Geddes Smith died in 1953; and Mildred C. Scoville retired in 1954, Harry E. Handley in 1958, Lester J. Evans in 1959, and Charles O. Warren, a medical associate, in 1960. John C. Eberhart, a psychologist, succeeded Scoville, but he resigned in 1961.[2] Despite predictably impending retirements in the late 1950s and 1960s, there was no effort to recruit younger staff members who might take the Fund into the next decades. At the time, however, these pending shifts in staff probably had little effect on the Fund's activities, as most of the projects then financed or under consideration were well known to the seasoned staff members who remained.

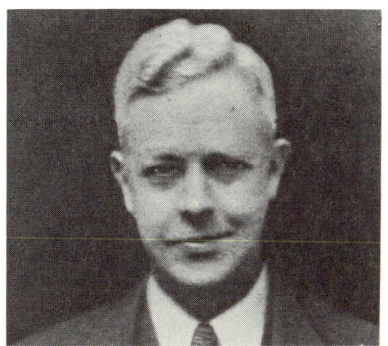

Figure 24. Geddes Smith
Reprinted from the Annual Report of the Commonwealth Fund, 1953.

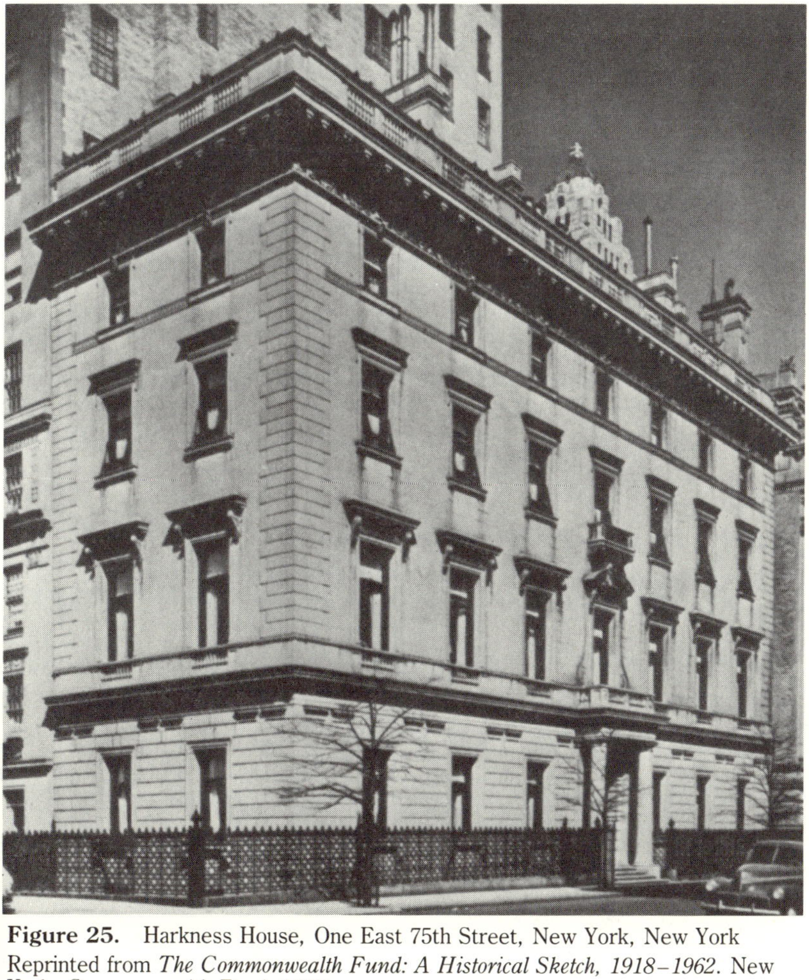

Figure 25. Harkness House, One East 75th Street, New York, New York
Reprinted from *The Commonwealth Fund: A Historical Sketch, 1918–1962*. New York: Commonwealth Fund, 1963.

Program Direction in the 1950s

By 1949 large federal subsidies to medical research and education (by the United States Public Health Service) and to rural hospital construction (through the Hill–Burton Act) caused the Fund to examine its programs and policies once again. Aldrich's report of January 5, 1950, to the directors of the Fund reflected months of deliberation with staff members and consultants about the Fund's future.[3] Suggestions for new fields of support had ranged from cultural anthropology, adult education and fellowships in literature and the physical sciences, to a survey of teacher training, but all appeared to be a rehash of former responses to similar inquiries. Aldrich's conclusion echoed Donal Sheehan's: The Fund's best plans for the future included a concentration on health and medicine, those areas in which it had already built up a reservoir of knowledge and staff experience—if in fact these areas were still fertile ground for exploration.

Aldrich approved of Sheehan's suggestion that the Fund withdraw from support of rural hospitals and of state and county public health units—concentrating public health work in communities by combining hospitals, medical schools, group clinics, and public health centers. Aldrich also wanted to develop Sheehan's plan to help one or more medical schools set up experiments in teaching comprehensive medicine. Two schools were under consideration: Western Reserve University and the University of Colorado.[4] The close relation of psychiatry to comprehensive medicine led Aldrich to suggest that the Fund continue to stress psychiatric work, to integrate it wherever possible with general medicine, and to search for more avenues to encourage psychiatric teaching and practice. Similarly, he would extend the Fund's fellowships for advanced training in psychiatry and public health.

The Fund's support of medical research needed reconsidering: Large federal and private sums were now available for research in cancer, heart disease, and other illnesses, and Aldrich thought that the Fund should turn to specific, relatively neglected areas (for example, dermatology and multiple sclerosis).

Finally, Aldrich saw continued support of the Division of Publications as a desirable course, as it enabled the Fund to publish the results of its work at prices below those of commercial firms.

Decision Making under Aldrich

The Fund's approach to individual grants was completely unlike the process used by a large federal agency. At the National Institutes of Health (NIH), decision making was clear and institutionalized. Outside experts, mainly from academic centers, manned study sections that assigned priorities to all research grant applications. This type of examination assured careful peer review by individuals outside the organization. From the study sections, the applications with their recommendations were sent to the council of each categorical institute, where final decisions were made and a priority number allocated. During Aldrich's tenure at the Fund, however, groups of outside experts were rarely convened. Consultation with outsiders was always relatively informal, through staff members who knew individuals with special expertise relating to a given program.

All grant requests were called "appeals," and were usually in the form of specific proposals. Although a staff member's interest would often stimulate an appeal, most proposals were entirely spontaneous. The fate of every appeal rested with the staff member to whom it was assigned for processing. If he thought the project should not be supported, he would draft an appropriate letter to Aldrich; if he felt the appeal had some merit, he would consult with his colleagues and prepare a memorandum for Aldrich. Once an appeal was accepted on preliminary review, a site visit was arranged. If the project was technical enough, an expert might be added to the visiting team or his views solicited and incorporated into the team's report.

At the NIH weekly staff meetings were occasions for thorough sharing of policy decisions and exchange of views. At the Commonwealth Fund, staff meetings took place only once a month. Aldrich went around the table, calling on each member of the staff in turn to review the appeals in his portfolio, describe their stage in the decision-making process, and give his recommendations for approval or disapproval. There was generally no discussion of administration, past decisions, or future plans. The informal discussions that took place between Aldrich and staff members concerned specific appeals rather than policy.

Approval of an appeal at a staff meeting would be followed by the preparation of a report to the board of directors. Before a board meeting, each director was given a portfolio with every project outlined in a six- to fifteen-page summary, which described the project in simple prose and always included a final section designed to convince the board members of the appeal's importance. Geddes Smith was a master at writing these reports, which had to persuade without giving that appearance. After Smith's death the Fund hired a writer from a popular professional medical magazine, but he never succeeded in producing reports as subtle and informative as Smith's: His were more like advertising copy, too flamboyant for Aldrich and the conservative members of the board.

Aldrich had no formal scientific background, and it was easier to get his approval for a project in medical education than for one related to scientific research. But if the experts said that a scientific project would yield important results, he would usually support it. The area of psychiatric research elicited his greatest reservations. He was always inclined to demur when confronted with programs stressing the psychological manifestations of disease—he had a strong dislike for the whole psychoanalytic concept as a framework for mental health research. One of the largest Fund-supported projects in psychiatric research was directed by Robert G. Heath, professor of psychiatry at Tulane University. Heath was able to obtain a grant because his program was moving in a strictly biological direction. On the other hand, psychoanalytically oriented projects such as those of Milton J. E. Senn at Yale University were difficult to sell to Aldrich, and Eberhart had to work hard to interest Aldrich in these studies.[5]

Throughout his tenure Aldrich struggled with the so-called founder's syndrome. According to Robert J. Glaser, later vice-president of the Fund,[6]

> At the Commonwealth Fund, there were no family members on the board because Edward Harkness had no children, but of course Mac Aldrich was essentially a substitute son for Mr. Harkness, and some of the trustees who were still on the Commonwealth Fund Board when I went on had known him. Accordingly, there was often an enthusiastic response in the case of projects where in earlier years the Commonwealth had given money on the basis that "Ed would have wanted to do this." That term applied particularly to proposals from Columbia–Presbyterian Medical Center and to certain projects at Yale. Mr. Harkness clearly was devoted to both institutions. . . . The problem of those who communicate with the founder and know exactly what they want is a difficult one for foundation officers. It is often very difficult, or indeed, impossible, to refute a statement that this is what the founder would have wanted, especially when it is stated authoritatively by a relative or old friend, but I consider it a detriment to foundation operation.

Except for George P. Berry or David P. Barr, board members seldom commented on the various reports. The board regarded them as Aldrich's recommendations, even though the primary authors were the other staff members. Because the reports had Aldrich's approval before the board saw them, members were in the position of repudiating the president's decision if they rejected an appeal. Board members were careful of Aldrich's feelings, as they recognized his long association with the Fund and had great respect for his opinions. Aldrich did consult with board members on any difficult or controversial issues before submitting a proposal to the board for action.

Berry, dean of the Harvard Medical School, joined the Fund's directors in 1951, becoming the second physician on the board.[7] Berry's invitation was issued in the railroad station in New Haven, Connecticut. Aldrich said that he would come halfway if Berry would meet him halfway—literally. After an hour's conversation, Berry agreed to accept the appointment. His administrative experience was vast: As dean at Harvard, he brought the various elements of the medical school and its associated hospitals together as the Harvard Medical Center. He worked extensively with the Association of American Medical Colleges (AAMC), serving on its council and as its president, and was largely responsible for creating the association's teaching institutes, which united the medical schools of the United States under the auspices of one organization.[8]

Berry never felt that directors tried to push pet projects of their own, but the question of conflict of interest hovers over decisions made by any foundation's board. Glaser, now director for medical science at the Lucille P. Markey Charitable Trust, speaks from years of experience as a foundation administrator:[9]

> In the purest sense, it is probably almost impossible to avoid some conflict of interest in a foundation, given the usual constituency of the board and senior officers. Almost without exception there will be members of the board—and some of the senior officers—who have some sort of relationship with organizations to which grants are made. Most foundations handle this reasonably well by simply having individuals acknowledge their affiliation with a given institution at the time a grant is being considered. In fact, competent legal counsel has indicated that it is perfectly proper for a board member to participate in discussion of a grant, and to indicate his or her view on the strengths of the institution for which a grant is being considered. In general, the individual should then leave the meeting when action is taken, although this is not done all the time.
>
> In some ways, the problem is most serious for a senior staff member, particularly the president or executive vice-president of the foundation. There have been occasions when we have considered grants to organizations with which I have had an affiliation. I have always made the matter known and have not participated in the voting. With a reasonably sized senior staff, one can delegate to his colleagues the responsibility of presenting the matter and can, therefore, at least to some degree, stay at arms' length from the transaction.
>
> My own view is that with care the matter can be handled fairly and without undue advantage being shown a given institution. There is, however, the potential for abuse.

George P. Berry served on the boards of several organizations, including the American University in Beirut, the Josiah Macy, Jr., Foundation, and Princeton University. In his opinion, "The Commonwealth Fund board got its work done about as quickly, as expeditiously, and as well as any."[10]

Aid to Programs in Medical Education

Medicine is an art practiced against a scientific background—a background that enlarges as new techniques and discoveries emerge. During Malcolm P. Aldrich's tenure as president of the Commonwealth Fund, American medical education was following the path laid out by Abraham Flexner in 1910, who believed that progress would be most rapid if the profession had its base in the university, where it could build on a sound foundation of scientific research. With scientific medicine as its objective and the university medical center as its focus, the predominant pattern of this first stage of American medicine was increased specialization.

By the 1940s seven scientific categories were recognized as the basic medical sciences: anatomy, bacteriology, biochemistry, biophysics, pathology, pharmacology, and physiology. To the practicing physician, each was important only as it added to his working knowledge of man as a living organism subject to many environmental influences. As specialized fields of knowledge, however, these sciences were training grounds for investigators and teachers. Newly responsible for developing not only embryo physicians but anatomists, biochemists, and other specialists, the university medical school had to accommodate both views. In the process medical schools acquired full-time faculty of great skill who nevertheless devoted an ever-increasing amount of energy to increasingly specialized disciplines. The result was a fractionation of undergraduate instruction. As the body of knowledge was augmented and the period of training for physicians and surgeons extended, questions were raised about medical education: its duration and content, and its ultimate effect upon the student in training and upon the medical care of the individual patient.

The changes in medicine and society after the close of the Second World War brought concomitant changes to medical schools. Research activities increased, as did financial support of research, particularly from agencies of the federal government; full-time faculties expanded; the nature of patients available for teaching changed as did the patterns of disease; the logarithmic growth of new knowledge was associated with increased specialization in graduate medical education; and the social and behavioral sciences began to win acceptance as legitimate areas of study. This climate of change led medical schools into an unprecedented period of reappraisal and experimentation in the late 1940s and early 1950s—ushering in a period of transition in which the concept of "comprehensive medicine" began to modify the scope and character of "scientific medicine."

The Fund's hope in the early 1950s was that a further phase would evolve, in which "scientific" and "comprehensive medicine" would be melded: The specialist and the generalist would be able to coordinate their individual efforts, and both medical education and medical care would be redesigned to meet the needs of a more sophisticated social demand for widely available, high-quality medical service. Instead, the increasing technological aspect of medicine was making it ever more difficult for the physician to maintain effective relationships with his patients. Because the hospital had become the center of care, medical service to the individual was episodic rather than continual and family-oriented. Intense efforts in medical research at hospitals and medical schools were leading to a lessened appreciation of the patient as the focal point of medicine.

Nor was the medical school able to reverse this trend. The standard curriculum in medical schools in the late 1940s had been built up by agglutination. The first two years were characteristically split into discontinuous fragments, and the student was given little help in putting these fragments together. In most schools one department neither knew nor cared what another taught. No school at the end of World War II had brought the basic medical sciences together as a comprehensive whole. In the clinical years as well, instruction consisted of the contributions of independent departments, which often differed in their pedagogical philosophies as well as in their approaches. Most instruction was given on the hospital wards: Although the majority of patients who were not sick enough to be in bed were seen in the outpatient department, the patients in this department were not as easily accessible to the student, nor were they receiving coherent medical care.

As the 1950s approached, individual efforts by medical schools to deal with the problems of medical education began to coalesce. Beginning at various points in the curriculum, under a variety of names, these programs attempted to provide the student with a better understanding of the complete human being. New aspects included an emphasis on the interrelatedness of the concepts on which modern medicine rests, continued contact with patients beginning in the first year of medical school, and study of the patient's social situation.

Because the medical center had several functions, including training and investigation, it could also be viewed as a laboratory of applied social research. Here the health needs of the individual patient, and of society, could be analyzed along with the relation of the doctor to other health personnel. Some universities were exploring this relationship by studying the medical center's connection to its parent university. The medical center was obviously dependent on the university for its existence, but it was also a vital part of the university's equipment for the study of man. Whenever this broad philosophy of the university medical center's function prevailed, the patient would receive comprehensive care in health and illness; the student would achieve the greatest intellectual, emotional, and social growth; and the teacher would find opportunity for creative expression.

Some schools instituted imaginative curricular revisions that attempted to unify medical disciplines and focus attention upon the patient. Most of these revisions integrated the basic and clinical years of training, and some shortened the training period. But for the most part, these attempts were ad hoc stabs at improvement that ignored the large body of information engendered by educational research during the previous half-century. Schools continued to base their curricular changes on traditional principles of teaching rather than contemporary knowledge of learning. The rigorous criteria applied to scientific research were set aside for "educational experiments" related to curricular revisions—"experiments" rarely developed with an experimental design and offered answers to implicit questions rather than presenting testable hypotheses.

As the university's interest in educational objectives and methods was growing, so was the Fund's appreciation of the need for even greater assistance to medical education as a key to the future of medicine. The Commonwealth Fund's approach to the process of learning in medicine contrasted with these unevaluable attempts at improvement. Fund-supported experiments were designed to improve faculty performance, as well as courses of instruction and the curricular framework of education for medicine.

The Commonwealth Fund's program in medical education represents the legacy of Lester J. Evans. From 1940 until his retirement in 1959, Evans was the senior and most influential member of the Fund's staff, the member most responsible for implementing the Fund's experiments in medical education during Aldrich's tenure. Evans had a real missionary spirit and a philosophy of medical education and health that permeated the thinking of the Fund's staff and of the larger world of American medicine. He pursued this philosophy with great energy, diligence, and patience. If one of his ideas did not at first appeal to Aldrich, Evans would not be discouraged but would put it on a back burner until he could recast it to give Aldrich another view. Through his persistence, he usually obtained approval for the things he considered important.

George P. Berry viewed Evans as an exceptionally creative force within the Commonwealth Fund: "I like to think of Lester as a sponge. He had the capacity to soak up and find out and then talk about different places. Lester would often talk about his last visit to Western Reserve. He knew more about that place than anyone at the school, I think. Lester would go in and track things down and fill up with ideas. Then he'd think about them and put them together. He would often come up to Boston to talk about what was going on in various places: Did I think the Fund would buy any of these things? Then he would get his ducks in a row and go to Aldrich who would buy some things, but not others."[11]

Evans was masterful at asking questions and stimulating conversation without manipulating events directly. Nor was he ever burdened with precommitments about the outcome of his inquiries. He would use a far-ranging dialogue to elicit an institution's capabilities to develop innovative programs: Because he was a good judge of what people would do in relation to what they said they would do, he could target areas and institutions in which the Commonwealth Fund might push the boundaries of inquiry just a little further. Evans also had a good sense of where the power for change lay in various institutions. After reaching an understanding with the institutional leadership, he would explore the possibilities in more detail with junior faculty members. His helpful appearance created an ambiance that led people to talk freely with him, confident that he would not use any information he gained to their disadvantage. This type of inquiry had its detriments, however: Each one of these conversations took a great deal of time. Evans himself had the time to spend because he used all available moments for work: On the train ride to the institution in which he would spend several days, he studied background material, his program of interviews having been worked out in advance by his secretary. During the train trip home, he would make extensive notes for the staff to review.

Evans also thrived on his contacts with other foundations. He was an avid participant in a confidential meeting called by Charles Dollard, president of the Carnegie Corporation, at which representatives of several foundations discussed the wisdom of conducting an independent study of medical education.[12] Evans stressed the utility of the Fund's "back-door" entrance into medical education: Its interest had arisen from a wide range of field activities, and the strength of its programs lay in its day-to-day contacts in the field. The distinguished group of foundation administrators agreed that the Commonwealth Fund's extensive field experience over the years had been one of its greatest assets.

"Medicine" to Evans and the rest of the Fund's staff meant no less than the broad description set forth by Lyle Saunders, an anthropologist at the University of Colorado: "a vast complex of knowledge, beliefs, techniques, roles, norms, values, ideologies, attitudes, rituals, customs, and symbols that interlock to form a mutual reinforcing and supporting system"—a system designated by the term "institution." Medicine as an institution, Saunders felt, was integrated with other major institutional complexes—government, religion, the family, art, education, the economy—into a functioning whole that was "culture."[13]

Evans worried that the "dazzling accomplishments of episodic medicine" were blurring the vistas of comprehensive medicine. If universities and their medical schools did not respond to social pressures for a better health-care system, they would be cut off from the mainstream of educational growth, and medical education would revert to its pre-Flexnerian proprietary status. He hoped that new knowledge of the fundamental aspects of disease mechanisms and of the process of life itself would force medicine to examine the circumstances under which disease and illness occur: "If more people are to live longer, if the threat of disabling illness is lessened because of reorganized rehabilitation activities, if chronic organic diseases are prevented or cured in the classical sense, if the meaning of good mental health is learned, it is natural to establish another set of guidelines pointing in the direction of the social and behavioral sciences. Relatively speaking, these sciences are young, dating from the early part of this century, but only through their integration into medical teaching and learning can the physician's basic service be advanced or even preserved."[14] The continuing advance of medicine depended upon specialization and compartmentalization of knowledge, but this knowledge had to be linked with the integration of university and medical education, improvement of premedical preparation, and teaching in the medical sciences. Evans believed that the Fund's crucial point of attack on the general problems of American medicine should be medical education.[15] There were very few other organizations whose work had taken them into as many varied fields of medicine and health, and over the years, the Fund had come to appreciate the close relationship between medical education and the quotidian distribution of health and medical services.[16] Despite its many-faceted nature, the Fund's overall program had attained exactly the integration that Evans considered most important. Its mental health program had begun as a somewhat isolated and specialized effort for the prevention of delinquency in children, but moved first into the broader field of child psychiatry and from there into general pediatrics and general medicine. Similarly, the Fund's regional hospital plan was its response to the realization that institutions could function alone only up to a point—that their effectiveness is enhanced by working with neighboring institutions. Public health activity had made the staff aware of the opportunities for medical service in the community and of the need to integrate the study of normal growth and development with the study of disease. By the 1950s the Fund's staff was well aware that the life history of the host was as important as the life history of the disease.

To the Fund's staff, correlation of teaching in the medical sciences was an important part of the integration of university and medical education and consequent improvement of premedical preparation. More important than the quantity of physicians being produced was the quality of medical education. To Evans "medical education" spanned the period from high school to the end of residency training, and the staff wanted to integrate the entire educational process, from college to preprofessional and professional education.[17] What kinds of doctors were needed and what was the best way to prepare them? Were there "best kinds" for different purposes and different individuals? Were the right people coming to medical school? How should students be chosen, and what prior educational experience should be required? How could medical teaching build on the student's experience and knowledge? How could the medical sciences be interwoven and related to the care of the patient? How could the break between scientific and clinical courses be repaired? Evans believed that the broadly based Commonwealth Fund program in medical education needed to help the medical schools take a fresh look at teaching methods, to learn more about teaching by studying the learning process. The dominant question was: How could this process become continuous and coherent?

A most pressing question was one of example: How could the medical school effectively demonstrate during the period of training the kind of medical care the student should be prepared to give, medical care that met the patient's needs without sacrificing the values of specialized skills? Furthermore, in providing such care, how could the medical school relate to its surrounding community? The Fund believed that the answers to these questions could emerge if each medical school could approach the problems of medical education in its own way. Certain values were appreciated, however: the necessity for education that focused upon the patient rather than the disease, upon learning rather than teaching, and upon an integrated curriculum rather than individual departmental responsibility.

The Fund was not content to leave the search for answers solely in the hands of the medical schools. Evans said, "As the activities in the field of medical education are developing, it becomes clear that we should not just simply receive proposals from medical schools and universities on which we are asked to act, but, rather, we should establish informal relationships with the universities and medical schools of such nature that we can participate in the early discussions of activities which we may be asked to support later."[18] He envisioned the Fund's staff in an active role, generating ideas for study and identifying the medical schools that might be capable of carrying them out.

A most important type of support was the planning grant, which was given to schools such as the University of Florida (see p. 277), Stanford University (see p. 274), and the University of Kentucky (see p. 298). The Fund hoped that improved facilities and educational programs at these schools would result in better community health care and that local support for medical school and university activities would increase.[19]

The Fund's support of medical education in the 1950s and 1960s focused on two aspects of the process. The first was the management of the increasing body of specialized information essential to the understanding and progress of modern scientific medicine. New technologies were rapidly coming onstream in such fields as immunology and biomedical genetics.

Advances in molecular biology in particular were linking previously separate segments of the biological sciences, and the Fund capitalized on this progress to support projects that integrated teaching among different basic disciplines. Teachers themselves were increasingly able to unify diverse scientific fields; many were well-trained clinical faculty members carrying out research in the basic sciences.

The second was the student's better preparation for his fundamental responsibility in medicine: dealing effectively with patients. Attempts to understand patients' needs were a major consideration in practically all the Fund-supported programs. Programs received grants to focus on the outpatient clinic as a vital area of patient care: a center for integrating community and hospital, for teaching continuity of care and concern for the patient in his social setting. In stressing both the emotional and physical well-being of the patient, all the Fund's programs attempted to shift student attitudes and values toward the patient rather than the disease. One measure of the success of these programs was their ability to establish an interdisciplinary team within the outpatient department of a teaching hospital and to educate students in the use of this team.

The Fund was one of the few organizations interested in what is now regarded as the basis of family practice in medicine—a body of knowledge and a way of thinking that Lester J. Evans saw as good basic training for all medical students. In speaking of the Fund's support of medical education in the 1950s and 1960s, Evans said: "Increasingly we had come to view health and disease in a holistic frame of reference in which the psychological, social, and cultural aspects of human behavior are appropriately related to the biological nature of man and the physical environment in which he lives."[20] This attitude was reflected in the Fund's focus on the ambulatory patient, training of paramedical personnel, and nursing education.[21]

In the 1950s, however, those raised in the tradition of "scientific medicine" saw their profession threatened by the rise of "comprehensive medicine." Many academicians feared that comprehensive medicine was advancing at the expense of the basic sciences. Many were also antipathetic to programs featuring home care and extramural preceptors. Active detractors of comprehensive medicine charged that programs incorporating this emphasis were anti-intellectual and unscientific, encouraging merely the application of compassion, humanitarianism, and common sense. Another frequently expressed criticism concerned the influence of "outsiders"—foundation staff and others who, not knowing the realities of patient care, wished to seduce the medical school deans with large grants to try out their pet schemes on innocent medical students and patients.

Yet proponents of comprehensive medicine were not trying to turn back the clock: No rational person wished to lessen the standard of patient care that had developed from the marriage of science and medicine. The intent was simply to apply knowledge from other areas (such as psychology, sociology, and preventive medicine) to the improvement of patient care. Humanitarianism needed no defense in medicine, but compassion for the welfare and comfort of a patient were not synonymous with an understanding of the social and psychological factors involved in illness. Failure to understand these influences was short-sighted and detrimental to the well-being of the patient.

The Commonwealth Fund was the target of criticism, but much of it was answered in Peter V. Lee's study of nine "experiments in medical education."[22] The "experiments" included studies on the integration of university and medical education (at Johns Hopkins, Northwestern and Boston universities), the teaching of comprehensive medicine (at Cornell University, the University of Colorado, Temple University, the University of North Carolina, and Boston University) (see app. E), the complete reorganization of the medical curriculum (at Western Reserve University), and the founding of a new medical school (at the University of Florida). In all programs, Lee pointed out, the most objective approaches had been used. The best response to the criticism, however, came from the Fund's own record of achievement.[23]

Comprehensive Care in Medical Teaching

The true physician must possess a dual personality, the scientific toward disease, the human and humane toward the patient.
—*James B. Herrick*

"Comprehensive medicine," an attempt to apply all available knowledge to the maintenance of health and the diagnosis, treatment, and rehabilitation of the patient, became part of the medical language of the 1950s.[24] An approach, a focus, an attribute, it implied the mobilization of every resource for the care of the patient; a primary concern for the patient, rather than the disease; a consideration of all factors affecting the patient's health; the application of preventive measures and the early detection of disease; and an understanding of factors that influence the relationship between doctor and patient. The object of comprehensive medicine was to minimize the gap between what was known and what was applied for the benefit of the patient.

Although the term had been coined by a Commonwealth Fund staff member in the late 1940s (probably Geddes Smith or Lester J. Evans)[25] and used extensively by Donal Sheehan, it was only during the 1950s that comprehensive care and medical education were linked: "Medical progressives use the word 'preventive' when they think of what medicine could do before disease develops; 'constructive' when they set positive health as their goal; 'comprehensive' when they, as doctors, deal with people whole instead of in part; 'social' when they feel the pressure of the human environment on the individual and want the doctor to be at least aware of it."[26]

Most of the experiments supported by the Fund attempted to delineate the areas of new knowledge applicable to better patient care, but they used varied approaches to define and teach comprehensive medicine. Cornell University's research-oriented group emphasized the sociology of medical education; the University of Colorado study used psychological techniques to evaluate an experiment located primarily in a general medical clinic of a city hospital; Temple University stressed psychosomatic medicine; at the University of North Carolina, preventive medicine dominated the interdepartmental clinic; and Boston University concentrated on home care.

THE CORNELL UNIVERSITY MEDICAL COLLEGE

Cornell's first program stressing the psychosomatic approach was the Fund-supported "Medicine A," a "Pilot Clinic for a Broader Medical Service." Directed by Harold G. Wolff, this clinic had stimulated better outpatient service and teaching in the late 1940s. Emphasizing the documentation of new clinical ideas by sound investigative procedures, Wolff and his group had raised the tone of medical teaching and practice.[27]

In 1949 David P. Barr, chairman of the Department of Medicine and a director of the Fund, thought the time was ripe to develop a more extensive program in comprehensive medicine. Barr had hoped that psychosomatic medicine would permeate all of medical education and teaching at Cornell. Instead, psychosomatic medicine was developing as a separate area within psychiatry. Care given in the highly specialized clinics of most teaching hospitals was compartmentalized and fragmented, tending to stress symptomatic, episodic treatment. Faculty members at Cornell, including Connie M. Guion,[28] were greatly concerned with what they saw as inadequacies in the treatment of ambulatory patients, and George G. Reader led the Cornell faculty in developing a statement of policy on clinical teaching: "Comprehensive medical care is basically the preservation of health and the prevention as well as the cure of disease. In practice this implies attention to emotional and psychiatric as well as physical factors, and continuing supervision of the patient in clinic, hospital, or home for a sufficient period of time to bring him through convalescence and rehabilitation to an optimal state of health and productivity, and to maintain him in it. . . . The unique features of comprehensive care are primarily related to a method and a point of view."[29]

Continuity was a cardinal principle of comprehensive care, and this required lengthening the time during which a student could follow his patients. Only through regular contact with the same patient over several weeks or months could a student learn how much could or should be done. This kind of patient care implied teamwork among the doctors, nurses, social workers, and medical consultants—teamwork that could be fostered only through frequent meetings and conferences.

In pursuit of a new approach, Barr talked to Lester J. Evans. It appeared to Barr that the Fund was ready to support a project in the area of comprehensive medicine. With Geddes Smith, Barr and Evans wrote up a prospectus presenting an extension of the original concept behind the Medicine A clinic that would reach out to the entire institution.

By 1952 the Comprehensive Care and Teaching Program at Cornell was underway. Directing the program was George G. Reader, later to become chairman of Cornell's Department of Public Health. Reader's longstanding ties to Cornell gave him a sensitivity to what could and could not be done at that institution. He began his career at Cornell as an undergraduate majoring in biology, with training in economics, sociology, and psychology, and he graduated from the Cornell University Medical College in December 1943. A fellowship with Bruce P. Webster and Walsh McDermott followed a tour in the Navy, after which he finished his residency training, working with Barr in the Department of Medicine. Reader next studied immunology with Robert F. Watson and then became a full-time instructor in charge of teaching fourth-year medical students in the outpatient department, the position he held when he was chosen to head Cornell's new program in comprehensive care.

The Fund's first grant was for a planning year, as time was needed to develop strategies for change. Additional grants were given first for teaching and an evaluation of the program and later to study the effects of the program on patients. The core of the program was the Clinic for Comprehensive Care, formed within the highly compartmentalized outpatient department to implement the overall plan of education, evaluation, and research. This new clinic had a full-time administrative and educational staff. It was not a true family clinic, but it focused the work of the general clinics in medicine and pediatrics, and of some specialty clinics, on the central problems of comprehensive teaching. Specialists usually came to the patient and the student, a revolutionary arrangement for all; as a result, the patient was cared for as long as possible in the general clinic instead of being shunted off to specialty clinics. All new adult ambulatory medical patients were first seen in the Clinic for Comprehensive

Care, and appointments were scheduled so that students at each clinic session normally saw one new patient and one or two patients making follow-up visits.

Conferences in psychiatry and comprehensive medicine were part of the program, along with home-care rounds and seminars in which each group of ten students met regularly with an instructor in medicine or pediatrics to review special topics or discuss the management of patients with unusual problems. The program's social worker and public health nurse were both teachers and participants in the clinic's patient-care and research activities. Each student was assigned a patient on the home-care service or a family in the family care program. The student saw the adult members of this family in the medical clinic and the children in the pediatric clinic, but most of the students were able to continue their contact with a patient who had been discharged from the hospital to the home-care service. In addition, some students had the opportunity to follow a pregnant woman through her prenatal period, attend the delivery, and provide postpartum and well-baby care.

The initial appropriation of $2,000 for evaluation had been inserted at the Fund's request. A Fund grant to a similar program at the University of Colorado also contained a provision for evaluation, and Reader was in close contact during this first year with a former colleague at Cornell, Frederick Kern, Jr., who was heading the project in Denver (see p. 231). Kern went to the Educational Testing Service to discuss the evaluation, and Reader to the Bureau of Applied Social Research at Columbia University, where he talked with Charles Glock, the director. Unenthusiastic about taking on an evaluation of Reader's project, Glock changed his mind when he learned about a grant application submitted coincidentally to the Commonwealth Fund by Columbia University's Robert K. Merton, who was requesting support for his studies on the process of professional socialization. Reader's program offered Merton the opportunity to investigate professional socialization in a medical context; Merton would give Reader the sound evaluation that the Fund required.

The sociologists developed a research design comparing students' attitudes before and after the course. Attitudes in each half of the class were compared as well, as one half of the class would take the course in comprehensive care first while the other half was taking surgery. After field work and in-depth interviews with staff and students, the sociologists devised questionnaires to tap attitudes and measure responses to the differential stimuli of the two curricular assignments. Later, these investigations were supplemented by interviews with students in each of the four medical school classes. A separate study of the Cornell faculty was done to determine the climate of faculty opinion.

According to this evaluation, the clinic clearly had the desired effect: For most students, it reversed the usual trend, from first through fourth year, of an increasing preference for patients with definable physical illnesses.[30] The students' professional objectivity and self-confidence were enhanced, and students exposed to the clinic developed greater appreciation for the significance of social and emotional problems of patients than those not so exposed. The effect was short-term, however, and when the students left the program, they tended to revert to concern with diseases rather than patients.

In launching the Comprehensive Care and Teaching program, the staff was wrestling concurrently with the practical operational problems involved in this new approach. Their research was intended primarily to assess the extent to which the program was providing truly comprehensive medical care for patients, but it expanded into many areas relating to the care of patients in general.[31] The program emphasized an objective appraisal of all methods and techniques, rather than a vocational or practical approach, the theory being that through this type of analysis the art of medicine might be made more objective. Investigations included studies of the cost of providing comprehensive medical care and problems in the management of patients with chronic illnesses—including nursing needs, nursing referrals, and the level of medical information among patients.[32] These studies were carried out not only by physicians on the clinic staff but by sociologists, social workers, public health nurses, statisticians, graduate students, residents, and fellows.

The program also dealt with problems of long-term care and support systems that extended beyond the immediate doctor-patient relationship. The home-care program proved to be a useful teaching instrument: Each student had several home-care patients and caring for them developed a great sense of responsibility.[33] Before the program was in effect, it was assumed that the doctor probably knew best about everything, but Evans's needling made Reader realize that others—for example, nurses and social workers—were able to contribute.

The Fund watched the progress of the clinic closely: Annual reports were required, and the Cornell group would meet at the Fund every three to four months. A conference at the Fund to evaluate this and other Fund-supported programs was attended by groups from Western Reserve, Cornell, and Colorado,[34] but nothing could substitute for personal, on-site visits. Although Charles O. Warren of the Fund's staff monitored the program, Lester J. Evans critiqued it. The Cornell group invited Fund staff members to view parts of the program that were going particularly well, but a constant stream of visitors also reported back to Evans. Evans himself spent a great deal of time visiting the project—popping in at irregular intervals to see for himself whether his suggestions were being implemented.

As a recipient of Evans's prolific ideas, Reader found this process helpful. Working with Evans was like working with a colleague; he contributed much that the Cornell group would not have arrived at on its own. Evans's style of "free association" would produce a range of notions, some relevant and some not. Yet Reader never perceived Evans's contributions as interference; when an idea did not fit, Evans did not insist on it. In fact, Reader reports, Evans's activity stimulated a kind of cognitive cross-fertilization. Evans recognized important concepts early and tried to inject them into the thinking of academicians. He was particularly concerned that the program at Cornell emphasize preventive medicine, and he was more aware of the public health model than most others then working in public health.

The program's progress led Joseph C. Hinsey (from Cornell), Ward Darley (from Colorado), and George P. Berry—all deans and active in the Association of American Medical Colleges (AAMC)—to spread the news around. Evans organized sessions at AAMC meetings for the groups involved in the practice of comprehensive medicine. In this way the Fund had a significant effect on medical education. In Reader's words, "A lot of people now would say that they were ahead of their time. They had a lot of seminal ideas, many of which worked out, but the Fund is not given the credit for them."[35]

The Comprehensive Care and Teaching Program's initial five-year experimental period was followed by three more years of support for the clinic's budget and an additional six years of funding for its research; from 1952 to 1966, the program continued almost unchanged. Until the Fund ended its support of the clinic's budget in 1960, the clinic's director had not only important financial resources but budgetary control over key personnel in the program as well. When the Fund's grant ended and the clinic's director lost control of the budget, part-time consultants from the various clinical departments no longer had a sense of allegiance to the program itself. Reader, for example, had a surgeon on his own payroll—a useful arrangement, as the surgeon came when scheduled. Later, when the grant was no longer available and the surgeon was paid by the Department of Surgery, it was harder to obtain his services on a regular basis. A critical coordinating element had been lost: Central control of the budget turned out to be important to the success of comprehensive medicine.

Faculty attitudes at Cornell also threatened the practice and teaching of comprehensive care: The program gave way to the faculty's demand for more time to display the specialties of medicine and surgery. Senior faculty and administration had concluded that early exposure to the various specialties could be accomplished best through electives, and in 1966 the curriculum was altered to allow a four- instead of a six-month rotation in the clinic. In 1969 the curriculum was changed again to make the entire fourth year in the clinic an elective period. One of the electives offered for the third year was in comprehensive care, but only an occasional student chose it and the home care experience had to be abandoned. Studies now under way have led at least one investigator to believe that had students participated in the program for more than one semester, it would have had more enduring effects.[36]

Evans was not discouraged by the program's erosion: He anticipated that the basic ideas of comprehensive medicine would return when social needs exerted a greater influence on decision making in medical schools and in government. The Comprehensive Care and Training Program influenced the attitudes of many student physicians, nurses and social workers, who became accustomed to delivering medical care as a team and saw their patients as individuals. The program was obviously successful in establishing these interdisciplinary teams within the outpatient department of a teaching hospital and educating members in the principles of team practice without detracting from their acquisition of knowledge about disease entities. Turning to social scientists for evaluation provided an early opportunity for the behavioral sciences to collaborate with sciences basic to medicine. Reader believed that the clinic was most important as an early experiment in patient-care research—a term and an area of study that did not become popular until years later.

The Cornell project today would be considered uneconomical. In view of the current emphasis on fee for service, the program's practice of sending the consultants to the patient was a bargain. The Cornell project was one of the first to act on the idea that people's problems were often those of living in society and could not be solved with a medication. The Fund recognized sooner than most that the doctor—and the universities—must be aware of the sociological and economic problems that influence the practice of medicine.

THE UNIVERSITY OF COLORADO SCHOOL OF MEDICINE

The program at the University of Colorado was an unusual attempt to prepare students to give comprehensive medical care through work in a clinic run by a nonuniversity hospital. Collaborating on the program were a state university trying to supply its geographical area with general physicians and a city health department responsible for medical care of the city's poor. The difficulties facing the program were formidable: the city hospital's administrative problems, the faculty's fear that their efforts would be diluted in a secondary teaching hospital, and the nature of the patient population.

Both halves of the team, the medical school and the health department, had improved greatly in the years just before the program began. Since 1930 the medical school had benefited from the cumulative influence of the Child Research Council, a Fund-supported program, which had demonstrated to the faculty the value of consecutive observations. Ward Darley, who became dean at the University of Colorado School of Medicine in 1946, had brought full-time teachers to the clinical departments, eliminating the proprietary atmosphere that had prevailed under the leadership of Denver specialists. Darley fought for the independence of the medical school and with the help of small-town doctors won the confidence and support of the state legislature. The strengthened faculty then began to reorganize the curriculum. The course for first-year students entitled "Medicine as Human Biology" dramatized the meaning of the life span and the problems of human adjustment by presenting growing children and troubled adults to the students. In Year 3 a coordinated course on human disease brought the departments together and eliminated much of the duplication found in clinical teaching. Preventive medicine was taught by a staff that kept in close touch with public health developments. By 1948 the school had decided to stress training for general practice and began to offer residency training in general medicine.

The rebirth of the health department occurred coincidentally. In 1947 a vigorous young man, James Quigg Newton, Jr., was elected mayor of Denver on a nonpartisan ticket. He brought into his official family Florence R. Sabin who, retired from the staff of the Rockefeller Institute for Medical Research, had successfully stumped the state for public health progress. He also placed the city's hospitals and public health services under James P. Dixon, a well-trained administrator. Dissatisfied with the medical care the city was providing, Dixon put forward a new plan, at the heart of which was a general medical clinic.

In 1951 a grant from the Commonwealth Fund allowed these two organizations—the medical school and the health department—to establish a clinic that would provide comprehensive medical services for ambulatory patients at the Denver General Hospital. The general medical clinic would apply concepts of psychiatry and preventive medicine to the individual, the family, and the community. It was also intended to improve the graduate training program for general practitioners and provide a setting for research and evaluation of both medical education and patient care. By 1953 the plans had been refined and the program's goal limited: In a pilot clinic at the Denver General Hospital, students would learn the principles of comprehensive medicine.

The clinic was intended to correct medical school deficiencies that had persisted despite Darley's efforts at reform. Although students were taught that the patient's environment was important, they had no opportunity to deal with it first-hand. Students saw mostly inpatients, and continuity in follow-up was lacking. There was much talk of comprehensive medical care, which Frederick Kern, Jr., the director of the Colorado program, defined as "ideal medical practice," but the school had no sample of it to show the students. The experimental clinic provided students with at least as much fundamental medical knowledge as the traditionally organized clinics, while allowing them to acquire additional skill in psychological and sociological areas. The cultural aspects of comprehensive medical care were not considered as separate entities but as component parts of its philosophy and practice.

The program was run as an experiment from 1953 to 1956. Fourth-year students were divided randomly into two groups: One-half of the class (the experimental group) was assigned to the general medical clinic at the Denver General Hospital and the other to a control group at the Colorado General Hospital. The program's planners attempted to provide a distinctly different experience for each group. Students in the experimental group were encouraged to develop a greater sense of responsibility for the patient and a closer doctor-patient relationship through continuity of student-patient contact and a thorough understanding of a few patients.[37] There was increased emphasis on all of the patient's problems and opportunity to deal with patients in their homes. One of the major differences between the experimental and control programs was an innovative activity in the general medical clinic: Whenever a new patient was assigned to a student, that student became responsible for the care of other members of the patient's family. The clinic itself stressed medical and pediatric problems, as about one-third of the patients were children. Because the clinic's primary purpose was the education of medical students, the number of patients was limited so that students would ordinarily see one new patient and one returning patient at each session.

The same faculty members responsible for ward teaching and clinical research programs in the medical school taught in the general medical clinic. Participating were faculty from the departments of medicine and pediatrics, social workers, and a public health nurse. Representatives of departments including obstetrics and gynecology, preventive medicine, psychiatry, and surgery served as consultants.

The goals of the clinic were reinforced in comprehensive care conferences, additional teaching sessions, conferences on psychosomatic medicine, and seminars on the management of ambulatory patients and the more common medical and pediatric problems. Groups of four or five students were assigned to two preceptors (an internist and a pediatrician), who provided guidance and an opportunity for the students to discuss the philosophy of comprehensive care.

The program's research component evaluated the differences between three classes of students, and the unique internal control used in the program evaluation applied to all three sets. Did the general medical clinic in fact enable its students to acquire as much medical knowledge as those in the control group? Had the experimental group acquired additional knowledge, skills, and attitudes not acquired by the group in the traditional program? What personality attributes held by students might relate to successful performance in the general medical clinic or in the control clinics? What were the reasons for any successes or failures in the attainment of the goals of the clinic? The objectives of the general medical clinic had to be specific and testable, the methods for testing developed, tests administered, and results analyzed. To understand the significance of differences between the two groups, planners had to determine how the experimental experience actually differed from that of the controls, and, if possible, which were the significant discrepancies. The research program also included a study of the individual differences among the students and the relationship of these differences to changes in test performance and to student performance in the general medical clinic.

Special methods had to be devised to measure the variables. One procedure involved a sound film showing a six-minute interview between a doctor and a patient; at its conclusion students were given a test that required the application of medical, psychological, and sociological knowledge. Recordings of student-staff conferences were also evaluated to determine how the teaching differed in the two groups. A number of tests were designed to measure the characteristics of individual students, so that the relationship between these qualities and the student's performance could be assessed.

The investigators concluded that time spent in the general medical clinic did reduce the students' development of increasingly negative attitudes toward comprehensive care without impairing the acquisition of traditional medical knowledge and skill.[38] A "scheduling effect" was also identified: Students were more resistant to the program goals during the second half of the senior year, when they were anticipating their internship, with its orientation toward disease. Both students and staff felt that the patients seen in the general medical clinic offered unsuitable teaching material for a comprehensive care program, as they often presented overwhelming social problems: Patients tended to be old and poor; they were often from broken families; and they were members of ethnic minority groups. According to the participants, these patients showed little motivation to get well and had a high rate of broken clinic appointments. They also had a limited variety of disease entities.

At the conclusion of the formal experiment, the control group was eliminated. Now most fourth-year students worked in the general medical clinic for a six-month period, but for only two or three half-days each week. The remainder of the time they spent in a program combining features of experimental and control curricula—in medical specialty clinics, pediatric clinics, ward work, and clerkships in obstetrics and gynecology. The staff began rigorous screening of patients for admission, opening another medical clinic and seven specialty clinics at the Denver General Hospital in July 1956. With these changes almost all student dissatisfaction disappeared. But after a dispute over finances in 1960 between the city of Denver and the University of Colorado, the hospital cut all ties with the university, ending the program.

In its nine years of operation, the program in comprehensive care at the University of Colorado taught many fruitful lessons. The general medical clinic had set the tone for a higher level of patient care at the hospital. Instead of diminishing the importance of specialty clinics, it had forced the creation of new ones. The faculty as a whole accepted the concept of the clinic as an appropriate environment for fourth-year outpatient teaching. Despite the termination of the hospital's contract, the clinic's influence persisted: The plans for the future university hospital called for the establishment of a similar clinic.

Of greater significance for medical education in general was the meticulous care given to the planning, execution, evaluation, and candid reporting of the research program based on the clinic's work. This work was well conceived and ably executed, and many of the techniques used became valuable to psychologists and medical educators: for study of individual differences among students; for the development of tests to determine changes in students' knowledge and attitudes relative to patient care; and for refining the techniques of observation and description of what actually takes place in teaching exercises.[39] The lessons learned, the solutions found, and the problems uncovered at Colorado would also prove valuable to other medical schools contemplating an evaluation of their educational programs.

The clinic and the research program at the University of Colorado School of Medicine could not have existed without the Fund's support. The general medical clinic was the product of the specific environment in the Colorado medical school between 1946 and 1956. This was a time of considerable change at Colorado; as a result, the clinic took a shape different from that originally visualized. Although not a perfect example of comprehensive medicine, the clinic led the way to improvement in the teaching of clinical medicine and altered the whole concept of patient care in the school. Later evaluation characterized the program as an important experiment in medical education, one that served as a nucleus for important research in the process of medical education and led to fuller acceptance of continuity of patient care, an appropriate student-patient relationship, and concern for the development of interdepartmental cooperation.[40]

THE TEMPLE UNIVERSITY SCHOOL OF MEDICINE

The Comprehensive Medicine Program at Temple University was primarily an intensive outpatient clinic experience for fourth-year medical students.[41] Based on the premise that medical care of patients can be improved by the use of psychodynamic and sociologic knowledge not ordinarily applied in most medical clinics, the program reflected twenty-five years of teaching in psychiatry and psychosomatic medicine by O. Spurgeon English and Edward Weiss.

Temple University's program began in 1953 as a weekly conference for fourth-year students in the medical clinic. Directed by internist William A. Steiger and psychiatrist A. Victor Hansen, Jr., it was unique among educational experiments in that its introduction required practically no modification of the existing curriculum. The change was made merely by introducing a comprehensive care staff into the University Hospital's existing general medical outpatient clinic. When a new outpatient clinic building was completed in 1956, the entire general clinic came under the direction of the comprehensive care staff.

The plan for evaluating the program included an assessment of students' performance and attitude development, but the program's effectiveness was to be tested by measuring its effect on patient care.

As in the Cornell program, the focus was on the patient rather than his disease, and the Comprehensive Medicine Clinic was staffed by a team of internists and psychiatrists. All adult nonsurgical patients came first to this clinic for diagnosis and care, and patients attended medical specialty clinics only by referral from this clinic. The student served as the patient's physician, and each student would see one new patient and a varying number of returning patients each day. Work-ups were reviewed by one of the internists or psychiatrists, depending on the student's assessment of the primary problem, and patients were usually seen at the first visit by both specialists. The faculty preceptors, often assisted by a social worker, helped the student to develop a clear idea of the patient's major problem and the cause of his disability. Because the emphasis was on diagnosis, evaluation, and application of practical methods of therapy, the psychiatrists did not spend a great deal of time exploring childhood origins of current conflicts; rather, they attempted to demonstrate the current manifestations of emotional problems and helped students work out short-term, immediately useful treatment. Comprehensive care conferences were held two or three afternoons a week; depending on the nature of the problem under discussion, the emphasis might be primarily biological, psychological, or sociological.

Although psychiatrists were participants rather than consultants, they made no attempt to emphasize psychiatric theory. Patients were helped to establish realistic short-term goals, and discussions stressed the need for the patient to solve his problems for himself rather than to use social difficulties or emotional background as an excuse for his disability.

As for the students, the staff observed early in the course of the program that they avoided examining their own feelings toward patients. Students were experiencing great difficulty in coming to grips with new patients' problems; they also spent an inordinate amount of time reviewing old patients' charts. Student-patient relationships would not be likely to flourish in the short time that students were assigned to the clinic, so a program was instituted to correct this difficulty. Each third-year student followed a patient with a chronic illness for the entire school year, seeing the patient at fortnightly intervals and discussing problems at conferences. This year-long relationship enabled the students to explore their own reactions toward their patients, and experience in the clinic proved to be useful in preparing the students for their fourth-year training.

Yet even the third-year program required additional preparation. Lectures and seminars on comprehensive medical care were started in the first two years of medical school, and the Department of Psychiatry gave a course entitled "The Doctor-Patient Relationship," in which second-year medical students were led to anticipate some of the interpersonal problems that would confront them in their relationships with patients during the clinical years.

In 1959 the program's emphasis shifted from the care of a single patient with a chronic disease to the supervision of the health care of a family in the immediate vicinity of the Temple University Hospital. The family program allowed the Department of Pediatrics to participate actively in the Comprehensive Medicine Program. The objectives of the family clinic program remained those of its predecessor: Students were encouraged to learn about dealing with patients rather than acquiring specific information about disease.

Studies indicated that the Comprehensive Medicine Clinic did lead students to develop positive attitudes toward the comprehensive approach. More important in view of the program's initial goals was the demonstration that patients cared for through this approach received more help with their physical and psychological disabilities than in the standard medical clinic. One of Hansen and Weiss's early studies involved the analysis of records of all patients whose charts weighed more than one pound. Not surprisingly, most of these patients had functional illnesses; they were being shifted from one specialty clinic to another, receiving symptomatic or supportive therapy for their most prominent current complaint. By spending more time with these patients during visits to the Comprehensive Medicine Clinic, students were usually able to define the basic nature of the patients' problems and in many cases to effect significant improvement in their personal well-being and social effectiveness. The comprehensive approach was eventually an economical procedure, since most patients required much less subsequent medical attention.

An intensive study of a sample of patients in the Comprehensive Medicine Clinic revealed, somewhat surprisingly, that although the student physician frequently felt that he had made little progress with his patients by the end of his six-week service, the patients themselves usually perceived definite improvement in their health within this period. Many of the patients, particularly those with psychological problems, could point to a specific clinic visit at which it became apparent that the doctor had communicated a real understanding of their problems.

THE UNIVERSITY OF NORTH CAROLINA AT CHAPEL HILL SCHOOL OF MEDICINE

In 1948 the state legislature authorized the conversion of the University of North Carolina School of Medicine from a school offering a two-year basic science program to a four-year medical school.[42] The new clinical faculty wanted an interdepartmental general clinic as the core of outpatient teaching and service. Because the Commonwealth Fund's two and one-half year grant in 1952 coincided with the beginning of clinical instruction and the organization of the outpatient department, its contribution was particularly important to the future of clinical teaching and patient care at North Carolina.

Operation of the General (comprehensive-care) Clinic[43] with Fund support began that year with the opening of the North Carolina Memorial Hospital. The clinic was directed by William L. Fleming, who was brought to Chapel Hill from Boston University as chairman of the Department of Preventive Medicine, and T. Franklin Williams joined the team four years later as a program coordinator. The program was staffed by a nucleus of faculty members based in the General Clinic, many of whom had carried their deep commitment to comprehensive medicine from their own residencies. Thomas B. Barnett, for example, was in charge of the pulmonary division in the Department of Medicine. He had been trained at the University of Rochester, where a traditional interest in general internal medicine was emphasized by Professor of Medicine William S. McCann. Students also benefited from the presence of residents in medicine and surgery, who used the clinic to follow patients whom they had treated in the hospital.

Medical students eventually spent half of their final year in the General Clinic and in the pediatric clinic. The General Clinic was the main entry point for new outpatients, and it emphasized continuity of teaching and service. The student learned as much as possible from each patient, following his own group of patients for his entire clinic rotation; the patient received the continuity of care that could be provided by a unified, comprehensively trained staff. On the home-care service each student was assigned one patient unable to attend the General Clinic.

Despite initial faculty enthusiasm, by 1956 the scope of the clinic's activities had begun to shrink as faculty members in this new school became involved in other projects. Many of the faculty (the surgeons, for example) complained that they were being asked to deal with problems outside their particular area of competence—problems that someone else could handle more effectively. Often these specialists were not good teachers of the comprehensive approach, and since the clinic required a staff of almost forty faculty members, the situation created a difficult logistical problem in a small school. Williams perceived a general withering of interest in the clinic, but he could not be certain whether this change related to the clinic's lack of funding.

Over the next two years the clinic changed its focus from teaching students and handling the ambulatory patient problems to health care research. Kerr L. White and T. Franklin Williams ran the clinic under Fleming's direction with the help of a smaller core group from the Department of Preventive Medicine with a commitment to comprehensive care. The clinic's projects included studies of patient referral patterns,[44] and a research workshop organized by the clinic's staff eventually became the basis for the Patient Care Research Section of the American Federation for Clinical Research. Despite the faculty's diminished enthusiasm, the clinic never lost its basic support; it retained about a dozen loyal, active faculty participants, many of whom later left to spread the ideals of the program to other schools.[45] During retreats held by the medical school faculty to discuss medical education, the General Clinic was often the base for discussion well into the 1960s.

Peter V. Lee, who assumed the task of evaluating the Fund's programs in medical education in the late 1950s, believed that the General Clinic at the University of North Carolina had a more significant and central role in its parent institution than any other he had visited.[46] Physically, it was the core of the outpatient department, and because Fleming considered patient care research and outpatient teaching legitimate academic activities, its intimate relationship with the departments of medicine, psychiatry, pediatrics, surgery, and preventive medicine had led to collaborative research activities and educational innovations. Students benefited greatly from this patient-oriented approach largely because all the departments impressed on them in their early years an intelligent appreciation of the doctor-patient relationship and the importance of social and environmental factors in medicine. The Department of Psychiatry participated in the teaching in all four years, and considerable progress was made in integrating the teaching of psychiatric principles with those of other clinical departments.

This Fund-supported clinic set the tone for clinical teaching in the school, resulting in enhanced interdepartmental communication and fewer barriers between the departments. It was unfortunate, Lee thought, that this was a new, small medical school in a predominantly rural southern state, because the lessons of its clinic might have been more widely appreciated had they come from a school whose experience was more widely followed. Still, he believed that the school had made a significant contribution not only to the welfare of the people of the state of North Carolina, but to medical education and patient care throughout the nation. Through a relatively small grant made at a critical time, the Fund helped this comprehensive care clinic meet and surpass its original objectives.

THE BOSTON UNIVERSITY SCHOOL OF MEDICINE

Home care closely related to medical education, another aspect of comprehensive medical care, was exemplified by this Fund-supported program.[47] For seventy-five years medical students at the Boston University School of Medicine had been treating indigent patients at their homes in Boston's South End District. In 1948, when the school established a Department of Preventive Medicine, the Home Medical Service—a four-week clinical clerkship for fourth-year students—was placed under the direction of the new department's head, Henry J. Bakst. The following year the Fund began a decade of support for the Home Care Program, intended to encourage a "consideration of the whole patient in his natural milieu." It also gave students greater responsibility in caring for patients under supervision; introduced them to the problems of general practice; emphasized social and environmental factors in patient care; taught preventive medicine at the level of the individual patient and family; instructed medical students in the use of public and private agencies and facilities in the care of patients; and coordinated medicine, psychiatry, preventive medicine, and other disciplines in a unified approach.

By 1954 several years' experience with improved teaching and patient care on the Home Medical Service led the faculty to introduce the student to a more prolonged relationship with patients and to better integrated clinical teaching. A new Human Ecology Program expanded the four-week rotation to four months by juxtaposing the fourth-year clerkships in pediatrics, psychiatry, obstetrics, and preventive medicine (the Home Medical Service). All four departments cooperated in releasing a few hours each week for the new exercise. The program coordinated approaches to growth and development and to environmental, social, and psychological factors in health and disease. Each student was assigned to a patient late in her pregnancy. During the four-month rotation, the average student was able to see his patient once or twice before delivery, observe the delivery itself, examine the new infant, supervise well-baby care, and participate in postnatal care, both in the clinic at Boston City Hospital and in the home.

When Lee reviewed the Human Ecology Program after five years of Fund support, it was still developing, still feeling its way. In a sense, it had originated prematurely, since for the first several years it received only token support from the Department of Pediatrics and less than full support from the Department of Obstetrics—two of the four participating departments. In addition, no single individual was fully committed to the program and able to give it the time and attention it needed. There was also little or no participation by members of the house staff at Boston City Hospital, nor by the Department of Medicine, and the program was not popular with the medical students, who felt that there was too much emphasis on social and psychological matters. Nevertheless, the patients received it enthusiastically. The students were more spectators than physicians, but for the first time in the patients' experience at Boston City Hospital, each had one doctor who saw him consistently over a sixteen-week period.

The Home Medical Service, in contrast, remained a well-established and valuable part of the medical school's teaching program. When the Fund's grants ended, the university assumed complete responsibility for the service's added supervisory staff. For American medical schools, it was the prototype home-care program. Lee felt that the change in the school in the short ten years since the Fund's first grant should have been a source of great satisfaction to the Fund's staff.[48]

In 1961 the home care and human ecology programs were incorporated into Boston University's new program of accelerated medical education. The combination of the dynamic leadership of Bakst and his staff and the Commonwealth Fund's timely support had set the stage for creative innovation at the university.

Yet the advent of neighborhood health centers in the 1970s led to difficult times for the home care and human ecology programs. The medical school's reorganization of the Department of Community Medicine turned much of its clinical responsibility over to a new Department of Sociomedical Sciences. Although medical students were no longer permitted to provide treatment themselves, the Home Medical Service endured: with a caseload of over nine hundred patients, the service accounts for about 10 percent of University Hospital's inpatient census. Since 1975 the Home Medical Service has provided fourth-year students with experience in adult and geriatric primary care. Its fifteen-member multidisciplinary staff includes nurses, social workers, pharmacists, physicians' assistants, chaplains, and students in the allied health professions. Residents in medicine at University Hospital also rotate through the service, as do geriatric fellows from Boston University and the Veterans Administration hospitals.

The future of the Home Medical Service seems secure: It has recently received a grant from the Robert Wood Johnson Foundation, and the Medicaid division of the state's Department of Public Welfare has approved its application for capitation funding for high-risk patients who would otherwise require nursing home care. Although the goals of the program have changed over the years, its present function is "indeed in keeping with the dynamic ebb and flow of health care and medical education."[49]

The Legacy of Comprehensive Medicine

The Commonwealth Fund programs in comprehensive medical care were innovative for their time, the first to recognize important deficits in medical education and health-care delivery. In emphasizing prevention and focusing on the patient rather than the disease, Lester J. Evans and the other members of the Fund's staff were swimming against the tide: the Fund was trying to develop programs in this area just when many medical schools were turning their backs on comprehensive care, family medicine, and health-care research. More glamorous areas, such as cardiology, were competing for students' interest, and medical faculties were seduced by federal research training grants in medical specialties.

Yet a small group of men and women in the United States, well known to the Fund, did persevere in keeping health-care research alive during the heyday of specialty development.[50] Kerr L. White and T. Franklin Williams of the University of North Carolina had obtained money for this type of research from the Hill–Burton hospital construction program. When a segment of the Hill–Burton program broke away in the 1960s to become the National Center for Health Services Research, White and Williams continued to receive its support. Even after the appeal of the term declined, the idea of "comprehensive medicine" continued to influence medical care and health legislation in the 1960s and 1970s. Principles to regulate levels of care, developed in the Fund-sponsored experiments, were incorporated into the Medicare amendments to the Social Security Act. In planning neighborhood health centers, the Office of Economic Opportunity also took advantage of the Fund's earlier experience in the teaching of comprehensive care. Tax-supported state medical schools developed family-care departments and programs to address the perceived imbalance between specialization and general patient care. Later, during the presidency of J. Quigg Newton, Jr., at the Fund, the concept was revived with the support of community-based health programs sponsored by university centers, with the emphasis once again on teaching comprehensive medicine in an organized ambulatory care setting. The present emphasis on "primary care" is a direct result of the assimilation of the concept of comprehensive care into the American medical system.

Experiments in Curriculum Reform

WESTERN RESERVE UNIVERSITY

In 1950 the Commonwealth Fund appropriated $434,000 to the Western Reserve University School of Medicine to rebuild the medical curriculum under the direction of medical school dean Joseph T. Wearn. The Fund singled out the Western Reserve experiment as "one of the most interesting undertakings" to which it had contributed.[51]

The Fund's leading staff member in this venture was, predictably, Lester J. Evans. Both Evans and the Fund had longstanding connections with the school. Wearn had become head of the Department of Medicine in 1929, and his department had received research project support from the Fund as early as 1930. Since then Evans had visited Western Reserve at least annually.

When Wearn became dean of Western Reserve's medical school in 1945, he presented the broad outline of a new program to President Winfred G. Leutner. A few months later, Wearn sent Evans his plan for a center of teaching, study, and research—what he called an "ambulatorium," a university-based community health center to train first-year medical students in the care of ambulatory patients. The center would offer services to patients living at home and was designed to facilitate care of the patient as part of a family rather than as an isolated individual. Wearn was also interested in the center's potential for prevention of unnecessary hospitalization as well as prevention of disease. Today it might be described as a "model family practice unit."

Roderick E. Heffron was struck by the "better morale of the institution" after Wearn became dean and by his interest in the development of a group practice at the Lakeside Hospital by the Western Reserve staff.[52] On a visit three years later, Evans termed the group of new young heads of departments "just as good as one might . . . find in any medical school."[53] Wearn responded, "A number of the boys have come in to say they enjoyed discussing the teaching of medicine with you and I think you may have sensed in them that we are just about ready for a pretty radical change of curriculum. Indeed, we had a spontaneous meeting the other afternoon and they wanted to know . . . why we can't start our plans right now."[54]

In early 1949 the Commonwealth Fund invited Wearn and his associate dean of student affairs, John L. Caughey, Jr., to a two-day conference in New York to expose the entire staff of the Fund to their plans.[55] The staff's key questions were: How did the Western Reserve faculty define comprehensive medical care and how did they propose to teach it? The group devoted much of the first day to definitions. Abandoning the question of comprehensive medicine, it tried to pin down the many facets of medicine in a wide-ranging discussion. The Fund's staff was pleased to find Wearn and Caughey comfortable with such terms as psychosomatic medicine, social medicine, preventive medicine, community medicine, family practice, clinical group practice, and prepaid group practice. Discussion rambled into many areas, but it was clear that Wearn and Caughey wished to make the curriculum and the entire educational experience subject-oriented and student-centered, rather than department-oriented and professor-centered. The Western Reserve faculty was churning out ideas, and the program needed a coordinator and a planner to capitalize on the readiness of faculty members to participate.

Another year of work was necessary before a budget for a coordinator of curriculum revision was approved, and another nine months passed before T. Hale Ham was on the job. Thomas Hale Ham, who did not have a department affiliation, was made chairman of a newly formed Education Committee, whose responsibility was to implement and guide the staff's thinking about curricular problems. Ham had come to Western Reserve from the Thorndike Laboratory at Boston City Hospital, where he had organized the Harvard Medical School's course in laboratory diagnosis.

Meanwhile, Lester J. Evans was insisting that Wearn and Caughey be very specific about what they proposed to teach and how they proposed to teach it. Granting agencies were not prone to act until they could see a budget, and the size and duration of the budget depended on the plan. Even when the applicant and funding agency had agreed on the feasibility of an experiment and the applicant had asked for planning money, the agency tended to press to see the plan, at least in broad outline, before authorizing the planning grant. When Evans and an associate, Charles O. Warren, made a three-day site visit to Cleveland in April 1949, Wearn was unable to provide details of the means by which Western Reserve would achieve the desired changes in its medical curriculum, even though he had settled in his own mind on the principles. After discussions with Harland G. Wood, the new head of the Department of Biochemistry, Warren was satisfied that curriculum revision was not just "a dean's office pet project" but had the faculty's genuine support.

Warren had difficulty understanding Wearn and the nature of his leadership:[56]

> There is a little something about the man that is enigmatic to me. He isn't the outgoing, extroverted type of person that one might expect in such a situation; rather, he accomplishes a great deal in a quiet and unassuming way. . . . I would expect to have a somewhat clearer notion than I have about his basic philosophy. . . . I have little doubt that the school will continue to develop rapidly under his leadership. . . . I think he makes a particular point of having the faculty arrive at their own major policy decisions whenever possible. . . . To implement his policy, he stimulates informal, frank discussions. . . . I get the impression that he makes a distinct effort to stay in the background as if his major work was done when he appointed these people to take the responsibility of these jobs.

Although Evans's long acquaintance with Wearn and his familiarity with Western Reserve affairs enabled him to offer a more secure view,[57]

Evans believed that the school's development might well consume a decade.

Two months later Wearn sent Evans a proposal that included a three-year budget amounting to $465,200. The new curriculum would be planned and introduced one step at a time. First would come a teaching program integrating the biomedical sciences taught in the first two years of medical school. The second step would integrate the sciences with clinical teaching in the last two years. Departmental barriers would be abolished, along with separations between preclinical and clinical faculty, as clinicians would join the teaching staff in the first and second years, and basic medical scientists would join clinicians in the third and fourth. A final plan was the reorganization of the outpatient departments into a university-based community health center, a portion of the proposal that would call for a new building to house the integrated program some seven or eight years later.

Evans found Wearn's report "not as clear and specific" as he had anticipated.[58] He thought that five years of support would be more sensible, and that the program should consume no more than $50,000 a year, or $250,000 overall. Had it not been for Charles O. Warren, the resolution of differences might have taken some time.[59] Warren's first reaction was that Wearn's proposal represented a long-overdue revolution in medical education: "The Western Reserve group seems to me to be the first to have the courage to tackle this major problem by methods commensurate with the scope of the undertaking." As to the proposed curriculum, he commented to Evans: "How is it supposed to proceed? What we need most at this point is a report of the curriculum committee which presumably deals with these varied questions. We do not know whether this report has been given to the faculty. If not, why not? Does this suggest less agreement on basic issues than we thought existed?"[60]

Evans arranged for Wearn and Caughey to meet with him in New York to work out final details. It was too late to draft a formal statement for the board meeting in October, so the matter would have to wait until the next meeting, in January 1950. In the fall of 1949, Evans had one remaining concern: "The principal . . . hazard I see in the program as proposed is the division between the teaching of the laboratory sciences and the social, psychological, and other aspects of . . . human behavior as steered primarily by Dr. Caughey. In spite of . . . arguments to the contrary, I still think there is a dichotomy here which may get them into trouble."[61] The formal proposal that Wearn intended to offer contained a revised budget totaling $50,000 for the first year; $87,000 for the second; and $100,000 for each of the next three years, for a total of $437,000. This was considerably more than the $250,000 that Evans had suggested earlier. The principal items were a $12,000 annual salary for the coordinator; $6,000 each for two physicians who would act as participant-observers, taking the entire course with the students; salaries of a physical anthropologist, a clinical psychologist, and a social worker-sociologist to teach in the introduction to clinical and social aspects of medicine; stipends for students' summertime participation in teaching experiments; money for revision of manuals; and salaries for additional instructors in the second year.

Evans felt that Geddes Smith, a nonphysician, should present the Western Reserve program to the board of directors. To prepare for his presentation, Smith made two visits to Cleveland to review all aspects of the Wearn proposal. Smith was not pleased with what he was being asked to defend: "I am puzzled by what appears to be the complete lack of any sort of tentative concrete program for the second year. The two memoranda sent us by Caughey are both defined as relating to a single year's work. I don't see where they go from there. Is this clear to any of the rest of you?"[62] Smith concluded that "because this has been taking place under the leadership of a dean who is a factual rather than philosophical man, there is strong emphasis on structure and method . . . and we are therefore presented with what might be called an instrumental rather than a philosophical approach to the reshaping of medical teaching."[63]

To the contrary, Wearn had strong ideas about the preparation of the student for his responsibilities as a physician.[64] He was devoted to intellectual freedom, and his philosophy of education centered on the long-neglected need to achieve a balance between humanism and science, to develop the student-physician's character along with his knowledge and skills. When the Western Reserve program was well under way, Wearn said in his presidential address before the Association of American Physicians:[65]

> It has been my experience that whenever medical educators grapple with the basic principles of teaching medical students, they inevitably are forced to ask themselves what kind of graduate they want to turn out. Until this question is clearly faced and answered, changes in curriculum content, methodology, etc. lose much of their validity. This ubiquitous question, seemingly simple, is a very baffling one, and was met in our discussions by a wide variety of answers. It was only when one of our hematologists came forth with the idea that a medical student at graduation should be the equivalent of the "undifferentiated blast cell" of the bone marrow that a starting point appeared to be found. . . . Endowed through its genetic factors, the cell probably develops enzyme systems enabling it to metabolize and synthesize at an extremely rapid rate. . . . With amazing speed it removes tagged amino acids from the bloodstream for the growth and development of the cells—among them the undifferentiated multipotential blast.

The medical student, said Wearn, enters as the counterpart of the primitive cell of the bone marrow and in medical school develops his "enzyme systems." Wearn noted the apparent increasing emphasis on arming the student with basic concepts; enriching his powers and skills; developing his capacity to obtain, integrate and critically analyze pertinent data; indoctrinating him in ideals, integrity, and moral responsibility, certainly in great part by example. And if, in addition, he is imbued with true humility, a spirit of service, sympathetic understanding, and compassion, he will have the vital factors for growth to the multipotential blast stage. These basic principles are as essential for growth in the student as the growth factors are in the cell, and they must be kept in sharp focus wherever the teaching is carried out—in laboratories, wards, and ambulatory facilities.

The most important "enzyme system" in the student is his S. E., or "self-educating enzyme." This, Wearn emphasized, is oxidative and requires potent catalysts and an enormous amount of energy to guarantee its continuation. Most students are resistant to it. It may be inhibited by other enzymes, particularly S. F., or the "spoon-feeding enzyme," which is fermentative rather than oxidative and requires little or no energy.

Wearn did not want to impose the dean's will on the faculty. While construction of Western Reserve's new curriculum was in progress, Wearn did not describe his model physician, nor did he state clearly the outcome he hoped for.

Smith recognized that once begun, this program would have to be seen to the finish. He was reassured that the medical school had committed itself to taking over the cost of the new teaching program when the Fund's grant expired. During December 1949 Smith completed a document for presentation to the Fund's board of directors, a thoughtful, perceptive outline of both the present and the future of the Western Reserve program. He stressed the complementary temperaments of Wearn and Caughey—one practical, the other idealistic. He also concluded that the faculty was young, vigorous, and united to an unusual degree:[66]

> The school has worked out a realistic plan—unique in the Fund's observation—which is well calculated to accomplish its ends: to relate medical education more closely to the patient's needs; to integrate the medical sciences with each other and with clinical training; to help students think. . . .
>
> The plan will not bring about the millennium in medical education. There are laggards on the faculty who, though they are in the minority, may dilute the effect of the changes that are seen to be needed. There may be overenthusiasm for certain strands in the teaching program. No revolution is wholly successful, nor is this the only way in which the teaching of medical schools can be made coherent and fruitful. It is a logical way for Western Reserve, as the school is now constituted, and shrewd planning has gone into it. . . . The essential fact is that Western Reserve offers a plan to do a

thoroughgoing job in modernizing medical education. Other schools have talked of such a job but have never yet attempted it on any comparable scale.

At its meeting on January 19, 1950, the Fund's board of directors approved a total grant of $434,000, only slightly less than Wearn's first request of $465,200.

The staff of the program at Western Reserve recognized that piecemeal changes were not going to solve the school's basic problem, and the coordinators of the curriculum committee had set about remaking the teaching program from the ground up. Subject matter was selected, arranged, and assigned to qualified teachers in accordance with their capacities and without regard for departmental classifications. The new plan required the entire rescheduling of the student's time for two or three years, the planning of new experiments, the rewriting of laboratory manuals and textbooks, and the redistribution of faculty time between teaching and research. The student was to feel that he was studying not anatomy, nor physiology, nor biochemistry, but medicine. Each part of his experience would reinforce all the others; nothing would be finished and cast aside. Theoretical work, laboratory work, and contact with patients would move forward together in a natural sequence that fitted the student's learning process, so that his growing understanding of people and his increasing sense of clinical responsibility would be his strongest motives for mastering the necessary scientific underpinnings.

Among the initial innovations was a course called "The Introduction to Clinical Medicine," taught by an internist long interested in individualizing the patient, a physical anthropologist concerned with constitutional differences, a psychiatrist, and occasionally a social worker. Together they trained the student to notice the differences between individuals, to learn something about the reasons for people's behavior, and to realize that the practice of high-quality medicine precluded treating patients by rote or routine. Patients were presented early in the course and frequently thereafter to help students learn how to appraise an individual, to illustrate problems studied in the basic sciences, and to show the impact of illness on both the individual and the community. The first two years in this integrative program taught the sciences in unit laboratories; laboratories in separate departments were abandoned, as were departmental lectures. Teaching and laboratory work were combined to facilitate the study of systems, as for example in the study of the circulatory system, which coordinated the work of several departments.

Because Wearn and Evans shared similar views of the ideal physician and the goals of medical education, this integrative program was an ideal blending of the philosophy and aims of the dean and the foundation executive.

Evaluation of the Program: The new teaching plan was put into effect for the class entering in September 1952, but the faculty at Western Reserve began to think about a means of evaluating the program as early as 1951. In April 1952 John H. Dingle, professor of preventive medicine, was appointed to head a Subcommittee on Evaluation. Although Harland G. Wood told the faculty that "Evaluation of the program is an integral part of the experiment," he appeared to be more concerned with operational than with experimental research, since he intended to study student and teacher performance in achieving "the objectives of correlated teaching."[67]

In November 1951, after a visit to Cleveland, Evans discussed the question of a controlled experiment: "Should Western Reserve under its new curriculum be compared with other schools? Should there be an experimental control within their program? Or, should it be judged as a matter of before and after . . . ?"[68] Perhaps a ten-year evaluation period was necessary so that a study could be made of graduates after they were established in their careers.

Wearn, Caughey, and particularly Ham were prone to refer to the new program as an "experiment in medical education" and to speak of a "research" approach to its evaluation.[69] But it was not specified whether this was a scientific or a social experiment, even though they were speaking mainly to scientists and physicians trained in the scientific method and accustomed to controlled experimentation.

Over the next seven years, the Fund's staff and Ham worked together on the evaluation process. The staff believed that T. George Bidder, a pharmacologist and a member of Dingle's evaluation committee, had the right approach to both the opportunities and the hazards of an experimental study. He favored comparing students of the class of 1956 with the classes of 1951 through 1955—the "before" group—and with graduates of other medical schools having curricula controlled by departments and taught by disciplines. In his view National Board examinations could be used to compare performance if Western Reserve could find cooperating schools and employ its own evaluation devices. He was well aware that the major problem was defining a suitable baseline from which to measure deviation, and he realized that this definition would be complicated by the shifting of any reference points as the curriculum continued to change.

In its first report, in May 1953, the Subcommittee on Evaluation considered the students' development in medical school, comparative studies, and career studies.[70] Development would be assessed by observation and description; comparison of performance through National Board examinations; and career studies through appraisal of the graduates' choice of career, medical performance, and skills. The general proposal was not acted upon by the committee on medical education or submitted to the general faculty, for within the next month the Fund opened up a "remarkable opportunity" for Western Reserve to join the Fund-sponsored program at Cornell in collaborating with Columbia University's Bureau of Applied Social Research (BASR) in a study of student behavior. The Western Reserve class of 1957, which entered medical school in 1953, was the first of three to use the BASR questionnaire.

The struggle between proponents of a scientifically rigorous evaluation and those supporting a more descriptive one continued into 1953. Wearn was not alone in his tendency to equate continuing change with progress and improvement, a reasonable reaction after many years of laboring with an undesirable system of authoritarian medical teaching. An objective study was needed, however, to evaluate the true worth of the changes. Dietrick and Berson elucidated the first point of view:[71]

> To the majority of medical schools, the curriculum is a matter of vital concern. Shifts and changes are constantly being made in the content and duration of the whole and of its separate parts. New programs are frequently tried, and it is claimed that they are experiments. Where, however, is there evidence of a planned, scientific approach, in which the results are measured by their effect upon the student in comparison with carefully established controls? Little or no evidence is to be found throughout the country of real experiments in medical education, even though experimentation and research are part of the armamentarium of medicine. Even when circumstances bring about a situation that would permit of a real experiment, with ready-made controls, the experiment is not carried out. . . . There is a real need for such experiments in medical education and in the study and testing of teaching methods. Too much reliance is placed on tradition and authority.

On the other hand, this appeal does not reflect a real understanding of the limitations of sociologists and psychologists in their studies of human behavior. Robert K. Merton was a spokesman for the other side: "For the most part, the continuing studies [in medical sociology] do not meet the strict requirements to which Dietrick and Berson refer. . . . Generally, the studies are more nearly like methodological studies in natural history and ecology than like laboratory experiments. But studies of this kind are far removed from casual impressions and, it is believed, provide a basis for sound estimates of processes through which the student develops into a physician. Inquiries of this kind can serve also as a useful prelude to more rigorous experimental study."[72]

Those responsible for the innovations in medical education were interested not in experiments in terms of process—to them evaluation meant judgment of outcome. So it was at Western Reserve. Fund staff members Charles O. Warren and John C. Eberhart were sharply critical of the activities of the evaluation committee. Warren met with the subcommittee in November 1953: "Everyone realized that the payoff is going to come some five years or so after the students have completed their internship and residency training and are firmly established in whatever fields of medicine they elect. Another point that is generally understood is that the term evaluation is best applied to this long-term assessment of the program. . . . The evaluative aspects of the program as one goes along are best described by such terms as description and analysis . . . I raise the question whether, in addition to . . . looking forward . . . there is also an immediate and recurring job in looking backward . . . and attempting to arrive at some provisional analysis of how things have gone."[73]

Warren returned to Cleveland alone in April 1954; on a second visit the following month, he was accompanied by Eberhart, who in a lengthy memorandum criticized the subcommittee's report to the Committee on Medical Education in May 1954 as lacking in "any very systematic review of the problems or objectives." He believed in the importance of this issue because a program can be strictly evaluated only in terms of what it seeks to achieve. Insofar as objectives are not known, not clear, or not agreed upon, it is difficult or impossible to assess the effect of change. Eberhart concluded that evaluation "has perhaps not received the single-minded attention which would be given to a research project of comparable magnitude. . . . There has not been enough organized and systematic thinking about this problem." He felt that the subcommittee had "persistently postponed the setting down of a list of specific objectives."[74]

In 1953 Milton J. Horowitz had begun a study of student behavior in the class of 1957; he intended to observe twenty students and their continuing relationship with their preceptors over a four-year period, reviewing the situation five years after graduation. With Joseph L. Brozgal, a psychologist, and Joseph W. Eaton, a sociologist, he also observed first-year students in preceptoral groups.[75] Eberhart had touched a sensitive area involving the conflicting viewpoints of academic physicians and social scientists as to the nature and function of research in the "applied social sciences." Of Horowitz, he said, "I was not entirely satisfied that his work was as tightly structured as I would like to see, even though I must admit at the same time that . . . we are by no means certain that any of the evaluation programs we are now carrying out will provide the perfectly clear and unambiguous answer to the question: Are these new programs worthwhile?"[76]

These conflicting opinions fell in the lap of Charles O. Warren, who was responsible for follow-up of the Western Reserve program. He concluded that all the evaluations in progress were centered on one biological truth: The student's response to the program depended on his individual make-up and background. "There was practically no effort to interpret these data in terms of the effectiveness of the program. . . . Furthermore, the data were not even presented in such a way as to make such interpretations easy for the reader. . . . I made a dozen or so notes on each of these papers and then went over them with Horowitz and Brozgal."[77] Warren aired his uncertainties with Ham and twelve faculty members from the Committee on Medical Education, the Subcommittee on Evaluation, and Horowitz and Brozgal. Warren later wrote: "I said, in effect, that it seemed to me there was some misunderstanding: The object was evaluation. Investigators were not attempting it. The committee was not attempting it. As might be expected, this precipitated a full and vigorous discussion, and about all that can be said for it at this point was that it got all the cards on the table."[78]

The outcome of this meeting was Ham's recommendation to the committee that the school set up a Division of Educational Research to continue the evaluation of the educational program; Wearn asked the Commonwealth Fund for additional support, and the Fund agreed to provide almost $80,000 for this expanded evaluative effort. The dedication of the Commonwealth staff to monitoring this program seems to have had a salutary effect on the Committee on Education: It was forced to come to grips with the problem of evaluation and the Fund's recommendations. Over the next year Wearn sought the right man to direct this new division, but none of the people that he thought desirable were available. More than a year passed before he turned to T. Hale Ham, who had wanted the job all along.[79] After a sabbatical leave, Ham returned in 1959 and began to tackle the problems of evaluation. His work in this area continued until his retirement in 1974.

Most of the original questions about educational research remain unanswered or unanswerable today. The small staff of the division published several studies under Ham's direction, many of which appeared in the *Journal of Medical Education*. Most were of no unusual significance. Ham and his staff did not play a dynamic role in Western Reserve's formulation of a second new curriculum between 1959 and 1968. As time passed, the division made its most important contributions by serving as a consultant to faculty members interested in improving their teaching methods through educational science, and particularly in its investigation of the relevance of the National Board examinations to the program.

The value of a system cannot be measured while it is changing, no matter how good the method of evaluation. Ham concluded that change had been built into the organizational structure of the school of medicine at Western Reserve largely because the general faculty had remained the policy group for instruction since 1946. He felt that change was inevitable, essential, predictable: a steady state itself. Although the architecture of change could be orderly and the basis of change could be objectives, results, and evaluation, the process of change was always difficult and frequently painful.[80] In the end, Ham and his group did not succeed in completing a satisfactory evaluation of the Western Reserve experiment, any more than did those evaluating the curricular changes that followed at other schools.

By 1964 further growth at Western Reserve hinged upon expansion and modernization of clinical facilities. Plans included two new buildings for the school of medicine, one of which would contain a health sciences library. The Fund made a contribution to the cost of new library space, contingent upon the school's raising the remainder of the $8 million needed.

The following year the Fund awarded a grant to advance the main projects of the Division of Educational Research, the first of which was a comparative analysis of the professional careers of the 771 Western Reserve medical graduates trained under the new curriculum. The second was a cooperative effort among twelve medical schools, including Western Reserve, to test and develop new teaching materials, while the third encouraged Western Reserve's plans to base the curriculum of all four years of medical school on the study of the body's systems.[81]

The program at Western Reserve was reviewed in 1959 by Peter V. Lee, who believed that as a whole it had succeeded, as its initial objectives had been fully attained and even surpassed.[82] Medical students were gaining experience in a family clinic, looking after mothers and children, some fourteen years before the Millis and Willard reports outlined a curriculum for the training of specialists in family practice, and attention to ambulatory care antedated by ten years Kerr L. White's introduction of the term "primary care." At the same time, the scholarly productivity of the faculty had kept pace, and the reputation of the school as an academic institution of the first rank had grown steadily.

Without Wearn's leadership, none of these changes would have come about. He, Douglas Bond, John L. Caughey, Jr., Thomas Hale Ham, and Harland G. Wood had the drive, the diversity of talent, and the loyalty to their mission to make the new plan work, at a time when the general attitude among medical educators was that "changing the curriculum in a medical school is like moving a graveyard." The new curriculum at Western Reserve began with the assumption that because it is impossible to learn everything there is to know in medicine, the product of medical school should be an undifferentiated physician educated to think scientifically and imbued with humane concern for the individual patient.[83] The result was the transformation of a dull, departmentally entrenched institution—where intense competition for grades created a hostile environment for students—into an exciting, vigorous, and intellectually stimulating place for students and faculty alike, a school where conflict between student and faculty gave way to a relationship in which students were treated as colleagues.

Several fortuitous circumstances made possible the sweeping curricular change at Western Reserve:

—The almost adversarial environment for both students and faculty was ripe for improvement. The faculty was remote from the students, and competition rather than comradeship prevailed among the students themselves.
—The dean was an especially sensitive and capable individual, who was able to perceive the need for change and implement it.
—One unique circumstance was assisting the idea of reform. The dean had the opportunity in a short period of time to replace almost all of the entrenched departmental chairmen with young, vigorous men who had the zeal and dedication to restructure the school's curriculum.
—The experiment was supported by a foundation whose staff was enthusiastic about the dean's proposals.
—The program's director was a capable and effective leader.

Even so, not all aspects of the program succeeded. Clinical and preclinical instruction was never integrated as thoroughly as the planners had hoped. The greatest failure was in the design of the basic medical, surgical, and pediatric clerkships intended to give the student clinical experience in a real-life setting. More successful was the group clinic, which took whatever ambulatory patients appeared for medical treatment, regardless of specialty; this clinic offered a more practical approach to the outpatient department as the intersection of hospital, community, and medical school.[84]

Western Reserve University received over $3.6 million from the Commonwealth Fund between 1950 and 1978. The university's program was a showcase for medical education, capturing the imagination of educators and leading the way to experimentation and change in almost every medical school in the nation. Lee believed that the faith and vision of the Fund's staff had been well rewarded by Western Reserve's record of achievement. The relationship between the Commonwealth Fund and the Western Reserve University School of Medicine was an example of what can come of philanthropic and institutional cooperation in an area of mutual interest.[85]

THE DUKE UNIVERSITY SCHOOL OF MEDICINE

In supporting the curriculum revision at Duke University, the Fund helped a new project build on the experience of a similar, earlier program. Planners of Duke's new medical-school curriculum were able to take advantage of Western Reserve University's experience, as Thomas D. Kinney, a member of Duke's medical faculty, had been at Western Reserve during its curriculum reform. He had come away with clear impressions of the system's practical deficit: Because most students were not familiar enough with the language of medicine used in the interdisciplinary courses, presentation of core material in traditional fields was necessary before students could be exposed to integrated teaching. (Duke's solution was to alternate preclinical with clinical years.) By building bridges between the university and the medical school, Duke's programs developed students' technical competence and proficiency, the proper attitudes peculiar to the practice of medicine, and an appreciation of the broader social and service responsibilities of the profession.

The basic-sciences segment of the first year was designed to meet the needs of a student body increasingly heterogeneous in its educational background. It offered clinical and basic science education simultaneously, permitted the student to explore his own intellectual preferences and capabilities, allowed study of selected areas in depth, provided greater freedom of course selection to encourage early career decisions, and achieved better integration of the medical school curriculum with residency training and the practice of medicine.

The Biomedical Research Training Program: In 1958 the Commonwealth Fund gave Duke University a grant of $225,000, principally for additional personnel in some of the newer fields of biomedical science such as biophysics, genetics, and neurophysiology.[86] Faculty members in these fields would join others from the medical school and science departments of the university in offering seminars on a wide range of topics and supervising the work of medical and graduate students in a new unit laboratory. This laboratory's facilities would supplement a program of intensive training and research in the natural sciences fundamental to medicine and biology.

At a time of increasing need for trained research personnel, Duke viewed its new Biomedical Research Training Program as an experiment in the integrated teaching of the basic sciences, a means of improving medical research and education, and a logical move toward closer relationships between the medical school and the university. To provide the physical facilities for this new program, the Fund's award had been preceded by grants from the Markle Foundation and the National Institutes of Health. This program gave a limited number of medical students and postdoctoral fellows an especially organized academic year without either delaying the student's graduation from medical school or increasing the cost of his medical education. Postdoctoral fellows could combine a year in the training program with a fellowship year in one of the medical center laboratories, possibly the first of a several-year investment in postdoctoral research training; the program also gave the clinical departments an opportunity to engage junior faculty members for a year or two before they undertook their clinical and teaching responsibilities.

Directed by James B. Wyngaarden, associate professor of medicine and biochemistry, the program quickly attracted graduates of other medical schools along with medical students from Duke. Within two years sixteen medical schools had sent visitors to observe the program and over 100 additional written requests for information had been received. The program became an important bridge between Duke's medical school and the university's science departments, and by 1961 it was considered an unqualified success at the postdoctoral level.[87] The postdoctoral fellow was a mature, serious, settled individual who had gained a measure of satisfaction and competence in a clinical area, had assessed various opportunities in medicine, and had decided to seek training to qualify himself as a clinical investigator or occasionally as a full-time worker in one of the basic sciences. Even students who eventually decided upon full-time careers in general or specialty practice were rewarded. They had gained some of the attributes of a good physician: a point of view and a sharpened ability to ask questions and think critically.

The enthusiasm of the postdoctoral fellows suggested that the program might serve as a model for the formal education owed by a university hospital to its resident staff. The impact on the medical students, however, was not readily susceptible to evaluation. The program was designed to offer prospective clinical investigators a degree of sophistication in the biomedical sciences that they would otherwise have to gain painfully over many years, to acquaint them with the thought processes of the biological investigator, to liberate them from the slavery—so common even among successful investigators—to a single technique. Their future success as investigators remained to be determined, but this aspect of the experiment was without controls, and evaluation even ten or twenty years later would be difficult at best. The Fund's staff hoped that at the very least, the postdoctoral fellows would be better prepared for an investigative career than their predecessors.

So striking were the program's secondary benefits that they threatened to eclipse its prime purpose. Reintroducing this group of students into the wards and clinics fanned the spark of inquiry and resulted in perpetual questioning of the validity of even the most routine clinical procedures. Also unexpected was use of the program by members of the faculty as a means of intellectual "retooling" during a sabbatical year.

Duke's faculty hoped that increased awareness of the problems of medicine among physicists, chemists, zoologists, and other faculty outside the medical school would also arouse their research interests while their special knowledge was transmitted to medical students and faculty. At a time when physics and chemistry permitted an increasingly rational understanding of the biology of man and when the application of these sciences had rendered meaningless the barriers between the classical biological disciplines, it was fitting that the medical school should truly be "of" and not merely "at" the university. The new research training program facilitated this process at Duke University.[88]

Curriculum Reform: Development of the Biomedical Research Training Program coincided with a general time of transition at Duke. The postwar growth of the medical school and the hospital had necessitated extensive planning for expansion of physical facilities. Between 1959 and 1961, Duke's first dean, Wilburt C. Davison, had retired along with several of the departmental chairmen. Davison's successor, Barnes Woodhall, had emphasized the need for a management consultant study, and when a report in 1961 stressed the necessity for strong basic science departments in a medical school of national reputation, Woodhall was determined to provide the leadership for its resolution. Deryl Hart, the university's new president, had been chairman of the Department of Surgery, and he too was interested in establishing closer relationships between the medical school and the university.

In this atmosphere of change at the end of 1961, a group of medical-school department chairmen turned their attention to the enduring problem of the curriculum. The group, which included Philip Handler (professor of biochemistry), Eugene A. Stead, Jr. (professor of medicine), Thomas D. Kinney (professor of pathology), and Jerome S. Harris (professor of pediatrics), agreed that the present curriculum was too rigid: Students were not allowed to vary their courses to suit their choices from among the many careers available to physicians, nor did they have the opportunity to learn one field in depth. The chairman also recognized that most medical students endured the first two years of the curriculum with frustration. A student's image of a physician was framed by his early contact with doctors, and he arrived expecting to learn something promptly about clinical medicine. For the students the basic sciences appeared less a preparation for clinical education than a series of hurdles to overcome on the way to becoming a physician. Only years later, after experiencing the realities of clinical practice and realizing the limitations of medical knowledge, did students recognize the importance of the material in the early basic science courses. By then, however, the demands of practice and family finances precluded any opportunity to return to scientific study.

To prepare a proposal for presentation to the entire faculty, Woodhall appointed an ad hoc committee of Stead, Kinney, Harris and the new professor of physiology, Daniel C. Tosteson. Many far-ranging discussions produced a revised version of the original plan, which was circulated among the faculty in the spring of 1962 and explored at a series of faculty retreats.

The new curriculum would condense the material of the first two years into a single year and emphasize the foundations of each of the medical sciences. In the second year, the clinical departments would offer students abbreviated rotations, each department determining for itself the best mix of didactic instruction with ward and outpatient clinical experience. Students would then return in the third year to the in-depth study of one or more areas of the basic sciences and in the fourth year would select clinical electives correlated with their career goals.

To make the curriculum as flexible as possible, this draft suggested that the student be free to arrange his work in the third and fourth years in any sequence of clinical and preclinical experience that he chose, so that these years would represent a single integrated learning experience if the student so desired. The third-year program might involve concentration on one or more basic-science electives, particularly through enrollment in the research-training program or in a basic-science graduate program. In the fourth year, the student was urged to engage himself in a field other than that of his chosen internship. At the very least, experience in two clinical fields was required. Although close contact between student and faculty advisor was considered essential to the success of the proposal, responsibility for the integration of medical knowledge rested with the individual student.

With the completion of this revised curriculum, the ad hoc committee was discharged, and the following year a Committee on the Curriculum chaired by Herbert O. Sieker began to prepare the final plans. Beginning in 1963 this committee coordinated departmental plans for curriculum revision with two subcommittees, one concerned with the first and third (basic science) years, and the other with the second and fourth (clinical) years. Next, a detailed curriculum was hammered out for outside criticism; finally, financial support had to be found. In 1964 William G. Anylan, the new dean of the medical school, approached the Fund's president, James Quigg Newton, Jr., for support of this proposal. Although the major funding for the elective curriculum would come from the continuing contributions of Duke University and the Duke endowment, new grants for additional faculty in the basic sciences were critical to the program's success.

The planners needed money for nine new positions during the first five and one-half years of the program's operation: The Fund was asked for $750,000. The Fund's staff sent the curriculum proposal to several medical educators, who turned in favorable reports. The reviewers recognized the quality of the faculty at Duke and the program's radically experimental approach to problems that medical educators had long acknowledged but not yet effectively addressed.

The Commonwealth Fund's staff paid particular attention to the critique of Joseph T. Wearn, by then dean emeritus of the Western Reserve University School of Medicine. He applauded the clearly experimental nature of the plan but wanted the Fund's staff to be certain that thorough planning had preceded the proposal's submission. Wearn cautioned that only such planning would allow the Duke faculty to cope with the many unanticipated problems that were sure to tax their creativity. He also questioned whether the curriculum would in fact encourage early career decisions, since many medical students were prone to vacillate. Recognizing that the majority of students would enter some form of practice, Wearn asked if the proposal provided the student with enough continuity in learning about the patient, his illnesses, and his health between illnesses. Some students, he argued, might need to be broadly prepared to take care of the sick. Wearn's conclusion was that if these questions and caveats (especially the matter of planning) could be heeded and resolved, the proposal should be supported.

When site visitors from the Fund presented these questions to Duke's faculty in December 1964, the resulting discussion provided satisfactory answers to Wearn's queries. Stead pointed out that the essential problem of any curriculum was finding a means of teaching students to learn and enjoy learning; one of the site visitors reported that "this program is so excellent that it is difficult to describe it other than in superlatives, but I shall try to restrain the wild use of these as far as possible."[89] In February 1965 the Fund's board of directors voted to provide the full $750,000 for the additional faculty members needed to inaugurate this elective curriculum.

By the mid-1960s expansion of biomedical knowledge was straining traditional courses beyond their limits. Extension of postgraduate medical education, most often as preparation for specialization, was raising questions about the proper scope of undergraduate medical education, and the increasingly wide variety of careers open to medical graduates was challenging the uniformity of course content and curricular structure. Demands by students for programs tailored to their individual abilities and plans were supported indirectly by competition for the best students from newly attractive programs in other scientific and technical fields, and social pressure mounted for the training of more physicians from more diverse geographic, racial and economic backgrounds. The program launched in the fall of 1966[90] was the first new model of medical education responsive to these social pressures for change.

In 1978 Duke analyzed its first ten years of experience with the new curriculum design.[91] During this first decade, the majority of the original planners remained in leadership positions. Enough time had passed to minimize the so-called Hawthorne effect—the impact of attitudes based primarily upon the experience of novelty—and the time span permitted a longitudinal analysis of students' feelings toward their education. The conclusion was that the curriculum needed no further revision: the existing one was adequate to produce future medical educators trained both in biomedical research and in practice of medicine. The Fund-supported revision had created a structure capable of responding simultaneously to several concerns, allowing the form of the curriculum to remain relatively unaltered as its content changed to meet the goals of individual students and the needs of society at large.

The revised curriculum at Duke was a drastic change from a previously successful model. A decade of experience had shown that a sweeping change in medical education need not dilute the quality of the education and that elective freedom is necessary if the student is to choose wisely from among many careers. Although final evaluation of the effectiveness of this restructuring was years away, provisional judgment was important, since national priorities in health affairs had shifted over the previous decade. Future shifts would undoubtedly come with similar rapidity. The new Duke curriculum appeared to be a successful model capable of accommodating the alterations made necessary by a changing society.[92]

THE INTEGRATED CURRICULUM AT HARVARD

Each year at Harvard University, embryo physicians and scientists—students following two different pathways—began the study of the basic sciences. Medical students were the larger group, which spent the better part of two years mastering the "preclinical" part of a four-year course leading to the M.D. degree. The smaller group, also college graduates, spent three or four years of study and research as candidates for the Ph.D. degree in their chosen area of the basic medical sciences. The two groups shared several common features: All students were taught by members of the medical school faculty; their work took place in the medical school laboratories; and at the beginning of their training they took some of the same courses in the school of medicine.

By the late 1940s, the medical faculty at Harvard was dissatisfied with the training of both groups. Doctoral candidates needed a stronger foundation in the basic sciences, and the entire medical school program needed greater coherence. Yet for Ph.D. candidates in particular, the tendency toward narrowness and specialization was increasing, as the practical purpose of the doctoral degree in a basic science was to establish qualifications for a research position or a teaching appointment. Nevertheless, those who completed the rigorous training were not necessarily effective teachers or investigators. Furthermore, not only was there a shortage of basic scientists in medical schools, but the basic sciences were taught individually, by men whose training and experience had given them a narrow point of view.[93] The first step in welding together the separate parts of the preclinical curriculum was to recast the education of the candidates for the doctor of philosophy degree.

When George P. Berry became dean of the Harvard Medical School in 1949, one of his goals was to unify its many independent units without destroying their individuality or diminishing their excellence. He wanted more emphasis on the students rather than on the subject matter, on the patient rather than the disease. To plan for an integrated course in the medical sciences, a faculty committee under the chairmanship of Eric Ball recommended the establishment of an experimental course to take the place of the first year of graduate training for all Ph.D. candidates.[94] In addition to improving the training of doctoral students, the course was intended as a pilot program for the reorganization of the medical school's preclinical curriculum. In this integrated course, the subject matter was not classified by discipline; instead, the contributions of the departments were interwoven to emphasize the central theme of the study of the living organism and its component parts. The course was organized by a small committee representing each of the medical science departments; a rotation system ensured that no one member remained active in the course for more than two years. Students were given a minimum of classroom hours and a maximum amount of time for study, and some were assigned to independent laboratory experiments. Finally, a new multidisciplinary laboratory was designed as the home base for the students in the course.

Berry was a director of the Fund as well as dean at Harvard, and in asking the Fund to support the new program, he was able to address the sorts of questions that he knew would preoccupy the other board members and the Fund's staff:[95]

> The primary job today of the dean of a medical school . . . is the creation at his school of a new kind of academic framework within which to train the "physician of tomorrow". . . . The embryo physician no longer has an opportunity for a broad approach to the understanding of man, which is, of course, the first requisite of a physician. We must discover anew how to bring "Human Ecology and Personality Into the Training of Physicians" . . . without making such training less "scientific. . . ." Tomorrow's physician . . . must have learned to see the *whole* man. He must have appreciated the concept that with increasing complexity of organization the whole is greater than the sum of its parts, parts limited to those now characterized in conventional physical, chemical and biological terms. . . .
>
> . . . What do I see at Harvard after two years in residence? I see a school in which there have been made, and are being made, tremendous contributions to scientific medicine. . . . We have produced many superb physicians, investigators and teachers, and are still doing so. Yet it is clear that our departmental "empires" and far-flung hospital "worlds" fall short of providing the best environment in which the physician-in-training can learn to see the whole man. . . . I think I see how to tackle the job. My present application to the Commonwealth Fund concerns support for the first step. Since this is mean-

ingful only when seen as part of a larger plan, let me sketch out the whole plan for you.

The Division of Medical Sciences has existed at the Harvard Medical School since 1908. . . . [It] brings together so effectively the so-called basic medical sciences and the natural sciences and other disciplines in Cambridge. When I came to Harvard . . . I was pleased to find considerable dissatisfaction . . . at how they were teaching the medical students and the graduate students seeking the Ph.D. degree. . . . I was able to create, and to participate later in the discussion of, several committees aimed at the various facets of the overall problem. From the Committee of which Professor Ball served as Chairman—Divisional Commitee to Plan an Integrated Course in Medical Sciences—have gradually emerged plans for a new course built around the living entity.

. . . What I have been describing is an experiment in education. It is one about which our whole faculty is excited. . . . It will permit our teachers to *learn by doing* . . . because the student will be permitted to explore problems for himself!

You have asked: "Why make the proposed experiment with graduate students? Why not with medical students?" The choice of graduate rather than medical students was made only after a lot of careful thinking. I am convinced for several reasons that this was the correct choice. The departments involved will have continuing responsibility for the graduate students who have been through the experimental year, because these students will be continuing for several subsequent years their graduate work for the Ph.D. in one or another department. Thus, the accomplishments and failures of the experimental program will come immediately and continuously under critical observation. The experimental procedures can thus be modified by experience. The legal restrictions, furthermore, which hem in the training of medical students are absent.

Please bear this point in mind: the same groups of teachers who will be working in the experimental program and observing—actually experiencing— its results are the same groups of teachers who teach the medical students. The "know-how" to re-orient the way we teach medical students will thus come from actual experience. . . .

When we have learned from the new program how to reorganize the teaching for our medical students . . . we will have "cleared" the way for bringing into the first two years an approach to understanding human ecology and personality. . . .

In a similar letter to Commonwealth Fund President Aldrich, Berry replied to a series of questions about the potential for re-orienting the training of future physicians: "We want to learn to build solidly and well on a small scale, i.e., by commencing with medical-science students. Then we want to enlarge the foundation for our medical students. We will have come to know what constitutes a solid foundation. On such we can design and construct an educational program extending throughout the whole period of medical study which will give full weight to medical sociology, the personality, dynamic psychiatry, and the rest of the 'humanistic' approaches so desperately needed today."[96]

In 1952 the Commonwealth Fund appropriated $197,748 toward the support of this experiment for three years.

By the end of the new program's first year, a second committee was at work studying the medical curriculum in the preclinical years, using the results of this integrated course in the medical sciences to prepare its recommendations. A year of experience had already revealed some of the strengths and weaknesses of the new program:[97]

> [With regard to the topics selected for the course] a rather fortunate decision was not to be complete. This was achieved successfully through careful selection and evaluation. Ample examples of theoretical and practical importance for the understanding of medical sciences and for the appreciation of research problems have been selected. However, the second objective, the eventual connection between medical sciences and medicine, has been poorly achieved. . . . The students have reacted favorably and some enthusiastically to this kind of course. The teaching . . . was a valuable experience for most of the instructors. For some it was the first time that they were exposed to all the disciplines of medical sciences and for the others it was a rare opportunity to modernize their knowledge in disciplines almost forgotten since the days they were medical students. . . .
>
> The present course cannot be adopted directly for a rewriting of the curriculum for the medical students. However, much of the experience can be exploited after one or more years of practice on the graduate student level.

The ad hoc Committee on Curricular Arrangements for Preclinical Teaching and Integration with Clinical Teaching had designed a course covering the first two postgraduate years. First, students would gain a firm footing in each basic science; then they would learn to apply the multidisciplinary approach to important problems in human biology. The first year would emphasize the normal; the second would stress abnormal and disease states.

In the first semester of the first year, students would take courses in the principles of biochemistry, physiology, gross anatomy, and histology. The study of histology would help unify the program and, conversely, would gain strength from the contributions of other disciplines. By focusing principally on enzymes, energy, and intermediary metabolism, the study of biochemistry would give students a solid general foundation in the basic sciences of medicine. The introduction to physiology would have the same goal, selecting a model for teaching the principles of the discipline. In the second semester, unified or interdepartmental teaching in several areas would be offered. Each topic would be taught by a team, which would allocate time and select material in consultation with the participating departments. The departments of biochemistry, physiology, and anatomy (histology) would be responsible for the program.

The second year would follow the pattern of the first, correlating the principles of pathology, bacteriology, and pharmacology. After students had obtained a good background in the dynamic and morphologic aspects of immunological reactions and infectious diseases, parasitology and chemotherapy would be introduced as interdepartmental courses. The main activity of the second semester would be a unified course called "Mechanisms of Disease," comprising special pathology, pathologic physiology, and elements of medicine and surgery—a logical development of the second-year course in medicine. Laboratory diagnosis would be an integral part of this major course.

The committee planned to incorporate unscheduled time into both years, allowing students to take elective courses or conduct research. Also spanning both preclinical years would be a course entitled "Growth and Development." A collaborative effort calling on faculty members from the basic sciences, obstetrics, pediatrics and psychiatry, it would include consideration of genetics and statistics, embryology, and somatic and psychic development from infancy through adolescence and adulthood into old age.

The committee did not see this rearrangement of the curriculum as a radical departure from the status quo. One of its chief merits was that it did not impose a complex reorganization on the departments. In addition, since the plans were flexible, the committee anticipated that the courses would change continually to represent the best ways of presenting the basic medical sciences to Harvard's medical students.[98]

The program for medical students was assessed in 1957 by Manfred Karnovsky, who had served as chairman of the ad hoc committee. Peter V. Lee's investigation two years later left no doubt that interdepartmental teaching in the basic medical sciences was feasible at the Harvard Medical School.[99] Yet he felt that it was still too early to evaluate Harvard's change in curriculum. Once the program was under way, the original ad hoc committee had given way to two separate committees, one for each year. The second-year faculty tended to underestimate the sophistication of the students and set their sights too low. Even after the program had been in effect for two years, Lee felt that very few faculty members had a clear idea of what was being done in the year in which they were not actively teaching.

There was also no faculty unanimity regarding the new curriculum. Some felt that integration had not gone far enough, while others took the view that there was too little opportunity for departments to expose the students to their disciplines. Many believed that interdepartmental teaching was not a desirable method for training graduate students: Research careers should be the goal of graduate student training, and medical school teaching should pursue its own specific goals.

When Robert H. Ebert succeeded Berry as dean, the program was experiencing increasing resistance from the faculty. Despite its success, individual department heads wanted more control over the curriculum for their graduate students. The spearhead for abandoning the integrated curriculum came from the Department of Microbiology, but the Department of Biochemistry also wanted to recruit and sequester its own graduate students. Strong departments succeeded in their efforts to control the destiny of their programs for graduate students, and Harvard's program of integrated teaching was abandoned.[100]

Lee wondered whether Harvard's program would set the pattern for the training of basic scientists, since few institutions had Harvard's faculty, students, or facilities. In later years, though, integration in medical school education survived and flourished. Accomplished without any great change in traditional departmental organization, integration did require a new level of interdepartmental cooperation. Teaching was already a primary responsibility of medical school faculty, and the increasing versatility of clinical department members added qualitative and quantitative faculty strength. The Harvard Medical School's plan, with its elective time for research, may not have been the best model for other schools, but the idea of integrated teaching secured a firm place in most institutions.

The Integration of University and Medical-School Education at Five Universities

Programs supported by the Fund at Johns Hopkins, Northwestern, Boston, and Stanford universities, and at the Albany Medical College in collaboration with the Rensselaer Polytechnic Institute, were intended to attract the gifted student to a medical career by pruning an eight-year curriculum that many considered wasteful of time and manpower. A program encompassing the years from college through medical school would enable faculties to assure continuity while minimizing repetition in the presentation of biology, chemistry, and the social sciences.

No documented evidence showed that the eight years of formal training discouraged well-motivated students from studying medicine, but the belief was pervasive. The desire of some students to begin their medical education at an earlier age was understandable. The medical degree itself was far from the end-point of training, and for almost all students, at least four years of residency and specialty education lay ahead. College faculties reported that the present medical admissions process had an adverse effect on the performance of premedical students, at least during their senior year, when applications and interviews were at their peak. Early selection would also avoid the competition for grades throughout the four years of college and the attempts by premedical students to select programs that might favorably influence admissions committees. Students armed with the assurance of a place in a medical school could concentrate on learning rather than on competing for high marks. On the other hand, early selection might merely shift the competition for grades to the high school or reduce the pool of capable four-year applicants.

What medical schools hoped was that the requirements for early admission would put pressure on secondary schools and colleges to strengthen their offerings. Boston, Northwestern, and Johns Hopkins universities also wanted their new programs to stimulate interest in careers in the basic medical sciences: The time saved through shortening the premedical years would allow students to pursue one or two additional years of study in a preclinical discipline. In addition, the rapid growth of knowledge in the natural and social sciences was leading the medical schools to acknowledge the practical contributions that university scholars could make to medical education. Through shared responsibility for the instruction of medical students, new curricula would bring medical and liberal arts faculties—and universities and their medical schools—closer together.

Although integration of medical and university education was a main goal of the new curricula at Johns Hopkins, Northwestern, and Boston universities, each school developed a program uniquely its own. All three offered the student the possibility of completing medical school in six years after graduation from high school, but this alternative was chosen by few students at Johns Hopkins, by about one-fifth of the class at Northwestern, and by the great majority at Boston University. Admission requirements varied as well: Students at Boston and Northwestern who had completed high school, usually with some advanced placement courses giving them college credit, were eligible for admission directly to the combined six-year curriculum; Johns Hopkins required two years of college and the completion of a year of chemistry and biology for admission to its five-year program. In comparison, the students who entered the regular programs (Year II of Hopkins or Year III of Northwestern or Boston) would ordinarily have the bachelor's degree and would have completed the usual premedical courses. The Johns Hopkins program provided generous amounts of free time for electives, and student research was emphasized, particularly in the preclinical departments.[101] Boston University was most interested in acceleration, so its program offered a limited amount of time for electives and independent work. While Boston University did intend to improve its premedical science coures, it planned minimal alterations in the existing medical phases of the curriculum.[102] At Northwestern the new curriculum was intended as a pilot study, stressing acceleration and new ways of teaching the biological and physical sciences. Elective quarterly courses were limited to the clinical years, suggesting that independent study would be encouraged primarily in clinical disciplines, and opportunities for special work in the basic science departments were provided during the summer.[103] At all three schools, students were encouraged to use the flexibility of the program to follow their own interests in the basic sciences (table 3).

THE JOHNS HOPKINS UNIVERSITY SCHOOL OF MEDICINE

The Johns Hopkins University plan, which received support from the Fund in 1954, was intended to integrate the liberal arts and medical education, offer a flexible curriculum so that students could plan individualized programs, give students an early start, and allow students to obtain their medical degree in less than four years.

Table 3 Shortening the Length of Medical Education: Comparison of Programs at Johns Hopkins, Northwestern, and Boston Universities

Feature	Johns Hopkins	Northwestern	Boston
Year instituted	1959	1961	1961
Student admitted after	2 yrs. college	high school	high school
Length of program	5 years	6 years	6 years
Minimum time from high school to M.D.	7 years*	6 years	6 years
Number admitted annually to special program	35	25	72 (whole class)†
Number admitted annually to traditional program	55	100	‡
Special courses offered:			
general chemistry	no	yes	yes
organic chemistry	yes	yes	yes
physical chemistry	yes	yes	yes
physics	yes	yes	yes
mathematics	yes	yes§	yes‖
biology	no	yes#	yes
Elective quarters	last 3 yrs.	last 2 yrs.	last yr. only
Total weeks of elective time (last 4 yrs.)	30 (3 × 10)	24 (2 × 12)	16 (1 × 16)

* For the occasional student who completed medical school in 6 years after high school, the M.D. degree was awarded on completion of the internship.
† Only 40 were admitted in the program's first year, but the plan was that the entire class would enter directly from high school.
‡ Only to replace those lost during the first two years: estimated 10–20.
§ With physics course.
‖ With physics and chemistry courses.
In second year, chemistry, physics, and mathematics were prerequisites.

Years I and II of the five-year program emphasized the unity of the educational process. In Year I the medical school offered certain "premedical" courses concurrently with liberal arts courses on the university campus. The intensive course in the history and philosophy of medicine and science in Year II was designed to provide a liberalizing influence during an otherwise heavily scientific year.

Acceleration, which attracted the greatest public interest, was only a minor feature of the Johns Hopkins program. A limited number of students in each class could take required clinical courses during the elective periods of Years III and IV and during one summer session. Although the student would complete the required course work twelve months earlier than his classmates, he would receive his M.D. degree only after finishing an additional year of study, in either an internship or research fellowship. Some students used the elective periods to catch up with their class after an extra year of study in a basic science department. Under special circumstances, permission to accelerate was granted to students who wished to begin their clinical training one year earlier than normal. The faculty at Johns Hopkins stressed that the accelerated program was not designed as a quick method for embarking on the practice of medicine after a minimal period of training; the student was required to justify his reason for acceleration in terms of his own career goals.

The total number of elective hours remained almost the same as in the standard Johns Hopkins program, while the amount of required work actually increased, the result of lengthening the school year from thirty-two to forty weeks in order to organize the elective time in ten-week blocks. Free time in day-long blocks or ten-week quarters was also useful for a student who wished to pursue independent study.

The Johns Hopkins program succeeded in turning able students of medicine toward the basic sciences. Students were attracted to the program by the free time provided early in the curriculum; by the block system of teaching, which exposed them to intensive study of one discipline for a ten-week quarter, and by the early start, which made it easier for them to drop out of school for a year of advanced study in one of the basic medical sciences. Because it was attractive to high-caliber students and offered a stimulating academic atmosphere, the program continued to meet what many of its faculty considered to be its main responsibility, preparing its graduates for advanced studies leading to positions in academic medicine.

THE NORTHWESTERN UNIVERSITY SCHOOL OF MEDICINE

In 1956 the Commonwealth Fund helped to unite Northwestern's medical school in Chicago with the university fifteen miles away. Part of an unrestricted grant was used for an experimental project offering the M.D. degree at the end of six years of intensive liberal arts and medical study.

Early that year a committee appointed by Northwestern's president, Roscoe Miller, developed a program that would eliminate the sharp division between premedical and medical education, introduce at the college level material more directly related to the study of medicine, include liberal arts courses in the professional curriculum, and reduce the length of time required to complete studies toward the M.D. degree. The entire integrated sequence of college and medical education was planned to train the mind rather than merely to impart information. The program was intended to be flexible enough to allow students in the early years to branch out without penalty into medical practice, teaching, or research; into one of several scientific specialties; or even, with some loss of time, into other branches of learning. The program also permitted students to be recruited into the study of medicine from schools other than Northwestern.

The premedical phase of the student's education was not the only area of change. For several years, the faculty had been modifying the medical curriculum to provide increased interdepartmental collaboration in the preclinical years. The clinical program itself was designed to offer greater opportunity for elective work, and comprehensive medical care was to be taught in a special clinic in the fourth year.

Acceptance into the first year of the new program implied that the student would complete his medical study. Without strong assurance of admission to medical school, it was unlikely that many applicants would choose the more rigorous program even though it promised a saving of one or two years.

A two-year curriculum on the Evanston campus prepared students for the transition to medical school. The acceleration in the experimental program of Years I and II was more apparent than genuine; the two real innovations in this program were the early acceptance into medical school and the coordinated premedical program in chemistry, physics, mathematics, and biology. The science component encouraged scholarly performance by bringing together small groups from the medical school and university. In addition, 50 percent of the curriculum was to be elective, so that students could construct for themselves a program that best complemented their individual interests in the arts, humanities, and social sciences. During the last four years, they would be required to register for five seminar courses in the humanities. The program's planners hoped that students with college standing in English and foreign languages, who were thus eligible for advanced humanities courses, would receive a broader educational experience than less talented students could attain in four years of college.

Minimum requirements for applicants included four years of high-school mathematics and four years of high-school English. Most students admitted to the program were expected to qualify for advanced placement in chemistry and mathematics, and in one of the humanities. At the end of Year IV (the second medical year) the student would be granted a B.S. degree in the medical sciences, qualifying him for admission into a doctoral degree program. Alternatively, a student could leave the new program and enter the usual bachelor's degree program after two years without serious loss of time, progressing at a pace dictated by his capabilities and interests.

The program was implemented in the fall of 1961 under the direction of John A. D. Cooper. Some changes have been made over the years, but the basic plan of the curriculum remains the same to this day. Because the program was attracting superior students, its name was changed in 1963 to the Honors Program in Medical Education. The size of the entering class has increased from twenty-five to sixty students, and the small science classes and laboratories have been enlarged to include students from other programs.

A grant from the Commonwealth Fund in 1960 provided for the detailed planning of the first-year course and for two years of operation beginning in 1961. A renewal grant in 1963 supported the operation of the program during its third and fourth years and contributed on a decreasing basis to the cost of the fifth and sixth years—that is, to the time of graduation of the first class in 1967.

Since the medical school continued to accept college graduates for medical training, the experimental program afforded an opportunity to compare the progress of the sixth-year group with that of the class entering the medical school after the usual four years of premedical preparation. An in-depth study carried out in 1976 to assess the effectiveness of the program included all students who had graduated from the program and those from the regular program in medical education for the years 1967 through 1974. Comparisons were made between the honors and regular graduates by year of graduation from medical school. The report of the study concluded: "The attraction of excellent talent to the program must be counted as one of the keys to its success. . . . In fact, this program is attracting talented scholars to Northwestern who would otherwise have enrolled at other more prestigious universities. It is safe to conclude, based on all the data analyzed in this study, that the Honors Program at Northwestern has been successful. The program has demonstrated that well-qualified high school graduates can be trained to be physicians in a shorter period of time and can successfully begin the practice of medicine at an earlier age."[104]

Other studies of this and similar programs have found that admitting students directly from high school to medical school has very few detriments. Results of these studies have been generally neutral to positive.[105]

THE BOSTON UNIVERSITY SCHOOL OF MEDICINE

The new program at Boston University, which began in the fall of 1961, was intended to provide an accelerated program and an improved educational experience. Students entered directly from high school and pursued a six-year course of study leading to the M.D. degree.

Planning for the program began in 1957, when faculty members from the medical school and the College of Liberal Arts first considered the possibility of shortening the period between secondary school and graduation from medical school.[106] A thorough study of the organization and content of the entire span of medical education, as well as the possibility of acceleration, was supported by a grant from the Rockefeller Foundation. A group at Boston University examined the American secondary school system, the English educational system, the principles of a liberal arts education, and various experiments in medical education. The faculty planning committees then developed specific objectives for combining the liberal arts and medical programs into an integrated unit to make medicine part of a general education.

The liberal arts phase of the program, conducted primarily on the university campus during the student's first two years, had the ambitious goal of providing the student with an understanding of human nature and an awareness of the range of human values, encouraging him to develop an orderly and scholarly mind, educating him in the responsibilities of the physician toward social problems, and giving him an appreciation of principles of ethical conduct. The new program featured a shorter period from high school to the M.D. degree, through special courses, full use of summers for course work, and a limitation of opportunities for elective courses at the undergraduate level.

The university originally intended to accept the new program's entire seventy-two-member class directly from high school. In the program's first year, however, only forty students were admitted: the additional students were accepted into the third year after completing the usual premedical courses. Students had to demonstrate outstanding ability in high-school work and high grades on entrance examinations, although advanced placement was not a specific requirement; required high-school subjects included four years of English and three years of mathematics. Students admitted to the first years of the program became provisional candidates for both A.B. and M.D. degrees. At the end of two years, the faculty assessed each student's progress, deciding whether each should continue toward the medical degree or drop out of the six-year program to seek a bachelor's degree in the College of Liberal Arts.

In the first two years, four courses in the sciences and humanities were offered during the regular school term and two courses during the summer. Especially designed basic courses in biology (including principles of genetics, embryology, bioenergetics, and physiology), inorganic and physical chemistry, and organic chemistry were also required. Mathematics was taught as part of physics and chemistry, rather than as a separate course. Biostatistics, given during the summer, completed the required science subjects. Every student had courses in English, history, government, psychology, sociology, and philosophy, in addition to a continuing tutorial program in a foreign language; this work in the humanities and social sciences was oriented toward the problems and opportunities of the physician. Later in the curriculum, seminars and tutorial work were emphasized, and during the summer between the second and third years, students took courses in literature or fine arts, and electives in the humanities, social sciences, or natural sciences.

The final four years of the program featured no radical changes in the teaching of either the basic sciences or clinical subjects. During the summer between the third and fourth years, there were seminars in the history of science and medicine, and opportunity for additional electives. The summer session between the fourth and fifth years offered seminar studies in health and society, and opportunity for electives in the humanities or sciences. In the sixth, or clerkship, year, sixteen-week trimesters in medicine and surgery were offered, as well as a four-month Human Ecology Program incorporating pediatrics, psychiatry, obstetrics, and home care (see p. 240). Throughout the six years of the program each student met weekly with his tutor, whose main function was to guide these younger and less mature medical students.

Two evaluations of the program were performed in 1976.[107] The six-year group's performance on standardized tests (Medical College Admission Tests and National Board examinations) was found to be higher than that of the regular group. In other aspects, such as class rank, honors at graduation, and grades in medical clerkships (as well as in postgraduate career choices), the two groups were similar. The conclusion, based on data for the first three graduating classes, was that qualified high-school students can succeed academically in an accelerated collegiate degree program, do well in medical school, achieve postgraduate certification, and begin the practice of medicine at an earlier age.

This program was followed by the introduction of the Modular Medical Integrated Curriculum (MMIC) at Boston University in 1977. As part of the Commonwealth Fund's Interface Program (see p. 485), the MMIC has since become one of three pathways available to students at Boston University who wish to obtain both A.B. and M.D. degrees.

THE RENSSELAER POLYTECHNIC INSTITUTE AND THE ALBANY MEDICAL COLLEGE

Another Fund-supported effort to reduce the time required to obtain the M.D. degree was the plan developed by the Albany Medical College and the Rensselaer Polytechnic Institute (RPI). In 1964 these two schools initiated a program that permitted qualified students to complete requirements for both the B.S. and M.D. degrees within six calendar years. Albany Medical College did not change its curriculum; it merely admitted a select group of students after two years of college.

The first program of accelerated studies to pair the faculty and physical resources of a school of medicine and a technological university, the Albany–RPI curriculum moved students rapidly through a sequence that normally required eight years. They acquired a science-based education not commonly experienced in liberal arts colleges and universities—one that was becoming increasingly relevant to the practice of modern medicine and to the research supporting it.

The student spent the first two calendar years of the program at RPI and the last four years in residence at the Albany Medical College. Rensselaer allowed course credit for many of the preclinical subjects taken at the medical school and for a research project, thus qualifying the student for the B.S. as well as the M.D. degree. Most of the science courses were mandated; the humanities courses were primarily elective.

The accelerated program offered a faster route to professional status for the qualified student. It made the profession more attractive and attainable for some who would not have followed the usual route, and it allowed careful direction and evaluation of the premedical portion of the student's program. It also tended to improve the quality of the student body.[108]

A progress report in the program's sixth year of operation revealed that on Part I of the National Board examination, the biomedical students scored higher as a group in every subject area than the regular medical students. Though achievement test scores are certainly not the only measure of success in medical studies, the biomedical group's performance was noteworthy in view of a college experience shortened by two calendar years.

In 1970 the Fund renewed its support of this program with a grant of $186,000. At the end of the three-year grant period, the program was expected to become a permanent part of the two schools' operations; it had been gradually expanded so that each class entering the Albany Medical College after 1971 would include at least thirty-six students in the accelerated program. From the very first pilot group, these special students were outstanding, winning most of the student research prizes at Albany and distinguishing themselves in their clinical clerkships.

THE STANFORD UNIVERSITY SCHOOL OF MEDICINE

The academic year 1959-60 marked the inauguration of the Stanford University School of Medicine's new program in medical education.[109] For many years Stanford's medical school had operated in two separate locations. Students were taught anatomy, biochemistry, microbiology, and physiology on the university campus near Palo Alto, while studies in pharmacology and pathology, together with all clinical work, were carried out in San Francisco. Communication between the two parts of the medical school, and between the school in San Francisco and the remainder of the university, was seriously handicapped by this physical separation.

The general increase in population in the West made Palo Alto a city with diverse clinical material, and in 1954 the university's board of trustees voted to move the entire medical school to the Palo Alto campus. This decision to bring the school of medicine into the university complex benefited all university departments. The ideal of medicine in a university setting fostered the development of an educational plan specifically designed to take advantage of this opportunity.

The primacy of education as a continuum was at the center of the new curriculum. The program's planners wanted to bridge the separation of medical and premedical work, encourage integrated teaching where it was likely to be most effective, and relate parts of the medical curriculum to the student's previous educational experience. They also believed that at the heart of the study of medicine lies a core of medical knowledge that should be presented to all students, whatever their eventual choice of medical career—even though the growth of medical science is so great and continues at so rapid a pace that it cannot be covered comprehensively. Core material was to be presented by subject area, rather than in isolated departmental courses, and would acquaint the student with the concepts underlying each of the major branches of medicine. For every student, core courses were to be supplemented with independent study.

The planners also believed that the student of medicine had passed beyond that stage of his education where the mere acquisition of "facts" could be defended. He was essentially a graduate student and should be encouraged to learn attitudes and approaches to problems in medicine, rather than merely acquiring techniques or accumulating data at the expense of interpretation. A tutor-advisor would help students plan individualized programs, and—in one of the most controversial parts of the program—students would be encouraged to undertake independent study and research[110] and to widen their medical and nonmedical horizons.

To combine cultural and scientific studies in the university with the specific program in the basic sciences of medicine, the faculty adopted a five-year medical curriculum in April 1956. Students entered this program after either three or four college years. An amount of time (designated "university time") equivalent to one academic year was distributed in equal segments through the first three years and might be spent in any department of the university. Simultaneously, the student began the study of the basic medical sciences. An introductory course brought him into contact with clinical problems at the start of his medical work, and in the third year, having developed some understanding of both the basic and the clinical medical sciences, he was introduced to the philosophical and historical aspects of medicine. The fourth and fifth years were devoted to a series of interdepartmental courses acquainting the student with clinical medicine, with the interdependence of the clinical fields, and with the patient as a member of society. Throughout the curriculum, a large amount of elective time was available, rising to a full third of the total time in the final year.

To fulfill the requirements for the A.B. degree, the student who entered the Stanford program after three college years was allowed to choose nonmedical work among the natural and social sciences, the humanities, and the fine arts, in accordance with his own interests. The student who entered with a baccalaureate degree was able to pursue an interest in his major field of college study or follow an interest in some other field. All students had the opportunity to complement work in medicine with work in related nonmedical subjects.

The faculty committee charged with developing the plan rejected any contraction in the program's total length, believing that the years of college and professional education represented the flowering of superior students' educational efforts and that these efforts should be unrestricted either by the need for longer academic years or by encroachment upon the educational interests of undergraduate colleges. The committee emphasized that medical education should provide a variety of possibilities, since no single arrangement would be suitable for all applicants.

The increasing cost of education and the social unrest of the time led to the plan's deterioration in the late 1960s and early 1970s.[111]

An Appraisal of Experiments in Medical Education

These Fund-supported "experiments in medical education" were assessed in 1977 by Carleton B. Chapman, then president of the Commonwealth Fund.[112] A knowledgeable participant and observer, Chapman was an enthusiast rather than an unbiased judge, and the main programs of his presidency were based on the Fund's earlier programs of curriculum reform. Chapman found no support for the common belief that after initial enthusiasm for experiment had waned, medical education tended to revert to established patterns. His study of curriculum content and sequence, particularly in the basic science years, showed extensive experimentation and considerable permanent change since the 1940s, including early exposure to clinical problems, a waning of emphasis on gross morphology, and updating of instruction in microbiology and biochemistry.

Some of the Fund-sponsored curricular experiments had been in operation long enough to permit methodological evaluation: The six-year programs at Northwestern and Boston universities, the Year I program at Johns Hopkins (actually a seven-year program), and the imaginative revision of teaching along integrated lines at Western Reserve. Chapman concluded that in this group of dissimilar experiments, all except the last operating in parallel with standard eight-year programs, comparisons disclosed no substantive difference between the graduates of the experimental program and those who traversed the traditional eight-year pathway. Dire predictions were unsubstantiated: Students taking the shorter route were not dangerously immature on graduation, and they were in fact given enough time to assimilate the vast amounts of bioscientific and clinical knowledge that they had encountered. It was true that the six- and seven-year programs were intended for gifted students; and perhaps because of this, some programs were at first beset by larger-than-normal dropout rates. Nevertheless, the faculties that designed and implemented these shortened programs seemed to Chapman remarkably reluctant to accept the positive results of their own experiments and at times were at great pains to discredit them. Some even put themselves in the untenable position of equating academic excellence with the passage of time: if eight years is acceptable, ten years should be better and twelve better still.

Chapman found it unfortunate that the feature looming largest in the minds of faculties and outside observers, both favorable and opposed, was the shortened curriculum. He believed that the most important feature was the collaboration of medical with arts and sciences faculties to improve the quality of the preclinical phases of medical education. This collaborative effort was, in Chapman's view, indispensable to the major purpose of premedical and preclinical education: to give the student a broad familiarity with the biosciences.

In the years since Abraham Flexner set out the now-traditional premedical and preclinical science requirements for students entering medicine, the concepts, the content, and even the purpose of the biosciences have changed enormously. One result is that previously accepted distinctions between the natural and the basic medical sciences are increasingly untenable. The initial course in biology in today's university, for example, bears little resemblance to the descriptive courses of the 1930s and 1940s. It now contains elements of cellular and molecular biology and of biochemistry, all of which are encountered again in the crowded curriculum o the first two years of medical school. It is possible, Chapman said, to identify institutions in which basic biology has been redesigned and redefined, while basic medical sciences such as microbiology and biochemistry still fit their descriptions in the Flexner Report of 1910. In other institutions it is the other way around: The old distinction between general inorganic and physical chemistry is no longer applicable, as the relevant principles of the latter are included, logically enough, in the study of the former. Yet it is not unusual to find in the catalogues of the same colleges a course bearing the label "Physical Chemistry for Premedical Students"— a course offered only because some medical schools require it.

Chapman found it difficult to avoid the conclusion that the premedical-preclinical sequence is academically and intellectually unsatisfying. If one adds the almost universal complaint that premedical requirements make it impossible for the student of medicine to obtain a liberal education (something that stubbornly defies implementable description), an educational problem of massive proportions is revealed. Yet Chapman was encouraged by the evolution of the experimental programs, designed and implemented by university faculty groups working in effective if not always peaceful collaboration—a process with the potential to upgrade education for the practice of medicine at its most fundamental stages to a degree that Flexner could not anticipate.

Founding New Medical Schools

The notion that the United States was suffering from a shortage of physicians was prevalent for many years after World War II. To train more physicians during the 1950s and 1960s, the Commonwealth Fund supported the development of new schools of medicine and the reorganization of existing ones, upgrading some schools from a two-year program in the basic sciences to a four-year program leading to the M.D. degree. The Fund also helped to create new departments in well-established schools and to rehabilitate other departments that had not kept up with advances in medical knowledge (see app. F).

THE UNIVERSITY OF FLORIDA

Standing in relief among the genesis stories of medical schools is the founding of the medical school at the University of Florida. Its start was marked by unusually extensive planning by both the state legislature and the university itself: Their mutual concern for the needs of a rapidly changing state and for education based on an understanding of patients influenced the design of the school's curriculum and facilities.

The germ of an idea for a medical school associated with the University of Florida had existed among local citizens of Gainesville for some time,[113] but it was not until 1945 that the Florida legislature authorized the establishment of the first schools of medicine and nursing in the state. The same year an executive order by Florida's governor empaneled a citizen's committee on education to make a comprehensive survey of education in Florida, and in 1947 a state congressional resolution directed a survey of the need, location, and cost of a medical school, nursing school, and teaching hospital. This project, directed by Vernon W. Lippard, then dean of the school of medicine at Louisiana State University,[114] had the support of J. Hillis Miller, the University of Florida's new president. The Lippard Report reflected their strong feeling that the place for a medical school was Gainesville, where it could be associated academically and administratively with the university.[115]

Once the location had been chosen, a federal grant of $10,000 enabled Lippard to submit a supplementary report in 1950.[116] In this he was assisted by Basil C. MacLean, director of the Strong Memorial Hospital in Rochester, New York, and a former Commonwealth Fund fellow. Little activity occurred until the next year, when the state legislature appropriated $100,000 for drafting of plans for a medical school.[117]

President J. Hillis Miller, a psychologist, envisioned a school integrated as closely as possible with the rest of the university and recognized that its establishment would be a project of greater magnitude than the mere drafting of architectural plans. He also seized the opportunity to involve the university in the planning and obtained a grant of $96,500 from the Commonwealth Fund to enable faculty and consultants to study the type of school that might be established.[118]

In June 1952 Russell S. Poor, a geologist with the Tennessee Valley Authority (TVA) and a former dean of the graduate school at Auburn University, was appointed director of a committee of university faculty members and outside consultants. Poor had no experience with medical education, and his position with the TVA gave him no responsibility for medical programs. John M. MacLachlan, professor of sociology at the University of Florida, was appointed as Poor's chief of staff; he recruited members of the university for specific projects and performed the statistical and demographic analyses of the study. Assisting the committee was Jefferson M. Hamilton, a retired architect on President Miller's staff, who had worked on housing projects for the federal government and had been involved in planning Duke University's West Campus. He toured several schools to study their architectural design and on these visits inquired about medical educators interested in physical facilities who might serve as special consultants. Wilburt C. Davison, dean of Duke's medical school, recommended George T. Harrell, Jr., an experienced medical educator and one of Poor's colleagues at the TVA. Assisting the committee were six faculty research committees, each assigned a different aspect of the problem, and a Medical Advisory Committee of practicing physicians. The research committees were supposed to ask all the questions essential to structuring the policy and facilities of a medical center and to report to the state legislature in the spring of 1953.

The plan the committee had in mind was so unconventional that few legislatures could be expected to view it sympathetically. The study reversed the traditional approaches: It explored the role of the university in medicine rather than the role of the medical school in the university. The committee focused on the education of physicians in the university setting and the care of patients in the local community. The resulting report wove the university's academic objectives into a pattern of medical education. The plan included a university college that would provide two years of general education as the foundation for many kinds of professional training; an agricultural experiment station producing studies of nutrition; and a small, independent cancer research laboratory affiliated with the biological sciences.

The committee's results were published in 1954, the same year the legislature appropriated $5 million to construct colleges of medicine and nursing, and Harrell was appointed the founding dean of the medical school. He brought to the job his experience in another new medical school, the Bowman Gray School of Medicine of Wake Forest University, as well as his service on Florida's planning committee.

With Hamilton, Harrell designed the medical school's physical plant.[119] Here Harrell and Hamilton were working in the dark: They had not been advised of shortcomings at other schools, and there was no published literature on the design of medical school facilities. As a result, they made several mistakes in projecting the engineering requirements—for example, soon after opening the medical school's building, it was realized that larger utility systems were needed. Harrell used his experience to educate others: After the Gainesville plant was finished, he chaired two committees for the United States Public Health Service on the design of medical school facilities and produced a book outlining the committees' work. As the first study of the subject and the only one for several years, the Public Health Service report was widely distributed so that others could benefit from Florida's early mistakes. When William R. Willard, the founding dean of the University of Kentucky School of Medicine, was planning that medical school (also with the help of a Commonwealth Fund grant), he used the University of Florida's architectural consulting firm and came up with a better design for the school's utilities. Harrell himself built upon his knowledge of the errors in scale and placement at Gainesville when he helped design the plant at the medical school in Hershey, Pennsylvania, a building that has been praised by architects all over the world.

Harrell next began the selection of faculty and the development of a curriculum. He chose the theme of human biology as a continuous thread in the university, running from the general educational program through specialized residency training in the hospital. Members of the medical faculty would emphasize basic concepts common to all living things, such as biological variability and adaptability. Medical examples in particular would illustrate that basic biological principles apply in the human species as they do in simpler forms of life. So that the educational theme of human biology might include social and behavioral points of view, the ambulant patient facilities were designed as a "laboratory of applied human biology," where any interested, qualified person in the university might work side by side with a medical student at a comparable level of educational training.

The program also stressed the relationship between physician and patient: the physician's understanding of people's behavior and problems and his personal responsibility for his patients' welfare.

The curriculum finally hammered out had three major goals: the education of practitioners, the integration of the health team, and the education of students for leadership. The development of thinking and reasoning, encouragement of habits of self-education, and experience with the use of the scientific method were emphasized in preparing students to become leaders in their professions.

The dean had decided that the primary function of the medical school was to educate family physicians for the future practice of medicine in Florida, whatever shape it might take. Florida's need for physicians trained for its specific problems, especially in small towns and rural areas, had been foreseen earlier by the Florida Medical Association, whose continuing education program had been linked with the University of Florida's graduate school. Since the responsibility for patient care rested with the family physician in the local community, he had to be aware of other health resources in his community and state. All members of the health team in the community were expected to be familiar with the same basic concepts; the talents of each person would be used more effectively if he understood not only his own role but also those of all others assisting in patient care. Planners of Florida's program envisioned a health center comprising three closely related schools—medicine, nursing, and pharmacy—which would be followed later by schools of health-related services and dentistry. The same common thread, the study of human biology, should run through the education provided by these ancillary schools.

The need for family physicians had been emphasized by the Fund-sponsored study and reinforced by Harrell's own philosophy, but the state legislature balked at recognizing it. Reflecting the opinions of the local county medical society, legislators feared that the medical school hospital would be the charity hospital for Gainesville and its county rather than a state-wide resource. Local physicians were concerned about competition and loss of patients, and J. Wayne Reitz, by then the university's president, denied permission for the school to offer a local program of primary care and family medicine. As a result, the school resorted to preceptorships with local practitioners outside Gainesville. (For further developments, see p. 455.) The medical school was also forbidden to have faculty members in either the humanities or the behavioral sciences, on the grounds that liberal arts disciplines had nothing to do with medical education. Harrell later rectified these errors elsewhere: As dean of the medical school at Hershey, he founded the first academic department of family and community medicine in the United States, the first department of humanities in a medical school in the world, and the first basic science department in the behavioral field. In a more sympathetic atmosphere, these pioneering programs, all of which had been suggested by the Commonwealth Fund's study, could have been established earlier at Gainesville.[120]

The Florida medical school decided to develop the ancillary field of health studies in 1970. Leading the way was the Department of Medicine, which with the help of a joint Commonwealth Fund–Carnegie Corporation grant of $150,000 had established a clinic in a nearby rural county. As the school's first teaching and research program in community medical care, this clinic rapidly crystallized the interest of the faculty and administration in problems of health service. Translating this interest into a formal program was an institution-wide Division of Community Health. The division was given a strong start in implementing the basic educational components of the program (including a curriculum to train physicians' assistants) by additional two-year grants in 1971 from the Fund and the Carnegie Corporation.[121]

A community-wide theme of human biology enabled the university to use its diverse resources in exploring education for all involved in patient care in a local community. Unforeseen circumstances delayed some aspects of the program, but the original concepts were eventually implemented.

THE UNIVERSITY OF HAWAII

Hawaii's distance from the mainland put it at a particular disadvantage in having no medical school. Residents of the state who wished to study medicine faced unusual expense and inconvenience; the percentage of medical students was considerably below the national average, and the islands had to depend upon physicians from elsewhere. To enable medical students to attend mainland medical schools for only their two final, clinical years, the Commonwealth Fund gave the University of Hawaii a grant of $120,000 in 1963 for a study of the feasibility of establishing a program in the basic medical sciences.[122] The twelve-month study was to be directed by a medical educator, with the help of national and local consultants, a lay advisory committee, and a faculty committee on medical education. It would include recommendations about curriculum, cost of facilities, administrative structure and personnel, administrative and operational policies, location, management, and financing of clinical facilities needed in the first two years of medical education, and programs of training in basic medical sciences leading to the Ph.D. degree as well as those preparatory to the clinical years in other medical schools outside Hawaii.

Among the university's assets were the Pacific Biomedical Research Center; graduate courses in biochemistry, human genetics, microbiology, and the behavioral sciences; and the East-West Center, which was supported by the United States Department of State. If the program in medical education was found to be feasible, its collaboration with the East-West Center in particular would help it to meet the great needs of the Western Pacific and Pacific Island areas for medical and other health personnel.

The study began in July 1963 under the direction of Robert D. Tschirgi, M.D., Ph.D., professor of physiology and anatomy at the University of California at Los Angeles School of Medicine. Although Tschirgi was initially given a leave of absence for this purpose, President Clark Kerr of the University of California later requested that he be released for only three-quarters of his time, so that he might become dean of academic planning for the entire University of California complex. As a result, Tschirgi supervised the study part-time, and in January 1964 it was completed by Richard A. Lockwood, an associate director of the study and a faculty member of the school of medicine.

Lockwood's report recommended the establishment of a six-year Biomedical Sciences Master's Degree Program, to be housed in a new College of Biomedical Curricula. The proposal had widespread approval: It was endorsed by the faculty committee on medical education, the university senate, and the board of regents, and approved by the Council of the Hawaii Medical Association and the directors of medical education of local hospitals. The governor of Hawaii gave his unqualified support, as did the 1964 state legislature. The university was instructed to continue its study of the program, to explore the possibilities of securing some of the necessary funds from outside sources, and to report its findings and recommendations to the 1965 session of the legislature. A supplementary grant from the Fund enabled the university to carry on planning and preparation through the coming academic year.

The plan made good use of existing facilities and personnel. The dean of the proposed College of Biomedical Curricula would also direct the Pacific Biomedical Research Center, and faculty members would hold dual appointments. Research would be conducted at the research center, and the college would administer the instructional portion of the program. The dean would also have overall responsibility for the existing school of nursing, as well as programs in public health, medical technology, and dental hygiene. These programs would be reorganized under an associate dean in each of the schools of biomedical sciences, nursing, and public health.

Yet the Biomedical Sciences Master's Degree Program turned out to be incongruent with the university's needs, and the College of Biomedical Curricula never materialized. Tschirgi and Lockwood originally envisioned three tracks for students—one leading to the master's degree in biomedical sciences, one continuing on to a doctorate, and one that would allow transfer to a four-year mainland medical school for the M.D. degree—but it soon became clear that although some students were interested in the first two alternatives, the real need was constituted by students who wished to become physicians. To satisfy the preponderance of demand, the university concentrated its resources on a two-year school of basic medical sciences.

This two-year program was intended for students financially unable to spend four years at a mainland medical school. Planners estimated that about twelve island residents were enrolling directly in mainland medical schools each year—a figure that remains stable today. Other island residents were enrolled in mainland colleges or universities directly from high school (or after one or two years at the University of Hawaii) in order to establish residency in another state and thereby gain preference for admission to medical school. To the extent that these students might remain in Hawaii for the first two years of medical training, mainland medical schools would be able to accept other applicants and increase the total number of doctors in training. Many mainland medical schools had clinical facilities for additional students in the third and fourth years, and it appeared that graduates of the University of Hawaii's program would have no difficulty in finding places for their clinical training. The small group of island residents studying on the mainland represented a privileged segment of the population, one that could afford the high cost of private schools.

The new program was also expected to bolster the continuing medical education of physicians practicing in Hawaii. It would strengthen both the university's department of public health, which would be developed into a school of public health, and the college of nursing; contribute to the national and international pool of biomedical scientists; attract to the university outstanding scientists and teachers through the promotion of training and research; greatly fortify an already well-advanced research program under the auspices of the Pacific Biomedical Research Center; and develop the University of Hawaii as the biomedical center for the whole Pacific Basin.[123]

Hawaii was not a wealthy state, and although the planners expected that legislative appropriations would eventually cover the new program's operating costs, the university needed help in meeting the initial expense. The new program increased the state's budget by $1,621,200 over the next five years. In addition, over the next three years the university would raise $6,836,000 for the program's buildings and equipment. It hoped to secure from private sources $1,269,000 of the total needed for operating costs and $1,912,000 of the total needed for capital costs. The Kellogg Foundation had made a grant of $1,250,000 conditional upon the university's ability to raise the remainder of the funds elsewhere; $500,000 was to be applied to the operating budget and $750,000 to the capital budget.

The university appealed to the Commonwealth Fund for an appropriation of $1 million, up to three-fourths of which might be used for capital construction. The Fund ordinarily did not contribute to capital or operating budgets of state universities, but it had aided the establishment of new medical schools in several state institutions. In view of the program's importance to Hawaii and its potential importance to the whole Pacific area, an appropriation to help meet the initial operating costs seemed warranted. A grant of $350,000, together with the $500,000 allotted from the Kellogg grant for operating costs, would cover the entire amount needed from private sources for operating expenses over the first three years and leave only $510,000 to be raised from private sources to meet the estimated operating budget over the first five years. In 1964 the Fund board of directors decided to award the University of Hawaii's program a five-year grant of $350,000.[124]

The University of Hawaii John A. Burns School of Medicine enrolled its first class in 1967. Three years later, at the instigation of the state legislature, the university studied the possibility of expanding its program to grant the M.D. degree, and in 1971 the Fund gave the university a grant to study the education of physicians and ancillary health professionals. The study team, headed by Walsh McDermott, chairman of the Department of Public Health at the Cornell University Medical College, included Carleton B. Chapman, dean of the Dartmouth Medical School; Rashi Fein, professor of the economics of medicine at Harvard; Robert S. Morison, professor of science and society at Cornell; and David E. Rogers, now president of the Robert Wood Johnson Foundation. The team was assisted by the International Council for Educational Development, headed by James A. Perkins, former president of Cornell University. The resulting report outlined the advantages of a degree-granting medical course at the university—including increased access to medical education for the state's college graduates, to continuing education for the state's physicians, and to more and better house staff for Hawaii's hospitals. The report also pointed out the university's potential to develop a unique M.D. program, one emphasizing ambulatory medical care in group-practice settings, which were more prevalent in Hawaii than in other parts of the United States.

On the other hand, the report advised that the university proceed with the formation of a degree-granting medical school only if an institution of distinct excellence could be assured. It set three conditions: a definitive plan specifying the goals of the school and the means of integrating them with the university's other professional curricula, such as public health; a system of hospital affiliations for quality clinical instruction under the supervision of full-time faculty; and a clear commitment from the state legislature for adequate capital and operating funds.[125]

With the fulfillment of these requirements, a full four-year medical school was begun in 1972 and graduated its first class of sixty-two students in 1975.

Terence A. Rogers, the present dean of the medical school, believes that the Commonwealth Fund's support of McDermott's study was crucial to the expansion of the two-year program: "The McDermott report convinced the legislature to authorize expansion in 1972 and to fund a four-year school the following year. . . . Its importance is far out of proportion to its cost of $20,000. . . . Dr. McDermott himself was a particularly convincing advocate of the expanded school with the state's legislative and executive leadership."[126]

Two aspects of the school's program were unusual: its focus upon primary care and its entire reliance upon community hospitals rather than a university hospital for the clinical segment of medical education. The first was intended to encourage graduates to practice in Hawaii and the Pacific area, as Hawaii's population of only 1 million required mainly primary physicians. The second was a matter of necessity: As Terence A. Rogers has said, "There is no way whatsoever that Hawaii ever could have afforded to build and operate a University medical center. Further, the new medical school could not have afforded, and probably not survived, the rivalry that would have been inherent in a University medical center where the facility itself and the faculty would be in direct competition with existing community hospitals and the community's non-academic practitioners."[127] Participating in the program were 524 community doctors as part-time, uncompensated clinical faculty, along with 38 full-time and 28 part-time paid clinical faculty.

The school of medicine was closely allied with the university's other health-professional schools (including the schools of public health, nursing, and social work). Collectively, they were designated the College of Health Sciences and Social Welfare. To improve the quality of preprofessional education within the university and its coordination with professional education, faculties of the professional schools and the undergraduate college proposed a core program in the college for the early years of all health-professional education; an interdisciplinary major in biomedical sciences for undergraduates preparing to pursue health-related careers; and review and improvement of the various majors currently pursued by health-science students in the undergraduate college. A $50,000 grant from the Fund in 1977 met the costs of released faculty time and other associated expenses.[128]

A final contribution from the Fund in October 1979 met the expenses of a two-day conference of the Faculty on Curriculum. The acting dean, John S. Wellington, characterized the conference as "a useful exercise well worth the time, energy and money expended on it."[129]

The University of Hawaii Integrated Medical Residency Program combined several free-standing, community-based residencies in internal medicine. The charge of the state legislature to prepare physicians for the practice of primary care medicine in Hawaii and the Pacific Basin led Hawaii's program to decline to offer residencies in the medical subspecialties. Says Rogers: "Events made a virtue out of what originally was a necessity. . . . The academic payoff has been that our students train in a setting similar to the one in which they eventually practice, rather than in the sometimes remoter world of a university medical center. I would emphasize that the full range of tertiary care is part of our students' experience in the community hospitals."[130]

Between 1976 and 1983, 119 residents completed their training. Of these, 30 continued their training in subspecialties, 73 went into the practice of general internal medicine (mostly in Hawaii and the Pacific Basin), and 16 elected military service, the university's master's degree program in public health, or some other option. As of 1984 approximately 185 residents were in training in the University of Hawaii system in six residency programs (surgery, psychiatry, pathology, pediatrics, obstetrics and gynecology, and internal medicine). There is also a one-year transitional program and a small program in orthopedics. In 1981 a primary care track was developed within the general internal medicine residency. Four residents participate each year, and evaluation of the new program's effectiveness indicates that it has provided excellent preparation for primary care practice.[131]

Rogers believes that "although funding was received from other sources as well, the timing and amount of Commonwealth Fund grants was absolutely fundamental to these developments and they have paid off handsomely."[132] Most of the fifty-seven medical students in each current entering class would not have had the opportunity to become physicians without this program.

Teaching the Teachers

THE UNIVERSITY OF BUFFALO SCHOOL OF MEDICINE

One of the physicians concerned with the education of medical students in the late 1940s was Edward W. Bridge, a member of the Department of Pharmacology at the University of Buffalo. Bridge had joined the University of Buffalo faculty in 1945 after establishing a sound reputation as a clinician and investigator in the Department of Pediatrics at the Johns Hopkins University School of Medicine. His major interest was in the pathophysiology of the functional disabilities of children with convulsive disorders, and his work in the laboratory of a basic science department brought him into contact with medical students who felt overpowered by the factual details of anatomy. The study habits they had learned in college were useless when thinking, reasoning, evaluating, and philosophizing were suddenly displaced by the need to learn the innumerable facts of anatomical structure. Bridge wondered whether the present standards for admission to medical school really favored the individual most likely to become successful in a profession based on physiological function and human relationships. He questioned the sequence of courses in medical education, which sharply separated the entering student from the interest in human beings that brought him to medical school in the first place.[133]

Bridge turned to Lester J. Evans for advice, and during the winter of 1949 Bridge and Evans met several times. Evans recalled that "Bridge asked what a school like Buffalo might do . . . to arouse an interest in medical education among the faculty. I suggested that they might simply divide the freshman class into small groups and pick from any place in the faculty where they could find them good young teachers who would be interested in meeting with these groups of freshman students once every two weeks."[134] Bridge seized upon this idea and by the following September had not only identified a number of potential participants but had also convinced the administration and faculty that such a program would be worthwhile. He proposed an elective course that would allow students to talk without inhibitions about themselves, their interests, and the medical curriculum, and would expose them to a variety of experiences illustrating the human and social aspects of disease.

This "Seminar on Medical Education" continued for five years and involved nearly 100 medical school faculty members. Reaction on campus was mixed. The medical school administration and the leading members of the faculty were not convinced that the program was accomplishing a great deal of good, but neither did they feel that it was damaging. In 1951 the program was expanded to allow the original tutors to follow their students into the second year while a new group of faculty members was recruited for entering freshmen. In the next five years, bedside teaching became central to this elective, and what began as an informal experience evolved into a more formal offering called "Introduction to Medicine." This course helped students to relate their first-year classroom and laboratory studies to the patients they would see during their careers.[135] Although a few other schools, such as Western Reserve University, were introducing first-year students to clinical medicine, this practice was still new and unusual. The unique feature of the Buffalo program was its accompanying seminar for tutors, in which the faculty—including professors of education, psychology, and sociology—exchanged reports of their meetings with students, debated institutional organization and policy, and heard each other out on issues of teaching methods, curriculum organization, and examination systems.

Bridge's next step was to reach out for help from professionals in education. At the suggestion of Benjamin Bloom, a distinguished educator from the University of Chicago, Bridge organized a collaborative study between professionals in education and teachers in medicine. In the course of this effort Bridge came into the orbit of Nathaniel Cantor, professor of sociology and anthropology at Buffalo, whose interest in the process of learning had spanned his professional lifetime. Cantor's ideas about the inextricable mixture of emotional, physical, and intellectual elements in learning, his personal performance as a seminar leader, and his illustrations of the differences between what teachers commonly do and what is required to facilitate learning had a profound influence on Bridge and his group.[136]

The promising results of these seminars for tutors led to a more elaborate training program for medical teachers. With the cooperation of the dean and of various departments of the medical school and with the support of the school of education, a five-year program for a "Project in Medical Education" was approved by the medical school's executive committee. Obtaining outside support for the program was more difficult: The Kellogg Foundation, the Rockefeller Foundation, the Fund for the Advancement of Medical Education, and the Hartford Foundation declined proposals for support.

The one foundation staff member who encouraged the group was Lester J. Evans. Evans filed the following note after a visit with George E. Miller, one of the key faculty members in this program:[137]

> About two years ago the university asked the Fund for a small grant . . . but at that time we felt the university really was not ready to go as far as we wanted and we had some doubts about the quality of the medical school leadership. Miller was, therefore, somewhat apologetic when he came in this time, saying he did not know how we felt about Buffalo but hoped that our attitude was more favorable than in the past. I immediately stated that our attitude had not been unfavorable but rather that in our judgment, and with the commitments we then had pending, Buffalo did not seem to offer the opportunity we wanted. . . .
>
> My interpretation of this proposal at the moment is something like this. That heretofore we have been asked to assist medical education by approaching it through study and rearrangement of the curriculum, for example, Western Reserve; the reorganization of subject matter, for example, Harvard Basic Science; the demonstration of a new type of patient care, for example, Cornell.

... Now Buffalo says they would like to concentrate on teacher training, so to speak, in the belief, from what they have seen over the last five years, that medical school teachers thoroughly familiar with such topics as listed in their proposal would quite automatically change course structure, course content, sequence of educational experience, and so forth to meet what they will have come to recognize as the students' educational or learning needs. ...

Even though there is much for the university to do in working out the detail ... of their proposal and much for us to do in appreciating this approach to the study of medical education, I hope that we can ... continue discussion with them.

Evans's cautious expression of interest led Dean Stockton Kimball to ask for a return visit by the Fund's staff, an invitation that precipitated a review by the Fund of the distant background of Buffalo's program as well as more recent efforts. The Fund's staff was ambivalent at first, as a flurry of internal discussion suggested, but eventually there was general agreement among the staff that the proposal deserved further consideration.

A final proposal was approved by the university's medical school executive committee in January 1955, and on February 1 Chancellor Clifford C. Furnas formally submitted it to the Commonwealth Fund. It advocated research into four questions: How important to the education of medical students was an awareness among medical teachers of fundamental educational principles? Can teachers be more effective if they are trained by other divisions of the university along with the school of medicine? What would be the effect of a teacher training program upon the education of medical students? How practical is such an approach to the educational problems of medical schools?

Two weeks after the proposal was submitted, Charles O. Warren of the Fund's staff suggested a formal site visit to review the program in detail. John C. Eberhart's notes from this visit in March reveal the care that the Fund devoted to evaluating potential projects:[138]

> This is a unique proposal, something quite different from anything in the field of medical education that we have been asked to consider previously. Its novelty, of course, does not of itself make the program good, but it is my feeling that the project is both novel and good. I base this on the following considerations: 1) the project is essentially a study of medical education, plus some experimenting with it, as a joint undertaking by medical and nonmedical professionals. Including the latter in the manner proposed is an excellent idea, since it is bound to bring new thinking into the field. These contributions from education, sociology, and psychology will meet the day-to-day discussion, criticism, and in some instances, actual testing by medical school faculty members.... The give and take that will inevitably result should be an almost ideal testing ground for new approaches to medical education; 2) Having the

focus on the learning process to the extent indicated in the prospectus is also a good idea . . . ; 3) While the ideas behind the proposal are attractive and seem sound, the project's most important asset, so it seems to me, is the quality of the people involved . . . ; 4) The fact that major curricular changes are not proposed at the outset should not be viewed with misgiving. This group realized perfectly well that a good curriculum is a vital part of any educational process, and they will certainly be analyzing curriculum structure to see what kinds of changes pretty much have to be made. But the fact that they want to start out finding out how much can be done within the present assignment of hours seems a perfectly sensible thing to do . . . ; 5) The program will doubtless have at least two general kinds of impact. In the first place, an activity of this magnitude and intensity cannot go on in a school like Buffalo without sensitizing pretty much the whole school to its educational program. . . . The other kind of impact will be on the participants, both the medical people and the others. The only question will be how much influence the participants from other medical schools will have on their own schools when they return; 6) The situation in which this program is to be carried out is a favorable one for the project. The University of Buffalo has the people, in and out of the medical school, to implement it, and they are strongly motivated to do so. . . . I view this project as potentially contributing importantly to medical education. It is almost a "natural" for the Fund at this time and I recommend its support in line with the above budget.

A delay of several months ensued, and it was not until November that Malcolm P. Aldrich informed Chancellor Furnas of the Fund's decision to appropriate $131,400 for this project from December 1, 1955, to August 31, 1958.

Once the University of Buffalo had been brought into the Fund's family, the university's staff was given the benefit of expertise attained by other Fund-sponsored programs: Each of the five seminar teams visited one or more of the other schools (Cornell University, New York University, Columbia University, the University of Rochester, and the University of Colorado) whose programs in medical education were supported by the Fund. In addition, all spent two days at Western Reserve University, which was then the scene of a sharp break with educational tradition in medicine.

After the program had been in operation for a year and a half, Eberhart assessed its progress: "I think the experience of this first year has demonstrated the wisdom of the decision of 18 months ago. This experience in the improvement of medical school teaching hits directly at a central problem of medical education, and it has shown that knowledge and skill in this important area can benefit through the assistance of those for whom the study of education is a life work. In view of the traditional isolation of schools of education from other units of universities, this is an important demonstration. We may well find that in the years to come, some of the young people who have participated in these programs will be among the leaders in medical education in the future."[139]

The project was designed as a five-year effort: a preparatory year followed by four one-year segments of a work-study program for local and visiting faculty. After the program had been underway for a few months, the administration applied for funds to complete the program during 1958 and 1959. New directions were proposed for these final two years: the medical school faculty should have more opportunity to meet with educational scientists; the school should find more economical methods of providing seminars and workshops for larger numbers of interested faculty from other schools; more emphasis should be placed on educational research to match the emphasis on educational programs; and reference materials should be developed for others embarking upon similar teacher training programs.

The Commonwealth staff responded favorably to this renewal application. Their report to the board of November 1955 stated:[140]

> The program is based upon the obvious but sometimes overlooked fact that the heart of all education, medical or other, is learning. Therefore in order to cope successfully with the problems of medical education, it is essential that the role of the teacher be both clarified and emphasized. This comment is as pertinent now as it was two and a half years ago. The Buffalo program, concentrating as it has on the function of a teacher in relation to student learning, has focused on a set of problems which in themselves are old but which have long needed new emphasis. The work of the project so far has been fruitful, and the activities proposed for the final year seem essential if the experience of this group is to be made available as widely as its merits suggest it should. In view of the Fund's continued interest in the improvement of medical education there seems ample justification for recommending continued support.

The Fund's board of directors approved a terminal grant of $60,000.

The first results of Buffalo's program were intangible. Educators saw how medical school instruction was carried out, and physician teachers saw their work anew through the eyes of colleagues who were more concerned with process than with subject matter. During its final years, however, the program was hampered by an unstable administration, and the venture consequently lacked real support. Through the tenure of two deans and one acting dean, most of the faculty saw the project as an interesting investigation more tolerated than sponsored by the school's administration. The program in Buffalo was never really a major influence on the general faculty; in this sense it had to be considered a failure. In the opinion of Donald R. Becker, the surgeon who headed the program in its last years, the final determination of the program's success would have to wait until junior faculty members had advanced to high administrative positions, where they could incorporate into their own medical education programs the knowledge gained during their years at Buffalo. Only then could it be determined whether the piecemeal gains had added up to final success.[141] Attached to the Commonwealth Fund file copies of the final report of the project is a handwritten note by John C. Eberhart: "A rather touching and somewhat sad final report on a noble experiment at Buffalo, a school with its troubles. It didn't set the Buffalo medical school on fire but that now appears not to have been very combustible. It did have some good wider influences."

Colonization of Buffalo's Program

Although the eventual assessment of the University of Buffalo's project in medical education was far off, its immediate influence was apparent. The stream of interested visitors led the staff at Buffalo to believe that others might profit from the expertise they were acquiring. The group's first public presentation took place at the June 1957 annual meeting of the National Institute of Health's Cardiovascular Teaching Grant coordinators; the Buffalo group described their program in tandem with representatives from the well-established Western Reserve experiment. In 1958 two of the project staff were asked to be consultants to the first teaching institute at the University of Michigan School of Medicine, and Buffalo's first summer institute in medical education spread the word of the program's activities through the enthusiasm of its participants.

The first offshoot of the Buffalo program appeared in a roundabout way. In December 1958 the Buffalo group submitted a grant proposal to the Commonwealth Fund requesting more than $36,000 for "A Study to Determine the Impact of an Educational Consultant on a Medical School." The study would have four stages: preparation, matching, implementation, and assessment. Although the Fund was sympathetic toward the proposal, it reluctantly concluded that it could not justify support for a program of this magnitude. The Fund's staff was prepared to discuss possible alternatives, however, and during the February 1959 Congress on Medical Education, Lester J. Evans and Charles O. Warren met with members of the University of Buffalo group and agreed to place a consultant in another school that seemed ready for the experiment.

Dean William Maloney of the Medical College of Virginia was eager to have Edwin F. Rosinski on his faculty as a lecturer in education and a consultant to the school's Committee on Medical Education. A site visit to Richmond by Warren and Eberhart in April 1958 produced a positive recommendation: "This proposal is a natural for the school . . . stemming as it does from their exposure to the Buffalo program."[142] In May the

Fund's board of directors approved the grant and Rosinski accepted the position.

Over the seven years of its existence, this first colony showed that a professional educator in residence could improve the educational program of a medical school. So effective was the program that in 1961 the college established a formal Office of Research in Medical Education, and when the Fund's grant was terminated the next year, the college assumed financial responsibility for the entire activity. The next year, however, the school instituted a completely new curriculum, and when Rosinski left the medical college in 1966, his position was not filled. His work at Virginia was nevertheless rejuvenated in 1972 through a newly established planning and development program that served the entire Virginia Commonwealth University Health Science Center.

The second colony was established at the Stanford University School of Medicine. When Stanford's medical school moved to Palo Alto, Stephen Abrahamson, one of George E. Miller's disciples at Buffalo, was given a temporary appointment to help establish the school's new education program.[143]

In the meantime a third offshoot of Buffalo's program grew up on the medical center campus at the University of Illinois in Chicago. During the late 1950s, Dean Granville Bennett had encouraged a group of young faculty members who were combining enthusiasm with scholarship to improve the institution's program of medical education. The faculty supported Bennett's idea that Illinois should undertake the kind of educational experimentation that until then had been carried out primarily by small, privately supported schools. When Bennett turned to the Commonwealth Fund for financial assistance in 1958, Lester J. Evans spent a week on the Medical Center and Urbana-Champaign campuses of the university. His long memorandum described the visit: "I am not yet able to understand fully why this school should have gotten such a good start in studies of medical education . . . but the fact remains that very few schools have done as wide a range of work as this. . . . Possibly the greatest single factor is in the quality of the faculty. They are faced with an enormous educational problem and are desirous of doing the best possible job as teachers. The nearest brief characterization I can give of the faculty group I saw and the enthusiasm with which they entered into the discussion of problems under consideration is that they are as much like the Western Reserve faculty of the early days of their educational program as any group I have seen."[144]

Six months later Evans's favorable impression had led to a formal proposal requesting support for the "Study and Evaluation of Medical Education at the University of Illinois College of Medicine." The proposal envisioned a center that would be regarded as an essential unit of faculty organization: "When one examines the present-day complexities of medical education, medical and biological research and patient care programs, and when one gives full recognition to the potential strength to be gained by a medical school that is truly integrated into the university, one cannot escape the conviction that a permanent center or Department of Educational Study and Research is a necessity.[145]

The Commonwealth Fund's board of directors was enthusiastic about the proposal; at their next meeting in November they made an award of $12,000 for a two-year study. In February 1959 Bennett set out to recruit George E. Miller to head this program; Miller accepted the assignment in May and installed as his assistant program director Lawrence Fisher, who had trained at the University of Chicago under Ralph Tyler, a professional educator interested in curriculum and evaluation. In September Miller and Fisher launched a pacesetting program that became a national center for the propagation of educational research in medicine: ORME—the Office of Research in Medical Education.

The system used to evaluate students at Illinois, as in most medical schools at that time, seemed designed to negate the goals of the teaching program. Rewards generally went not to independent thinkers and critical analysts of complex problems but to students best described as "dependent memory banks." ORME's first effort was not a curriculum change in the conventional sense but an attempt to change the climate for learning by modifying the system of student appraisal. The idea of separating learning from certifying examinations may seem to be no great advance today, but in 1960 it ran against the grain of faculty skepticism that examinations that "did not count" could serve any useful purpose. ORME soon learned that the task of creating examinations to probe the many cognitive, psychomotor, and affective goals of medical education was not work for amateurs. To its office were added experts in testing who encouraged the use of examinations as tools for educational research as well as for judgment of academic progress. ORME also recognized that neither the medical faculty nor the student body could afford to give precious time to fruitless manipulation of courses. Until basic questions about institutional climate and methods were answered, mere shifting of hours had little permanent value.

After ten years of work, the staff of the Office of Research in Medical Education wanted the medical school's faculty to evaluate its progress: Was ORME moving in a manner in keeping with faculty understanding of its original purposes? Should these purposes be modified during the continuing years? Should long-range opportunities be seized and developed? The medical school's executive committee endorsed the character of the program, the emphasis that had been established, and the importance of grasping these long-range opportunities. With this support the pace quickened, and extramural as well as intramural challenges began to receive the attention of the growing staff.

The next organized institutional unit deriving from the Buffalo experience appeared in 1963, with the establishment of the Division of Research in Medical Education at the University of Southern California (USC). After one year at Stanford University, Stephen Abrahamson had returned to the University of Buffalo, then moved west again to head USC's new division, which became one of the leading American centers for this type of educational research.

Abrahamson's influence extended to the founding of the Michigan State University College of Human Medicine. Andrew Hunt, its first dean, was committed to making this new school different. After working closely with Abrahamson at Stanford, Hunt was convinced that he needed the help of someone professionally skilled in educational programs, planning, implementation, and evaluation. He called on Lester J. Evans for advice, and once again the Commonwealth Fund provided financial assistance, establishing what was to become the Office of Medical Education, Research, and Development at Michigan State. Hunt invited another of the original Buffalo group, Hilliard Jason, to become the first director of the new unit, which was an independent entity rather than an arm of the dean's office.

For the first time experts in science and education had jointly planned a medical school curriculum from the very beginning. The result was a program that emphasized individualized learning and student responsibility for achieving defined professional competence, deemphasized conventional grades, and highlighted the attitudinal goals of medical education and the interpersonal skills essential to the delivery of optimum health care. The program included early clinical experience and stressed equal emphasis on behavioral and biomedical sciences.

Reflecting upon the program in 1977, Dean Hunt observed that recruitment of faculty—particularly of new clinicians—was enhanced by the presence of the office and its well-known director. The college's generally acknowledged reputation was at least partly due to this unit's contributions to the school's educational philosophy and instructional practices, as well as to the wider field of research and development in education. Given another opportunity to design a new medical school, Hunt said, he would again include this educational resource as an integral component.[146]

Without the Fund's generous support to the earliest units of research and development in medical education, it is unlikely that the emerging science of education would have gained a foothold by the mid-1960s. By mid-1977 there were seventy-two medical schools in the United States and Canada that had established some type of unit for educational research and development.

The Teaching Institutes of the Association of American Medical Colleges

In 1957 the Fund gave the Association of American Medical Colleges (AAMC) $100,000 to support a series of teaching institutes, which reexamined medical education, emphasizing the social and behavioral sciences.[147] Participating in the 1959 institute was Paul J. Sanazaro, then an associate professor of medicine at the University of California Medical Center in San Francisco. His suggestion that the AAMC become a central resource for schools wishing to initiate programs in medical education was funded a few years later by the Carnegie Corporation.[148]

Two years later the Fund renewed its grant to the AAMC, enabling the organization to extend its comparative study of student selection, medical school performance in relation to college grades, and personality characteristics of medical students. The renewal also provided for a two-year continuation of the annual teaching institutes, emphasizing clinical and graduate instruction.

In January 1962 Thomas Hale Ham proposed to AAMC president Donald G. Anderson that "report meetings" be scheduled during the Association's annual sessions so that those doing research in medical education could share their findings with interested colleagues. These meetings were eventually integrated into the association's development program for research in medical education and evolved into the well-known Annual Conference on Research in Medical Education.

Teacher-Training Programs in Perspective

It was unfortunate that Fund-supported projects to "teach the teachers" never gained the sort of acceptance enjoyed by its other efforts in medical education. This type of program was most successful at new schools that were building a faculty and curriculum de novo and at old schools undergoing major reorganization. Successful teacher-training programs in this country and Canada usually find their home in the less research-oriented schools of medicine; in the more research-oriented schools with well-articulated traditional mechanisms for curriculum design, formal programs to train teachers are notably absent. Faculties in established, stable schools are more concerned with scientific research than with the study of teaching or the improvement of the teaching skills of individual faculty members. In these schools the student-faculty ratio is small, the variety of talents available does not encourage formal attention to this aspect of medical education, and faculties assume that their firsthand experience cannot be greatly improved upon.

Most schools have considered programs to educate teachers as outside the medical school's basic budgetary responsibility. When external funds are readily available, these programs continue to function, but when funds diminish, moneys available to "teacher-training programs" fall at a faster rate than those for less peripheral programs. This circumstantial evidence attests to a lack of wide-scale acceptance of teacher-training programs as essential ingredients in the basic medical school structure: The attitude of faculty is often that these programs should not usurp funds intended for biomedical research.

As one observer commented: "The new discipline moved into the medical milieu as did Cortez on the Indians. The educationists sometimes seemed to possess intuitively a greater truth far above the ineptness of the jugglers of hours and schedules. They used a language which though new and appealing was in essence meaningless to the uninitiated. Such phrases as 'the learning environment,' 'information versus knowledge,' 'data base versus facts,' 'behavioral endpoints,' 'educational objectives' were often abrasive rather than soothing. The lack of communication created by the jargon polarized the opinions of the Indians. A few were attracted; a few were hostile; but most were unimpressed, skeptical, or indifferent."[149]

The problem of recognition and acceptance was magnified by the rapid turnover of deans—even if a dean was supportive, his tenure might end before the educational research and development program could get off the ground. Since these programs were somewhat peripheral to the traditional administrative and departmental structure, securing academic appointments and a departmental home was frequently a source of difficulty. Nor was lack of enthusiastic acceptance confined to problems of funding, recognition, and rewards. Miller described the attitude of the basic and clinical scientists on the faculty as one approaching arrogance. They saw nothing inconsistent in their insistence on devotion to scientific inquiry in the laboratory and their rejection of carefully planned educational studies whose findings might "fail to match their educational preferences."[150] They readily accepted data that supported the traditional views about teaching but were unresponsive to findings that suggested better ways to carry out their pedagogical responsibilities.

Perhaps even more influential was the question of departmental autonomy: A department would vigorously defend its curriculum time and guard against any invading ideas about improving the educational process for which it was responsible. Once a department was assigned a piece of the curricular pie, it decided what was taught and how. Yet faculty contributions to a better educational mix could be achieved without fracturing the traditional departmental structure, as the program at Western Reserve University demonstrated. Few schools were able to imitate Western Reserve's success, however. "A lifelong commitment to learning, a sense of personal responsibility for that learning, a spirit of critical inquiry, a sensitivity to individual human needs, and a willingness to share decision-making with patients rather than denying them an opportunity to have a voice in determining how their health shall be maintained or their ill-health managed"[151] must not be the property of any one individual segment of the medical school, but should permeate the whole institution. "It is here that the medical educationist, charged to assist faculty in designing a curriculum, instructional materials, or evaluation procedures that address such goals, often experiences the greatest frustration."[152]

Medical Education and the Community

THE UNIVERSITY OF KENTUCKY SCHOOL OF MEDICINE

The new medical school at Kentucky was also supported by the Commonwealth Fund, with a series of grants beginning in 1957.[153] One of its most exciting experimental programs stressed the place of the individual and the family in the ecology of the community by providing each medical student with a community medicine clerkship, which included a field placement. This required course, a central part of the medical school curriculum, was designed to demonstrate the basic principles of public health, preventive medicine, epidemiology, and organizational patterns of medical care.

The program included clinical and laboratory studies, experience with public health nursing, and social service consultation, but its essential feature was the six weeks that each senior medical student spent in a Kentucky community.[154] Here the student became an observer and special health worker under the general guidance of a local physician, who might be a private practitioner, health officer, or industrial, mission, or group clinic physician. Students felt the close interrelationship of the problems of medicine, preventive medicine, public health, and family and community life. The clerkship also gave them a first-hand acquaintance with facilities available for handling health, social, and environmental problems. Introducing students to the nature of medical practice in these communities, the clerkship benefited the communities as well: As it actively and repetitively involved the medical school in community health problems, it became a type of postgraduate education for the local physicians involved. The key figure in both aspects of the program was the student, who served as a liaison between the patients on the one hand and the local physicians and medical school staff on the other.

A pilot program allowed four senior student volunteers from other medical schools to take an extramural clerkship during the summer of 1961. In 1962 twenty-four senior students from Kentucky's new medical school participated, and the following year the first class that would graduate from the University of Kentucky College of Medicine took the required course.[155]

The organizer of this innovative department was Kurt W. Deuschle. After receiving his M.D. degree from the University of Michigan in 1948, Deuschle pursued postgraduate training in internal medicine and oncology at the University of Colorado and the Syracuse School of Medicine (now the Upstate branch of the State University of New York).[156]

Early in the Korean War, Deuschle applied for a position in the Public Health Service, requesting an assignment in India. What he received was an assignment to the Indian Service on the Navajo reservation. He was given charge of the tuberculosis hospital, although he had never treated a case of the disease. Also on the reservation were Walsh McDermott and Carl Muschenheim, who were working at Many Farms, in a community health demonstration project developed by Cornell University; emphasizing primary care, it was the prototype of today's neighborhood health centers.[157] McDermott and Muschenheim exposed Deuschle to the role of the behavioral sciences in medicine; from them he learned the importance of understanding cultural differences when treating patients. During his time on the reservation, he also collaborated with John Adair, an anthropologist. His experience in the Southwest amplified the knowledge he had acquired in medical school: new ideas about the behavioral sciences, epidemiology, and biostatistics led to his interest in what he called "community medicine." Deuschle was ultimately put in charge of the Many Farms project, where he documented patterns of disease among the Navajos and conducted research on the interplay between the tribal faith healers and modern medicine. He developed an intense desire to find a medical school setting in which he could continue this type of work, refining the solutions to questions that depended on the study of a population base.

In 1960 Deuschle received an offer from William R. Willard, dean of the University of Kentucky College of Medicine, whose interest in community medicine was as strong as Deuschle's. Four years earlier Willard had suggested, in a memorandum outlining the philosophy of medical education for the new school, the founding of just such a department at the University of Kentucky: "To know the health problems of the area, some members of the faculty must study them. . . . To accomplish this the community must be utilized as a laboratory in which the medical school studies certain problems just as the hospital ward or physiological laboratory must be utilized for the study of other problems."[158] What Deuschle hoped to do at Kentucky was to develop a replica of the Many Farms project.

Deuschle's approach was to study the community surrounding the university. He found that the local physicians deeply resented the new medical school: They felt that it was taking money away from the University of Louisville—their own school, the school from which they had graduated. Coupled with this resentment was a certain lack of sophistication in the ways of academic medicine: Some thought that the beneficiary of a grant received the money personally. A demonstration project, Deuschle concluded, would be the worst approach, leading these doctors to believe that he was talking down to them. His plan was instead to assign students to work on specific problems with these physicians; the choice of problem would be the student's, but the problems would be ones that the physicians or the community wanted pursued.

In devising this plan, Deuschle had consulted with George G. Reader, a colleague at Cornell, and Reader suggested that he approach the Commonwealth Fund for support. Although Roderick E. Heffron liked Deuschle's ideas, he recognized his inexperience; the Fund's three-year grant reflected Heffron's belief that the plan would require a larger budget than Deuschle had in mind.

Deuschle gave a great deal of thought to naming his new department. He did not like the idea of including "public health" in the title, as public health activities were looked upon as second-rate and politically oriented among the physicians he dealt with. "Preventive medicine" did not seem exactly right either, as preventive medicine was already a recognized part of each doctor's responsibilities. Deuschle finally chose the term "community medicine" to represent the department's dual interests in medical care and the recipient population, because he felt that the department should stress the scrutiny of populations and should train its internists to be not only good doctors but good epidemiologists as well.[159]

Deuschle recognized the close relationship between health and the other factors that can hamper or facilitate the development of a community. Medical education traditionally emphasized diagnosis and treatment of individual diseases, and responsibility for families and communities was relegated to professionals in other fields such as public health or sanitary engineering. In his new department, Deuschle wanted to combine these two closely interrelated functions. To prepare practitioners to use all the health sciences, the first step was to give the student a basic familiarity with the field of epidemiology. Later the student was sent into the field to learn how to apply this knowledge to the health problems of a particular community. The community medicine program began in the medical student's second year, with classroom exercises and discussion of the distribution and determinants of disease in human populations. The fourth-year clerkship allowed each student to identify strongly with a community in the same way that he identified with his patients in the hospital. The student spent several hours each day with his sponsoring local physician, but most of his time was dedicated to obtaining a complete picture of health care in a community. He studied the family not merely as a collection of indiviudals but as a dynamic group in which health was seen to relate to a multitude of physical, biological, and cultural variables. (Deuschle initially required each student to keep a field diary, a technique he had learned from his association with anthropologists.) The student learned how the community was organized and how its major institutions functioned politically, economically, and educationally. Most important, he learned how to work with personnel in other fields as part of a team.

As a link between the medical center and the established medical practice in the local area, the student was able to inform the university medical center about health conditions in the local communities and, on the other hand, to convey to the local physician information about the work of the medical center. The medical student was also able to encourage new practices in the physician's office and a new look at the community—for example, in promoting the use of new diagnostic tests. When a student screened patients for carcinoma of the cervix in the doctor's office or health department, he usually turned up a significant number of abnormal test results, encouraging other practitioners to intensify their own screening. In one case a practitioner had abandoned the cervical cytology test because he was not obtaining any abnormal findings. Once the student had tactfully demonstrated the proper technique, he and the practitioner were soon finding the expected number of abnormal results.

A long-established precedent encouraged university consultation in communities throughout Kentucky. Since the university was a land-grant college, providing agricultural extension services to all parts of the state, the people were familiar with a university functioning at the "grassroots" level. Just as the agricultural agent provided information on the latest development in his field, so the student provided the local physician with information about medical advances.[160] The agricultural extension agent was traditionally the most popular public servant in most rural areas, and the warm reception accorded the Department of Community Medicine may have been partly a bonus, spillage from the community's respect for the agricultural program.

To develop more teachers of community medicine, a graduate training program was essential. Deuschle's program incorporated a first year of hospital-based clinical training and a second, or academic, year equivalent to that spent acquiring the master of public health degree in a school of public health. Each year one or two postdoctoral fellows also joined the department as teachers and investigators.[161] The physicians in the Department of Community Medicine also held appointments in clinical departments, and the state commissioner of health and three of his division heads held teaching appointments in the department.

The program was a great success: The new department's work was effective, and the students were enthusiastic about their clerkships. After two years Deuschle suggested to the medical school's dean that the president of the university assure the program's support after the

Commonwealth Fund's grant ended. In 1963 President John Oswald provided him with this guarantee.

When the University of Kentucky requested a final two years of support in 1964, the Fund commissioned an evaluation from Henry J. Bakst, professor and chairman of the Department of Preventive Medicine at Boston University. Bakst interviewed members of Kentucky's Department of Community Medicine, administrative officers of the medical center, students, and graduates of the program. In all, twenty-three faculty members participated in the evaluation, including Willard, the medical center's vice-president. Bakst concluded that the program was enhancing the continuing education of physicians in Kentucky and would have a wider influence on medical education in general. The Fund's staff was also enthusiastic about the program. Roderick E. Heffron, the Fund's program monitor, had been a particularly valuable resource—a frequent visitor and an experienced advisor with whom Deuschle could discuss his progress and air his ideas. Bakst's favorable appraisal led the fund to meet the university's request for a grant of $190,520 to the Department of Community Medicine.[162]

Bakst's review of the program's progress had been preceded by evaluations built into the program itself. The field physicians appraised the entire clerkship program along with each student's work. The program's staff also used several carefully selected techniques—students' performance on the National Board examinations, follow-up reviews of students' work and career choices, and student and faculty evaluations of the program.

The multiplier effect of the Fund's grant was well illustrated by the later positions held by the members of Deuschle's staff. Hugh Scott Fulmer set up a department of community medicine at the University of Massachusetts; M. J. McNamara became chairman of the Department of Community Medicine at the University of Ohio at Toledo; Jesse W. Tapp, Jr. joined Herbert K. Abrams at the University of Arizona, where a similar program was founded; and Anthony Adams returned to the University of Sydney, Australia, where he later became a leading policy maker in the national health deparment. A department of community medicine at the new medical school in Marshall, West Virginia, was also modeled after Kentucky's program.

When Deuschle left Kentucky in 1968 the clerkship in community medicine was one of the most popular and respected courses in the curriculum. The program in community medicine had been developed at a time of rapidly accelerating scientific progress. With the resulting new social, economic, and political problems in health care came a new concept of comprehensive health care. Community medicine emerged as a cooperative field integrating medical and biological disciplines. In the ensuing years, emphasis on the preservation of health, not just the treatment of disease, has become a part of our culture, fortified by legislation. The physician must now share the health-care turf with the social worker, sociologist, cultural anthropologist, industrialist, economist, and politician, and the result has been many significant changes in medical teaching and practice.

In coining the term "community medicine" and creating the first formal department, Deuschle put comprehensive medicine out into the field. He transferred the concept of comprehensive care, which he had gained by participating in George G. Reader's clinic at Cornell, from the tertiary care center to the rural field situation. His efforts could never have come to fruition without Commonwealth Fund support—in this case, support of an idea never before tested.[163]

THE MOUNT SINAI SCHOOL OF MEDICINE

In 1968 Kurt W. Deuschle was asked to head the Department of Community Medicine at the Mount Sinai School of Medicine. He was considering this offer when Colin M. MacLeod, the Commonwealth Fund's vice-president, gave the commencement address at the University of Kentucky, and Deuschle had the opportunity to discuss the potential move with him. MacLeod was obviously interested in an attempt to adapt the rural experience in community medicine at Kentucky to an urban area. The Curriculum Committee at Mount Sinai had included a six-week full-time clerkship in community medicine as a required rotation during the last clinical year, hoping that Deuschle's successful model could be transplanted to urban soil.

Established in 1852, the Mount Sinai Hospital was known for its notable clinical scientists and prominent specialists. Yet it was not until 1968 that Mount Sinai was reorganized as a medical school and medical center. Most of the clinical faculty was on the scene, but a second faculty in the basic sciences had to be recruited from the outside academic community. A unique feature of the Mount Sinai plan was the addition of a "third faculty," which would run the school's planned programs in the social aspects of health. The selection in 1965 of George James as dean, president, and the first director of this third faculty reflected the aspirations of its administration and trustees to establish the institution as a ranking center of medical learning. James was a national leader in community health and preventive medicine and an advocate of an interest by urban medical centers in ongoing community health problems. Mount Sinai was located in East Harlem, a community ideal for this sort of liaison. James incorporated the third faculty as the Department of Community Medicine, an integral part of the total group responsible for creating professional problem solvers in the fields of health care delivery and environmental health.

James also recognized the importance of affiliation with neighboring community hospitals, as academic collaboration might lead to improved health services for a much broader segment of New York City's population. Links with the Hospital for Joint Diseases in upper East Harlem, the Beth Israel Medical Center on the Lower East Side of Manhattan, the Elmhurst Municipal Hospital in Queens, and the Bronx Veterans Administration Hospital rapidly swelled the bed capacity of affiliated hospitals to more than four thousand.

One of James's first missions was to move Mount Sinai into a university complex, and he succeeded in establishing the Mount Sinai School of Medicine within the City University of New York (CUNY). The school, which admitted its first students in September 1968, represented the union of a large voluntary hospital and a public university. Its commitment to community health was overtly expressed through the establishment of a Department of Community Medicine and its allocation of teaching time for community medicine in all four medical school years. CUNY underwrote the full support of ten professorships—a link between its graduate school and the medical center—and James assigned two of the ten to the Department of Community Medicine, one in medical sociology and a second in health economics. Adequate endowment and operating income were still to be secured, however, and the school needed short-term funding to see it through its early years. Money for a sound basic science faculty was particularly important, and a grant from the Commonwealth Fund helped meet this cost.

As he had done at Kentucky, Deuschle began his tenure at Mount Sinai by learning something about the community his department was to serve. He felt that the request for Mount Sinai's technical assistance should come from the community itself. Deuschle did not ask physicians to go out into the community, and he resisted the opening of "storefronts"; his feeling was that one does not win any battles by simply giving without asking the community to contribute as well. His approach was to work with the community if it wished help and was willing to accept reciprocal responsibility. In 1970 the Commonwealth Fund gave the program $600,000 for a preliminary study of the community and its needs.[164] This grant enabled Deuschle to survey East Harlem's health problems and to identify community organizations concerned with health.

One of his first targets was an organization created under the Model Cities Program, in the so-called triangle area of East Harlem. The executive of this program had demanded medical care from Mount Sinai doctors, but Deuschle suggested that before committing the hospital to such an effort, they look at the area's overall situation. Deuschle discovered that although no physician practiced in this area, its residents lived fairly near hospitals that could provide medical service. What the area really needed was transportation: Its inhabitants were in a cul-de-sac and had difficulty in reaching the sources of medical care. Deuschle directed the organization to a source of funds for the purchase of a van, trained a van driver in emergency medicine, and gave workers training in health procedures. This community did not need an influx of physicians—it needed the opportunity to identify its problems. Once Mount Sinai's studies had documented the problems, the department could help community organizations compose a grant proposal to secure the funds they needed. The grant proposal could in turn include requests for the services of Deuschle and his staff.

A second grant from the Fund three years later enabled the department to investigate the possibility of developing a health maintenance organization for the area.[165] To head this project, Deuschle recruited Samuel J. Bosch, who brought considerable experience in developing prepaid health insurance plans. Although Bosch concluded that a health-maintenance organization would not be practical in Harlem at that time, the Fund's grant cemented him into place in the department, and over time Bosch became a major influence on Mount Sinai's efforts to improve community health.[166]

Deuschle had also recruited Michael M. Stewart to head an academic unit at a Mount Sinai affiliate, the Elmhurst Municipal Hospital in Queens.[167] The unit was intended as a research arm of Mount Sinai that would study problems of a city hospital and its surrounding community. The city's financial situation worsened considerably just as it was planning to take over the support of this unit, and the municipal government had to back out of its commitment. The project's work had progressed well, however, and the group was highly respected, so the Fund awarded the unit a large grant to compensate for the city's default.

Deuschle's faculty also obtained a federal grant to train internists in primary care. Once again, the program was oriented toward community medicine, even though it came under the umbrella of the Department of Medicine and was directed by Harry Rubin, a nephrologist.

The Fund's grants enabled Deuschle to organize his department so that it could influence the systems of public health, and coordinate health and hospital work and prepaid health-care group practice. Managing the department's program for the health department was Nicholas Cunningham, who set up a model comprehensive clinic for the care of infants and young children. The health and hospitals work was the responsibility of Stewart's unit at Elmhurst, and the group practice was managed by Bosch and his group.

Deuschle was also able to apply strategic flexibility to training students. A required clerkship occupied each student full-time for four weeks in his third year of medical school. This clerkship in the clinical years enabled the student to obtain first-hand experience in establishing the relationship of population data to clinical problems. The program was modified by

Bessie S. Dana and her staff in the Education Unit to reflect the urban situation. At the University of Kentucky, the students had been sent out into the community for their clinical clerkships; in the East Harlem community sensitivities and the dangers of the street—drugs and crime—prevented students from working directly in the ghetto community. Instead, each student developed an epidemiological definition for a problem in East Harlem, and worked the problem through to the stage of a written thesis. Theses could explore any of six areas:

1. Health care delivery to a specific community or population group (e.g., the elderly, children, adolescents)
2. A past or present epidemiological problem
3. A current health care delivery organization, such as New York Blue Cross, New York's Health Insurance Plan, or Mount Sinai Hospital (emphasizing, for example, quality of care, financing, or structural issues in health care delivery)
4. Human interaction in a medical setting, such as a doctor's office (e.g., compliance, patient education, behavior)
5. Patient-physician interaction
6. Important issues and organizations in national health care (for example, the National Institutes of Health, Medicaid, Medicare, government policy, the Professional Standard Review Organization

The range of topics selected by students for investigation reflected the department's emphases. In early years projects dealt largely with East Harlem's health problems and resources, in keeping with the high priority the department gave to understanding its neighboring community. Later projects expanded to include systematic studies of child abuse, alcoholism, and teenage pregnancy, and of the epidemiology of chronic illnesses (especially hypertension, coronary heart disease, and cancer). Subsequently students surveyed the efficacy of health education programs, patients' preferences in the selection of physicians, differing modes of clinical intervention, and, with increasing frequency, the systematic study of the phenomena of rising health-care costs, quality-care assessment, and new forms of health-care delivery and payment. The theses generated much excitement among the students, and many of the manuscripts were published. Dean Thomas C. Chalmers, an epidemiologist in his own right, was so impressed with this work that he personally funded a prize for the best paper.

The transplantation of community medicine from a rural to an urban setting could not have happened without the Commonwealth Fund's support. The Fund's grants allowed Deuschle to focus on what he felt was important and to set up his program efficiently.[168] His success can be measured in part by the expansion of his department, which eventually had fifty-five full-time members and a budget of over four million dollars a year. Commonwealth Fund seed money was transformed into an ongoing, sustaining budget for the Department of Community Medicine—a department whose budget now includes approximately $200,000 a year for community services. The Commonwealth Fund's essential contribution was to provide the money for high-risk ventures not funded by the school or the community. Had the Fund not supported this idea at the start, the community medicine program at Mount Sinai would have died without seeing the light of day.[169]

THE UNIVERSITY OF VERMONT SCHOOL OF MEDICINE

As the only four-year medical school in the tri-state area of Vermont, New Hampshire, and Maine, the University of Vermont School of Medicine had traditionally emphasized the training of general practitioners for this sparsely settled region. When George A. Wolf, Jr., was appointed dean in 1952, he decided that the school needed to assume greater responsibility for providing high-quality medical care to the upper New England area.[170] He appointed Leon R. Lezer, a former Vermont practitioner with a master's degree in public health from Harvard and experience in administration, as director of health studies and head of the planned Department of Preventive Medicine. The programs that evolved from Lezer's investigations reflected the philosophy of the school and the department. In his words, "A department of preventive medicine must reach into the environment if it will effectively understand and teach environmental medicine."[171]

Lezer's program featured, in addition to the basic work of the new department, a teaching program in preventive medicine for medical students; the Total Family Care Program (actually a part of the teaching program); and the Regional Medical Needs Program, the department's major service and research arm. All four parts were intended to teach the concepts of comprehensive medicine and demonstrate the application of paramedical resources to the care of patients and the evaluation of medical needs, encourage students to enter general practice in the tri-state area, bring better medical care to rural areas and develop rural health centers, foster interdisciplinary teaching activities, and extend the philosophy of the New England Higher Education Compact to medical education and medical care.

The medical faculty accepted the idea that designing better local programs required the skills of sociology, public health, and nursing, and in 1956 a grant of $24,000 from the Commonwealth Fund enabled the Department of Preventive Medicine to begin planning and organizing community health facilities.[172] The grant was extended the following year to provide $124,000 for the regional medical care project under development and $60,000 for a family care project.[173] August B. Hollingshead, chairman of the Department of Sociology at Yale University, provided the program with two medical sociologists; the Fund's grant also allowed Lezer to arrange legislation creating a tri-state Regional Medical Needs Board, a forerunner of similar national legislation.[174]

By the time Peter V. Lee evaluated the program in 1959, the department included, in addition to Lezer, an assistant physician trained in public health, a social worker, a nutritionist, a health educator, a public health nurse, two part-time general practitioners, and the full-time director of the new rehabilitation unit. Lee concluded that the Department of Preventive Medicine had fulfilled the intentions set out in its initial grant proposal to the Fund. Although the school's success in achieving one of its long-range objectives—encouraging students to enter rural general practice—would not be known for many years, all the other goals had been reached on schedule. The teaching program in preventive medicine had been expanded from a few lectures in sanitation and epidemiology to a four-year program including sociology, patient care, preventive medicine, rehabilitation, and a family care clinic. The Total Family Care Program, a program exposing fourth-year students to ambulatory patients, grew out of a reorganization of the Burlington City Dispensary, an affiliate of the school for several years. This program improved the quality of patient care for the indigent population of Burlington, demonstrated high-quality general practice to medical students, and coordinated teaching for students of medicine, nursing, and other paramedical disciplines. Medical students worked for one month in the general practice clinic and home care service and were also assigned to supervise the long-term health of families. At a time when few medical schools were studying the particular problems of practicing medicine in an aging population, the University of Vermont's program also included a rotation in geriatrics at the St. Joseph Home for the Aged. On the debit side, a severe handicap to the Total Family Care Program and the school as a whole was the lack of an effective program in psychiatry (still a division of the Department of Medicine).

In the Regional Medical Needs Program, the Department of Preventive Medicine consulted with medical societies and health agencies throughout the tri-state area. Over a score of communities had been studied as candidates for rural health centers, and several centers had been established. A unique arrangement of grass-roots community support for these centers had been crucial to their success. To Lee, the most striking feature of the program was the school's central role as a consultant to communities with problems in health care.

The volume of consultation requests had so increased that the work of the Regional Medical Needs Program had become the department's largest single activity. While community service was undeniably important, the demands of this program prevented the members of the department from engaging in research. Lee came down hard on this problem: the school of medicine had a basic obligation to approach preventive medicine from a research point of view (rather than merely to find no more than currently appropriate solutions).

After Lee's evaluation the Fund continued to help the University of Vermont School of Medicine stress comprehensive medical care at reasonable cost. A three-year grant of $225,000 assisted the school in developing a campus-based group medical practice for patients from a cross-section of the community; opened in 1971, this operation grew into a model teaching center. The most innovative part was its structured approach to medical care, known as Problem-Oriented Patient Care. The patient would fill out a detailed questionnaire before his visit; next he would undergo a standardized series of examinations and laboratory tests conducted by trained medical aides; finally, he would be examined and interviewed by a physician. Physicians would analyze the resulting information to identify the patient's problems, including psychological and social stresses, determine the priorities of these problems, and formulate a plan of treatment for each item. Through these steps the patient's record was organized as an active document presenting the full spectrum of his needs.

Lawrence L. Weed, who had come to the University of Vermont from Western Reserve University to head an operations research laboratory, assessed the ratio of treatment cost to benefit. His unit determined whether the most economical plan was being followed and applied his concepts and methodologies to the redesign of medical services.

The problem-oriented approach was also used to teach students how to conduct the office practice of medicine—to show them how operations and records could be structured to ensure that patients received comprehensive, economical care. The first step was to involve students directly in constructing and using the patient-oriented record. The entire freshman class participated; in subsequent years these students studied the management of patients with specific diseases and participated in the care of patients with the group's physicians. Hospital-based training had long been the dominant form of the doctor's clinical education, but the staff saw as a long step forward their effort to elevate ambulatory medical care to the same level and to use it in the instruction of future physicians.

Five years later five additional centers had been established in Vermont and nearby areas of neighboring states. The six facilities comprising the university's program in primary care were governed through the college's Departments of Family Practice and Internal Medicine. The major center serving Burlington and Chittenden County alone handled 20,000 patient visits each year and was adding from 200 to 250 new patients each month.

Up to this point, the problem-oriented approach seemed to be an economical, reliable system for providing ambulatory care. Rational and evaluable, it was able to compete in quality with other types of practice. Program directors nevertheless identified obstacles to the system's wider distribution. The problem-oriented approach conflicted utterly with the system of reimbursement set in offices for ambulatory medical care, a system whose economy was based on the volume of patient care as the chief measure of productivity. Its use of nonphysician personnel and the participation of patients in their own treatment had also contributed to reducing the cost of care, but put it at odds with the office-based physician's traditional economic incentives. To reconcile this discrepancy, the Health Care Center was negotiating with New Hampshire–Vermont Blue Cross/Blue Shield (which covered more than 50 percent of the center's patients and handled Medicare and Medicaid payments) to develop reimbursement systems consistent with the problem-oriented approach. Considerable study of these issues was needed during the next few years, and the center turned to the Fund for support. A grant of $100,000 in two equal annual installments was provided to evaluate the center's accomplishments and develop financial systems consonant with the problem-oriented approach to primary medical care.[175]

By August 1977 five years of experience with the Problem-Oriented Record System had enabled the Given Health Care Center at the University of Vermont to demonstrate substantial improvement in the quality of care and a similar reduction in its expenditures—the result of changes in the behavior of both patients and physicians.[176] The next step was to connect the use of the problem-oriented medical record to payment for care. The center intended to provide financial incentives for physicians and patients to use the system wisely; the resulting savings would be used to further expand the center. To carry out this plan, the center's staff obtained a further grant from the Commonwealth Fund to develop:

—An advisory board made up of owners of businesses in the county served by the center
—A network of practice sites that would be willing to implement the problem-oriented system and, in collaboration with the center, form a prepaid health program
—A management team and data base system that could be used in work with insurance companies or a third-party carrier such as Medicaid or Medicare

All three programs were completed during the span of the Fund's grant. The head of the project wrote: "Without the award from the Commonwealth Fund it is doubtful whether these steps could have been taken. Certainly this work would have taken a lot longer, and may have been seriously abridged without the award."[177] This final grant from the Fund prepared the way for the next phase of the program, the actual planning and implementation of a prepayment program, which was begun with the support of the Kaiser Family Foundation.

The Problem-Oriented Health Care Program continues today as an important part of the medical school. The centers originally supported by the Commonwealth Fund's grant have grown substantially. Full-time faculty at three internal medicine practice sites and the Family Practice Center log over fifty thousand patient visits per year, and provide primary care to about twenty-two thousand people in Chittenden County. More outlying centers also continued to thrive as part of the medical school's referral network, and the Blue Cross/Blue Shield reimbursement plan now involves all of the university practice groups.[178]

Teaching Community Medicine

The teaching of community medicine, among the most innovative of the Fund's programs in medical education, represented further efforts by the Fund to integrate its programs. An extension of comprehensive care, it brought forcefully to the medical student's attention the necessity of integrating principles of public health with those of preventive, diagnostic, and curative medicine. In the original program, at the University of Kentucky, the teaching of community medicine was an excellent type of continuing education for the practitioner; for the medical school, it served as a listening post in their efforts to evaluate the preparation of students and house staff for general practice. Most important, it had the capacity for self-perpetuation, as when, for example, members of the pioneer program at the University of Kentucky left to found similar departments in other schools.

Each Fund-supported program in community medicine had a slightly different cast in its relationship with its parent university and surrounding community. The Mount Sinai project was a broker in the provision of health care, guiding the community to make its own arrangements. This department became a sort of mini-school-of-public health and ultimately played only a modest role in the planning for the larger medical center. The University of Vermont was active in putting educational principles into effect in the community, whereas the program at the University of Kentucky focused on educating its medical students. The strength of the Department of Community Medicine at the University of Southern California was its ability to combine government support with the innovative use of foundation funds.

The Fund regarded projects in community medicine as promising trials of the belief that medical schools should turn toward their surrounding communities. Begun during Aldrich's presidency, this aspect of the Fund's program was continued by James Quigg Newton, Jr., Aldrich's successor, who was deeply committed to encouraging universities in applying their considerable resources to problems of health care. His hope was that schools would be able to create efficient models applicable on a national scale. Although these early attempts may have failed to reach some of their lofty goals, they provided a base of information for later efforts.

Financing Medical Education: The Use of Capital Funds

Until 1947 the Fund's only contributions to medical schools had been grants that enabled them to try out some specific but small-scale approaches to improve their teaching. Subsidies in twenty medical schools during the academic years 1946 and 1947 related primarily to the Fund's mental health and public health programs. By March 1951, however, the Fund's staff was ready to present to the board a formal statement of policy on support of medical education, extending the Fund's concern with the medical school alone to the school's relationships with the parent university, the surrounding community, and the nation.

The Fund's staff believed that professional education for physicians was in danger of reverting to a proprietary status. They attributed this trend to increasing control of medicine during the first half of the twentieth century by the physicians themselves. It was movement in the wrong direction. Throughout its history medicine's role in society had called for vigorous and unbiased social leadership. The university alone could provide some of this leadership, but organizations like foundations could help the university to exert even greater influence. The historical importance of the medical school's association with a university had long been recognized,[179] but the Fund's staff believed that when universities accepted the responsibility for an annual expenditure of $80 to $90 million in the name of medical education, they were obliged to do more than simply keep intact a vocational training program granting medical degrees.

By 1955 the Fund had already aided half of the eighty established medical schools in the United States. Its targets had spanned schools private and public, of national and local importance, distributed around the country. Some projects focused on the early part of the medical curriculum, some on the latter part, some on intrauniversity integration, and others on extramedical school and university-community relationships. Emphasis in education after high school had shifted from the natural sciences to the social and behavioral sciences, and this shift was echoed in all of medical education. Although the Fund's initial grants had been limited to relatively small, isolated segments of the total educational sequence, with experience the staff came to realize the importance of considering relationships between the segments. Three focal points of interest were converging: the learning process, comprehensive patient care as a basis for clinical teaching, and integration of medical education within the university.

The president and staff of the Commonwealth Fund believed that the future of medical education was being decided at this critical time. An injection of philanthropic dollars, wisely applied at strategic points, could be most effective in strengthening the present and shaping the future of medical education. The Fund considered several alternative approaches. It could give a large unrestricted sum to an organization such as the National Fund for Medical Education, the American Medical Association, or the Association of American Medical Colleges for distribution to schools of their choice. With this type of program, however, the Fund's staff would learn nothing, since they would have no control over the selection of recipient schools and thus no opportunity to study the schools under consideration. Another possibility was the use of unrestricted awards to individual universities. Earlier the Fund had considered giving block grants totaling between $50,000 and $100,000 to universities for "human biology" programs: integration of teaching and research in the basic sciences. Lester J. Evans now favored an initial modest expenditure of $300,000 to $400,000, to be apportioned among ten or so schools to use as they wished, but with the informed understanding of the Fund.

Between February and April 1955 the Fund's staff came around to the idea that money might be drawn from capital, making possible much larger grants to individual schools—a timely plan, since congressional committees were scrutinizing the activities of private foundations and the market value of the Fund's endowment had increased greatly over the years. Large unrestricted grants would be of immediate help to schools and might also encourage other foundations to greater support of similar projects. The policy of making unrestricted grants from capital to medical schools was formally adopted by the board of directors at its meeting on May 26, 1955. The new grants would supplement, rather than replace, the Fund's current activities in medical education.

In line with its previous policies, the Fund's staff felt that the objectives of unrestricted giving should be consistent with the Fund's interests and experience. These new grants were intended to enable schools to institute or maintain creative programs in medical education, adopt what they saw as the best in current educational experiments in other institutions, enlarge the impact of current medical educational experiments, clarify their educational objectives and take greater initiative in deciding the direction and rate of change in their educational programs, and stimulate giving from other sources.

Rather than dwelling upon details of implementation, the Fund's staff decided to ferret out the distinctive characteristics of the leadership in applicant schools and the inherent capacities of the institution. The Fund's staff had set itself an enormous task in studying the institutional needs of even the short list of schools already developed. To investigate a school, the staff would scrutinize its objectives, its concepts of teaching and learning, the implementation of its philosophy in the curriculum, its commitment to educational research, its present or potential points of growth (such as interest in the sequence of university and medical school education, integration of basic science teaching, improved or comprehensive teaching and patient care, and integrated psychiatric teaching), and its relationship with the surrounding community. The skill of the Fund's staff in judging both the potential of an institution and the school's ability to follow through would probably be more important than a detailed program outline (unless the outline demonstrated the institution's insight into its own problems). Often an institution envisioned its growth only around some new activity, when the revamping of an old one might be just as valuable.

For a grant to be most effective, however, it should be used as the institution saw fit—for staffing, for equipment, or for remodeling of laboratories—and it should be made in several large aggregations or spread over a period of years. This new flexibility represented a shift in the Fund's policy: The institution's judgment of its needs became more important than the Fund's insistence on some set of established requisites. The public announcement of the new program reflected this change. It said that the objectives of an applicant's program should be consistent with the Fund's interest and experience, the gifts should meet the needs of the institution, and the money should be spent as the institution judged best for its purposes.

Grants would be made on the recommendation of the president and staff and after approval by the board of directors. Appropriations for this program were expected to total $12 million, and individual grants would range from $300,000 to $1 million. The proposed program of capital grants would in no way militate against the ongoing programs of the Fund.

Financial considerations and the time needed to evaluate each applicant school led to the Fund's decision to spread the expenditures over three years. The schedule of appropriations and expenditures permitted three types of activity: immediate gifts of substantial size from the 1954–55 allocation to complete the Fund's assistance to major projects already underway in institutions well known by its staff; immediate discussion with institutions about the possibility of assistance in the coming year; and scouting among institutions that might be satisfactory prospects for future awards but were now largely unknown to the Fund.

The staff knew that grants of this size would focus national attention on the Commonwealth Fund. For the country at large, the grants would be evidence that the Fund was willing to complete programs that were progressing successfully. The staff worried, however, that to professionals in the field, large capital grants might create the erroneous impression that the Fund was finishing off its interest in medical education, shutting the door to opportunities not yet visualized. To allay these fears, the Fund's staff wanted to extend the Fund's support into new fields over the three-year period as well as to round off some of the Fund's present commitments.

In the six months between the formal adoption of the program and the next board meeting, the members of the staff investigated thirteen of the twenty-seven schools that appeared to qualify for consideration and made recommendations for grants to ten. Former Fund gifts to each institution were taken into consideration in arriving at the amounts recommended, but greater weight was given to the soundness of the school, its potential for medical training and leadership, and its current programs.

Between November 1955 and February 1956, the staff investigated another seven schools. Two (Northwestern and Tufts) had recently undergone major shifts in administrative leadership at both university and medical school levels. The result was fresh, creative thinking that had produced a number of imaginative proposals covering a range of educational activities. The Fund believed that these two schools, at this strategic point in their growth, would benefit more from fluid grants earmarked for certain broad areas than from a completely unrestricted grant. The grants proposed for Northwestern and Tufts would come from the unexpended balance of the Fund's regular medical education budget and would combine elements of both project and capital grants. While limited to general areas, they could be applied within these areas as the school saw fit. For the Fund this type of award would exemplify the principle of fluid support.

Soon after the board voted the first ten grants from capital funds, the Ford Foundation announced a plan of awards to each of the country's privately supported medical schools. At the same time, Congress was considering legislation to aid medical school construction, and it appeared likely that industry and other foundations would make still more money available for medical education. The president and the staff of the Commonwealth Fund were delighted: This additional support would free more medical schools from the pressures of meeting day-to-day demands. Schools could then begin to think creatively about the future, enabling them to do an even more effective job of educational development.

The final allocations from capital funds were made at the board of directors' meeting in May 1956. In the past six months, nineteen medical schools at private universities had received grants totaling $11,500,000 from capital and $1,000,000 from income (see app. G) The Fund's staff saw no uniform pattern in the disposition of the grants. Some schools placed the funds in permanent endowment, using only the income; some planned to use both principal and income over a period of years. A few allocated the grants for construction and equipment. Many schools added faculty members and increased the salaries of their present staff; some set up pilot experiments in medical education; some strengthened and enlarged programs already installed. In the group as a whole, every aspect of teaching function was aided in one way or another in both the basic sciences and the clinical areas.

It is difficult to generalize about the value of these grants to the recipient institutions. The psychological effect was a marked boost in faculty morale. The general public also appeared to be developing an increased understanding of the problems of medical schools. Editorial comments indicated that these grants from the Fund helped to focus attention at a crucial time on the serious problems facing university medical education. In retrospect the timing of the gifts appears to have been fortuitous, not only for schools such as USC, Emory, Northwestern, George Washington, and Tufts—where opportunities at the time were unusual and pressing changes were needed—but for the country in general.

Lewis Thomas recalled the Commonwealth Fund's grant to New York University:[180]

> A year before the end of my term in pathology, the NYU medical school received a major grant of $750,000 from the Commonwealth Fund, with instructions to use the money in whatever way seemed best for the future of the school. The preliminary discussions with the foundation, and within the faculty, had concerned the possibility of installing some new educational programs for paramedical personnel—physiotherapists, occupational therapists, medical social workers, and other professionals who work in close collaboration with physicians. We did a lot of arguing, and a rump session of the chairmen, led by Colin MacLeod, began meeting to discuss alternatives. We emerged several months later with a different plan, for which I had the job of drafting the initial proposal, a new program to be called the Honors Program, under which all of the new money would be set aside for the single purpose of providing new opportunities for selected medical students to undertake fundamental research while still in their student years, with fellowship support, ample time off from the regular curriculum, and the requirement of a formal, full-scale thesis before graduation "with honors." The Honors Program won the day, after much debate, and was initiated with its base of operation and offices in the Department of Pathology. It was the first program of its kind that I am aware of, and later received support from NIH as the precursor of similar programs set up at other universities, culminating in the combined M.D.-Ph.D. training programs now under way in about twenty medical schools. Looking back, I think this was the most interesting experiment of all the ones I had a hand in during my time at NYU.

Vernon W. Lippard, then dean of the Yale University School of Medicine, discussed the unrestricted grant to that institution:[181]

> [It] came just at the time when medical schools were becoming more and more dependent on federal research grants. This made it very difficult to make up a solid budget before the end of the year due to the fact that a final decision on many of the grant requests was still in limbo. So we put the Commonwealth Fund capital grant money in the savings bank. Thus, if we wanted to start a subdepartment of otolaryngology, we could support the cost in the budget against the Commonwealth Fund grant. Then by the end of the year, funding would become available from another source, making it possible to put the Commonwealth Fund money back in reserve, ready to come to the rescue when another similar contingency arose. We used this fund many times over in just this way. It gave us a tremendous boost and was, in my opinion, one of the most constructive things ever done by a foundation.

Lester J. Evans was particularly pleased with the University of Rochester's use of a substantial portion of its capital grant to establish a department of preventive medicine.[182] Rochester received the Fund's capital grant at an especially propitious time, as it had in hand a small contribution from a private source for this purpose. With Robert L. Berg as its first—and present—chairman, the new department's focus changed from the classical interest in control of infectious disease to health care delivery. At first the Commonwealth Fund's capital grant was applied to salaries; later the Fund's money was used to build a model teaching unit for ambulatory care.[183]

From the Fund's viewpoint, these grants led staff members to become more aware of the needs and potential of many hitherto unfamilar medical schools; they benefited from the process of studying recipient schools before and after the awards. This series of "unrestricted" grants was an important and integral part of its established program of help for medical education and greatly increased the Fund's general knowledge of the field.

Experimental Health Services

There are perhaps few things upon which men are so agreed as that the problems which beset them today surpass in difficulty those which confronted any previous generation. It is maintained that never has knowledge been so complex nor the pace of life so insistent; that never has it been so difficult to take thought on those larger considerations which allow men to appreciate the trend of events and the measures by which they might be controlled.

—*Harold Himsworth, 1953*

The study of specific diseases, a drug's mechanism of action, a new surgical procedure, more accurate diagnostic tests—all these were worthy of support, but the Commonwealth Fund superimposed the principle that in the attack on the broader problems, definition and practical solutions required trained individuals from many different areas. Only cross-fertilization of diverse areas of knowledge could produce the wise, innovative counsel that would lead to practicable solutions to the many vexing problems facing medicine in the United States.

Greatly increased government spending in public health had made sanitation, control of communicable disease, and ordinary public health activities the direct responsibility of federal, state, and county agencies. The Hill–Burton Act had provided money for rural hospitals, and grants for research and training were liberally available from both governmental and nongovernmental institutions. Although the Fund made no formal study of the opportunity for large-scale projects in community health care, its experience led it to try out new forms of service at the frontiers of public health, hospital programs, and medical education. In the late 1940s, regional and community health efforts and activities without other sources of support were consolidated in a new classification: "Experimental Health Services." These experiments, however limited, were the points at which new concepts were tested and stepping stones laid down toward an integrated community health service. Progress was necessarily slow, because all features could not be fully mapped at the time.

The Experimental Health Services projects were varied in subject and scope. They included the medical care of indigents by the Richmond Department of Public Health; a study of family experience with medical care by the Health Insurance Plan of Greater New York; aid to the mental health program of the Rip Van Winkle Foundation of Hudson, New York; a survey of chronic illness in Baltimore; and a program of continuing professional education sponsored by the Rochester Regional Hospital Council. Among the most notable was the pioneering program at the medical center in Hunterdon County, New Jersey, a facility that went far beyond the usual community hospital in its smooth coordination of all the private and public medical care in a community.

THE HUNTERDON MEDICAL CENTER

At the height of the Fund's Rural Hospitals Program, the director of welfare in Hunterdon County, Rose Z. Angell, approached the Commonwealth Fund's staff about the possibility of building a hospital in the only county in the state without one.[184] Although her request was turned down, she would not be discouraged. With the help of Mrs. William F. Leicester, a county resident experienced in organization and public relations who was married to a New York corporation executive, Angell took her proposal to the Hunterdon County Board of Agriculture. Although this quasi-official organization represented the agricultural interests of what was at that time a very rural community, it included representatives of other community institutions, including schools, churches, and the chamber of commerce. Angell was not a member of the board, but this organization appeared to be her best hope, since it was the only one that represented the county as a whole and it had a record of giving early support to programs that later proved to be nationally important. The board was at first reluctant to involve itself in Angell's project, but in 1946 it agreed to appoint a committee to investigate her idea. Lloyd B. Wescott headed the committee, which included Mrs. Leicester as well as a half dozen community leaders. Once the support of the Board of Agriculture was obtained, the Commonwealth Fund was again approached for assistance.

From the outset, the Hunterdon project's true "spiritual leader" was Lester J. Evans, who recalled this initial period: "We began to hear about it from Mrs. William F. Leicester, a very flamboyant woman in dress, jewelry, style of hat, outspokenness—all in all a most attractive individual. Some of the staff were not in sympathy with the idea and since a previous request for a hospital had been turned down thought that things should go no further. Mrs. Leicester came to see me at the suggestion of James Alexander Miller so I was very willing to continue talking to her. We had known Miller through his sponsorship of the outstanding research program of Richards and Cournand which we were supporting. As I listened to Mrs. Leicester, I felt that they had something going that was worthwhile."[185] The Commonwealth Fund's usual policy prevented it from contributing to construction costs, but it agreed to consider support for other specific aspects of the project.

With the continued encouragement of the Commonwealth Fund and the state health department, the county's board appropriated $500 to hire an expert consultant, E. H. L. Corwin, of the New York Academy of Medicine. Corwin submitted his report in mid-1948, stating: "To sum up, if Hunterdon were to build just another hospital, I would be lukewarm to the proposition, but if this hospital is projected in terms of a progressive institution with a university affiliation, a model of its kind, aimed to bring what is best in medicine to the residents of a rural county and has associated with it an active, full-fledged health center and good follow-through social service, I would be strongly for it. The opportunity is here and there is unquestionably enough civic pride and business enterprise in this community to bring the plan for a hospital and health center to a successful consummation."[186]

An affiliation with New York University was available as part of a project directed by Clarence de la Chapelle to upgrade medical care in smaller voluntary hospitals in and around New York. Hunterdon Medical Center was incorporated and in 1949 opened a fund drive with a goal of $1,200,000. Before the contract to build was signed in 1951, gifts had been obtained from over 75 percent of the families in the county.

Evans then received an invitation to attend a dinner sponsored by Mrs. Leicester and Wescott, who as president of the medical center's board was the community leader in the movement to establish the hospital. No other foundation representatives were present, although representatives of the New York Academy of Medicine and New York University attended, along with Willard C. Rappleye, dean of the Columbia University College of Physicians and Surgeons. What was needed at this point was money for planning and administration. The following day, Evans wrote a memorandum recommending a grant of $25,000 from the Fund that was quickly approved by the board of directors.[187] This project fit perfectly with Aldrich's recent recommendation that the Fund support the development of an overall community health service that would unite hospital, medical school, public health, and medical clinic groups.[188]

The Commonwealth Fund's grant allowed Hunterdon County to recruit an outstanding staff, including Edmund D. Pellegrino in medicine, Andrew Hunt in pediatrics, and Ray E. Trussell in administration. Formerly an epidemiologist with the New York State Department of Health, Trussell came to Hunterdon from the Albany Medical College, where he was professor of preventive medicine. Through his influence, public health became a prominent interest at Hunterdon, implemented through countywide programs to reduce the incidence of such illnesses as rheumatic fever and rheumatic heart disease.[189]

The Fund deviated from its customary policy and appropriated an emergency construction grant of $250,000; Hunterdon needed quarters for special programs that required 10 percent more floor space than was usual in hospitals of its size. In 1951, $50,000 was allotted for programming, consultation, and other expenses connected with the center's opening, and $60,000 for the planning, direction, supervision, and field work necessary for a health inventory. Two years later the Fund added $158,100 to its earlier appropriations, and in 1954–55, a renewal grant of $118,250 was made to underwrite two-thirds of the cost of the center's community mental health program.[190]

Winthrop Rockefeller, chairman of the New York University–Bellevue Medical Center, secured $150,000 to provide the Hunterdon Medical Center with senior medical staff consultants and house officers. Affiliated with the New York University School of Medicine, the consultants were accessible to outpatients as well as to bed patients, and with the house officers carried their share of responsibility for the preventive and clinical service ordinarily associated with the health department. Hospital and health department were under unified direction. Home visitors and sanitary engineers worked out of a common center, and as new kinds of care were developed—for example, education and preventive mental health activities—they, too, spread from the same source.

Lloyd B. Wescott commented on the early phase of the project:[191]

> To sell so visionary a dream to a rural community was difficult but somehow it did arouse the most remarkable degree of support. One basic promise that we made the community was that if we were not able to raise the money to build the project it would be abandoned and everybody's money would be given back except for one or two gifts from individuals who had funded the drive.
>
> As we neared our goal, an architect was hired and the plans for the building were designed. As is almost always the case, estimates of our costs were unrealistically low and as the elapsed time had included the period of the Korean War, prices had escalated enormously. When the bids came in, we found we were $950,000 short and our options seemed to be to abandon the project and hospital. The Commonwealth Fund (I am sure at the urging of Dr. Evans) told us that they would give us a building grant of $250,000 if the community would accept the responsibility for going ahead with the project with the belief that the money could be raised or borrowed to complete the project by an opening date of 1953.
>
> The community accepted the challenge. Immediately after the groundbreaking, The Commonwealth Fund pointed out that we had to have an administrator and as our local funds had been pledged to construction, they funded the salary of Dr. Trussell. One year before opening in 1953, they suggested that we employ five key physicians to not only prepare the hospital for opening but to consolidate the concept with the general practitioners in the community and the community itself. These included Dr. Pellegrino as head of medicine and Dr. Hunt as head of pediatrics.
>
> Although Dr. Trussell deserves great credit for seeing the hospital through its construction and opening, and through the subsequent two years, I believe that credit for implementing the fundamental concepts on which the Medical Center was founded should be given to Dr. Pellegrino and Dr. Hunt. Frankly its development followed much more closely the concepts enunciated by Dr. Evans than it did those of Dr. Corwin. Dr. Corwin thought of two separate institutions: one a hospital and one for public health.

Medical Care at Hunterdon

The medical center began with 125 beds; twenty-five general practitioners, who had been in the community before the start of the project; eight specialists; and no family health centers. In its early years Hunterdon offered hospital privileges to any general or family practitioner in the county, an experiment that gave the patient the benefits of his own family physician as well as ready access to hospital specialists.

Eventually the medical center comprised a well-equipped hospital with

200 beds, including 15 for psychiatric patients; and four family health centers, which opened in areas distant from the medical center and were used as training centers in Hunterdon's Family Practice Training Program. Primary care was provided by twenty-five family physicians, most in private practice in towns scattered throughout the county. The closed, full-time staff of thirty-two specialists had offices only in the center. These physicians had been recruited with the help of the New York University–Bellevue Medical Center and provided a secondary level of care in sixteen specialties, with the number in each specialty related to demonstrated community need. The composition of the staff was determined by board action upon recommendation of a committee of staff and board members.

Hunterdon's specialists accepted county patients on referral from family physicians and returned these referral cases to the care of the family physician as soon as possible. Patients needing so-called tertiary care were referred to other hospitals, usually university centers. Family physicians did not have offices in the center, but they had admitting privileges in medicine, pediatrics, and obstetrics, and could retain responsibility for hospital care of their patients, ask for consultation, or put their patients under the care of the indicated specialist.

Teaching Programs

This rural hospital's intimate affiliation with a large urban university medical center (at New York University) was a unique feature of Hunterdon's program. While it lasted, the arrangement provided the local physicians with professional development and brought health services of the highest quality to the residents of a rural county, as each full-time Hunterdon specialist maintained contact with academic medicine by spending one day a week at Bellevue Hospital.

The affiliation was eventually replaced by Hunterdon's own family practice program, in which students rotated through Hunterdon from medical school at the University of Pennsylvania and from Albany and Jefferson medical colleges; interns came from St. Vincent's and Lenox Hill hospitals in New York, and residents from Lenox Hill. This program was one of the first of its type in the nation, and most of the physicians it trained were eventually certified by a medical specialty board.

Hunterdon Medical Center was next affiliated with the Rutgers Medical School of the New Jersey College of Medicine and Dentistry. All Hunterdon staff members had faculty appointments, and twelve third-year medical students at a time rotated through Hunterdon on clinical clerkships. Six residents a year served in the three-year Family Practice Training Program, giving the center one of New Jersey's largest and most capable residency training staffs. In collaboration with a nearby two-year college and a local high school, Hunterdon also provided clinical experience for registered and practical nurses and classes for x-ray and laboratory technicians.

Another important part of the Hunterdon educational mix was its program of continuing education. Daily contact between full-time specialists and general practitioners provided informal continuing education,[192] third-year medical students at Rutgers still come to Hunterdon Hospital for their clinical clerkships, and Hunterdon has always been able to fill the six openings in its family practice program with graduates from outstanding medical schools in the United States.

Financing Medical Care

Lester J. Evans had urged the group to consider a prepayment program, but since lack of subsidy required the center to limit its members to those able to pay, the planners' commitment to the entire community made them reluctant to follow this suggestion. With the inauguration of Medicare and Medicaid in 1969, however, they were able to consider such a program. In 1970 a $29,000 grant from the Commonwealth Fund supported a study of the feasibility of establishing a prepaid health-care plan that would offer all the residents of the county complete coverage under a unified system of medical service. This grant covered statistical, operational, and other studies and included the participation of experts from two groups at the University of Pennsylvania—the Leonard Davis Institute of Health Economics and the medical school's Department of Community Medicine. The Prudential Life Insurance Company made a key contribution by assigning top members of its actuarial staff to the project.

The Hunterdon Medical Center's physicians played a central role in establishing the criteria that would govern the plan. Since transition to prepaid medical service was being advocated through such measures as the formation of health maintenance organizations, implementation of the Hunterdon plan could have had national significance. But as the plans developed, the physicians raised more and more questions about financial risk, governmental domination, and the corporate practice of medicine. The hospital was ready to implement the plan on a capitation basis, with the support of a large number of the family physicians, but many of the specialists resisted it. In March 1972 the staff voted against the proposal by a two-to-one margin.

Despite the absence of a health-maintenance organization, the Hunterdon project was cost-effective. A Fund-supported report in 1971 by McKinsey and Company showed that the number of inpatient days per thousand population was 768 at the Hunterdon center, as compared to 1262 in New Jersey as a whole, 1212 in the United States as a whole, and 524 at the Kaiser Health Plan. The report concluded: ". . . the HMC [Hunterdon Medical Center] care system substantially outperforms the traditional system in New Jersey and the U.S.; the health of the population HMC serves is comparatively good; and the center's emphasis—through a variety of actions—on keeping people well and out of the hospital lies at the heart of this performance."[193]

In 1973, with the Fund's support, the Hunterdon Medical Center and Princeton University sponsored a symposium to celebrate the center's 29th anniversary. Medical educators and health-care planners at the symposium attested to the importance of the Hunterdon model. Edmund D. Pellegrino, the center's medical director from 1955 to 1960, said: "Almost all the principles upon which Hunterdon is built were hotly disputed two decades ago. . . . Today, most of the ideas that constitute the Hunterdon plan are considered essential to proper community planning for comprehensive health services. . . . Hunterdon's great contribution was to take a group of relatively new ideas, implement them in one institution, and unite them around a common mission—to provide the highest possible care for the people of a rural community."[194]

As the staff grew and personnel changed, the early sense of common interest decreased, productivity declined, and it became very difficult to attract physicians in the higher-income specialties. An "incentive plan"—a professional service fund—instituted in 1964 increased incomes and improved productivity, but dissatisfaction did not disappear. To distribute this fund, the president–medical director determined each specialist's salary for the ensuing year by estimating his contribution to the fund in fees and appraising his contribution to the overall operation (patient care, teaching, administration). The search for a solution over the next few years nevertheless failed, leading to a court suit and finally to a settlement negotiated by lawyers at vast expense to the center. At this time net income for the specialists after expenses ranged from $45,000 to $80,000; fringe benefits were offered but excluded malpractice insurance.

The settlement necessitated a new set of by-laws, which allowed the specialists to practice either in the medical center or in the community. They could be completely free of any formal commitments to the center or could continue under some negotiated agreement. Although Hunterdon's original goals were abrogated, the final settlement left in place of the unique rural center something better than just a good acute-care hospital. Wescott commented:[195]

> The ratio of board certified family physicians to hospital specialists has not changed significantly. Actually the community programs have continued to expand in areas such as patient education, predischarge planning, day care centers, programs for the elderly, a unique program in training retarded children at a very young age, programs to deal with both alcohol and drug

abuse, an extremely active home care program providing a wide variety of services, to mention just some of the more obvious ones. Community support continued to be very generous on an annual basis. We do have a trust fund provided by Mrs. J. Seward Johnson which produces about $325,000 a year. The income is to be used *exclusively* for programs that keep people out of hospitals. It also helps fund our Family Practice Training Program.

The DRG [Diagnostic Related Groups] Program oddly enough has worked in our favor. We always had a short length of stay and we never did take out every pair of tonsils that existed. Consequently, relating the case load to the length of stay is beneficial.

What interests me is less the extent to which Hunterdon has changed than the extent to which other hospitals seem to be following similar paths. The number of hospitals which train family physicians has increased enormously. I am inclined to think that it is to produce patients for the specialists. From the less cynical point of view, a great many are calling themselves "medical centers" and are indeed undertaking a broader community responsibility.

In 1977 the Hunterdon center proposed to document and evaluate its twenty-three years of experience, so that other rural communities across the nation could examine their health-care problems and choices.[196] The lack of access to medical care in many predominantly rural communities was a significant deficit of the nation's health-care services. Approaches to this problem had been proposed and tried, but none with outstanding success. In contrast, a self-sustaining health-care system was providing residents of Hunterdon County, rich and poor alike, with comprehensive health-care services that were in some respects without parallel in this country. In 1977 the Hunterdon Medical Center was the focus of nearly all local health services. Its hospital maintained 152 acute-care beds, 15 beds for the mentally ill, and facilities for newborns. More than thirty full-time, salaried specialists practiced at the center, providing postgraduate medical education as well as regular medical services; the county's twenty-seven general practitioners were affiliated with the center's hospital. The center also maintained a large department of physical medicine, a visiting nurse service, and clinics for speech and hearing therapy, well-child evaluation, mental health care, and drug and alcohol abuse. Three satellite clinics had recently been set up to increase access to care by residents farthest from the medical center. It also attracted federal money, receiving the highest priority in the state of New Jersey for support through the Hill–Burton Act. The experience of Hunterdon County obviously needed to be examined fully and objectively, the elements of the medical center's success identified, and the findings made available to health-care planners in other areas of the country and in government at several levels.

It was natural for the Hunterdon staff to turn to the Commonwealth Fund for assistance with this evaluation. Henry E. Simmons, a physician and health-care administrator of national stature and experience, had recently become president and director of the medical center. He proposed that the center recruit a small, highly qualified research staff to conduct a three-year, in-depth evaluation. For this purpose Hunterdon requested and received approximately $100,000 a year for three years to support the cost of a full-time research director, a junior research associate, secretarial assistance, travel, supplies, and overhead expenses.

An assessment of the Hunterdon center posed the question: "Is Hunterdon an idea whose time has passed? Has it been by-passed as a result of technology, astronomical costs, health-maintenance organizations, state rate regulation, federal cost-containment and the whole complex of increasingly centralized, increasingly bureaucratic controls that are emerging to cope with runaway costs?" In reviewing the failure of the original plan for the Hunterdon center, A. R. Somers pointed out that the national "commitment" to prevention, primary care, health-care planning, cost control, and the like was more rhetorical than real. There was no major accompanying effort, even through programs like Medicare and Medicaid, to redress the long-standing differentiation between specialists and family or general physicians, so that much of the "primary-care educational push" had been canceled out. As Somers indicated, we have continued to direct resources toward high-technology and tertiary care services by blank checks for such services written into Medicare, Medicaid, and most private health-insurance programs. "Many of the Hunterdon specialists felt that they were left behind in the nationwide race for the newest and fanciest technology that our multibillion dollar health-care economy would buy; that they were denied unrestricted access to all patients in the use of the technology, and the status, earnings and excitement that accompanied these developments."[197]

Although economists tended to dismiss Hunterdon as an isolated rural "happening" with little or no relevance to general national problems, Somers hoped that Hunterdon could turn out to be an idea whose time had not yet come. Perhaps a generation from now, when the limits of our health economy are more clearly understood, when the cost-effectiveness of prevention and primary care is more adequately documented and the experience of less affluent countries is fully assimilated, Hunterdon will be remembered and its wider potential applicability reexamined. This will depend in part on the values of the statesmen of the medical profession—on their voluntary acceptance of some sacrifice of personal freedom for the sake of a community program that may help to avoid eventual participation in a monolithic national system.

Edmund D. Pellegrino commented on the sequence of events at Hunterdon:[198]

The demise of the Hunterdon plan and vision is a complicated story which, of course, you cannot detail. The anatomy of that dissolution is yet to be made. . . . A few observations might be of interest. . . .

I am not sure there ever was genuine difficulty in attracting physicians in the "higher income" specialties. Many of these would be in the tertiary care specialties which were not appropriate to Hunterdon's mission. Moreover, the added attractions of an opportunity for full-time medicine, in a teaching hospital, and an attractive setting, compensated for differences in income. As director I always found recruitment much easier than the later staff wanted to believe.

In my opinion, the "incentive plan" was a major factor in the deterioration of the Hunterdon experiment. As soon as compensation was related to "units" of teaching or service, the whole idea of full-time medicine collapsed—as it has in so many medical schools. . . .

I was there when these thoughts first began to surface. We were successful in opposing them by the simple device of reasserting Board policy as a condition of employment. We urged those who wanted primarily to expand their incomes not to stay. Only one left and he was quickly replaced. . . .

A major factor was the fear that full-time physicians would leave en masse. . . . My answer always was, and is, that the Hunterdon staff was well compensated. Their base salaries plus fringe benefits . . . plus opportunities for teaching, research, and attendance at meetings would be hard to match. The specialists would have had to work much harder to net the same total compensation in private practice. Interestingly, few if any of the full-time specialists had had any experience with private practice. Those who did were the least dissatisfied.

The central issue was not really income but the kind of physician we wanted, and who could be attracted to the Hunterdon idea. Such physicians always sought us out. My problem as medical director was wishing I could employ some of the fine young specialists who wanted the kind of medical life we could offer them.

As you know, departments of medicine and pediatrics always have excellent clinicians and teachers who want an academic career but do not have the interest or capacity for clinical investigation. These people seek just the kind of situation Hunterdon offered. Even the surgical specialties are attracted. After all, we did recruit excellent full-time specialists in the "higher" income categories at the outset. And this was at a time when full-time salaried practice was in bad favor outside medical schools.

I was sorry the Board decided to settle out of court. Hunterdon would, I believe, have been a landmark case on the point of whether a community through its hospital Board may not employ physicians and establish the conditions of their compensation. We are certainly moving in this direction today in the for-profit, corporation-controlled hospitals. . . .

I believe that the ideas being tested out in Hunterdon County and the reasons for their being compromised have much to teach us that is relevant for the future of medicine. . . . The original Hunterdon plan may well turn out to be the middle position between corporate for-profit medicine with salaried physicians responding to corporate order, on the one hand, and laissez-faire practice in a so-called free market that so many medical entrepreneurs seem to prefer on the other.

. . .The Commonwealth Fund in its support for Hunterdon exhibited an uncommon prescience. Its leadership detected the significance of Hunterdon and enabled the most unusual community rural hospital in the nation to get off the ground.

THE MONTEFIORE HOSPITAL

The pioneering program supported by the Fund at the Montefiore Hospital in New York City was an experiment in the coordination of hospital and home medical care to relieve pressure on hospital facilities.[199]

In the late 1940s, the accepted place for a seriously ill person was a hospital, where medical, nursing, and technical services were available for his care. This course had obvious advantages: It put the patient in a controlled environment; it made both diagnostic and therapeutic facilities quickly available; it permitted each doctor to care for many patients without loss of time in travel; and it spared the patient's family the inconvenience of caring for the patient at home.

These advantages were bought at a price, however, and part of the price was psychological. The patient who accepted hospital care had to give up his normal relationships and submit to the ministrations of strangers; particularly if he were old, poor and sick unto death, he had to reckon with the overwhelming loneliness of dying among these strangers.

There was also a heavy financial price. The cost of building and maintaining hospitals had risen so much that community resources were severely strained. In the Fund's own experience, the cost per bed of building hospitals of approximately fifty beds in rural or semirural communities had risen since 1927 from $3,995 to $10,556. In 1949, for example, the $1 million promised by the Fund for hospital construction around Rochester, New York, would build perhaps one and one-half hospitals of fifty beds. Moreover, the survey made in 1946 by the Commission on Hospital Care indicated a need for 195,473 additional beds in the country as a whole. As for maintenance, figures compiled by the American Hospital Association indicated that in 1947 the average patient-day cost in short-stay hospitals for general and special purpose in the United States was $11.09. Even with federal aid for construction, it had become critically important to discover some way to lessen the burden hospitals imposed on public and private funds—perhaps by changing the way in which hospitals were used.

In 1924 Ephraim Michael Bluestone, the director of the Montefiore Hospital, had published a plea for the individualization of medical service in hospitals. He deplored the method of ward service that cared for patients en masse and identified them as bed numbers.[200] His search for a corresponding construction plan led six years later to an integrated hospital service in which the care of short-term (acute) and care of long-term (chronic) patients was completely united in the general hospital on a continuing basis, as long as the need for a hospital bed could be proved.[201] His plan emphasized continuity of responsibility at all times and under all conditions. Two years later, after completing a survey of health and hospital activities for the Associated Jewish Charities of Baltimore, Bluestone presented a plan that explored the possibility of using the home as an additional resource during illness.[202] As he pointed out, the demand for more hospital beds was nationwide, and it was clear that these additional beds would be prohibitively expensive. Bluestone's formula of home care for selected patients was a new idea in social medicine. With grants from the New York City Cancer Committee and the Greater New York Fund, Bluestone and his staff were able to plan a one-year demonstration project that offered an extension service on an extramural basis, with a free interchange of patients between the hospital and home under identical management.[203]

Bluestone was a theoretician, able to conceptualize programs that challenged the basic organization of medical care. During the time when hospitals were becoming an increasingly dominant force, he was developing the idea of "home care" in response to suggestions from doctors with terminal cancer patients. He chose Martin Cherkasky, the chief resident in medicine, to implement the idea at Montefiore, recruiting and training workers, rounding up equipment, and establishing routines that were to bring quality hospital care to patients at home.

Montefiore's Home Care Unit was the country's first hospital-based home health service, established as a separate department of the hospital on a par with the outpatient department. A medical home-care executive drawn from the visiting staff was placed in charge, and the project began on January 1, 1947. The plan returned to their homes—after the home and family situation had been studied by a social worker—carefully selected indigent ward patients who no longer needed surgery or x-ray treatment. There they continued to receive medical care from members of the hospital staff, nursing care from the Visiting Nurse Service of New York (under contract with the hospital) and social service from the hospital. They were given the use of movable hospital apparatus and supplies (hospital beds, foam mattresses, wheel chairs, and the like as well as syringes, bandages, crutches, and medication); from time to time, as needed, they received the attention of a physical therapist; and their families could have the help of a paid housekeeping aide. Specimens needed for laboratory analysis were secured in the home and taken to the hospital. When a patient needed the use of facilities that could not be brought to him, he was taken to the hospital in an ambulance or taxi and then returned to his home, a procedure not very much more difficult in crowded urban neighborhoods than putting a patient on a stretcher in a ward of a hospital and taking him to the x-ray room.

In the first year, 121 patients were selected for this service, and the average number under care at any one time was 31. Again, on average, these patients were visited by a doctor a little more often than once a week and had a little more than one-half hour of nursing time each week. Those whose conditions deteriorated were readmitted and they had priority over new patients on the waiting list. Cherkasky and Bluestone called the experiment a success. The patient-day cost to the hospital for service rendered in the first year was $2.25, as compared with a ward patient-day cost of $11.59.

During this initial period most of the patients selected had terminal cancer. Obviously, each new disease group presented fresh problems and the clinical feasibility of the plan could be fully tested only when a variety of diseases was represented. Many other questions called for study: What were the psychological effects of the plan on the patient's family? What auxiliary services were needed and how could they best be provided and coordinated? What were the implications for the long-term care of patients in the hospital? How could a continuous flow of service to the patient be maintained whether he was in the hospital, at home, or in the outpatient department? In particular, how should home care be related to the care of ambulant patients? Where, if anywhere, could home care for insured patients be instituted? Were there other, better methods of supplementing hospital care for patients with chronic illnesses?

As a step toward obtaining information of this sort, the hospital asked the Commonwealth Fund for a grant of $40,000 a year to permit the care of approximately thirty additional patients with various diagnoses and provide for the measurement, analysis, and evaluation of the work done under the entire plan. The Fund saw the proposed evaluation as an opportunity to gain information that might be of great significance in the future planning of hospital service and health services in general. Granted that Montefiore was not a typical institution: It appeared to be the only voluntary hospital in the country devoting itself chiefly to the care of the chronically ill, as more than half the patients admitted in 1947 were fifty years of age or older, and ward patients spent an average of 116.9 days in the hospital. Chronic disease represented so heavy a load that the success of community planning rested on finding some way to lighten it. Montefiore was a logical place to begin such investigations, starting at a relatively simple level—the care of the chronic patient—and working gradually into the more complicated field of aftercare for patients admitted to the hospital for acute conditions.

The Montefiore Hospital had 791 beds divided between two plants, a general hospital in the Bronx and a tuberculosis sanatorium in Bedford Hills, New York. It was affiliated for teaching purposes with the Columbia University College of Physicians and Surgeons. For its home-care experiment, the hospital had to look to outside sources for funding, but Bluestone was convinced that the cost of this sort of service, if it stood up under evaluation, would be borne by the hospital from its own funds. In his opinion, there was likely to be a direct relation between home care and decreased hospital needs for future expansion of physical facilities.

To learn to meet the manifold needs of patients requiring long-term care, to link the hospital more intimately with its environment, and to relieve the present pressure on hospital facilities, the Fund's staff felt that this experiment would be sufficiently instructive to justify fully the proposed appropriation. The Commonwealth Fund therefore gave Montefiore's Home Care Program $40,000 for each of three years.

The Home Care Program, which held a unique and valued position within the Montefiore Medical Center, became a prototype for other programs throughout the country. The original physician-oriented program reduced the rehospitalization of cardiac and cancer patients, and the resulting publicity led to the investment of both public and private funds. The program grew steadily through 1966, when it served over four hundred patients. A plateau in the number of patients served between 1967 and 1974 appears to have been associated with the development of Medicare, and the subsequent inception of a new "coordinated" model for the delivery of home health services resulted in a need to reevaluate Montefiore's program.[204] Although home-care services became available to more patients through Medicare benefits, the program at Montefiore continued in its traditional ways. Health-care professionals were also finding it difficult to adjust to Medicare regulations, and the introduction of governmental funds led to a decrease in the availability of private philanthropy.

The Home Care Program experienced a dramatic surge in the demand for its services after 1974, and from 1980 through 1982 it showed an increase in patient census of 3 percent, 50 percent, and 35 percent for each year, respectively. Three factors related to this growth were the advent of formal utilization review procedures for the inpatient service, the active participation of home-care staff in discharge planning, and the development and general acceptance of criteria necessary for expanded home-care services. The entire department increased by 24.75 full-time equivalents during 1982, and the staffing pattern in that year called for five direct-care nurses. This addition made it possible to obtain state approval to designate nursing as one of the direct services, resulting in substantial savings and better coordination of services.

The Division of Social Medicine

Montefiore's Division of Social Medicine was established in June 1950 by two men who were able to unite concepts from the worlds of philanthropy and medicine. The concerns of this division often ran counter to the mainstream of American medical care, education and research, but they arose naturally in an institution involved over many years with patients and families struggling with the complex medical and social problems caused by chronic disease.[205] "When I was in medical school . . . we were taught that it was important to think of a patient as a whole, and not just to examine a limb or an eye. We have now come to a point in the practice of medicine where we must broaden that point of view. When we think about a patient, we should think about him not only as an organic and spiritual whole, but also as a whole in society. It is no more fair or useful to separate a man from his environment than it is to divide him into separate and independent parts," wrote Martin Cherkasky in 1949 while chief executive of Montefiore's department of home care.[206] He was describing the philosophy behind the modern model for the provision of out-of-hospital care for patients whose well-being would be better served in their own homes than in an institution. He was also stating the rationale behind a series of experiments in the delivery of medical care that took place at Montefiore in the five years immediately following World War II, experiments that culminated in the formation of a department of social medicine of equal rank with the traditional hospital disciplines.

These two physicians—E. M. Bluestone and Martin Cherkasky—were at a hospital with a long tradition of social concern. The social service department was probably the second oldest in the United States, preceded only by its counterpart at the Massachusetts General Hospital, and Montefiore's experience with chronic diseases had made the recognition of family and social problems a dominant factor in its program of medical care.

Political activism was, furthermore, part of the tradition of the leadership at Montefiore.[207] Ernst P. Boas was a practicing cardiologist and director of Montefiore in the 1920s, who crusaded on behalf of the chronically ill, most of whom were still receiving totally inadequate care at home or in local workhouses and poorfarms. In 1939 Boas became one of the founders of the Physicians' Forum, an organization designed to provide an arena for discussion of the social aspects of medicine, especially the extension of medical care to those unable to pay their own way. The national climate was not conducive to any action in this regard: It was during these years that the American Medical Association bitterly opposed President Roosevelt's tentative approaches to the inclusion of health insurance in Social Security legislation.

Bluestone had come to Montefiore with his own history of social concern. In the early 1920s, he had worked with George Baehr, head of the Department of Medicine at Mount Sinai Hospital in New York. Baehr's most original work in medicine may have been his efforts to develop new ways of delivering medical services to people who could not afford care for themselves and their families. In the 1940s Baehr and Bluestone responded to Mayor Fiorello La Guardia's desire to insure New York City employees against the cost of medical care, a cost that had driven many of them to borrowing from loan sharks. Bluestone persuaded the board of trustees to set up a health insurance plan (HIP) based at Montefiore. The Commonwealth Fund assisted the HIP by making funds available for special studies, but did not help in establishing the program, a reflection of its desire to stay away from anything that might be called "socialized medicine."

Although Montefiore had been able to accept the idea of home care as an extension of services to its traditional constituency, its board of trustees was less ready to welcome prepaid group practice. A controversial idea at the time, this type of practice would make a fundamental difference in the structure of the hospital, since admission was offered to the membership for acute as well as chronic conditions. Henry Moses, at first the president of the board of trustees and then the head of the Committee on Social Medicine, helped persuade the more reluctant board members and contributed a large part of the $25,000 donation from the board that, together with a grant from the Josiah Macy, Jr., Foundation, a loan from HIP, and $7,500 from David Heyman of the New York Foundation, made possible the start-up of the Montefiore Medical Group. (Another hospital board member who supported the idea of a prepaid group practice, George Kirstein, later became director of the Health Insurance Plan of Greater New York.) Bluestone was again able to rely on Cherkasky to give form and substance to the program, and he appointed Cherkasky director of the group in 1948.

The Home Care Program and the Montefiore Medical Group were discrete entities that had in common a driving leader and an attitude toward the uses of medicine shared by social reformers in the United States and Great Britain. Yet another program at Montefiore, the Family Health Maintenance Demonstration, had its roots in an article by George Baehr in 1944 describing the Peckham Experiment, a pioneer health center set up in London in 1926 to provide preventive medical services not just to individuals but to families as units: "The Peckham Experiment, then, was really a combination of a health center, a club, and the settlement activities with which we are familiar in this country. Its significance for the maintenance of health and the prevention of disease is far greater than that of any other form of preventive medicine that has as yet been attempted experimentally, because it was designed to guide families and help them to guide one another in all medical, social, and environmental relationships which have an important bearing upon disease.[208]

The paper greatly impressed Bluestone and Cherkasky, who were interested in extending and studying the effect of the care offered to families through the medical group. Both were heavily involved in the negotiations that brought the Peckham idea to Montefiore. Participating families and medical staff came from the medical group, and money was donated by the Community Service Society (the offspring of one of the earliest private philanthropic welfare groups in the United States) and the Milbank Fund. This experiment to judge the impact of long-term social and medical services on family life in the Bronx was conducted under the guidance of a governing board, with members drawn from the Society, the hospital, the Health Insurance Plan of Greater New York, and the Columbia–Presbyterian Medical Center. Bluestone asked his board of trustees for permission to consolidate Montefiore's programs in a division of social medicine. As a result, Martin Cherkasky became full-time chief of the division with responsibility for social services, home care, the medical group, the Family Health Demonstration Center, social statistics, education and research in social medicine, and cooperation with all other divisions and independent services of the hospital.[209]

Social medicine was a discipline especially difficult to delineate, and the activities of the new division, whether in teaching, research or service, varied according to patients' needs, the dictates of available knowledge and funding, the concerns of society, and the character and interests of the incumbent chairman. George Silver, the second chairman of the division, struggled with the problem of definition in an article he wrote with William L. Kissick, a former house officer in the division and by then a surgeon in the United States Public Health Service. They concluded that: "Social medicine . . . at Montefiore . . . concerned itself with social factors as they influence medical practice" and meant "principally the concern for problems relating to the organization and administration of medical service."[210] Equally important was the growth of the formal Division of Social Medicine, not from theory but from programs already in place: "From the standpoint of the Montefiore Hospital the 'action' qualities of social medicine are paramount, and social medicine is rather like the technology of clinical medicine—the application of clinical medicine to society."[211] This department survived the fears of the 1950s about socialized medicine, the revolutions of the 1960s, and the soul-searchings of the 1970s, and it gave to an entire hospital a philosophy and a purpose.[212]

Recommendations for the Future

Malcolm P. Aldrich's review of the Fund's activities in 1957 was an effort to guard against complacency by review of the past and anticipation of change. A look at both prior experience and future trends, the report reflected the accumulated wisdom of Aldrich's thirty years with the Fund, but it was also the product of meetings with staff members, informal talks with individual directors, and conferences with prominent individuals.[213]

Aldrich favored the continued support of medical research. Although the federal government had greatly increased its resources for research, he felt that the participation of foundations was still needed, particularly for pursuit of worthwhile leads. Long-term projects should be phased out at the Fund, he believed, as investigators could obtain adequate support from governmental agencies. Aldrich recommended allocating $100,000 for fluid (as opposed to restricted) research grants. To combat the increasing duplication of effort by the Fund and the federal government, Aldrich suggested making grants to nongovernmental, nonuniversity research institutions, such as Cold Spring Harbor and Woods Hole.

Comprehensive medicine should remain an important focus for the Fund, Aldrich believed, and opportunities still existed for the Fund throughout medical education. The Fund should work for full-time teaching in clinical and basic science departments; better salaries; experiments in curriculum reform and in the teaching of comprehensive medicine; emphasis on interdisciplinary teaching; a more logical sequence between college and medical school programs; integration of preprofessional and professional education; aid in original planning of medical schools and in continuing evaluation of their educational programs; new teaching and communicative devices, including television; new buildings; and planning aid, especially in new state institutions where it was difficult to obtain legislative appropriations for this purpose. Stronger educational programs, physical facilities, and community relationships all depended on the right kind of preliminary planning, and the success of planning programs at the medical schools of the University of Florida, and at Johns Hopkins and Stanford universities supported Aldrich's view. Over the next three to five years, a few larger grants should be given to carefully selected institutions, and the results of the recent capital grants program should be appraised. In the meanwhile, he advocated giving some schools partially restricted grants for more general purposes, in addition to regular project grants.

Aldrich also suggested consolidating the Fund's Experimental Health Services and medical education programs under the title "Medical Education and Community Health." The results of these projects had ranged from excellent to not entirely satisfactory (in a relatively few cases).[214] Aldrich did not want to eliminate this field entirely, since he considered it important to support programs integrating and reorganizing health services in the community.

Mental health was also an indispensable part of comprehensive medicine, and psychopharmacology and exploration of the biochemistry of the nervous system were becoming important tools in the effort to learn more about mental disease. Aldrich saw a continuing need for improved psychiatric teaching within the medical school curriculum; research to discover cures for emotional disturbances; and improved systems of patient care for the mentally ill. Here, too, because increased federal aid was reducing the need for the Fund's support, he recommended giving fluid funds to a few outstanding departments of psychiatry as a valuable type of assistance seldom provided by other agencies.

Sufficient funds appeared to be available for training in psychiatry. The National Institute of Mental Health had allocated $12 million for psychiatric training in 1956, and the Ford Foundation had appropriated $3.7 million for the training of investigators. Once again, Aldrich and the Fund's staff felt that its support was no longer greatly needed. They planned to remain active in the field of mental health without organizing a formal program, by considering research requests for studies of neuroendocrinology, neurochemistry, and psychopharmacology; studies of emotion and personality, and of the genetics of mental disorders; experiments in patient care; travel grants for directors of mental health institutions; and miscellaneous activities relevant to the Fund's interest.

The staff saw human ecology and the sociology of medicine as neglected areas of research important to the development of comprehensive medicine, but Aldrich could not recommend that the Fund take up support of the social sciences as a major program, a step that would have required building a staff with experience in this field. He did suggest backing good projects involving the sociology of medicine and health, the training of sociologically oriented health professionals, and the teaching of the behavioral sciences in medical schools or schools of public health. Otherwise, he believed, the field of the social sciences should be left to already interested organizations such as the Ford Foundation, the Russell Sage Foundation, the Brookings Institution, the Institute for Advanced Study at Princeton, the Social Science Research Council, and the Rockefeller Foundation.

The large increases in governmental spending in the health field made it difficult for private philanthropies to pioneer and experiment. Health remained so important to society, however, that Aldrich and his staff wanted the Fund to continue its search for innovative approaches not covered by formally structured federal programs. The study of genetics had gained visibility, but the Fund decided against supporting this field. Two attractive possibilities were programs designed to raise the quality of health personnel in foreign countries through education, and programs in postgraduate or continuing medical education. Another important area singled out for future interest was research in patient care. Some of the current grants in medical education, mental health, nursing, and community health projects touched on this area; but new, more specific programs might be found, involving general clinics, community hospitals, service areas such as home care, or new types of team approaches to medical and mental health care. Here the Fund was not concerned with duplication of effort but was alert to innovative approaches that could be expanded by the larger sums available from governmental and other sources.

Aldrich also concluded that the time had come for the Fund to abandon its reluctance to give grants for construction. Medical schools needing new facilities for programs in medical education and research were dependent on a source of matching funds. The Fund's altered policy should nevertheless remain conservative: These grants should be infrequent and given only for buildings that facilitated innovation or represented useful experiments in medical education.

The Fund's intention to give fewer but larger grants required fewer staff members. The sales and distribution operations of the Division of Publications had been eliminated, several staff members had retired or resigned, and a few had died, so that the staff had already decreased in the past decade from sixty to thirty-nine. In 1957 it was composed of relatively older men, several of whom were to reach retirement age in the near future—Lester J. Evans, E. K. Wickman (director of the Division of International Fellowships), Harry E. Handley (an associate in public health), and Robert Jordan (an administrative associate). Aldrich felt that the Fund's needs could be met by adding no more than two or three young replacements, who would be in place before their predecessors retired. The type of individual chosen would depend on the fields selected by the Fund for future activity.

By 1962 Aldrich was considering stepping down; the search for this successor was conducted partly by the board, but primarily by Aldrich himself. Malcolm P. Aldrich retired on September 1, 1963.[215]

8

The University and the Community

The habit of apprehending a technology in its completeness: This is the essence of technological humanism, and this is what we should expect education in higher technology to achieve. I believe it could be achieved by making specialist studies the core around which are grouped liberal studies which are relevant to these specialist studies. But they must be relevant; the path to culture should be through a man's specialism, not by-passing it. . . . A student who can weave his technology into the fabric of society can claim to have a liberal education; a student who cannot weave his technology into the fabric of society cannot claim even to be a good technologist.

—*Eric Ashby*

The Third President: James Quigg Newton, Jr. (1963—1975)

Malcolm P. Aldrich and James Quigg Newton, Jr., met in the Navy during World War II, and Newton had joined the Fund's board of directors in 1951 at Aldrich's invitation. In 1963 George P. Berry, another board member, suggested Newton as the next leader of the Fund, and Aldrich broached the idea to Newton. The proposal came at a propitious time: As president of the University of Colorado, Newton had finished most of the projects on his agenda, and he was looking for an interesting challenge.

J. Quigg Newton, Jr. (fig. 26) brought the Fund the benefits of his varied career. Born in Denver, Colorado, in 1911, he received both bachelor's and law degrees from Yale, and had served as secretary to William O. Douglas when he was chairman of the Securities and Exchange Commission. Newton had also practiced law in Denver and served as the mayor of that city, vice-president of the Ford Foundation, and president of the University of Colorado.[1]

When Newton assumed the presidency of the Commonwealth Fund on September 1, 1963, Malcolm P. Aldrich remained as chairman of the

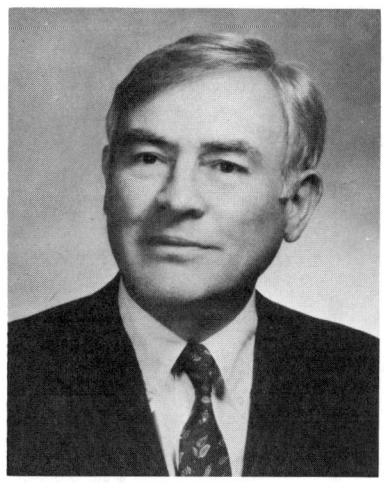

Figure 26. James Quigg Newton, Jr.

board and John A. Gifford, a partner in the law firm of White and Case, stayed on as vice-president and treasurer.[2] Most board members were long-standing close friends of Aldrich and Gifford; all were distinguished in business, finance, and law. Aldrich did not give up the reins of leadership entirely. For the first few years of Newton's term, he retained an office at Harkness House, expecting Newton to bring him all proposals before presenting them to the board. Because of his close relationship with Edward S. Harkness, Aldrich felt responsible for making certain that the Fund operated as he believed Harkness would have wished were he still alive. Newton recognized Aldrich's integrity, his devotion to the Fund, his experience, and his contribution to its successful past programs. He was able to collaborate with Aldrich, and in the early years of his presidency their work together preserved what was useful in the Fund's tradition and paved the way for the implementation of new projects.

Aldrich had felt that the chief executive officer of the Fund should be a generalist, relying on his staff members for technical expertise. Lester J. Evans had provided Aldrich with the specific viewpoint of a trained physician, but he had retired in 1959. Newton's solution was to select physicians with academic training—Colin M. MacLeod, Robert J. Glaser, and Carleton B. Chapman—to serve in succession as vice-presidents of the Fund, and each influenced the Fund's programs through his individual enthusiasms and outlook. For the first three years of his presidency, however, Newton worked alone, and grants given in the mid-1960s reflect his own particular interests and policies.

In 1965 Newton did hire Terrance Keenan to augment the Fund's staff as senior executive associate and recording secretary. Keenan had majored in English literature at Yale University, and after graduation had worked as a financial writer for Merrill, Lynch, Fenner, and Bean. Keenan met Newton during his nine years as director of the Ford Foundation's Division of Reports and speech writer for the foundation's president, Henry T. Heald. Keenan eventually decided that he had little opportunity for advancement in that position, and he had almost agreed to return to Yale when Newton offered him the job of interpreting the Commonwealth Fund's work to its directors and the public.

The Transition: 1963—66

Newton began his presidency by attending the meetings of many groups related to medicine and by holding membership in umbrella organizations such as the National Committee for Health Manpower. He wanted to broaden his background and sharpen his views, to spread the word that the Fund was still interested in supporting innovative programs in medical education and health-care delivery, and to generate new ideas for the Fund's consideration.

Newton's philosophy was that a foundation is only as good as the expertise it mobilizes, and the role of the foundation as a kind of clearinghouse for ideas was particularly well-developed during Newton's presidency. At the intersection of the foundation's resources and its requests lay the essence of the private foundation's responsibility: identifying priorities so that its funding targets could be critically selected from hundreds of projects. To know the history of the constituency it serves, to identify the strengths and weaknesses of various institutions, to be familiar with the finest leaders in special areas, to be cognizant of the experiments that have been tried and to recognize which have succeeded, to be practical in pursuit of the ideal: This seemed the essence of wise foundation management. Newton believed that the professional foundation must specialize by carefully defining a role and trying to grow within its boundaries; the key to its success would be the creation of a network of expert consultants. In this way the foundation could become useful even to the applicants it must turn down.

Within the Fund, Newton relied heavily on the opinions of his board members, but from the time he assumed the presidency until Macleod's arrival in October 1966, his most trusted advisor came from outside the Fund. Robert J. Glaser was dean of the medical school at the University of Colorado when Newton was the university's president; together they had worked on the plans for the university's new medical center. With his broad base of knowledge, Glaser excited Newton's interest in medical education, encouraging him to active participation in the affairs of the medical school. The two found that they worked effectively as a team, and they grew to have great confidence in each other. Newton felt comfortable in accepting the presidency of the Commonwealth Fund because he knew that he would have the benefit of Glaser's advice, and the programs of Newton's first three years as president owed much to Glaser's influence.

The Fund's appropriations in the first year of Newton's presidency maintained the pattern of recent past years: 70 percent ($3,341,432) supported projects in medical education, and 12 percent ($574,000) supported fellowships and awards in the health field—primarily to strengthen medical schools. Emulating his predecessors, Newton reviewed the Fund's programs and policies at the start of his tenure, but he relied more formally upon consultants than had Smith, Sheehan, or Aldrich. With Glaser's help Newton organized a meeting of a small group of distinguished academicians to assess the Fund's present position and plot its future directions.[3] The meeting emphasized the current needs of medical schools—a focus in keeping with the Fund's major interest in medical education. Newton also talked informally with each board member[4] and with distinguished individuals outside the Fund[5] to discover whether they thought changes in the Fund's programs were desirable. Newton kept detailed notes of these interviews, and each began with a detailed presentation of Newton's own view of the Fund's position. By the end of his first year in office, Newton had developed a position paper, which he presented to the board in November 1964.[6] The Fund's long experience and its good connections with medical schools led Newton and the board (especially George P. Berry) to conclude that it should continue to support projects in the field of medicine.

Newton's tenure was marked by the widespread public perception of a health care "crisis,"[7] a line of thought encouraged by some legislators and physicians to bring about reforms beyond the provisions of Medicare. In a press conference in 1969, President Nixon said that "unless action is taken in the next two to three years. . . .we will have a breakdown in our medical systems."[8] Six months later the editors of *Fortune* magazine presented a special issue on medical care, in which they declared that American medicine stood upon the brink of chaos. "Much of United States medical care," they said, "particularly the everyday business of preventing and treating routine illnesses, is inferior in quality, wastefully dispensed, and inequitably financed. . . . Medical manpower and facility are so maldistributed that large segments of the population, especially the urban poor and those in rural areas, get virtually no care at all. . . . The time has come for radical change."[9] The focus of public attention had shifted from scientific progress to the economic and social problems facing medicine, and the public's main concern was providing the best quality medical care to all at the lowest possible cost.

The national response was to demand precipitate action: Public and private organizations were analyzing the system's defects and suggesting varied solutions. Newton's response was to continue the Fund's emphasis on the nation's systems of medical education. He felt that the Fund would be exerting the most leverage on the nation's health if it remained knowledgeable about the operations, plans, and needs of medical schools and answered their requests to support innovative programs.

Medical schools in the early 1960s were rapidly growing institutions standing at the intersection of medical research and health care. Health care itself had become highly sophisticated and very technical, but it was distributed unevenly between economic groups, among races, and between urban and rural areas. The medical schools themselves could not directly meet the nation's entire need for health care, but they could set standards for the nation, devise innovations, develop and test new systems of delivery, and introduce and then perfect new methods of medical treatment. Most medical schools depended on major universities to sustain them and to provide expertise in the natural and social sciences; in all the medical school's tasks, the resources of its parent university could help the school to understand the social implications of its work.

Medical research was now a multi-million-dollar enterprise, supported primarily by the National Institutes of Health and producing discoveries that had to be translated as quickly as possible into general use. Most of the federal government's awards had been given to the great medical centers for research, and nonresearch areas—particularly the advancement of education—received inadequate funding. The result was an imbalance between research and teaching in many medical schools and hospitals. Although the federal effort offered great advantages for American medicine, the significant problems it created offered the Fund unique opportunities.

Two complementary paths presented themselves to Newton: The Fund could continue its long-time role of accepting applications from individual investigators or institutions, or it could initiate studies and other projects intended to solve the major problems of biomedical institutions, particularly their problems in education.

Newton believed that medical education had to become more efficient so that students could accomplish more in the same length of time. The curriculum revision at Western Reserve had had a marked effect on medical schools across the country, but rapidly increasing knowledge in the basic medical sciences was calling for further change and experimentation. The accumulating store of medical knowledge not only impinged upon the design of the medical school curriculum but created problems for premedical education as well. The Fund had already supported some attempts to integrate premedical and medical education by decreasing the time between a student's entrance to college and his graduation from medical school. Preliminary evaluation of programs at Johns Hopkins,

Northwestern, and Boston universities suggested that they had been successful, but Newton wanted the Fund to search for further modifications in the pattern of premedical education.

Postgraduate medical education was another area of concern, as no effective methods had been developed to ensure the continuing education of physicians. Newton saw the Fund's involvement in this area as a continuation of the fellowship awards similar to those in its public health and rural hospital programs. If the right proposal appeared, he felt that the Fund should pursue this area again.

Newton also advocated supporting unbiased studies of different methods of financing medical education—through, for example, the use of professional fees from insured patients in teaching hospitals. All medical schools—especially the privately supported institutions—were underfinanced, and although the Fund could not rectify this hazardous situation through its own resources, it could help in delineating the problem and in proposing solutions.

Money for bricks and mortar was a point of controversy. The Fund had traditionally been reluctant to provide grants for construction of medical school facilities, but Newton wanted to consider this type of application, especially on a matching basis. Although the Public Health Research Facilities Program allowed institutions to expand laboratories for health-related research, matching funds for private medical schools and teaching hospitals were frequently unavailable, and institutions often had to turn to foundations or private donors for half the sums needed for construction.

Newton also identified other grave problems in American medicine less directly related to medical education. One was the lack of uniform quality in medical service. The lag continued between the discovery of new knowledge and its translation into better medical care—the basic reason for biomedical research. The role of the individual doctor was diminishing, in contrast to the growth in group practice and the widening services rendered by hospitals. The health needs of a large segment of the population in New York City, for example, were unmet, and this area offered broad opportunity for study. Preventive medicine was not adequately emphasized—and, like postgraduate medical education, this was a field in which the Fund had pioneered in the past. One of the most vexing social problems in this country was the continuing increase in the cost of medical care and insurance, and Newton believed that the Fund should be prepared to support projects designed to control the seemingly neverending rise in these costs. In addition, despite the Fund's accomplishments and the huge sums available from the National Institute for Mental Health for the training of personnel and for psychiatric research, the field of mental health still needed attention. Continued support was also required for senior faculty fellowships and for properly designed conferences.

Newton had no single solution for each of these problems; his leadership was marked by a willingness to test many approaches to a single issue (see app. H). Like those of other philanthropic foundations, the Fund's resources were small relative to the nation's pressing needs but the Fund's independent judgment and relative flexibility could greatly enhance the effect of its grants. In planning the Fund's future course, Newton did not choose in advance a fixed agenda of specific activities. Instead, he and his staff identified a number of major topics whose study would form the basis for the future.

Support of Basic Resources in Medical Education

Large allocations for faculty endowment and facilities to Harvard, Western Reserve, and Rutgers universities, the Columbia–Presbyterian Hospital and Medical Center, and the Cornell University Medical Center during 1964 and 1965 reflected Newton's belief that the best use of philanthropic funds was support of quality programs in quality medical institutions, especially those setting the educational standards and providing most of the faculty for other medical schools.[10] Like his predecessors Edward S. Harkness and Barry C. Smith, Newton foresaw a "trickle-down" effect: Spread throughout the country's medical schools and medical institutions would be well-trained individuals who would improve the quality of medical education, medical research, and medical care at all levels.

Several special grants strengthened basic resources of the nation's system of medical education. The Fund's grants for libraries and endowed professorships also showed other institutions the value of timely, well-placed awards. Further growth of Western Reserve University, for example, hinged upon its expansion and the modernization of its teaching and clinical facilities. The Fund's early support of basic library resources at the Rutgers Medical School, the new branch of the state university of New Jersey, helped it expand to a full, four-year program. Although the Fund rarely supported hospital building costs, a grant to the Columbia–Presbyterian Hospital was an understandable exception, in view of the Harkness family's well-known and longstanding interest in the Columbia University medical center's development.

By Newton's third year in office, there was a growing belief among medical educators that university medical centers were responsible not only for teaching, research, and patient care, but for taking the lead in identifying and solving the complex problems of the nation's system of health services. The university setting provided opportunities for medical scholars to work with nonmedical faculty in fields bearing crucially on these problems—economics and sociology, for example. The university medical center was seen as the crucible for experiments and demonstrations that would lead to improved arrangements for health care. During 1965 the Fund supported programs in health-care delivery at seven university medical centers: Harvard, the University of Washington, the University of Southern California, Albert Einstein, Colorado, Stanford, and Columbia–Presbyterian. To train more medical school faculty and biomedical investigators, the Fund made appropriations to eleven medical schools and institutions: Brown University, the Albany Medical College, the Rensselaer Polytechnic Institute, Columbia University, the Columbia–Presbyterian Medical Center, Vanderbilt University, Yale University, the Massachusetts Institute of Technology, the Bowman Gray Medical College, the Illinois Board of Higher Education, and Oxford University. (Behind this unusual grant to a foreign medical school was the hope that Oxford's immense prestige would encourage the universities in Great Britain to emphasize medical sciences as a branch of learning and to assume fuller responsibility for the professional preparation of physicians. The success of this grant showed once again the importance of an infusion of seed money into an institution of quality.)[11] Although more physicians were needed, Newton felt that physicians could not do the job alone. During his presidency the Fund supported several programs to educate ancillary medical personnel.

Training New and Established Health Professionals

The Background: Fellowships for Nurses

As key performers in any medical or public health program, nurses had received constant attention from the Fund since the 1920s. In 1928, under the Fund's Rural Hospital program, the first fellowship was given to a nurse at the Farmville Rural Hospital in Virginia; during the next twenty years, hundreds of nurses received fellowships as part of this program. By 1936 dozens of scholarships for public health nurses in Tennessee, Mississippi, and Massachusetts had raised standards of nursing practice: two-thirds of the nurses in full-time county units in Mississippi and Tennessee had taken at least four months of postgraduate training. Over the next fifteen years, nurses who had received fellowships from the Fund were beginning to surface as leaders in the profession—for example, the new dean of the Vanderbilt University School of Nursing.[12]

Parallel to the Fund's support of individual nurses was its interest in the standards of the profession as a whole. In 1937 it commissioned a study of "the best current thinking about the mental hygiene aspects of public health nursing."[13] The Fund's fellowship program for nurses also gave preference to individuals with responsibility for training other public health workers: in 1949, for example, county supervising nurses in

Tennessee were put at the top of the list; and in 1950 two teachers of nursing and a nurse responsible for the field training of university nursing students were given fellowships for postgraduate study at the London School of Hygiene and Tropical Medicine, the Harvard School of Public Health, and the Michigan School of Public Health.[14] But these were piecemeal efforts, and the Fund soon recognized that "unfortunately, nurse training and nurse education in this country [left] much to be desired."[15] Many nursing schools were small, with limited curricula and low standards. A number of schools were maintained by hospitals chiefly as a cheap source of semiskilled help.

One means of raising standards of nursing education was through accreditation of nursing schools. The profession had tried to set up a national accreditation program, but the six separate national nursing organizations could not agree on membership qualifications, standards, or objectives. In 1951 these six groups decided to concentrate their leadership by merging into two national organizations. The transition would be handled by a series of joint committees; the major temporary committee in this process, the National Committee for the Improvement of Nursing Services, appealed to the Fund for help.[16]

In 1951 there were about 1,150 schools awarding undergraduate diplomas in nursing, only 150 of which were accredited. A grant from the Fund would enable the committee to propel many hopelessly substandard schools out of existence—in some cases by combining schools—and to help the remaining schools in improving their programs. The Fund gave the committee a three-year grant of $75,000, conditional upon its raising the remainder of the total budget of $307,103 from other sources.[17]

The Fund's staff wanted to immerse itself even more deeply in the problems of the profession, and while the initial grant was in progress they talked with nursing educators and administrators. Three main types of nurses were needed: administrators and teachers, consultants and supervisors in clinical areas of nursing education, and nurses who would perform research in nursing problems. The staff concluded that "under existing policies the board would be receptive to proposals from the nursing field that conform to these general principles and clearly tend to further the development of comprehensive health care. Such proposals might be for assistance (including fellowships) for nurse education on an exploratory or experimental basis, or for new approaches to the organization of nursing services, or for the coordination of nursing and other services."[18] Much of the Fund's assistance did take the form of fellowships to the National League for Nursing, to the Southern Regional Education Board, and to six university schools of nursing.

By 1952 the merger into the National League for Nursing, Inc., was complete, and by October 1953, 218 nursing education programs enrolling 31 percent of all student nurses had been fully accredited.[19] The best estimate was that 20 percent of the positions held by registered nurses required a master's degree, and for an additional 30 percent, preparation at the baccalaureate level was desirable. But in 1953 only 1 percent of all nurses held the master's degree, and 7.2 percent the bachelor's. Worse still, not all of these degrees had been awarded for work in nursing. The number of institutions offering graduate programs in nursing had almost doubled between 1947 and 1953, but the number of graduate nurses enrolled in these programs in 1953 was exactly the same as in 1947.[20]

To improve these dismal statistics, the National League for Nursing planned to select a number of nurses for fellowship aid, the amount of the individual fellowship to be determined on the basis of each candidate's plan of education. Decisions would be made by a Committee of Award, which could comprise directors of academic schools of nursing and professors of nursing education throughout the country. Older nurses exerted substantial influence on the field, and the Fund intended to enlarge their effectiveness. The plan was to select candidates in the following order:

1. Students who were already doctoral candidates.
2. Students who had master's degrees and were interested in specific types of advancement.
3. Students who had academic qualifications but needed a residency in some nursing specialty.
4. Students with great promise who were working toward master's degrees.

The Fund appropriated $158,200 for a one-year fellowship program providing between ten and twenty awards. The league solicited applications from 132 fellowship candidates the first year; 70 applied and 8 awards were made. At the end of the year, $74,400 remained in the league's budget; the Fund renewed the grant, allocating $120,560 for another year. Fellowship awards for about twenty nurses already progressing toward the doctorate totaled $114,400; the remainder was given to five younger nurses beginning graduate study.

In 1958 the Fund voted an additional $170,000 to the National League for Nursing. In extending the fellowship program for three more years, the Fund added about 66 more fellows, bringing the total in this program to 138. Before the initiation of the league's project, there were only about 80 nurses in the entire country with doctorate degrees; now there were 128.[21] The goal was to provide at least one nurse with top training for each of the 185 college and university schools of nursing. A final grant was given in 1961, bringing the sum allocated over the seven years of the program to $1,511,823.

The Fund also supported the Southern Regional Educational Board, a public agency established by fourteen southeastern state legislatures to focus on master's-degree training in nursing. Through this organization six of the thirty-odd collegiate schools of nursing in this area were able to establish or improve their programs at this level. Each of these schools—at the Universities of Alabama, Maryland, North Carolina, and Texas, and Emory and Vanderbilt universities—developed a unique course of instruction in the field of its greatest interest and resources. Vanderbilt, for example, offered courses for the master's degree with majors in maternal and child care, and medical and surgical nursing; North Carolina concentrated on psychiatry, nursing administration, and public health nursing; and at Texas majors were offered in maternal and child care, medical and surgical nursing, psychiatry, and nursing administration.[22] The Fund did not believe that the regional nature of the program would limit its usefulness. On the contrary, this experimental project was seen as a pilot demonstration.[23] A $67,200 grant made in 1954 was renewed the following year and again in 1957, when $12,000 was allocated to each of the six schools for between forty and fifty fellowships. The Fund permitted some flexibility in administering the grants by allowing portions of the grants to be transferred, for similar fellowship purposes, among the six schools as their individual needs suggested.[24]

Three other Fund-sponsored fellowship programs assisted undergraduate programs in nursing education. In 1957 the Fund gave the University of Vermont a two-year grant for initiating sound classroom teaching and field experience in public health nursing. The Yale University School of Nursing was given $24,000 for graduate fellowships in 1956; renewal of this grant in 1959 allowed the school to continue to train students in three specialty fields—maternal and newborn nursing, mental health and psychiatric nursing, and public health nursing—as well as to develop a fourth specialty, pediatric nursing. In 1964 a grant to Northeastern University's nursing school permitted it to offer combined college education and nursing training to individuals who could not otherwise afford to attend college.[25] Throughout the 1950s separate grants were given to the National League for Nursing and the Southern Regional Educational Board for seminars and other activities built around the problems of accreditation and standards.

At the same time, the Fund was interested in stretching the capabilities of the nursing profession. The idea that certain activities in medicine are the exclusive province of the physician is embedded not only in tradition but in law. Contrary to this notion are ideas of change and flexibility in the roles of professionals who provide health care. Newton supported the second philosophy, and in the mid-1960s the Fund began to assist programs intended to demonstrate that nonphysicians could do many of the things previously done only by physicians. The Commonwealth Fund's awards for the training of new health professionals, especially in nursing, are of historic significance. It was the first foundation to support the nurse practitioner, staying with the new group until it became part of in-service and graduate nursing. This quiet revolution in the status of the nation's health-care professionals started in 1965, although the change was not recognized as revolutionary at the time.

Nurse Practitioners

The first program for nurse practitioners began in 1966 at the University of Colorado Medical Center with the aid of $253,998 from the Commonwealth Fund.[26] This three-year grant supported an experiment to train public health nurses for increased responsibility in the care of children from low-income families. The program was intended to provide adequate medical attention to groups most likely to be affected by the increasing national shortage of physicians—the rural and urban poor. It was also a demonstration that the reach of doctors might be extended through the use of nurses with advanced clinical training. When the Commonwealth Fund approved the plan, it was taking the risk that a small group of people with limited experience would be able to change the standard methods of providing health care. Most doctors and nurses predicted that this concept could not succeed, and the federal government agreed: Before receiving the Commonwealth Fund grant, the Colorado group had been turned down by a number of federal agencies (including the Children's Bureau, the Office of Economic Opportunity, and the Bureau of Health Manpower).

The program, which was conducted by the Department of Pediatrics, prepared public health nurses holding the master's degree to handle much of the routine pediatric care ordinarily performed by physicians.[27] Graduates of the program served in public health departments under the supervision of public health doctors and local practitioners. They were trained to recognize conditions requiring a physician's attention; routinely, guided by physicians, they carried out normal pediatric procedures, including physical examinations, medical histories, laboratory tests, immunizations, and family counseling on nutritional, behavioral, and other matters affecting child health and development. The program offered four to six months of intensive clinical training by senior faculty of the Department of Pediatrics and the nursing school, which was collaborating in the program, followed by eighteen to twenty months of faculty-supervised field experience. The field training was centered initially in Trinidad, a rural community in southern Colorado, and was conducted in cooperation with local public health and medical practitioners. Later, the medical school established a field training station in a low-income neighborhood of Denver.

The experiment, which had the endorsement of the state health department, was directed by Henry K. Silver, professor of pediatrics in the medical school, and Loretta C. Ford, a professor on the nursing school faculty.[28] The Fund's grant was used primarily for staff costs, training stipends, and field office expenses, and the original grant called for the preparation of some thirteen pediatric nurse practitioners (PNPs)

The first class spent four months in a variety of clinical settings—doctors' offices and community and public health facilities in rural urban areas. Central to the program was not the teaching of new skills but a new concept of nursing—the nurse as an independent decision-maker who could provide primary health care. In evaluating and managing healthy children as well as those with acute and chronic disorders, the nurse became proficient in performing a complete physical examination, assessing a child's overall status to decide whether she should manage the illness alone, obtain a physician's advice, or refer the patient. She acquired the ability to evaluate hearing defects, speech difficulties, visual impairments, congenital and acquired orthopedic deformities, and dental problems; she learned to obtain some laboratory specimens and to perform urinalyses, hemoglobin determinations, and other tests; and she was trained to assist in the management of such emergency situations as poisonings, accidents, hemorrhage, and apnea. Included in the program were seminars on parent-child relationships, variations in growth patterns, physical and psychosocial development, infant nutrition (including breast feeding, the preparation and modification of formulas, introduction of solid foods, vitamin and other nutritional supplements), and immunization procedures and schedules with individualized modifications. Also covered were the dynamics of physical, psychosocial, and cultural forces affecting health; the salient features of personality development; and techniques of counseling parents in child rearing, including bathing, toilet training, and accident prevention.

The attitude of the physicians was the key to success, since they had to be willing to share tasks that they had always performed themselves. For a new patient, the nurse would take a complete history, do a thorough physical examination, make a tentative assessment of the patient's condition (differentiating normal from abnormal findings), and offer a preliminary interpretation. The nurse practitioner could also handle many phone calls for the physician. The physician was then free to focus on items needing his particular expertise. Although individual state laws varied, nurses were generally permitted to observe, care for, and counsel the ill, injured, or infirm. The nurse practitioner's responsibilities stretched tradition, but her activities remained nursing functions.

Silver and his colleagues found that his program's graduates could, by themselves, care for about three-fourths of all pediatric outpatients. They could provide almost total care to well children (slightly more than one-half of all patients) and could evaluate and manage the problems of half of all sick and injured children seen in an office. Most parents found the combined care acceptable or even preferable. As for the quality of care, there was a high degree of agreement between pediatric nurse practitioners and pediatricians in assessing the health of children. A significant difference in evaluation occurred in only 1 percent of cases—probably as good a concordance as would have been found among different physicians. Rather than compound the nursing shortage, as some critics claimed it would, the nurse practitioner program helped solve it by giving greater job satisfaction to nurses and retaining more of them in an active role. This combination of services probably offered better primary health care at less cost than physicians alone could provide.

The gamble that Newton and his board of directors took in supporting this program at its inception paid off handsomely. The Fund's initial grant was instrumental in preparing more than 150 nurse practitioners at the University of Colorado as well as more than 2,000 PNPs throughout the United States. Graduates of the program at Colorado developed other nurse practitioner programs, wrote books, and became involved in a variety of associated activities;[29] federal legislation eventually made the nurse practitioner an integral part of the health-care system and provided for many additional training projects. The Colorado PNP program became the model for more than fifty other programs as well as for programs training nurse practitioners in the specialties of geriatrics, family practice, obstetrics and gynecology, and industrial health.

An additional grant to Silver and Patricia R. McAtee enabled them to help with the preparation of state legislation that provided for additional undergraduate nurse practitioner programs; ensure that the faculty teaching in these new programs were themselves trained as nurse practitioners; develop an internship as the terminal part of undergraduate nursing training; and establish an assistant nurse practitioner program to train more refined counterparts to the Chinese "barefoot doctor"—individuals with a limited medical background working in rural physicians' offices.

For the nation's health-care system, the training of nurse practitioners has emerged as one of the most important developments of the past thirty years. The value of nurse practitioners is now widely recognized, and nurses are seen as a key group in meeting the need for well-trained professionals to provide primary care. By now, nurses have skills previously considered the exclusive province of physicians; accreditation of nurse practitioner programs and certification of qualified graduates have also contributed to an improved identity for nurses and acceptance of their expanded role by other health professionals and the public.

Child Health Associates

In 1968 the Fund awarded $236,725 to the University of Colorado School of Medicine to establish an experimental curriculum for the preparation of child health associates—a wholly new type of professional practitioner in medicine at the baccalaureate level.[30] After two years of preparation in college and three years in the Child Health Associate Program (less than half the time it takes to train a pediatrician), the graduates of this program were able to provide comprehensive health care to at least 90 percent of the children seen in a pediatrician's office.

The Child Health Associates Program had been planned by Henry K. Silver and members of the nursing faculty with the held of a Carnegie Corporation grant. An outgrowth of the Fund-supported program to train pediatric nurse practitioners, it was incorporated as part of the Department of Pediatrics at the University of Colorado School of Medicine. Legislation backed by the Colorado State Medical Society, the state chapter of the American Academy of Pediatrics, and other medical organizations permitted the introduction of child health associates into the state's medical-practice system and set out the terms governing educational requirements, certification by the state Board of Medical Examiners, and the scope of the associates' activities.[31]

Two chief safeguards affected the associates. First, each was supervised by a physician who reviewed the associate's work and was available for consultation at all times. Second, the associate was mainly concerned with well-child care—for instance, scheduling physical examinations, performing immunizations, and providing routine hospital care for the newborn—and with minor ailments and injuries. Although acute illnesses were handled by the physician, the associate was trained to recognize symptoms for early detection of disease. One of the most important aspects of the training was to provide these associates with background and experience sufficient to teach them what they could *not* do. For recertification, a provision built into the child health associate law required the associates to participate in postgraduate programs for at least fourteen hours each year.[32]

Students spent the first two of the five years taking liberal arts courses and premedical studies at the University of Colorado at Boulder or at other institutions. Students accepted into the program then transferred to the University of Colorado Medical Center in Denver for three years of intensive professional education leading to the bachelor's degree—two years of basic medical sciences and clinical education, and one internship year. By 1974 twenty-three associates had graduated from the program and forty students were in training.

An evaluation carried out after the program had been underway for several years indicated that the child health associates had a good understanding of basic-science material relevant to the practice of pediatrics. Second-year associate students were equivalent to senior medical students in their knowledge of clinical pediatrics. A further study showed that diagnoses were not significantly different in more than 97 percent of 143 cases seen separately by child health associate interns and practicing pediatricians. It seemed clear that graduates of the program would be able to identify the problems of ambulatory pediatric patients. A measure of the program's long-range success was its receipt of the Outstanding Teacher Award in 1982 from the Ambulatory Pediatric Association.

The child health associates' assessment skills, acceptance by parents, and overall performance in caring for patients were found to be comparable to those of pediatricians. They could provide a wide range of diagnostic, preventive, and therapeutic services to children and could write prescriptions for many drugs. In public health facilities, they were able to help 65 to 95 percent of the patients usually seen by pediatricians, for one-third to one-half the cost. Most of the graduates of this program were practicing in rural and other underserved areas having a desperate need for primary health care.

School Nurse Practitioners

In 1970 the University of Colorado Medical Center, in collaboration with the Denver public schools, received a grant of $84,540 from the Fund to train and later to evaluate a third new category of health professional—the school nurse practitioner—whose duties would extend far beyond the traditional scope of school nursing, including many tasks ordinarily performed by physicians.[33] This program was intended to overcome this country's neglect of school children's health, the result of the separation of educational and health-care systems. With the Fund's help, the two principal professions concerned with the well-being of the child—education and medicine—combined their efforts to create more effective school-centered systems of health care.

This experimental program was also directed by Henry K. Silver and was jointly implemented by the schools of medicine and nursing of the University of Colorado Medical Center and the Denver public schools. When the program was started, failure to capitalize on the skills of approximately twenty-nine thousand school nurses in the United States represented a major loss to the health-care system at a time of sharply increasing demand for service.

The grant to the University of Colorado built on a pilot grant to the University of Rochester School of Medicine two years earlier. By the 1970s an additional three-year grant was enabling the University of Rochester to train pediatricians to work with school teachers in the school setting. The Rochester program had expanded to include four inner-city schools, four suburban school districts, and two nursery schools. Medical faculty at the University of Rochester taught school teachers to deal with child and adolescent growth and development and with drug abuse and narcotics addiction. Pediatricians conducted regular evaluation sessions at the schools for children with learning or behavioral difficulties; they also provided medical treatment and follow-up. These pediatricians were also able to refer children with problems too complex or serious for school-based treatment to the university medical center's specialty clinics. The Rochester program also gave medical students and house officers a firm grounding in the dimensions of child health and enabled the medical school to employ the range of educational specialists needed to augment the extensive medical and hospital resources already committed to the program.[34]

Like Rochester's project, the program at the University of Colorado was designed to relieve the strain on the country's increasingly short supply of physicians. Colorado's program was limited to experienced school nurses with a bachelor of science degree; the curriculum consisted of four months of intensive training at the university medical center in the theory and practice of child care and school health, followed by eight months of supervised experience in a cooperating public school. The training was designed to equip the school nurse practitioner to serve as the first line of defense in identifying and managing the basic health problems of the children in her school. The practitioner arranged prompt care by a physician when needed, but otherwise handled most problems independently. She took medical histories; screened children to detect acute or chronic disorders, speech, sight, and hearing impairment, and congenital and acquired orthopedic deformities; immunized children and treated common illnesses such as mild upper respiratory infections and skin rashes; gave emergency care; and assessed psychological, neurological, nutritional and other problems affecting normal development, behavior, and the ability to learn. The school nurse practitioner also worked with teachers, helping them handle students with behavioral problems and other disabilities that affect performance in school. In addition, she met with parents in regular conferences and home visits. Because the scope of her work was carried out in consultation with school physicians, family doctors, and the medical staffs of hospital outpatient departments and public clinics, the nurse was able to form new links among community medical care resources, the public schools, and the children's homes.

To give health professionals, other health workers, and the lay public a clear idea of the role and function of these nurse practitioners, a concise description was developed:[35]

> Nurse practitioners are registered nurses who have the competence to provide a broad range of direct primary health care services. They were prepared to assess health status; perform physical examinations, initiate and provide plans of care, counselling and anticipatory guidance; make decisions and assume

responsibility for management and follow-up care; refer patients and coordinate services; and work toward continuity of care for patients. Nurse practitioners have acquired advanced knowledge in clinical skill and nursing by completing a formal program of study representing a collaboration between schools of nursing and medicine, the program meeting guidelines established jointly by the two professions. Nurse practitioners provide primary health care by combining the services of registered nurses with services traditionally provided by physicians, but their new responsibilities are carried out under the direction of physicians. Finally, they function as associates and colleagues of physicians and work collaboratively and independently with them and other health personnel.

By 1977 the Colorado medical center had graduated approximately two hundred pediatric nurse practitioners and one hundred school nurse practitioners. Between 1965—when the first pediatric nurse practitioner completed the program—and 1976, about fifty other pediatric nurse practitioner programs were established in the United States, graduating more than three thousand pediatric nurse practitioners. Since then at least seven other school nurse practitioner programs have been initiated. The concepts that emerged from this program were later incorporated into the graduate and undergraduate nursing programs at the University of Colorado and at many other nursing centers throughout the United States.[36]

In addition to getting the three nurse practitioner programs at the University of Colorado underway, the Fund's initial support enabled Silver and his group to obtain grants, for these and later programs, from the Carnegie Corporation, the Bruner Foundation, the Robert Wood Johnson Foundation, and federal agencies. The Fund's awards also allowed Silver and his collaborators to build naturally on each preceding endeavor.

Physicians' Assistants

Duke University's experiment to train physicians' assistants began in 1965 with a grant to Eugene A. Stead, Jr., by the Josiah Macy, Jr., Foundation. Duke's program emerged as the most important single prototype for introducing these new health professionals into American medical practice. To speed the pace and set standards for establishing this new health profession, Duke increased the size of its entering class in 1969 from twelve to forty students. At the same time, Duke designed an experiment to test its graduates' effectiveness in delivering primary care in rural communities and inner-city neighborhoods. The Commonwealth Fund, the Carnegie Corporation, and the Rockefeller Foundation each made grants to Duke to cover the cost of establishing this new level of activity; the Fund's contribution was $150,000.[37]

The program began in the Department of Medicine but later moved to the Department of Community Health Sciences, a previous recipient of grants from the Commonwealth Fund and the Carnegie Corporation. This department led the medical school in work on problems in delivery of medical care. Under the leadership of Harvey Estes, Jr., the physicians' assistants program became a central activity of the Department of Community Health Sciences, but it drew in participants from the departments of surgery, medicine, pediatrics, radiology, pathology, psychiatry, and obstetrics.

The curriculum spanned two full calendar years and provided rigorous training in the principles of human biology, the elements of clinical medicine, and the procedures of medical care. Previous experience in the health field was required of all candidates accepted for the Duke program, and most of them had met this condition in one of the military medical services. The graduates of the program were equipped to carry out measurements, tests, and treatment, most of which were customarily done by physicians. Graduates took medical histories; examined patients; performed electrocardiograms and chest films, diagnostic tests involving serological determinations, urinalyses, and lumbar punctures; immunized patients, changed dressings, started and regulated intravenous infusions, and sutured skin lesions.

When Duke decided to augment its program in 1969, twenty-nine graduates were assisting physicians in many settings—including solo and group general practices—and in specialties such as internal medicine, surgery, and ophthalmology. In addition, physicians' assistants were helping to supervise hospital units for cardiac monitoring, renal dialysis, and respiratory support. In every instance, the productivity of the supervising physicians and institutions had been greatly enhanced. Requests for Duke-trained physicians' assistants from the country at large consistently exceeded the number of graduates at a ratio of 5 to 1—another reason for the school to increase its class size.

Estes also believed that physicians' assistants could provide a simple, economical means of bringing adequate health and medical care to the many families in rural areas and urban ghettos who did not have regular access to physicians' services. To test this premise, Duke set up two teams of physicians' assistants, one in Durham and the other in the city's rural environs. Each team comprised two physicians' assistants and three health aides—neighborhood residents who would be trained by the physicians' assistants to register and maintain close, supportive relations with the families within the team's area—and each team provided first-line care to about one thousand people. The physicians' assistants provided twenty-four-hour coverage in their communities, making house calls and examining patients in community-based dispensaries. A backup doctor was always available and referrals were made as necessary to designated physicians in Durham public health clinics, in the Duke outpatient department, and in private practice. The work of the teams was continuously monitored by Duke faculty members.[38]

Public and professional interest in the new health professionals grew rapidly, although in 1971 fewer than two hundred physicians' assistants had been graduated. In an address in February 1971 about the nation's health, President Nixon called for $15 million for the training of these professionals, and, following the president's lead, Congress passed the Comprehensive Health Manpower Training Act, which included specific provision for the education of physicians' assistants. Moneys authorized by the Health Training Improvement Act and the Nurse Training Act were also designated for this purpose. To assure a unified approach, funding for these programs was combined in the National Institute of Health's Office of Special Programs, in its Bureau of Health Manpower Education.[39]

Since 1973 physicians' assistants have been represented by the American Academy of Physicians' Assistants, which provides public information and legislative support and maintains close relationships with major medical organizations. The National Commission on Certification of Physicians' Assistants, organized the following year, has representatives from medicine, nursing, the federal government, and the general public. By 1984 fifty-four accredited training programs in the United States had trained over sixteen thousand physicians' assistants.[40] Approximately 75 percent were employed in family practice, general internal medicine, emergency medicine, pediatrics, or obstetrics and gynecology.

Physicians' assistants are not licensed and must depend largely on supervision by physicians; licensed nurse practitioners, however, have at times sought a more independent role in the practice of medicine. The increasing number of physicians has caused concern about the future of these ancillary professionals, since their training began in response to a perceived shortage of primary-care physicians. The continuing shortage of medical manpower in many areas of the country, the expanding clinical role of these groups, and the economics of medicine nevertheless make it likely that their services will continue to be in demand, particularly in group practices such as health maintenance organizations and nursing homes.

Surgical Assistants

In 1972 a three-year grant of $425,000 to the Cornell University Medical College established a program to train surgical assistants, who would provide the country's hospitals (particularly its community hospitals) with qualified supporting staff for highly technical, large-volume patient services, including emergency rooms. Most hospitals were using interns and residents almost exclusively to meet requirements for supporting staff, and foreign medical graduates were often recruited as residents, even though the institutions lacked the capacity to offer high-quality specialty training to these young physicians.

In introducing the idea of a mid-level health professional in one of the largest hospital-based specialties, the Cornell program served as a model for similar programs in other specialties. The program offered two major advantages over the existing system. First, by reducing teaching hospitals' reliance on house staff, it allowed the redesign of house-staff programs to emphasize the educational component, and, as a crucial adjunct, it provided community hospitals with a stable source of well-qualified personnel.

The Cornell program was designed and administered by Paul A. Ebert, chairman of the Department of Surgery. Students received two years of in-hospital training emphasizing closely supervised, direct clinical experience with surgical faculty in the emergency room, the operating rooms, the intensive care unit, and the hospital wards. The surgical assistant was also able to pursue some specific interest in depth, such as cancer chemotherapy, renal dialysis, or intensive care for patients with postoperative cardiac problems.

Recruitment was on an individual basis, and prior experience, often in the armed forces, was accepted in place of more formal college preparation. This substitution offered upward mobility for many health workers, including nurses.[41]

Sex Education in the Medical School

Parallel to the Fund's large programs in its main areas of interest had always been a number of smaller, autonomous "inquiry programs." No fixed percentage was allotted to this type of program, but its support had become a permanent part of the Fund's overall philosophy. The neglect of sex education in the medical school curriculum had attracted Newton's attention, and the Fund's grants in this area continued even beyond Newton's presidency. Curricular neglect, Newton believed, was transmitted to the patient: Although physicians were expected to function authoritatively in practice, they largely ignored this aspect of their patients' well-being.

Formal training in human sexuality in the nation's medical schools was the exception rather than the rule. In 1965 the Fund supported an informal study committee led by Frank R. Lock, chairman of the Department of Obstetrics and Gynecology at the Bowman Gray School of Medicine, which included representatives of the American Medical Association, the

Association of American Medical Colleges, the Sex Information and Education Council of the United States (SIECUS) and senior faculty and deans from several leading medical schools. The Committee's position was that "faculty responsible for these [sex education] courses are dealing with an essentially new subject in medical education and share a common need to develop effective syllabi, texts, case materials, and methods for teaching them. It has become apparent that if duplication of effort is to be avoided and the best knowledge and experience made widely accessible, a scholarly center in the field should be established."[42]

This report led the Fund to give grants to several organizations concerned with sex education. The first recipient (of $50,000) was SIECUS, which was just organizing its program. Established in 1964 as a national center for discussion of all aspects of sexual behavior, SIECUS was managed by a board of professionals in teacher education, family life, the ministry, medical and health education, and the social and behavioral sciences. Its executive director was Mary S. Calderone, a physician with a master's degree in public health. A second grant to SIECUS the following year funded a community service unit to consult with local groups; a national conference for lay and professional leaders about the content of sex education programs; a pilot teacher-training workshop for school teachers, school administrators and health officers; and an arrangement enabling the Mental Health Materials Center, Inc., a nonprofit organization, to edit, produce, and distribute SIECUS publications.

The Bowman Gray School of Medicine, in 1965 one of the few medical schools in the country with a program in sex education, was given a three-year grant to develop an experimental teaching program in marital health, family life, and human sexuality. Bowman Gray's existing program, devised by Lock, had been in effect for eight years and included courses for first- and third-year students and seminars for interns and residents. The faculty was composed of teachers from other medical specialties in addition to a professional marriage counselor and a sociologist. The Fund's grant enabled Bowman Gray to extend its program to all four undergraduate years, forming a full-scale experiment in the education of physicians for patient care and guidance in problems of marriage and sexuality. In 1967 the original grant of $180,000 was amplified by a renewal award of $121,000. The first year of funding was used for faculty positions, and two more years of support attracted scholar-teachers through a longer period of assured tenure. Bowman Gray's experimental curriculum was already interesting medical educators across the country, and the school was sharing its experience through a series of summer training institutes for faculty members from other universities.

The following year the University of Pennsylvania School of Medicine received a grant of $143,774 from the Fund to establish a Center for the Study of Sex Education in Medicine, a part of the Division of Family

Study within the Department of Psychiatry. Under the leadership of Harold I. Lief, the program trained medical school faculty in human sexuality, developed and disseminated materials for medical school sex-education programs, and conducted research in sex education and sexual problems.

When the center opened in 1968, only 30 of the nation's medical schools were offering their students some formal instruction in human sexuality. By 1975, 106—almost all—had established formal courses, and most were using the center's syllabi, tests, case materials, and teaching methods. The Fund gave the center renewal grants of $240,000 in 1969 and $308,569 in 1971, enabling it to build on its successes. By 1975 the center was shifting its emphasis to improving the quality of sex education in medical schools. It became a clearinghouse for the production and distribution of teaching materials needed to keep medical-school programs current in this rapidly expanding field of knowledge. In conjunction with the Marriage Council of Philadelphia—among the largest clinics for marriage and sex counseling, training, and research in the United States—the center provided treatment for approximately eighty-five couples each month, a total of 8,000 therapy sessions a year. In addition, it developed models for influencing the education of primary care doctors; established a new health career in sex and marriage counseling; and constructed a "sex history reporting system" for patients. These new projects received a total of $476,343 from the Fund.[43]

The Department of Psychiatry at the Stanford University School of Medicine received a three-year grant of $174,000 in 1972 from the Fund to support an integrated approach to complex medical problems. Designed by Herbert Leiderman of the Department of Psychiatry and Ben Z. Tabor of the Department of Obstetrics and Gynecology, Stanford's experimental program focused on sexual dysfunction, treating it as a model multifactorial medical syndrome. Therapeutic teams consisting of a social worker and a specially trained nurse—backed by residents, medical students, and nursing students—worked with the patients either as couples or individuals, depending upon the particular clinical problem presented. The research component of the project evaluated the team concept—its use of paramedical and parapsychiatric personnel and its cost efficiency.

In the same year, the Fund joined other foundations in supporting a program in human sexuality at the University of Minnesota. Under the direction of Richard A. Chilgren, the program was established as an independent academic and administrative unit of the university; Chilgren was directly responsible to the dean of the medical school and was empowered to carry on a full range of activities in teaching, research, and service. Like the other programs, the University of Minnesota's was intended to correct a serious common deficiency in medical education: the lack of formal training in the techniques of counseling and therapy required by physicians to manage their patients' sexual problems. The program's thirty faculty and staff members were assisted by consultants and voluntary workers in conducting a wide range of activities. The Sexual Attitude Reassessment Seminar, designed by the National Sex Forum, was adapted to the needs of the human sexuality program and became an integral part of its teaching service and research activities. Education in human sexuality, sexual dysfunction, and management of sexual problems was made a part of the core curriculum of the medical school, and health professionals were taught to deal with the sexual problems and potential of the physically disabled. A sexual health services unit within the medical school offered several approaches to individual and group therapy. Finally, research evaluating the plan's components and analyzing the extensive data collected permitted modifications crucial to progress in this new area.

In 1973 the Fund gave the Columbia University College of Physicians and Surgeons $75,633 to implement a plan in sex education for medical students that would eventually be extended into the residency training program. The directors of the program were Robert Michels of the Department of Psychiatry and John F. O'Connor, director of reproductive behavior at the International Institute for the Study of Human Reproduction. This modest grant made the teaching of human sexuality a part of the core curriculum for medical students, correcting a well-recognized, long-standing deficiency in medical education at this school. Since many of Columbia's medical students entered academic medicine, their improved education ensured that the teaching of human sexuality would be carried to other schools of medicine.

A final, one-year award for programs in sex education was given to the University of California at San Francisco in 1974. The Human Sexuality Program was directed by Herbert E. Vandervoort, a psychiatrist, who was also director of the medical school's training program in family medicine. This was not an entirely new undertaking for the university: the program's predecessor was a course for medical students first given in 1967, which two years later became part of the medical school's required curriculum. In 1972 the program established a Sex Advisory and Counseling Unit, which treated thousands of couples during its first two years of operation. The unit had also instituted in-practice training programs, ranging from specialized education for M.D. and Ph.D. students to preparation of paramedical personnel—such as the family planning worker—as assistants in sexual counseling. The Fund's grant enabled the program to enlarge its permanent staff to include personnel who would develop and test a large body of printed, audiovisual, and graphic materials. In 1975 the program received one of the few, very competitive "innovative teaching" awards from the University of California system.

The success of the Fund's investments, when combined with the efforts of many other institutions and individuals, established a sound base in this neglected area of medical education. The three renewal grants in 1975 were the last made by the Commonwealth Fund for programs in sex education in medical schools and brought the Fund's total investment in these programs to more than $1,600,000.[44]

THE NATIONAL BUREAU OF ECONOMIC RESEARCH

In 1966 the National Bureau of Economic Research (NBER) appealed to the Commonwealth Fund for support that would enable it to enter the field of health economics. The nation's investment in health and medical care had become one of the largest, fastest-growing elements of the total economy: The annual outlay for medical services had reached $35.4 billion by 1964—a tenfold increase over thirty-five years—and was expected to exceed $50 billion annually before the end of the decade. Employment in the health field had grown 54 percent between 1950 and 1960, and by 1966 more than three million persons were employed in health professions and institutions, not counting an estimated additional million who were manufacturing and distributing pharmaceuticals. (Employment in construction work, in contrast, had increased only 10 percent, and in agriculture had declined 38 percent.)

The economic aspects of the field had nevertheless received relatively little scholarly attention. Although a handful of universities—among them Harvard, Chicago, Michigan, and Columbia—had economics departments with a professed interest in health studies, fewer than six doctorates in health economics were awarded each year throughout the country. The relative lack of academic interest in the economics of health had implications beyond the limitations it imposed on the nation's ability to understand the impact of medical enterprise upon the economy; it also impeded the country's capacity to advance health care itself. Many of the larger problems on the current health scene were not wholly medical questions but economic ones as well. Yet soaring costs throughout medicine—for facilities, staff, equipment, education, and research—were forcing attention on the efficiency of the whole field. As the proportion of the gross national product devoted to health (then over 6 percent) began to compete with such other primary needs as education, society would insist on a financially efficient health-care system. Analysis of the best use of the system's resources would require sophistication, new economic insights and a larger number of qualified economists.

Yet economists found the health field more intractable than other areas of economic research. There was no generally accepted definition of the "product"—that is, what constituted the entity of health. Consumer choice was relatively circumscribed, pricing was largely determined by nonmarket factors, data were sparse and incomplete, and the whole system was conducted through a complex array of institutions and arrangements derived primarily from social rather than economic demand. These characteristics peculiar to the delivery of health care probably helped to explain the dearth of economic research in the field—it required scholars who combined high competence with a flexible and imaginative outlook.

The bureau was founded in 1920 as a private, nonprofit research organization dedicated to the impartial compilation and interpretation of economic facts. Over the years it had helped to transform economics into an empirically oriented discipline, equipped with scientific tools for handling the problems of the real world. The results of its research, embodied in more than four hundred books and papers, had been a major influence on the improvement of economic decision making: Some of its basic contributions were the development of principles and techniques for measuring the gross national product and related national income statistics; the measurement and analysis of business cycles; and studies of the growth of output, employment, and productivity. More recently the bureau had undertaken pioneering research on "investment in human capital" and the economic benefits of education, and on ways of measuring productivity in industries such as retail trade and finance. Many of the statistical measures developed by the bureau (for instance, estimates of the volume of consumer credit) had been taken over by departments of the federal government.

A cardinal feature of the bureau's work was its refusal to make policy recommendations. In the words of its 1965 annual report, "By issuing its findings in the form of scientific reports, entirely divorced from recommendations on policy, the National Bureau hopes to aid all thoughtful men, however divergent their views on public policy, to base their discussions upon objective knowledge as distinguished from subjective opinion."

The bureau was governed by a board of directors from industry, banking, labor, agriculture, academic scholarship, law, and journalism; the board also included scholars and professionals in economics and management. The bureau's research program was carried out by forty full- and part-time general and specialist economists. Its budget, which amounted to $1,500,000 a year, was financed largely from private sources, including foundations; each year more than $350,000 was received from hundreds of business firms in amounts ranging from one hundred to several thousand dollars. Only about 10 percent of the bureau's income was derived from federal grants.

The distinguished work of the National Bureau of Economic Research in other areas of economics led the Fund's staff to conclude that the bureau was capable of comparable pathfinding contributions in health. In 1966 the Fund awarded the bureau a three-year grant of $150,000.[45]

The award was not intended to cover specific research but to be expended entirely on program planning and development; partial support of the director's salary; the salaries of economists experienced in health research; secretarial assistance; publication costs; and space, equipment, and computer charges.

The bureau was allowed discretion in allocating the grant among the specified purposes. Since the program was new, this degree of flexibility would be advantageous to staff recruitment and other initial operations. The bureau was confident that once the program was staffed and a research plan worked out, it could obtain funds from other sources (particularly the United States Public Health Service, which had recently begun to support research in health economics).

The program was supervised by Victor R. Fuchs, an associate director of research, who devoted almost half his time to the new program. Fuchs was a first-rate economist who had joined the bureau in 1962, leading its work on the economics of the service industries. He had long been interested in health economics, and at the bureau he had managed to carry out a considerable amount of exploratory work in the field. Fuchs expected the new program to be concerned with factors affecting decision making in the allocation of resources for health; the economic structure and dynamics of the health-services system, with emphasis on major trends and means of economic measurement; and the implications for health, and for costs, of alternative institutional arrangements for producing and financing health services.

As the grant came to an end, Fuchs summarized the results of the Fund-sponsored work:[46]

— Ten publications in as many professional journals including the *New England Journal of Medicine* and the *Journal of the American Medical Association*.
— Six studies well along with completion expected within one year.
— Recruitment to the health field of several excellent young economists at predoctoral and postdoctoral levels.
— Active participation of NBER researchers in the Mount Sinai School of Medicine, advisory committees of the Department of HEW, and other health-related activities.
— Receipt of a grant of $327,000 plus overhead for a four-year period from the U.S. Public Health Service for continuation and expansion of our program of research in the economics of health.

The Commonwealth Fund's initial grant encouraged other foundations to support the bureau, and, after a decade, Fuchs was able to report to Newton that the program in health economics was "flourishing . . . both in terms of its ability to attract bright young investigators to the field, and in attracting financial support. . . . Subsequent support has been obtained from the National Center for Health Services Research, the Robert Wood Johnson Foundation, and the Kaiser Family Foundation. The National Bureau has also invested a substantial amount of its unrestricted funds in this area. My colleagues and I have produced more than 60 published papers, four books and monographs, and have participated in a very large number of conferences, advisory committees, and other public activities.

"I will always be grateful to you and the Commonwealth Fund for getting us started in this important area."[47]

Colin Munro MacLeod: Vice-President for Medical Affairs (October 1, 1966–September 30, 1969)

Robert J. Glaser had been a somewhat shadowy figure at the Commonwealth Fund since 1963; he was not a member of either the staff or the board of directors, yet as Newton's informal consultant and sounding board, he had exerted a great influence on the Fund's programs and policies. Wanting Glaser's expertise full-time, Newton tried to persuade him to become the Fund's vice-president. Glaser had just taken on the presidency of the Affiliated Hospitals Center in Boston, however, as well as a professorship of social medicine at Harvard, and he was loath to leave his new positions.

Newton's next choice was Colin M. MacLeod, who was deputy director of the President's Office of Science and Technology. MacLeod had an impressive background: He had been deeply involved in the development of the New York University School of Medicine, and he had formidable scientific skills coupled with an interest in innovative approaches to medical education. MacLeod came highly recommended, and Newton himself believed in his abilities.

Colin M. MacLeod (fig. 27) was born in Nova Scotia in 1909 and educated at McGill University. After receiving his medical degree, he became first an assistant and later an associate at the Rockefeller Institute for Medical Research. During his seven years at the institute, he worked primarily in the laboratory of O. T. Avery, where he participated in the clinical studies of pneumococcal pneumonia and the development of rabbit antiserum as a therapeutic agent. With the discovery of the sulfonamides as bacteriostatic agents applicable to the treatment of pneumococcal disease, he made the first observation on the occurrence of "sulfapyridine-fast" strains of pneumococcus and of natural inhibitors of the sulfonamide drug. Other studies with Avery clarified the nature of C-reactive protein and identified the "transforming factor," which turned out to be DNA. In 1941 MacLeod became chairman of the Department of Microbiology at New York University; a move to the University of

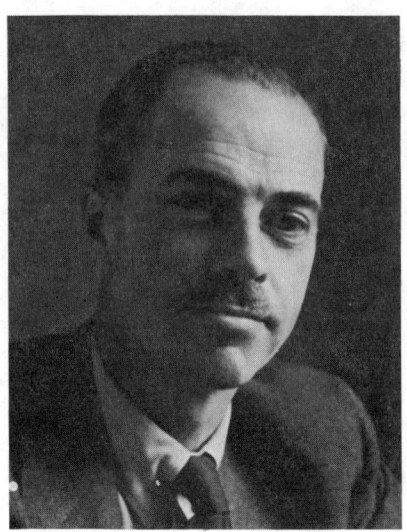

Figure 27. Colin Munro MacLeod
Photograph courtesy of the National
Library of Medicine, Bethesda,
Maryland.

Pennsylvania as professor of research medicine was followed by his return to New York to set up the Section of Genetics in New York University's Department of Medicine. During these years in academic medicine, he also served as director of the Commission on Pneumonia of the Army Epidemiological Board, consultant to the Surgeon General of the Army, chief of the Preventive Medicine Section of the Committee on Medical Research of the Office of Scientific Research and Development, and first president of the Armed Forces Epidemiological Board.

Six months into his new position with the Fund, MacLeod had come to believe that the Fund should support substantial changes in the structure of American medicine. Its central concern should be the relation of medical education to the nation's entire system of health-care delivery.[48] The Fund's staff and directors agreed: As the only foundation in the country heavily committed to helping medical schools improve their educational programs, the Fund had a unique responsibility. Its programs should concentrate on responding to the ideas of schools in order to sift out the most creative proposals, those that would affect the quality of either medical education or medical care. MacLeod talked with leaders of many medical schools, letting them know that the Fund would welcome their proposals. The result was a group of important programs that attest to Newton and MacLeod's insight in identifying the most potentially fruitful applications (see app. I).

MacLeod's main influence was in matters of policy rather than philosophy. He reinforced Newton's commitment to involving academic institutions in problems and issues of medical care and especially in reengaging the

Fund in medical education for minorities.[49] His academic experience enabled him to encourage good academic standards through programs combining the skills of disparate types of scholars at excellent universities. But MacLeod's most important contribution as vice-president of the Fund may have been the philanthropic coalition.[50] A joint effort was the solution to the funding of larger projects, as no one foundation had or wished to invest the total sum required for one project. A coalition also overcame the problem of limited manpower, enabling foundations to pool their staffs as well as their financial resources. MacLeod recognized that Meharry College was an institution for the times, and it was MacLeod who put together the coalition of foundations—Kellogg, Carnegie, Rockefeller, Macy, and Commonwealth—that gave $3 million for Meharry's rehabilitation.

Medical Education for Minorities

NATIONAL MEDICAL FELLOWSHIPS, INC.

The Commonwealth Fund's history of assistance to minorities in the United States extended back to the 1920s, when the Rural Hospital Program was put together partly to improve medical-care facilities for southern blacks. In advocating aid for Meharry Medical College, MacLeod could point to the Fund's tradition of support for the only national organization devoted specifically to helping minorities become physicians: National Medical Fellowships, Inc. (NMF).

NMF was established in 1946 as the Provident Medical Associates, a nonprofit corporation taking over the assets of the Julius Rosenwald Fund, which was then in the process of liquidation. NMF's board was made up almost entirely of physicians and included representatives of Chicago's four principal medical schools; its part-time staff operated at a modest cost of approximately $2,000 a year; and its volunteer secretary—and guiding spirit—was Franklin Chambers MacLean. At its inception, its primary purpose was to break the barrier to residency-level training for black physicians. In addition to giving fellowships for advanced study, NMF provided consultants for Provident Hospital's training program for black physicians.

MacLean had been chairman of the Department of Medicine at the University of Chicago, and director of the university clinics. He preferred the laboratory to the desk, however, and in 1933, at the age of 45, he left medical administrative activities completely to become professor of pathological physiology. From then until his death in 1968, his full-time activity was the study of the metabolism of calcium and the physiology of bone, and he made notable contributions in this field. Although he had terminated his formal administrative responsibilities at the university, MacLean retained a lifelong devotion to upgrading medical education for black students, and NMF honored him on his eightieth birthday by creating the Franklin C. MacLean Fund for Blacks in Medicine. Over twenty years some six hundred black pre- and postdoctoral students received financial assistance through NMF (including Lloyd Elam, who later became president of Meharry Medical College).

In its first four years, the Provident Medical Associates concentrated on fellowships for black house staff preparing for National Board certification in medical subspecialties. It also offered to help fellows in planning their programs of training and their future placements.

The Rosenwald Fund's assets were entirely distributed by 1949; by the time this support ended, the Provident Medical Associates had spent more than $76,000 for fifty-nine fellowships to thirty-seven individuals. Some replacement funds were found: the Field Foundation agreed to continue its support if other groups would participate, and the National Foundation for Infantile Paralysis had made a grant of $50,000 for seven awards for graduate study in neurology, pediatrics, and orthopedics. Stipends were small and qualified candidates were few, and MacLean felt that an additional $20,000 a year would allow the organization to fill all its requests. To make up the shortfall, MacLean appealed to the Commonwealth Fund for $10,000 yearly for the next three years. The Fund's board of directors realized that although their contribution represented only a fraction of what might be done in medical education for members of minorities, it was a useful fraction. Although the best ways to increase the number of black physicians were far from clear, it seemed appropriate for the Fund to extend the umbrella of its fellowship program to help the Provident Medical Associates, which in the early 1950s changed its name to National Medical Fellowships, Inc.

Between 1949 and 1961, the Fund gave NMF three grants totaling $140,000. A grant from the Fund's Division of Publications in 1962 helped the organization to produce *New Opportunities for Negroes in Medicine,* a booklet designed to interest black high-school and college students in medicine as a career to inform them of NMF's program of financial assistance.[51] An increase in governmental and private funding for advanced studies in medicine during the late 1950s allowed NMF to shift its attention to the medical-school years, and it became the main source of financial help for black students admitted to medical school. During the early 1960s, grants from a dozen foundations, notably the Sloan Foundation, enabled NMF to keep pace reasonably well with the demands upon its resources, largely because the number of black medical students remained relatively small. Excluding students at Howard and Meharry, only about 175 blacks were enrolled in medical school—and NMF was able to assist about 100 of these annually.

The situation changed greatly in the mid-1960s. The nation's colleges increased their enrollment of blacks, and many medical schools followed. By 1969 a report from the Association of American Medical Colleges was calling on medical schools to bring minority enrollments to parity with the number of blacks in the population. As a result, for the academic year 1969–70, NMF received applications for assistance from 366 eligible medical students—nearly three times as many as in 1966.

To make matters more difficult, NMF was barely in a position to meet even its normal level of support. MacLean had been in ill health since 1965, and Irving Graef, a member of NMF's board, had been elected to succeed him as secretary-treasurer. The organization had also appointed Robert C. Stepto to fill the largely honorary position of president, and the new staff required time to adjust to the new demands. Before 1968 the only paid member of the staff was the executive secretary; in 1969 NMF expanded its staff to include William E. Cadbury, Jr., as executive director. Cadbury worked only part-time at NMF in his first year, however; after serving as dean and premedical adviser at Haverford College, he became the director of Haverford's postbaccalaureate fellowship program for minority students preparing for graduate and professional school. NMF moved its office to New York in 1970, and that year Cadbury shuttled between New York and Pennsylvania as he phased out his relationship with the college's program.

On the national scene, 1969 was a year of critical change. In the fall, 501 minority students had been accepted in United States medical schools, twice as many as in 1968. Simultaneously, federal aid to minority students in individual schools, available since 1965, was cut back by the Nixon administration. The medical schools were in a very difficult position, since they had accepted these 501 students with the anticipation that financial aid would be available. NMF stepped in to help, joining several other foundations in making emergency grants to students entering medical school that fall. The Commonwealth Fund's grant of $25,000 to NMF came with the provisos that this was a one-time award and did not imply future support; and that for each student aided by these funds, NMF would ask his medical school to contribute the maximum feasible amount so that the Fund's grant could be used to assist as many students as possible.[52]

At the same time, there was an urgent need for NMF to complete its administrative reorganization so that it could raise additional funds. That fall Graef and Cadbury met with J. Quigg Newton, Jr., John Bowers of the Josiah Macy, Jr., Foundation, and Robert N. Kriedler of the Sloan Foundation. None was enthusiastic about giving further help until the NMF's structure was sound, but the reorganization could not be accomplished without an infusion of funds. The circle was finally broken when the three foundations agreed to contribute money for NMF's administrative programs. The Fund's staff recommended an award of $70,000 for 1969–70—$50,000 toward the 1970–71 scholarship drive[53] and $20,000 toward the operating budget through NMF's 1970–71 fiscal year. The key portion of the budget was this $20,000; it was one of the Fund's most important grants to this organization, making it possible for NMF to recruit Rufus Smith, a professional fund raiser. In early 1970 Smith left his position as top member of the fund-raising staff of the National Association for the Advancement of Colored People to become associate director of NMF.

The Fund's emergency grant did not turn out to be a one-time allocation. In 1971 the Fund supported NMF's expanded effort to cope with the increase in black students entering classes in the nation's medical schools, and to undertake a new project: an intense search for suitable black students and other minority students, primarily Mexican–Americans. Building upon its experience and its broad base of acceptance, NMF designed a program to help medical schools increment their enrollment of minorities. A major hindrance to progress, however, was the lack of financial aid for students, as few blacks could consider medical education without scholarship assistance. NMF's approach had been to raise as much money as possible and then distribute it among the eligible applicants who had been accepted to medical school.

Until 1969 awards had been made to a limited number of students on the basis of academic ability. Cadbury changed this policy, believing that any student who was accepted to medical school was worthy of support, whether he was at the top or the bottom of his class. Now need replaced academic status as the criterion; the amount given to each student was related to his family's ability to help and to the money available from his medical school. NMF gave the schools with the most minority students the most funds, as a stimulus to enroll more minority applicants.

In this first year of its new national drive—1970–71—NMF had expanded its contributors from twenty organizations and individuals to 113, and increased its scholarship awards from 270 to 598; 36 of the awards were financed by the Commonwealth Fund. These gains brought the proportion of NMF scholars to 40 percent of the country's minority-group students studying for the M.D. degree. In the second year of its expanded program, NMF planned to concentrate its assistance primarily on freshmen and sophomores, since upperclassmen could use loans to complete their training without accumulating an intolerable burden of debt. The momentum it had achieved and the projected need led NMF to anticipate doubling its first-year record: It hoped to award 1,170 scholarships, including 120 to third-year students. The Fund contributed $95,000 in 1971 toward NMF's $2,220,000 goal.[54]

That year 6 percent of first-year medical students were from minority groups. A five-year goal had been set in 1970 by the Inter-Agency Task Force on Medical Education of Minority Students—that by 1975–76, 10 percent of freshman medical students should be from minority groups. Obviously this goal would not be met without strenuous efforts to find financial support, yet NMF was showing laudable gains. In 1970–71 the organization had raised $923,750 in scholarship funds; in 1971–72 it raised $1,687,950, representing donations from thirty additional foundations and corporate donors and many more individual donors. In 1973 its funds again increased, to $1,730,438, and its base of support expanded. Corresponding to this increase, scholarship awards increased greatly between 1970–71 and 1971–72, and again the following year. Sixty-five of the 1,518 awards in 1973 were financed by the Commonwealth Fund's contributions, and NMF's goal was to raise $2,700,000 for 1,800 scholarships in 1974.

The Robert Wood Johnson Foundation had set aside $10 million for the medical-school education of women, students from rural areas, and members of minority groups. But benefits for minority students were largely offset by sharp cutbacks in federal funds, which were affecting the overall budgets of most medical schools. The Commonwealth Fund provided some stability by renewing its support at the level granted in previous years—$75,000 for scholarships and $20,000 for operating costs.[55]

NMF's plans for 1974–75 called for 1,970 scholarships at a cost of $2,743,000. Although the Comprehensive Health Manpower Training Act of 1971 authorized substantial federal scholarship funds for medical schools, of which $14.9 million was intended for scholarship aid to minority students, the actual amount provided for this purpose in 1974 was $6.8 million, some 6 percent less than the previous year and nearly 45 percent less than originally specified by the Act. Compounding the problem was the medical schools' 9.6 percent increase in student enrollment in 1973. Once again NMF's role in directly and specifically supporting minority-group medical students remained crucial. Equally important was its attempt to increase the average amount it could give to each student—an amount that had decreased significantly in recent past years because of the rapid rise in the number of medical students from minority groups. The Fund again recommended that a grant of $95,000 be appropriated to provide $75,000 toward NMF's scholarship drive and $20,000 toward its operating budget.[56]

In 1974 NMF again reviewed its overall program and reorganized its financial structure and fund-raising procedures. Its current president became chairman of the board, and the presidency was redefined as an active staff position. Now the president would run the board meetings and consult with Graef and Cadbury about the organization's day-to-day operation. Jerry Lewis left his job as special consultant in charge of community health for the American Lung Association to take on NMF's presidency in October 1974.

Grants from the Commonwealth Fund amounting to $620,000 and

support from many other private foundations had helped NMF since 1969 to lower the hurdles—financial and otherwise—that tended to limit the number of minority students in medical schools. NMF officers believed that scholarship funds for minority students allowed medical schools to recruit them more actively with less fear of straining their own limited funds for student aid. The nationwide push to expand minority enrollments allowed most well-qualified minority applicants to be accepted, and NMF saw active recruitment through financial assistance as the key to increasing the enrollment of minorities in medical schools.

Twelve percent of American physicians and twelve percent of American medical students would have to be black for the percentage of black physicians and black medical students to correspond to the percentage of blacks in the population at large. At the end of World War II, approximately 2 percent of American doctors were black; in 1978 the percentage was the same (i.e., 8,000 black physicians out of a total of 400,000), and it was clear that this part of the goal could not be reached during the twentieth century. To increase the number by 10 percent during the next ten years would require training 58,000 additional black physicians. Similarly, the medical schools would have to graduate 5,800 black physicians each year (about 38 percent of each graduating class). This goal, while not within reach, was at least being approached: In the academic year 1968–69, about 2.6 percent of first-year medical students were members of minority groups (predominantly blacks), but by 1975 minority representation had increased to 7.5 percent, with a later decline to 7 percent.

In the academic year 1976–77 NMF awarded $1,558,833 in scholarships to 12,495 students in 112 American medical schools. The average scholarship, $1,043, covered one-fifth or less of the average cost of a year of medical school. Total resources available to NMF in 1975–76 would have been far less, but the Robert Wood Johnson Foundation made a special grant of $500,000 late in the year, increasing the organization's available resources from less than $1,400,000 to $1,897,200. In 1977 the Commonwealth Fund gave an additional $70,000; in 1978 and again in 1981 the Fund awarded NMF a grant of $150,000.

Despite financial support and increasing enrollment of minority students, in 1981 there were only 480 blacks, 245 mainland Puerto Ricans, 66 Mexican-Americans, and 21 American Indians among the 31,000 M.D.-level medical-school faculty members in the United States—minorities accounting for less than 3 percent of the total.[57] When reports implicated the scarcity of role models for minority students in addition to the well-known financial problems,[58] the Fund added a new feature to its support of National Medical Fellowships: in 1983 it paired each fellowship recipient with a mentor. Many distinguished men and women in academic medicine today say they chose their careers because an older individual guided their path and encouraged them at crucial points. The Fund hoped that this type of personal guidance would help surmount the critical barrier to the development of minority faculty and minority academic leadership.

MEHARRY MEDICAL COLLEGE

Meharry Medical College, in Nashville, Tennessee, was founded in 1876 and named for the family that provided its initial support.[59] It came to national attention in 1909, when Abraham Flexner identified Meharry and Howard University as the two black medical schools in the country worthy of development. Flexner's assessment led to long-term support by the Rockefeller Foundation's General Education Board, which was primarily responsible for Meharry's move in 1931 to its fourteen-acre campus near Vanderbilt and Fisk universities. Although Meharry received support until the 1960s from the General Education Board, and from the Rosenwald, Ford, and Danforth foundations, its ability to survive remained in doubt. An ambitious fund drive launched in 1960 resulted in a new wing and a three-story clinical research area for the George W. Hubbard Hospital, the college's teaching institution, but failed to increase the college's small endowment, which stood at only $9 million. The college remained in difficult straits—poorly financed, with substantial need for more facilities and an improved and enlarged faculty.

Despite its needs and weaknesses, the school had two important assets: First, it was a lively institution serving black higher education, jointly accredited by the Association of American Medical Colleges (AAMC) and the American Medical Association, with a nucleus of full-time faculty of professional excellence and rare dedication. Second, it represented one of the country's best hopes for improving health opportunities for the black community, particularly in the South. Predominantly black institutions had a crucial role to play in collegiate and professional education. The ratio of black physicians to the black population was about 1 to 3,800, compared with one doctor for every 670 persons in the country as a whole. In the South the disparity was much greater. Mississippi, for instance, had one black physician for every 18,000 blacks in the state, only slightly better than the physician-to-population ratio prevailing in Africa. While it was assumed that all physicians—white and black—were bound by ethics, training, and custom to assist any person requiring their help, it was also true that few white doctors practiced in black communities. Until this pattern was changed, the health status of the black population would depend in large measure on the number of blacks trained for medicine and on the quality of education they received.

Inadequacies in educational background and economic, cultural, and other deficits limited the ability of many blacks to attend predominantly white institutions, even when many of these institutions were striving to increase their black enrollments. Because of increased opportunities for professional careers in other fields, fewer blacks were enrolling in medical school in the 1960s than in the 1950s. In medicine, although roughly one-third of all black medical students attended the nation's predominantly white institutions, the remainder of blacks aspiring to medical careers had to look either to Howard University College of Medicine in Washington, D.C., or to Meharry. Of the two schools, Meharry had fewer financial resources. Howard, a federally chartered school, received government support for its basic operations; Meharry, wholly private, depended largely on nongovernmental funding, except for annual support for students enrolled from member states of the Southern Regional Education Board (SREB).

By the 1960s Meharry had trained half the black physicians and dentists then in practice in the United States. Authorities in health care from medical schools, private foundations, and governmental agencies agreed that it was an institution of fundamental importance to the nation. Federal officials worked with the medical college's administration to help it qualify for a larger share of funding under national legislation for health and higher education. Locally, the SREB was exploring ways to increase its contributions. Most important, Medicare payments received by the Hubbard Hospital, as well as the anticipated activation of Medicaid in Tennessee, were expected to eliminate the hospital's large annual deficit, which had long been a severe drain on the college's slim financial resources. In the mid-1960s the prospects for Meharry's future were more encouraging than they had been for many years.

The medical college had recently completed a comprehensive plan for academic improvement. Clinical instruction was to be completely reformed to include the innovations introduced over the past decade at other schools— for example, early exposure to patients and clinical problems; interdepartmental planning, teaching, and testing; and elective clerkships and basic science studies in the fourth year. Community and family medicine would be part of all four years of the medical course. Although these studies would be directed by the new Department of Family and Community Medicine, all clinical departments would participate. The new department would also manage a Neighborhood Health Center, where medical students would spend part of their clerkships.

This plan, the work of a group of Meharry's ablest faculty members and key trustees, had been studied by representatives of the AAMC; deans and senior faculty of leading medical schools, such as those at Duke, Vanderbilt, and North Carolina, and officials at the highest level of public service, including James A. Shannon, director of the National Institutes of Health. In addition, the plan was thoroughly reviewed at a meeting of foundation representatives convened in June 1967 by the

Commonwealth Fund and the Josiah Macy, Jr., Foundation. At this meeting were representatives from the Ford, Rockefeller, Kellogg, Sloan, and Markle Foundations; the Carnegie Corporation; the Milbank Memorial Fund; and the Maurice Falk Medical Fund. All who saw the plan agreed that although the school needed both a sharper delineation of priorities and a specific operational process for putting the plan into effect, the proposed program offered a sound design for the medical college's overall improvement.

Meharry's faculty and trustees gave first priority to the development of the basic sciences: They worked out a detailed program of implementation, including the aspects that needed financing from private sources. The plan called for thirty-five new faculty members over the next five years and construction of a basic sciences teaching and research building.

Meharry proposed to begin the course with ten students and gradually expand the enrollment to thirty. Because of the additional year involved, scholarship support would be essential, and funds for erecting and equipping a prefabricated teaching laboratory would also be required. Medical educators regarded the course as a prototype enabling all schools to admit bright black applicants whose inadequate premedical education would otherwise lead to their exclusion—an experiment with national implications. The program would also enhance the college's ability to compete for able faculty, which in turn would strengthen basic-science education for undergraduate students.

Since the basic sciences flourished best in an atmosphere of graduate education, the medical college also proposed to develop a graduate-level teaching program, first at the master's and eventually at the doctoral level. To cope with the frequently encountered problem of the exceptionally able graduate student with a defective college background, the master of medical science course would offer three years of preclinical training instead of the usual two. The program would build on the college's twenty years of experience in master's-degree education in physiology, microbiology, and biochemistry. Work in these fields would be expanded, and new master's-degree curricula would be added in other disciplines—including anatomy, pathology, pharmacology, and the behavioral sciences. The challenging course would include all the requirements for the master's degree in a particular discipline, as well as instruction in cell biology, physiology, and pathology; it would enable the college's most capable students to obtain a sound scientific background for their subsequent clinical studies or for doctoral studies at another institution.

Also included in Meharry's application to the Fund was a proposed collaboration in premedical-preclinical studies with Fisk University intended to correct deficiencies in science education and to interest students with superior intelligence in medical and biomedical careers. Fisk University was among the best black universities, with a growing graduate enrollment and faculty strength in biology, chemistry, mathematics, and physics. The two institutions would identify and work with eighteen promising freshmen and sophomores in black colleges in Tennessee and nearby states gradually expanding the program to include about fifty students. A Meharry faculty member would serve as a full-time director of the experiment, and four Meharry teachers would counsel the students, visiting their campuses for discussions and seminars. Laboratory teaching sessions would also be arranged at the Meharry campus during the year, but the most intensive instruction would take place during the summer, when students would study at both schools. The beginning of formal academic collaboration between Meharry and Fisk, this program would help set new standards for premedical education in black colleges and provide medical schools across the country with a group of black students with a substantial preclinical background who were well prepared and motivated for medicine.

Funds were needed for student scholarships, the program director's salary, released time of faculty counselors, salaries of Meharry summer-session faculty, renovation of laboratories, and equipment. Finally, because of the importance of library resources to the other aspects of the plan, Meharry included in its proposal to the Fund a request for support of a new central library building and an expanded staff and collection of books and periodicals. The existing library was entirely inadequate for even the medical college's current needs.

The budget submitted for Meharry's basic-science developmental program covered the four elements in the college's request: expansion and improvement of graduate-level teaching; the master of medical science course; the premedical-preclinical program with Fisk; and library improvement. Nearly $2 million was required for building renovation, construction, and equipment; $394,673 in annual operating funds was required for the first two years, and $578,173 for each year thereafter. To obtain this substantial amount, the medical college was seeking the participation of several foundations. The Fund's staff had learned from staff members at other foundations that a number planned to contribute. The Kellogg and Macy foundations, for example, had already expressed interest in supporting Meharry's plan.

The Fund's staff believed that their most effective contribution would be help in financing the first and largest item in the budget: the expansion and improvement of graduate-level teaching. The staff saw this as the keystone to the medical college's academic improvement, since it would result in a significant increase in faculty competent to provide first-rate instruction in the underlying sciences of medicine. Not only would this added strength benefit all Meharry students, but it would also ensure an adequate academic base for the second and third projects in the college's proposal.

The Fund's board of directors approved a grant of $700,000 to Meharry Medical College in 1967 in support of the medical college's proposed developmental program in the basic sciences.

The president of the college, Lloyd C. Elam, summarized the effects of this grant:[60]

> A major strength of the Fund's support of the College during the past five years has been its integrative character. Assistance in the revitalization of Meharry's basic science offerings, both for key faculty support and physical facilities, came at a time when this program area of the College badly needed upgrading. . . . The Fund's long acquaintance with Meharry enabled it to make what was in essence, I believe, the right contribution at the right time. . . .
>
> A one and one-half story biomedical sciences facility, covering 12,000 square feet, was erected in 1970–71 and the Commonwealth Fund's support made its construction possible. This is the building that houses some 12 biomedical scientists who engage in cross-disciplinary research and teaching. . . .
>
> Again, the timeliness of the Fund's gift is important to emphasize. Between 1969 and 1973, plans were advanced and finalized for the construction of a new, larger basic sciences facility. This structure was to be of such a size (about 190,000 square feet) that ample room would be available for a vastly expanded program of teaching and research in the basic medical sciences. Also, it would need to accommodate larger class sizes. In 1973, construction of the six-story facility started and we are hoping now that it will be ready for occupancy in 1975.
>
> I would stress that being able to develop our program in a manner that such a new structure will truly meet and fit our needs goes back to our being able to work and experiment in the smaller facility. Three departments, for example, have started fledgling Ph.D. programs the past two years and these disciplines will very much appreciate the resources of new surroundings. . . .
>
> We feel, then, that most of our objectives to date have been realized in revitalizing and strengthening our basic science program offerings. Finding and retaining good faculty is a perennial problem and we will continue to need assistance and imagination in meeting that need. However, the Commonwealth Fund's early support gave us a visibility which helped to attract other friends. And it was the Fund's singular foresight and willingness to act which has done the most to give our efforts in the basic sciences a sense of permanency and direction. For all these things, we remain deeply and respectfully grateful.

In 1972 Meharry Medical College received a five-year grant of $5 million from the Robert Wood Johnson Foundation—the largest ever given to the college—to expand its training of health professionals for front-line service in "under-doctored" communities. This was pioneering work: developing new teams to provide the full range of medical care for both urban and rural disadvantaged communities. By providing a teaching base for Meharry's students, the teams also strengthened Meharry's national role in medical education.

COLLABORATION BETWEEN HARVARD UNIVERSITY AND THE MASSACHUSETTS INSTITUTE OF TECHNOLOGY

During MacLeod's vice-presidency at the Commonwealth Fund, Harvard University and the Massachusetts Institute of Technology (MIT) began a joint enterprise to apply modern science and technology to medical problems. The Fund helped to develop this program, the Division of Health Sciences and Technology, which continues today, combining the strengths of two schools to educate physicians.

MacLeod's efforts began in 1966, when he was still in the President's Office of Science and Technology. He and James A. Shannon, director of the National Institutes of Health, visited MIT's president, Howard W. Johnson, and its provost, Jerome R. Wiesner, to urge the establishment of a medical school emphasizing science and engineering. Their message was that the federal government was prepared to give $50 million to a medical school offering this unorthodox type of program. The offer was tempting, but after exploring the idea thoroughly over the next few weeks with faculty members, potential recipients, and consultants, Johnson and Wiesner demurred: The cost of establishing and running such a school would greatly exceed any possible government contribution. To develop additional teaching hospitals in a city already well supplied with schools would be difficult, and MIT did not wish to jeopardize its excellent relationships with Harvard and the other schools of medicine in Boston. Yet although they rejected the offer, Johnson and Weisner remained interested in engaging MIT in the fields of medicine and health.

Across the river, Robert H. Ebert, the new dean of the Harvard Medical School, was being urged by David D. Rutstein and other faculty members to commit Harvard to a major program combining medicine with the physical sciences and engineering. Ebert knew that it would be difficult to attract good engineers and physicists to a medical-school setting, but conversations with Wiesner soon revealed MIT's interest in a collaboration. A joint Committee on Engineering and Living Systems appointed by the two university presidents met over the next two years to explore the possibilities for projects in education, research, and health care. The committee recommended that the great enthusiasm of both schools for a collaborative program be harnessed, and its first recommendation was for a detailed design of a joint institution and its programmatic objectives.

Meanwhile, Irving M. London, professor and chairman of the Department of Medicine at the Albert Einstein College of Medicine, had been asked to consider a professorship at Harvard. He did not find the lateral move attractive, but he was interested in the developing relations between Harvard and MIT. From 1967 to 1969, he was a consultant to the Harvard–MIT project under study. When it became clear that the joint effort would receive a strong positive recommendation, London was asked to serve as chairman of a planning committee to develop a detailed design.

It was then that the two universities applied to the Commonwealth Fund for support. The Fund granted a total of $655,000 for development of a detailed programmatic design and its early implementation.[61] London took a sabbatical from his position at Einstein in 1969, intending to spend no more than one year on the project. Matters progressed more rapidly than he had expected, however, and the committee quickly came up with a program incorporating education, research objectives, health-care policy, and management programs. By the spring of 1970, this program had been presented for discussion to the faculties of both universities, including the faculty of the Harvard School of Public Health. At the Harvard Medical School, a resolution to establish a Harvard–MIT School of Health Sciences and Technology was passed overwhelmingly, with the provision that new financial resources be obtained. A similar resolution was passed at MIT without dissent.

In June 1970 the corporations of Harvard and MIT endorsed these resolutions and decided to establish this enterprise as a formal program of the two universities. As soon as a nucleus of $10 million was available in endowment, a permanent joint institution would be established.

London accepted the invitation to direct the program. The Commonwealth Fund's support was crucial in allowing the first part of the joint program—a curriculum leading to the M.D. degree at the Harvard Medical School—to get off to a very fast start. This new curriculum was designed to emphasize a strong science background in the education of physicians. The program would offer a wide range of scientific material calling upon the strengths of the entire university, not just those departments ordinarily found in a school of medicine.

London wanted the program to develop several kinds of health scientists:[62]

1. Physicians and public health experts with a strong base in the social sciences and with a knowledge of management, administration, and planning
2. Physicians and dentists with a strong scientific base in engineering and the physical sciences, e.g., a cardiologist with a knowledge of electrical engineering, an orthopedic surgeon with mechanical engineering skills, or a dentist with a knowledge of biomaterials science
3. Health-care planners and operations research and systems engineers
4. Economists, political scientists, and public administrators concerned with public policy for health and medicine
5. Biomedical engineers engaged in the application of engineering to

      biological systems and to the solution of health problems, e.g., bioengineers concerned with control systems and instrumentation for life support mechanisms or biomaterials scientists involved in the development of materials required for artificial organs and prosthetic devices
6. Biologists oriented toward human biology and concerned with human evolution, human genetics, human behavior, and population biology

In London's view the Fund's support was critical to getting this program underway. Not only did it provide the essential money to recruit faculty from within the institutions, allowing the two schools to "buy" the time of key individuals, but it also represented a large vote of confidence that impressed other potential donors.

An additional $600,000 was requested from the Commonwealth Fund in 1971 to get the program airborne while fund-raising efforts were being organized by a national sponsoring committee of distinguished individuals. The $600,000 was granted, but not without resistance from some members of the board.[63] The Fund stressed to the two universities that they were expected to take their fund-raising very seriously, as the Fund would not be receptive to pleas for further support if their efforts were unsuccessful. As long as the Harvard–MIT effort was a program and not a permanent institution, the schools were to consider this second Commonwealth Fund grant a terminal one.[64]

Although the Fund gave no further financial support to the Harvard–MIT program after August 1972, the program and the Fund maintained contact; when the Fund began its Interface Program in the mid-1970s (see p. 463), its staff drew on the Harvard–MIT project's experience in engaging all the scientific resources of the university in medical education.

The Fund permitted Harvard and MIT to stretch out expenditures for its second grant, so the close-out expenditure report was not submitted until 1974. Newton appraised the venture a few years after the Fund's support ended:[65]

> Although the objectives of the health sciences and technology program are being realized, it is much too early to attempt to render a definitive judgment on its success or importance to the world. Whether the special training these rather elite students receive, with emphasis on the quantitative sciences, will result in their making a unique contribution to the teaching and practice of medicine, and whether the enhanced collaborative research between the MIT and Harvard faculties will result in major advances in scientific knowledge only time will tell. It is worth noting that several universities throughout the world have indicated interest in this program's emphasis on the quantitative sciences in medical education and research. But it is too early to judge whether this approach can or will be replicated elsewhere.
>
> I recommended these grants to our Board because outstanding members

of the faculties and administration of two of America's strongest institutions, in whom I have great confidence, believed that it was highly important for these institutions to undertake this collaborative effort in education and research. Now, six years later, I believe this joint enterprise is on target in terms of what we hoped would be accomplished. Our recent site visit reaffirms my earlier view of this program in health and science technology as an important project, one eminently worthy of Commonwealth Fund support.

Over $8 million in endowment was raised in the five years after the Fund's support ended, and by 1977 the program was on a sound financial basis. That year presidents Derek C. Bok of Harvard and Jerome B. Wiesner of MIT agreed to establish the program as a formal institution. The joint institution was originally to be called a "school," but the term has different meanings at the two universities. At MIT a school is a constituent of a single university faculty; at Harvard a school generally represents an independent faculty. The term "division" was deemed sufficiently ambiguous to serve the purpose, and the program became known as the Harvard–MIT Division of Health Sciences and Technology.

The program suffered at first from organizational asymmetry: the Harvard–MIT division was anchored on the Harvard side in the faculty of medicine, but at MIT health-related activities were diffusely spread throughout the institution (this despite the often unappreciated fact that one-third of MIT's total research activity is in the life and health sciences). The solution suggested by MIT's administration was a home for their components of the division. Since these areas transcended the interests of any single department or school, their idea was to establish a College of Health Sciences, Technology, and Management—a center for health-related activities that would also allow MIT to continue its independent pursuit of aspects of human biology, experimental medicine, biomedical engineering, and health policy and management. The term "college" was used for the first time in the history of MIT, presenting the concept of a multidisciplinary academic unit in which faculty members throughout the institution could participate in common programs of education and research related to health. This idea was based on the experience of the multidisciplinary Harvard–MIT division, whose faculty members also held appointments in departments of the two universities.

Until 1977 the sum of the division's physical facilities was only a small amount of teaching space at MIT and one office at the Harvard Medical School. As a result, the division was finding it difficult to recruit faculty members. The College of Health Sciences, Technology, and Management at MIT (Whitaker College) was designed to consolidate health-related activities at that school and provide the joint program with facilities of its own.

In London's words, "We would not be here, we would not have the

Harvard–MIT Division, which has led to the creation of Whitaker College, were it not for the support of the Commonwealth Fund at a very critical stage in development. The Commonwealth Fund can take pride that its support was a major influence in establishing these institutions."[66]

Collaboration with Other Foundations

The Carnegie Corporation's main liaison with the Commonwealth Fund was Margaret E. Mahoney. Adept at obtaining help from outside experts, she depended on MacLeod for advice on medical programs. Her education in the medical field was greatly enhanced by her contacts with him, and their collaboration was an important contribution to the Fund's future, as Mahoney later assumed the presidency of the Commonwealth Fund. Newton was pleased to collaborate with the Carnegie Corporation, a conscientious partner.

Although the Carnegie Corporation had been involved primarily in higher education, its chief executive officer, Alan Pifer, believed that the deepening problems in American medicine required his foundation's attention. In 1966 he deputized Mahoney to develop plans and budgets for a program in medical education and health care. The Carnegie Corporation could not devote much of its resources to new interests, so Mahoney's program received only a small annual allocation and had to compete for a relatively small amount of money from general funds. She consulted with Newton and MacLeod in a search for a clear-cut issue that the Carnegie Corporation might address, and together they defined the area in which the two foundations might collaborate: Since medicine offered a broad window on many social problems, how could medicine manipulate the social and economic factors affecting the health of individuals without mounting a frontal attack?

The first tangible result of the collaboration was a jointly sponsored conference in Fort Lauderdale, Florida, which was attended by professionals from universities and the National Institutes of Health (NIH). The agenda for the conference was prepared by John Z. Bowers, president of the Josiah Macy, Jr., Foundation. For an entire week in February 1966, participants talked about what were then important topics: problems in medical education and the delivery of health care. For many of the participants, it was a frustrating meeting: "Some were hearing things they had heard many times before, and others were hearing things they didn't want to hear at all."[67]

The participants concluded that whether or not the current situation could be termed a crisis, there was sufficient reason to be disturbed at the poor match between the requirements of patient care and the imbalances resulting from the effects of widespread specialization in medicine.

The role of nursing was especially ill-defined: Nursing schools were producing managers rather than people taking care of patients. On a larger scale, badly differentiated roles plagued all the allied health professions. The conference served as the starting point for discussion about patient care at the community level. How could the academic climate be altered so that medical students and house staff would think in terms of total patient care rather than specialization?

Also emerging from a collaboratively sponsored meeting was the idea of the "clinical scholar." In 1968 the Carnegie Corporation and the Fund invited five physicians—Julius R. Krevans from the Johns Hopkins University, Austin S. Weisberger from Western Reserve University, John C. Beck from McGill University, Halsted R. Holman from Stanford University, and James B. Wyngaarden from Duke University—to a meeting in Swampscott, Massachusetts. There they developed the notion of a uniquely trained individual: clinically based, sponsored by a department of medicine, but concerned with the organization, assessment and cost-effectiveness of medical care. He would be a new force for public health in medicine, a person still practicing clinical medicine and therefore likely to be a future department chairman or head of an ambulatory-care program. Wise in the ways in which administration and management were linked to the organization of medical care, he would be clinically and intellectually competent to deal with the issue of quality in medicine and trained to deal with the grosser issue of cost. Responsible for all the staff work that pulled together the Clinical Scholars Program was Margaret E. Mahoney.

The Clinical Scholars Program

The Clinical Scholars Program was a response to the high cost of health care, the paucity of general physicians, and the widening gap between advances in medical knowledge and technology and the quality of care available to most Americans.[68]

The federal government had tried to eradicate these inequities with the Medicare and Medicaid programs of 1965, which increased access to medical services and brought the elderly and indigent into the mainstream of private medical practice; the Heart Disease, Cancer, and Stroke Amendments of 1965, which linked academic medicine with community groups and medical practitioners in regional medical programs; the Office of Economic Opportunity's Health Centers Program, which developed community-based medical care facilities in areas of poverty; the Community Mental Health Centers Acts of 1963 and 1965; and the Comprehensive Health Planning and Public Health Services Amendments (the Partnership for Health Act of 1966).

Yet even this spate of programs was not enough. By the late 1960s, the American public—including medical students and house officers—had become vocal about social issues, and academic medical centers were struggling with their communities' demands for general medical care. These demands represented a new interpretation of the medical centers' usefulness, a sharp contrast to their traditional self-perception as tertiary-care, referral institutions. Philanthropic foundations as well as medical centers agreed that a new type of physician was required, a highly qualified clinician with the skills to translate the results of medical research into medical care. The Clinical Scholars Program was designed to train these physicians.

The idea of the Clinical Scholars Program evolved through several exploratory conferences and seminars. In 1965 the Carnegie Corporation joined with the NIH and the Richard King Mellon Foundation to sponsor the Endicott House Summer Study on Medical Education. Organized by Oliver Cope, professor of surgery at the Massachusetts General Hospital, and Jerrold Zacharias, professor of physics at the Massachusetts Institute of Technology, the workshop stimulated discussion between the presidents of the Carnegie Corporation and the Commonwealth Fund. The two foundations subsequently undertook joint sponsorship and funding of an additional series of conferences: the Exploratory Conference on Medical Services and Medical Education, in February 1966; the Swampscott Study on Behavioral Science in Medicine, in November 1966 (also chaired by Cope); and a Swampscott conference on internship and residency training for physicians, in April 1967.[69]

It was at the second Swampscott meeting that the five professors of medicine first discussed their common interest in revising postgraduate medical education at their respective institutions. The conference was followed by several meetings with the Carnegie and Commonwealth staffs. These five institutions were already in the Commonwealth Fund's family of grant recipients through their programs of curricular experimentation.

In 1968 the five presented a joint application to the Carnegie Corporation and the Commonwealth Fund. They intended to develop new approaches to medical residency training and experiment with continuing education for practicing internists. Their program intended to use graduate medical education to incorporate the application of the social sciences and all other nonmedical academic disciplines into every phase of medicine and medical education; to produce a new type of physician, a "clinical scholar," who would be taught to apply both nonmedical and medical knowledge to the exercise of innovative leadership in medical and health affairs; and to enable practicing physicians to draw upon the medical school and its university in rearranging their pattern of practice, so that they would have the time and opportunity to include professional growth as a continuing element in their lives.

The two foundations agreed to a two-year grant: The Carnegie Corporation provided $250,000 and the Commonwealth Fund $298,100 for planning and implementation of the Clinical Scholars Program. At first the program was conducted under the joint supervision of its five original architects. The Fund underwrote the employment of a full-time program director in each school, and the Carnegie grant provided support for an overall coordinator and stipends for training activities in each institution.

Departments of medicine were able to produce a significant number of Clinical Scholars with the advanced clinical skills required for certification as specialists in internal medicine. These physicians also undertook studies in a variety of academic and professional fields relating to delivery of health services. What skills were taught depended upon the physicians' specific career goals, but the Clinical Scholars were able to study the application of programmed instruction, audiovisual presentation, and other advanced educational techniques to medical education; the use of applied mathematics in conjunction with computers and other technologic aids to design clinical experiments evaluating patient care; and the application of economic analysis, systems engineering, and other nonmedical disciplines to health services. As this range of studies suggests, the two foundations anticipated that Clinical Scholars with varying interests and capabilities would become leaders in hospitals and group-practice clinics; in programs and agencies planning national, state, and area-wide public health services; and in medical schools and teaching hospitals.

Four of the five schools asked for renewal grants in 1971. (Case Western Reserve University had suspended its participation because of Weisberger's death.) The Clinical Scholars Program had developed into a pilot program of fellowships attempting to establish the field of health-services research as a serious discipline within academic medicine. The program's current purpose represented a significant departure from that articulated in the original application for funding three years earlier, when the principal emphasis was medical residency training, the training of academic clinicians, and continuing medical education. Now applicants were expected to be good clinicians with at least two years of internship and residency training. For prospective academicians subspecialty training usually followed two years of postgraduate work in internal medicine, and the Clinical Scholars Program was designed to take advantage of this natural fork in the road.

In the second (and probably final) round of funding, the two foundations together provided a two-year total of $480,000, $144,000 each to Duke and Johns Hopkins and $96,000 each to McGill and Stanford. By the time the Carnegie–Commonwealth sponsorship ended, the program had trained twenty-eight Clinical Scholars, and the Carnegie Corporation suggested that the program be presented as a national model to the federal government.

The torch was passed in 1972 to the Robert Wood Johnson Foundation, which emerged in that year as the second-largest foundation in the United States and the largest with a commitment to improving health care. Many of the Clinical Scholars were working on aspects of health care that the Robert Wood Johnson Foundation had identified as its principal targets, and the revitalized foundation's officers included persons familiar with the Clinical Scholars Program: President David E. Rogers, formerly vice-president for health affairs and dean at the Johns Hopkins University; Vice-President Margaret E. Mahoney, formerly of the Carnegie Corporation; Terrance Keenan of the Commonwealth Fund; and Robert Blendon, who had also been at Johns Hopkins during the program's early years. In its first year, the Johnson Foundation embarked upon a series of national programs, which were managed by outside groups. When Mahoney indicated her interest in the Clinical Scholars Program, the new foundation undertook to continue it almost immediately.

The Clinical Scholars Program originated by the Carnegie Corporation and the Commonwealth Fund produced a new type of clinical scientist, one with special capabilities and training that had not previously been combined. Some of the Clinical Scholars have gone on to assist the Robert Wood Johnson Foundation with new programs. Other program alumni are now serving as directors of primary-care residencies and developing faculty for family practice, academic departments of general pediatrics, rural infant-care, and other outreach projects. Several graduates are now directors or faculty members of the present Clinical Scholars programs. The program was also a harbinger of fellowship projects sponsored by other agencies, such as the Institute of Medicine, the Milbank Fund, and the Kaiser Family Foundation.

The Robert Wood Johnson Foundation was able to expand the original Clinical Scholars Program to support important clinical research on medical practice and the delivery of health care. The growing tendency for departments of medicine to carve out divisions of general internal medicine is an obvious legacy of the Clinical Scholars Program, as are projects to identify potential leaders in academic medicine.

Other Collaborative Projects

Additional jointly sponsored programs attempted to cope with increasing student unrest, the intensifying demands of minority groups for better health care, and general problems of community medicine. In the early 1970s, the Rockefeller Foundation joined the Carnegie Corporation and the Commonwealth Fund in supporting a plan at Johns Hopkins for health care in East Baltimore and a similar program at Duke University. With the Carnegie Corporation, the Fund initiated the ambulatory care program at the Beth Israel Hospital in Boston (see p. 423) and supported a program uniting the efforts of Harvard University's Department of Pediatrics and the Judge Baker Foundation to orient pediatricians toward behavior and psychiatrists toward growth and development. The initial activities of the Drug Abuse Council were sponsored by the Commonwealth Fund, the Carnegie Foundation, and the Ford, Rockefeller, and Kaiser Foundations.

Not only collaborative projects but the Fund's individual efforts reflected Newton's conviction that American medical schools were on the threshold of a new phase of social responsibility. In 1967 the Fund supported socially important programs at seven university medical centers—Harvard, the University of Washington, the University of Southern California, Albert Einstein, Colorado, Stanford, and Columbia–Presbyterian. The prototype of assistance given to these schools was a three-year grant to the Harvard Community Health Plan, an award that permitted the Harvard Medical School to expand its study of better arrangements for the provision of health care.

Another socially important project, the Yale Trauma Program, received one of the largest grants ever given by the fund—$2,000,000. Developed by Yale's Department of Surgery, the Trauma Program made a concerted attack on accidental trauma, the leading cause of death and a major cause of disability in the first half of the normal American life span. It was one of the first efforts to design a regional organization to solve an important health problem. More directly, the Yale Trauma Program was the medical community's first organized attempt to cope with trauma as a challenge to the nation's system of health care.

THE HARVARD COMMUNITY HEALTH PLAN

As the nation's largest single source of medical teachers and scientists, Harvard University had been preeminent in transforming medicine into a science-based profession. Yet the Harvard Medical School was not only a research and educational institution of international stature, it was the hub of a large health-care complex of immense regional importance. The Harvard Medical Center, organized in 1956, included seven hospitals, the medical school, and the schools of public health and dental medicine, and it was affiliated with municipal, state, and Veterans Administration hospitals.

For sixteen years George P. Berry, a director of the Fund, had been dean of the medical school. During his tenure Harvard had received several grants from the Fund, including an unrestricted grant of $1 million in 1955; help in developing a course that would integrate studies in the first two years of the medical curriculum for Ph.D. students in the Division of Medical Sciences; support for a program in comprehensive pediatric medicine; a large sum toward the development of the Countway Library; and the endowment of two professorships in the medical school, one named after Berry himself. In 1965 Robert H. Ebert was chosen as Berry's successor.

Ebert was interested in programs that would use Harvard's resources to meet social needs. During his first year as dean, Ebert and Henry Meadow, the associate dean, developed a two-pronged prospectus including a plan for prepaid medical care and a center that would bring economists, sociologists, and other professionals together to discuss health policy in a broad social context.

Ebert and Meadow approached the Commonwealth Fund for support. Newton was enthusiastic, although there was some feeling among staff and directors that Harvard had received more than its share of the Fund's grant money. In the end, the Fund gambled on Harvard's ideas—concepts that at the time were far from detailed, offering little substance on which the Fund could base its decision. Ebert was not surprised at the Fund's willingness to support his still-unformed project: The Fund characteristically took chances on promising ideas. A planning grant of $125,000 in 1966 ($25,000 for each of five years) enabled Ebert to work with the head of the Department of Preventive Medicine, David D. Rutstein, in delineating central problems of medical education and health care as well as possible solutions.[70] Ebert intended to give particular attention to the discipline of social medicine, which embraced such concerns as the influence of social factors on illness, the influence of illness on the structure of society, and the use of social resources in preventing and treating disease. The grant would also help Rutstein expand his department, which was primarily responsible for the study of the interaction of health and social problems.

Harvard decided to go ahead with its study of health-care systems, and the Fund's planning grant was followed the next year by a three-year award totaling $600,000 ($200,000 a year) to help Harvard get its project under way.[71] Now Ebert led the medical school in enlisting Harvard's exceptional resources in a concerted attack on the complex problems of the nation's pluralistic and sorely pressed system of medical services. Aimed at bringing these problems into the mainstream of teaching and research, the program represented the growing recognition among university medical centers that they must provide the intellectual base for the action demanded by a society that increasingly regarded access to comprehensive health care as a basic right.

Between 1965 and 1966, Ebert added to his principal staff Jerome Pollack, a medical economist, as associate dean for medical care planning; Sidney S. Lee, a former general director of the Beth Israel Hospital, as associate dean for hospital programs; and Leona Baumgartner, a former commissioner of health in New York City, as visiting professor of social medicine. Along with Rutstein and others at the Harvard Medical School, these experts held extensive discussions with individual faculty members; service chiefs in the affiliated hospitals; administrators; deans and chairmen of various university graduate departments; deans and faculty of other Boston-area medical schools; and city, state, and federal government officials.

The process of intensive consultation resulted in the outlines of a plan to create a new university center, the Center for Community Health and Medical Care, which would expand Harvard medicine into a new dimension: research, education, and demonstration projects in health. Centered in the medical school, the proposed program involved the school's associated hospitals, the School of Dental Medicine and the School of Public Health, the departments of economics and social relations, the graduate school of public administration, the Law School, and the graduate school of business administration. A joint venture of the Medical School and the School of Public Health, the new center was intended to facilitate collaboration among medical and nonmedical disciplines in the university and the Boston community.

In his proposal to the Fund, Ebert commented:[72]

> There is universal awareness of the exponential increase in medical knowledge, and of the role played by medical schools in the acquisition of new scientific knowledge. It is perhaps less apparent that modern technology and sophisticated methods of diagnosis and treatment have been imposed upon a system of health care that was designed for another age. This system is ill-equipped to adapt to radical change. While universities have profoundly influenced the provision of health care by their contributions to biological knowledge, they have expended little effort to evaluate thoughtfully or attempt to reconstruct the health-care system that has had to absorb these changes.
>
> Yet, the fact remains that medical schools, together with their parent universities and related teaching hospitals, represent the only force which can successfully bring quickly to bear the intellectual and physical resources necessary to study and to modify existing methods for the provision of care. If they are to assume a role in medical-care planning commensurate with their ability, there must be a major shift in emphasis within these institutions from the present preoccupation with the problems of the individual patient to the broader social and preventive issues of health care. Critical examination of the problems of how to deliver health care with respect to the total health needs of a community or population, and of how to use our manpower and our funds efficiently and effectively is imperative.
>
> Thus, involvement in medical-care planning can no longer be a peripheral activity for academic medicine. The modern medical center must become a laboratory for experimental approaches and a training ground for the several kinds of professionals needed in today's world of medicine. The Harvard Medical School has a special responsibility because of the unusual opportunities for experimentation made possible by the breadth and diversity of its clinical

and academic resources and those of the University of which it is a part. For this reason, the Harvard Faculty of Medicine must exercise leadership in providing new ways of looking at patient care and in developing the principles and techniques that can be widely applied to the organization of comprehensive health care programs for the benefit of the American people.

The center organized new educational programs, research efforts, and experiments and demonstrations in health care. It also performed an essential advisory role, making sure that all available talents and resources were used to best advantage within a coherent framework. In the beginning the center was administratively free-standing, its director reporting directly to Ebert; eventually it was folded into the Department of Community Medicine.

This grant from the Fund financed the planning and implementation of four other demonstration projects as well. Their aim was to illuminate the factors that shape health services—educational, professional, institutional, social, and economic—and to modify these factors to improve the medical profession's capacity to prevent disease and cope with illness. Experiments of this kind required a defined population of individual patients for continuing care and study in a sociomedical laboratory of a sort whose characteristics could be quantified. Harvard's five projects involved several such laboratory settings, each with different features: a population enrolled in a prepayment, group-practice system; a patient-care research laboratory; the health system of a specific community; the maternal and child health system of Boston; and a community-extension program of a large-city hospital (at the Cambridge City Hospital).[73] The Fund ensured that this grant would be used for projects consistent with its own overall goals: its interest in community participation in health plans led it to stipulate that priority be given to the group-practice project and the project at the Cambridge City Hospital. Although part of the appropriation might be allocated to the three remaining projects, individual proposals would require the Fund's approval.[74]

New staff members recruited to run the five projects included Paul Denson, who had been deputy commissioner of health for New York City. An epidemiologist and biostatistician, he was placed in charge of health planning. Others brought to Boston were Rashi Fein, an economist, and Robert Weiss, professor of psychiatry at Dartmouth Medical School. Joseph L. Dorsey and H. Richard Nesson were added to the staff in 1967; as the first medical advisor to the Community Health Plan, Nesson helped to devise the system for delivering health care.

The Community Health Plan was the most important of the five projects. Its corporate structure linked it with Harvard, but it was separate, autonomous, and fiscally accountable, so that Harvard could determine whether the plan would survive without subsidy. Jerome Pollack developed the plan's original benefit package and negotiated contracts with third-party payers and with the Harvard hospitals. He also took care of the nuts and bolts: Through his efforts Harvard rented several empty floors of a partially vacant apartment building as a home for the plan.

The plan began in 1968 with physicians recruited from the Harvard faculty. Patients in the beginning were few in number, and financially the situation deteriorated rapidly. Ebert, Lee, Meadow, Newton, and Keenan met at the Commonwealth Fund to discuss the plan's problems. Newton felt that at this stage that the financial responsibility for the plan's operation should be diffused, and he adroitly acquired additional support by organizing a meeting at the Century Association so that Ebert could present his program to representatives of the Rockefeller Foundation, the Ford Foundation, and the large insurance companies. The Rockefeller Foundation made a grant to the plan, and later a large award came from the Ford Foundation. The Commonwealth Fund itself gave the plan additional money in 1970.[75] Support also came from the Surdna Foundation, money loaned to the plan and eventually repaid. These foundations allowed the Community Health Plan to stay afloat without federal funds—which, in any case, were not available at that time.

Help in marketing the plan was also needed, as insurance companies had no incentive to support it. To develop a marketing strategy, Robert L. Biblo joined the Harvard team in 1970. The following year he replaced Pollack as chief executive officer. It was Biblo who, more than anyone else, turned the plan around, and by 1974 it was in the black. When Biblo left in 1978 to become head of New York's Health Insurance Plan, he was replaced by Thomas O. Pyle.

The Harvard Community Health Plan eventually acquired a patient clientele of over 150,000. Centers were developed in Boston, Wellesley, and Cambridge, and two additional centers were planned. A separate foundation administered the money set aside for the support of research, teaching, and community health—1.5 percent of the plan's premiums each year. At first, the plan's resources for teaching and research were not fully exploited. Fellowships in community health for residents were first offered in 1974, but there was little participation by medical students. Part of the problem was the difficulty of integrating medical students into a prepaid plan. (Gordon Moore, who succeeded Joseph Dorsh as the plan's medical director, has recently relinquished that position to develop a new teaching unit for medical students; the current president of the Commonwealth Fund, Margaret E. Mahoney, has helped to find support for this new activity.) The plan's research component eventually merged with the Center for Analysis of Health Practices (see p. 445), and the combined center is now directed by Howard Frazier.

The Commonwealth Fund's support was crucial to the start of this successful health maintenance organization. By mobilizing a consortium of potential supporters, Newton created the setting in which the plan could obtain the additional financial aid necessary to maintain it through its critical period. The Harvard Community Health Plan is intended to provide high-quality medical care at the lowest possible cost, but, in addition, it creates an opportunity for Harvard to apply its resources to the study of the features that shape health services.[76]

THE YALE TRAUMA PROGRAM

The Yale Trauma Program began as an analysis of emergency treatment services in New Haven and outlying communities. It was supported at its inception in 1967 by the Travelers' Research Center, which donated $3,000, and the Connecticut Regional Medical Program, which paid the salary of a full-time systems analyst. The program was continuing hand-to-mouth when in 1969 Jack W. Cole, chairman of Yale's Department of Surgery, requested a grant from the Commonwealth Fund. What developed was a prototype regionalized system of emergency medical service featuring a central call number and medically controlled dispatching.

Cole envisioned a program that would reduce the number of deaths from trauma, particularly automobile accidents. With Kristaps J. Keggi, assistant clinical professor of orthopedic surgery at Yale, he devised a plan based on Keggi's year as a military surgeon in Vietnam. The military system for evacuating battlefield casualties to field hospitals was based on daily computerized predictions of the number of combat casualties and the number of helicopters and hospital beds needed to care for the wounded. Staged emergency medical care established a line of priority stretching from the combat line through medical corpsmen and battalion aid stations, and eventually to hospitals for surgical care back in the United States. This system had reduced the death rate of wounded reaching a hospital to 1 percent, compared to 3 percent in Korea and 8 percent in World War II.

When Keggi left Yale, Cole remained to pursue their plan. He set out to establish a base for research and education as a catalyst for reform and recruited an able young team—twin brothers, Blair L. and Alfred M. Sadler, Jr., and Ann Bliss, a clinical nurse with training in psychiatric social work. In his proposal to the Fund, Cole advocated a program that would embrace all phases of emergency medical care rather than trauma alone:[77]

> Although most schools have devoted a great deal of time toward achieving a better understanding of the biological, physiological, and biochemical derangements of the human organism resulting from trauma, insufficient effort in research had gone into the . . . psychological, sociological, medicolegal, rehabilitative, and transportation fields. In short, to the best of our knowledge,

no medical school has seen fit to embrace . . . all of the areas that go on in the health care system dealing with the postaccident phase of injury. To develop such a broadly based, multidisciplinary unit under the aegis of a leading medical school would indeed be unique, and its capacity to enlist the help and cooperation of responsible groups in government, industry and lay community should eventuate in model systems for the care of the trauma victim.

The Fund decided to support the Yale Trauma Program with a grant of $2,000,000.

By 1973 the program had greatly increased public awareness of emergency medical service.[78] Public response in turn prompted a shift in the program's emphasis. State legislation requiring tighter control of ambulance personnel, improved communications, and certification of emergency medical technicians also required improved hospital emergency departments and physicians who could cope with the severely injured patient. After its initial tooling-up, the trauma program concentrated on educating medical and paramedical personnel, evaluating its efforts, categorizing the ability of emergency departments to deliver specialized trauma care in the state, and implementing a centralized communications system in south central Connecticut. The Fund's grant was designed not to underwrite laboratory research projects but to provide "seed money" for a multitude of initial investigations. Additional funding was expected for ongoing improvements, based on the merits of each individual project. By 1974 the program had been able to use this seed money to generate funding from independent sources.[79] A flow sheet shows the progress made in emergency medical services, health manpower, communications, education and research related to the management of trauma (fig. 28). It clearly demonstrates the power of the Fund's seed grant to bring projects to fruition and lead to funding from other sources.

The trauma program used a portion of its grant from the Fund to construct a laboratory for surgery, obstetrics and gynecology. As space for biomedical research in the field of trauma became available, a full-time research assistant was added to the core staff. In addition to housing the biomedical research of the trauma program, the laboratory allowed the entire Department of Surgery to expand its trauma-related research. By 1974 the laboratories were in full use.

Parallel to Yale's interest in the investigation of trauma was the state of Connecticut's interest in the same field. In December 1970 a group of citizens formed an ad hoc Committee on Emergency Medical Services (EMS) to improve emergency medical services in Connecticut. This committee grew and diversified, until at the request of the state health commissioner and one of the governor's representatives to the state's Department of Transportation, it became the Connecticut Advisory Committee on EMS, assigned to advise both departments in this field.

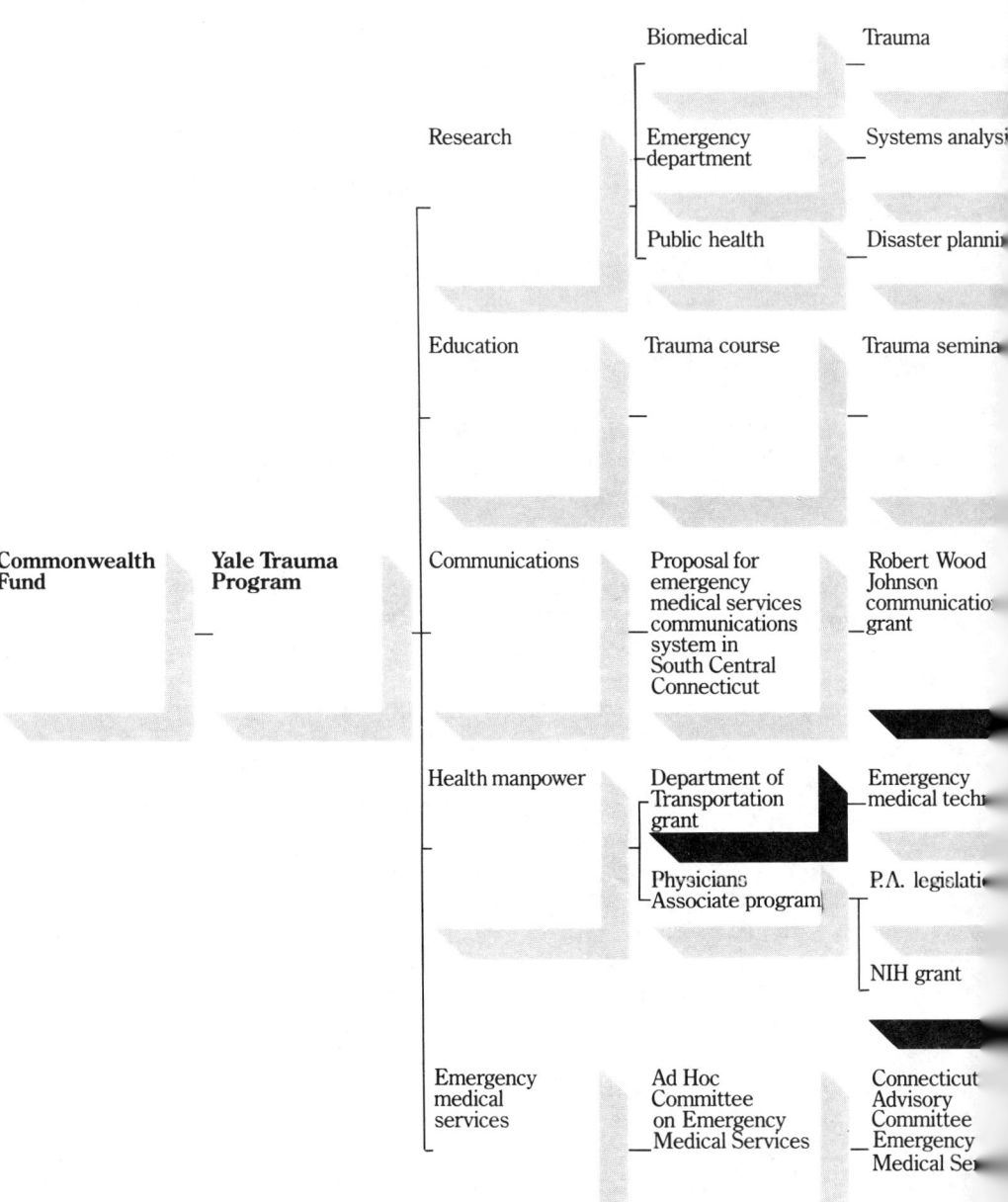

Figure 28. Offshoots of the Yale Trauma Program
Adapted from the Third Progress Report of the Yale Trauma Program, June 1974, Commonwealth Fund Archives.

Burns — NIH spinal cord trauma grant

Time = effort study

Standards of care

Emergency department consultants — Emergency department trauma book — American College of Surgeons symposium — Emergency medical services education and evaluation center grant

Training grant — Evaluation grant

P.A. employment — Trauma care

Legislation — Movie "EMS in Connecticut" — Television — Public Law 74-305

Child abuse

The University and the Community

The information necessary for effective planning did not exist, so the committee granted top priority to conducting the necessary background studies. A federal grant was obtained in 1971 to support part of the cost. The governor of Connecticut, Thomas J. Meskill, characterized the investigation as "the first step in the creation of an adequate emergency medical system, a system which we have so far been lacking."[80] The seven-hundred-page study received the full support of the advisory committee on December 4, 1972,[81] and was submitted to the governor on the following day. A fifty-page summary informed the citizens of the state about the priorities developed by the study team and offered specific recommendations. Wide distribution of the summary raised the public's level of awareness and encouraged public support for legislation. Three months after the report was issued, the draft of a bill was submitted to the Connecticut Committee on Public Health and Safety, but the committee decided against reporting on any bill concerned with emergency medical services in 1973.

This setback focused the efforts of the advisory committee and the Yale Trauma Program: their joint goal became the passage of legislation that would encompass their recommendations to the governor. To gain public support for this legislative effort, a movie produced by the Yale Trauma Program, "Emergency Medical Service in Connecticut," was shown throughout the state at meetings of civic organizations, municipal governments, and professional societies, as well as on public television. Reinforcing the movie's message were forty thousand pamphlets, and on May 30, 1974, the governor signed into law the act establishing emergency medical services in Connecticut. When the new law became effective on July 1, the Connecticut Advisory Committee on Emergency Medical Services was officially dissolved. It was replaced by a twenty-five member panel, the State Emergency Medical Services Council, intended to advise the Council on Hospitals and Health Care. The director of the Yale Trauma Program was given a permanent position on this council.

One of the committee's main interests had been that interval between the patient's injury and his arrival at a medical facility. This is a critical period, when the successful use of lifesaving measures depends upon trained and equipped personnel. Approximately 20 percent of the trauma patients who died at the scene of an accident or en route to a hospital could have been saved by simple measures delivered by appropriately trained paramedical personnel. The most obvious deficiency in Connecticut's EMS system was the lack of adequately trained manpower for ambulance work. With the collaboration of several national groups, the trauma program instituted an eighty-one-hour program to train Emergency Medical Technicians (EMTs) in 1970 and made the course's training manuals available to similar programs. The recently passed state legislation required EMT training for all ambulance attendants, and in 1971 the program obtained funding from the United States Department of Transportation and the state health department for the training of two hundred emergency medical technicians. A twenty-hour refresher course was also instituted, and a continuing education program for ambulance-riding EMTs was established in 1973. Monthly lecture-seminars dealt with topics such as thermal burns, treatment of open wounds and open fractures, treatment of difficult orthopedic emergencies, cardiac failure, arrhythmias, and drug and alcohol abuse.

To justify the continued support of these programs, in late 1972 the Yale Trauma Program organized its first evaluation of the EMTs' performance.[82] The study tested the diagnostic accuracy and overall quality of the EMTs' therapeutic intervention, compared the performance of graduates of the EMT course with nongraduate personnel, and determined which aspects of the curriculum should be revised or should receive additional emphasis. A federal grant to enlarge this pilot study was awarded to New Haven Health Care, Inc., one of nineteen experimental health-service delivery systems operating in the United States. The studies now offered a way to survey continuously the overall effect of the EMT training program on the delivery of emergency care.

Through the efforts of the trauma program, a second federal grant was awarded to the Yale–New Haven Medical Center's EMT program to allow it to continue its basic course, institute more refresher courses, and train dispatchers in centralized emergency medical communications.

One of the trauma program's first priorities was training individuals to assist physicians in caring for critically injured patients. The state's failure to provide for such training was considered one of the greatest defects in the health delivery system. Blair L. Sadler, the program's co-director, lobbied to give physicians' associates the legal right to practice. In 1971 Governor Meskill signed into law Public Act 717, which stated that the provisions of the Connecticut Medical Practice Act should not apply "to any person rendering service as a physician's trained assistant, a registered nurse, or a licensed practical nurse, if such services are rendered under the supervision, control, and responsibility of a licensed physician."

Once this law was in effect, the trauma program began to supply the state with well-trained associates, and the Yale Physicians' Associate Program was split off administratively from the trauma program. Independently funded by the NIH's Bureau of Health Manpower Education, the associate program graduated its first class of five students in January 1973. Eight months later the trauma program employed its first two graduate physicians' associates, who worked in the emergency department of the Yale–New Haven Hospital alongside surgical residents, and on the inpatient trauma service, where they filled the gap between nurses and surgical house officers.

Another legislative effort of the trauma program concerned child abuse.

Work by the Child Abuse Advisory Committee and member Blair L. Sadler led to the passage of the State Act Concerning the Correction of Child Abuse, which became effective in October 1971. Under the new law, medical examiners, police officers, and clergymen, as well as physicians, surgeons, hospital residents, school teachers, and social workers, were required to report suspected child abuse, and reportable abuse was no longer limited to abuse by a parent or other person responsible for the child's care. The trauma program later sponsored a study to help pediatricians in Connecticut evaluate the effectiveness of this law.

Improving communications systems was a particularly complex goal of the trauma program, since several towns and counties were involved, along with diverse organizational entities (for example, police, fire department, and hospitals). Regional change was initially found to be more feasible than state reform. A detailed proposal entitled "A Communication System for Emergency Medical Service for South Central Connecticut," developed by Thomas Brask and the Sadler brothers in 1971, led to a $15 million national program of grants for regional emergency medical communications systems. Administered by the National Academy of Sciences, the program was sponsored by the Robert Wood Johnson Foundation, where Blair L. Sadler had become an assistant vice-president.[83] The program encouraged central dispatching as well as regionalization and integration of hospital and ambulance services.[84]

In 1973, at the urging of the trauma program, the Yale–New Haven Hospital and the Hospital of Saint Raphael received about $400,000 from the Robert Wood Johnson Foundation to defer the cost of establishing a regional emergency medical communications system for the south central Connecticut region, including the municipalities of New Haven, East Haven, and West Haven, with a total population of 400,000.[85] The grant provided for immediately available access by citizens to medical dispatching; well-equipped ambulance and rescue vehicles available at all hours; dispatch of the nearest and most appropriate rescue apparatus to the emergency site; highly trained ambulance rescue and dispatch personnel; hospital emergency facilities offering a uniformly high level of general and specialized care on a twenty-four-hour basis; fully coordinated regional emergency and other medical services; and ongoing data collection for assessment of the program's effect on regional medical care.

The trauma program also spearheaded educational efforts within the state. One of its first was a day-long seminar in 1973, "The Emergency Department Care of the Injured Patient," produced in collaboration with the Connecticut Committee on Trauma of the American College of Surgeons, the Connecticut Chapter of American Emergency Physicians, and the Connecticut Advisory Committee on Emergency Medical Services. The response was so favorable that such programs became an ongoing part of the trauma program. The following year Yale University was chosen as the site for a national symposium entitled "Lifesaving Measures for the Critically Injured," sponsored by the American College of Surgeons. The trauma program was also involved in this symposium; Martin Robson, the program's director, chaired the symposium along with Cole and Thomas J. Krizek, chief of plastic and reconstructive surgery.

A twenty-week core course developed in the medical school was well attended by students, nurses, and house officers, and a panel including all the surgical specialties was put together to teach the practical aspects of trauma care in the emergency department. To enable the large house staff to deliver consistently first-rate treatment, algorithms were developed for problems including burns, soft-tissue injuries, upper extremity injuries, and infection. Whenever the routines used did not fit with these algorithms, the case record was pulled and the situation reviewed. Since 1975 this effort has been successful in solving the problems deriving from frequent changes in rotation of residents through the emergency room.

The trauma program also supported the preparation of a concise training manual for medical students, interns, residents, and other health personnel in the Yale–New Haven Hospital emergency department. *Diagnosis and Early Management of Trauma Emergencies: A Guide to the Emergency Service,* by Robert Touloukian and Thomas J. Krizek, was later expanded into a textbook. A prehospital care manual was developed over several years by the Advisory Committee on Emergency Service, which is composed of all the emergency room directors in the area. Paramedical personnel were enabled to perform a number of life-saving procedures in the field—including treatment of cardiac arrhythmias, anaphylactic shock, and traumatic shock due to spinal cord injury—using well-established protocols in their "bible." These professionals, who receive more training than EMTs, are requalified yearly in their field.

Finally, to correct continuing deficiencies in training of EMTs, the trauma program established an Emergency Medical Service Education and Evaluation Center.

Research continued on trauma, particularly as it related to epidemiology and public health. A multimillion dollar contract from the NIH in 1971 allowed Yale to establish an Acute Spinal Cord Research Center under the direction of William Collins. Other areas of research interest were thermal injuries, traumatic soft tissue infections, and the effectiveness of current emergency measures to decrease contamination of open wounds.

The Yale Trauma Program's interest in prehospital care—identification of treatable problems that could be dealt with at the site of the emergency (for example, airway control, hemorrhage, support of breathing, and lack of circulation) was stimulated by William Frazier. A plastic surgeon, Frazier was one of the organizers of the Emergency Medical System

Council and was responsible for training EMTs and paramedical personnel. He was also instrumental in obtaining the grants that grew out of the original award from the Commonwealth Fund.

Today most of the trauma program's support derives from a block grant from the state, awards from several foundations, private gifts, and NIH grants. In addition, the army has directed a grant toward research in prediction of outcome after trauma. The Yale Trauma Program, now under the direction of Christopher C. Baker, recently shifted its emphasis from the emergency room per se to the overall care of the trauma patient—what happens in the field, the emergency room, the operating room, and the intensive care unit.

A large training program in trauma management for physicians' assistants and associates is concentrated in the surgery department at Yale. The initial two years are based at Yale University and a one-year residency is shared between the New Haven and Norwalk hospitals. About a dozen individuals become qualified each year to give surgical care, especially care relating to trauma and burns.

Formal protocols for the care of the trauma patient have been instituted in the emergency room and in the early phases of hospital care. Beginning in July 1983, a trauma service was established to coordinate care for all multiply injured patients. Demographic data and comparisons of mortality rates, while historical and not randomized, reveal a significant reduction in the mortality rates for trauma patients admitted to the intensive care unit: from 25 percent before to 6.4 percent after institution of the service.[86]

Other recent projects of the trauma service include a weekly conference directed to discussions of specific issues of patient care; a study of decision making and hospital admission from the emergency room for critical conditions, including chest pain, respiratory insufficiency, and closed head injury; and the establishment of a volunteer paramedical service, the first of its kind in Connecticut. The C–MED communication system now extends through all twenty towns of south central Connecticut, and advanced life-support service are available to most parts of the region. Finally, the emergency room of the Yale–New Haven Hospital now has a system of full-time attending physicians, which has already resulted in significant improvement in documentation, decrease in patient complaints, and greater consistency in patient care.[87]

Plans for the future include research on prevention of mortality; the functional outcome of rehabilitation—especially in the elderly, a population that seems to be particularly debilitated by relatively minor traumatic injuries; and a training program in endotracheal intubation for paramedics.[88]

The Yale Trauma Program has accomplished all that it set out to do:

—A regional emergency care system has been developed to organize hospitals according to their individual capabilities and to link them

in a common transport and communications network (which includes experimental use of television to assess casualties on the scene)
— Medical education is preparing physicians to lead in improving the delivery of care to trauma patients: new types of paramedical personnel are being trained, including surgical associates, who are skilled in managing patients from the site of the accident to the emergency room
— Research has been conducted in clinical care and physical and psychological rehabilitation
— Biomedical research is improving the understanding of biochemical and physiological effects of trauma
— Social science studies investigate the problems of injury, such as the effectiveness of social agencies in dealing with accident victims and their families
— The adequacy of the legal system in handling accident cases has been evaluated, particularly with respect to medical evidence

The Fund's First Half-Century

"It is a characteristic of an advancing civilization that its aspirations should become progressively more inclusive as the attainments of one generation open up new horizons of possibility to the next,"[89] said the Fund's annual report in 1968 as it reviewed the Fund's objectives at the half-century mark. The advances of the past fifty years in medicine were what the Fund's staff termed underlying factors in the evolution of health as a dynamic value in American society. "The history of the Commonwealth Fund," they said, "is a chronicle of continuous participation in this process."[90] The nation's aims in medicine were reflected by the Fund's activities in child guidance, child health, the mental health movement, rural public health services, community hospitals, and medical research. In the 1950s the Fund was able to emphasize medical education and delivery of services because its previous programs had become part of the nation's definition of health care.

Now, in 1968, the Fund would have to cope with what it saw as a large and unprecedented process of change in the American social system: "Scientific and technological advancement have, in effect, generated a second industrial revolution—accelerating the transition of the social structure from rural to urban, and providing a powerful new economic base that has not only sustained an expanding population but also nourished a rising standard of living and level of expectations. . . . No segment of our people will now accept exclusion from the mainstream of our national development. Equality of opportunity in employment, housing, education, and health care are considered to be entitlements to be secured by society for each individual."[91]

This goal of universal accessibility to effective health care was based largely on the brilliance of the biomedical community's record; yet other aspects of medicine, such as the nation's system of medical education and medical service, were so deficient as to pose obstacles to future progress.

As in the 1950s, the Fund turned to the nation's universities and their medical schools for solutions. Now, however, the Fund's strategy was to link medical schools with their surrounding communities. Model programs such as the Yale Trauma Program and the Harvard Community Health Plan used the university as a base for improving health services.

Questions about the nation's health were inevitably related to medical education: How could more physicians be produced to serve impoverished population groups? How could medical student enrollments be expanded generally in a professional field increasingly dependent on preceptorial instruction? How could the curriculum both assimilate the expanding body of biomedical knowledge and accommodate and nourish students' individual learning interests? How could the long, complex, and expensive enterprise of medical education be properly financed? Grants to Meharry Medical College, the Mount Sinai School of Medicine, Boston University, the Association of American Medical Colleges, the National Board of Medical Examiners, and the University of Pennsylvania School of Medicine in 1968 supported studies in these areas. Important grants in 1969 to study planning of the medical teaching institution and its future role were given to Tulane University and to the Boston University Medical Center.

One means of fortifying medical education was to develop programs that would make the best use of the country's limited supply of doctors. During 1968 experimental and developmental programs were supported through grants to Duke University, the Johns Hopkins University, the National Academy of Sciences, Northeastern University, Alderson–Broaddus College, and the College of Physicians of Philadelphia.

With the Carnegie Corporation, the Fund assisted an intensive examination of the nature and dimensions of the medical schools' financial plight—a study carried out by a stellar committee led by Lewis Thomas, dean of the New York University School of Medicine. The committee's report, "The Crisis of the Medical Schools," stressed that the teaching functions of medical faculties—the heart of the educational enterprise—were being conducted on a restricted and precarious financial base. The Fund also awarded $54,000 to the Brookings Institution of Washington, D.C., for an analysis of the financial aspects of the entire system of educating medical manpower, part of a comprehensive inquiry sponsored by the Carnegie Corporation into higher education in the United States.

The Fund's objectives were further evidenced by grants for new medical schools and for existing schools revising their four-year medical curricula. The surge of biomedical discovery and recognition of the effect of psychological and social factors on health were both making the prevailing pattern of professional training obsolete. A key grant was the $75,000 given to Dartmouth University in 1969 to expand the medical school from a two-year program in the basic sciences to a full four-year, degree-granting program.

Despite the prevailing emphasis on the university, the Fund's program in the late 1960s remained flexible enough to leave room for special grants to organizations such as the Urban Coalition, which was working for social change outside the university structure.

In 1969, a year beyond the Fund's half-century mark, Colin M. MacLeod left to become president of the Oklahoma Medical Research Foundation.[92] The next year Robert J. Glaser resigned from his position as dean of the Stanford University School of Medicine and joined Newton as vice-president of the Commonwealth Fund.

The Vice-Presidency of Robert Joy Glaser (September 1, 1970–June 1, 1972)

Robert Joy Glaser (fig. 29) was born in St. Louis, Missouri, in 1918. He received the bachelor of science and medical degrees from Harvard University and honorary doctor of science degrees from the University of Chicago, Temple University, and the University of Colorado. His medical residency was spent on W. Barry Wood's service at the Barnes Hospital in St. Louis, and he also served as an assistant resident physician at the Peter Bent Brigham Hospital in Boston. After two years as a National Research Council fellow at Washington University, Glaser became an assistant and then an associate dean at the medical school. In 1957 he moved to the University of Colorado School of Medicine as dean and professor of medicine, and it was there that he met J. Quigg Newton, Jr.

Glaser left Denver in 1963 to take a position as professor of social medicine at Harvard and president of the Affiliated Hospitals Center, Inc. He held this post for only two years, moving to Stanford as vice-president and dean of the medical school, and as professor of medicine. In 1967 he became a member of the board of directors of the Kaiser Foundation Hospitals and the Kaiser Health Plan and, in 1969, a member of the board of directors of the Commonwealth Fund. The following year, when he moved to New York to join the staff of the Commonwealth Fund,

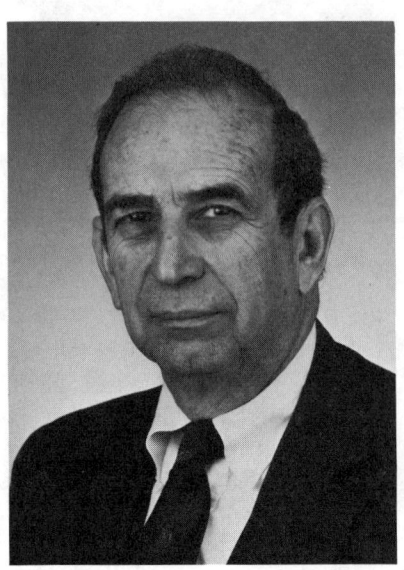

Figure 29.   Robert Joy Glaser

Glaser maintained his academic affiliation by becoming clinical professor of medicine at the Columbia University College of Physicians and Surgeons.[93]

Glaser's arrival at the Fund precipitated a conspicuous change in the atmosphere at Harkness House, even though he was there only five days every other week during the first year of his vice-presidency. Glaser and Newton instituted an open-door policy, welcoming people who dropped in to talk over both their own problems and the Fund's programs. Coupled with the staff's visits to leading educators, the Fund's new accessibility continued to keep its staff abreast of the news at medical centers throughout the nation.

The Fund's expanding programs in medical education required additional staff, and in September 1971 Newton and Glaser recruited Reginald H. Fitz, one of their associates at the University of Colorado. Born in 1920, Fitz was a graduate of Harvard College and the Harvard Medical School. Interning at the Faulkner Hospital, he came under the influence of Channing Frothingham, a member of the staff of the Peter Bent Brigham Hospital with a broad interest in the social aspects of medicine. After his discharge from the Army in 1948, Fitz became a resident in medicine at the University of Colorado under James Waring. Two years of residency were followed by promotion first to junior head of the medical service at the Denver General Hospital and to chief of service in 1956. The influence of Gordon Meiklejohn, chairman of the Department of Medicine at the University of Colorado, led to Fitz's decision to remain in academic medicine.

Glaser appointed Fitz his assistant dean for student affairs and head of the admissions committee at the University of Colorado, positions that encouraged Fitz's interest in medical education. After four years Fitz moved on to become dean of the new medical school at the University of New Mexico in Albuquerque. There he installed a curriculum modeled after the one at Western Reserve University, giving first-year medical students experience with patients. In 1968 Fitz left the university to become head of the New Mexico Regional Medical Program, and three years later, attracted by the Fund's interest in medical education, he moved to New York to join the staff.

Fitz directed the Book Program (see p. 525), participated in many of the site visits, and worked on a variety of problems with the other staff members. In addition, when Newton and Glaser recommended a change in the Fund's procedure for managing grants, Fitz revamped the process and supervised its implementation. Before Fitz took over, expenditures were not checked systematically, and abuses did occur. Sometimes the Fund's grant was used to obtain money from other sources; in other instances, the Fund would award a grant to get a project underway and then discover that none of its money had been expended by the end of the grant period. Perverting the intention of the original award, the recipient would then request permission to spend the unused money. Fitz instituted a system that would prevent this accumulation of unspent funds without evaluating the investigator's work itself. He set up a review file to ensure that the Fund would receive periodic progress and expenditure reports in a fashion consonant with the federal regulations governing philanthropic programs, so that approval of funds for the next period could be based on up-to-date budgetary information. More detailed follow-up also aided the Fund's officers and staff in assessing decisions retrospectively, offered perspectives useful for future judgments, and led to the quarterly, rather than yearly, provision of grant money.

Another new staff member was Walter Donway, who came to the Fund as Terrance Keenan's assistant in November 1971;[94] when Keenan resigned in March 1972 to join the staff of the Robert Wood Johnson Foundation, Donway became an executive associate and took over Keenan's position as recording secretary of the Fund.

During Glaser's vice-presidency the Fund's method of dealing with grants was improved without changing significantly. Glaser and Newton did not solicit specific proposals, so all applications were given the same initial consideration. After an application was received by the president or vice-president of the Fund, a staff member would meet with the applicant to discuss his proposal in detail. The staff would then decide whether the applicant should proceed to a more formal proposal. Keenan, who saw all of the proposals, would summarize for senior members of the staff those he felt should be rejected. Summaries of projects that seemed of interest would be discussed at the weekly staff meetings.

These meetings eventually became iterative, no more than a means of scheduling work on projects as they progressed from their arrival at the Fund to their presentation to the Board.[95] In deciding which proposals should be pursued, the staff considered the amount of money available for the remainder of the fiscal year, so that each grant could be weighed against the funds still open for commitment. If a formal grant application was being prepared, the staff would often make a site visit, and the recording secretary—first Keenan, then Donway—would prepare a summary for discussion.

The recording secretary had plenipotentiary powers concerning staff work. He did all the day-to-day labor on the grants, participated in all the meetings, and took detailed notes in the form of a play script (he said, she said, and so forth). After shaping all the background material into a report for the board, he supervised its printing.

As an item gradually moved up at subsequent staff meetings into the "probable" category, it would be scheduled for presentation to the board. Time and dollar amounts would already have been decided so that the item could be inserted into the funding cycle. The staff was careful not to commit the board prematurely, but since the university's fiscal year began in July, school authorities were often told that the project would be recommended to the board and that recommendation usually meant approval.

Before the thrice-yearly board meetings, Newton would discuss the upcoming proposals with Malcolm P. Aldrich. Keenan would write up the projects in memoranda to the board, including budgetary data. Keenan's writing was meticulous, but Newton had considerable influence on wording. Both were aware that the members of the board responded best to a low-key approach that did not try to sell the project.

For rapid decisions the board's executive committee could be called into action. In one case, money was needed quickly to support the formation of a commission to reformulate the New York City Health and Hospitals Department—a successful program that created the city's Department of Health and Hospitals. Within three days the Fund's executive committee had made a commitment to support the project.

The decisions of the board could carry enormous weight in unexpected directions. One proposal from the Mount Sinai School of Medicine requested a grant of $500,000. The school's lack of an academic affiliation caused the board to reject the application, and this rationale precipitated consultation between Mount Sinai and the City University of New York (CUNY). The Fund's initial rejection led the hospital's board to reconsider its plans, and it established a firm affiliation with CUNY. When a revised proposal was resubmitted to the Fund's board of directors, a grant was approved.

A good working relationship between the president of the Fund and the chairman of the board was critical to the Fund's smooth operation.

Frequent discussions between the chairman and the board members prepared the way for grant proposals, so that discussion at meetings might be fairly brief. To an uninformed observer, the board might have appeared to be reacting in a pro forma manner, but in fact the real discussion had been held pro cathedra. The more controversial the proposal, the more thoroughly it would be discussed among the interested individuals before the meeting. The result was that there was seldom any delay at board meetings, and relatively few items were ever tabled.

More weight in the decision-making process was given to individuals with good track records who were well known to the staff. The quality of the institution, the importance of the programmatic area, and the reliability and talent of the individuals submitting the grant were the major determinants of a proposal's outcome.

Newton and Glaser believed that in addition to maintaining the conventional policy of making grants throughout the country, the Fund should establish its own in-house program on a modest scale. Harkness House was a unique asset, insufficiently enjoyed. They hoped to invite three to five individuals as visiting fellows of the Fund in Harkness House each year. The group might include a well-established scholar, someone at the junior or middle level in his career, and a student or house officer. During the year-long fellowship, they would be asked to study a specific topic of import to medicine. Although Eugene A. Stead, Jr., served as a visiting fellow for one year, this recommendation was not carried out as originally conceived; yet selected groups of distinguished individuals did assemble at Harkness House for a day to discuss key issues of the time, such as the organization of medical faculties and compensation plans, the interrelation of theology and medicine, and the problem of health care in prisons. At each conference, from twelve to eighteen outstanding professionals from fields including medical education, law, government, and social sciences gave a day of their time to freewheeling discussions. The Fund's staff found these meetings useful in clarifying basic issues and in suggesting potentially promising areas for support. In this small way, Harkness House became a center of intellectual activity that not only improved the background knowledge of the staff but gave the participants an opportunity to discuss important problems informally in a setting in which no vested interest was involved. No formal records of the proceedings were kept, but either Keenan or Donway took extensive notes.

Recommendations to the Board of Directors: Programs for the 1970s

One of Glaser's first projects at the fund was a review of the programs of the past seven years. Although he and Newton assumed that the Fund would continue to support programs in medicine and health, they wanted to begin to plan for the years ahead. By early 1971 Newton and Glaser had prepared an extensive list of recommendations from which the board could choose the most promising for support.[96] Invaluable assets were the flexibility of private foundations in general and the particular flexibility of the Fund as it operated under a broad mandate. The suggestions to the Board reflected Newton and Glaser's deep sense of responsibility for continuing the Fund's history of innovation.

The same areas advanced in the 1964 report to the board seemed to provide important opportunities for the Fund in the 1970s. Not all received the same measure of attention: The mounting crisis in health care led Newton and Glaser to recommend substantial grants to medical schools for projects that would improve the delivery of health care. Fund-supported programs over the past four years had focused on the disadvantaged populations of major cities. Health care for these individuals was only part of their unmet needs, but improvement in this area would ameliorate other problems as well, including lessening the tension that characterized the metropolitan ghettos. A rational system for delivering health care would also lead to opportunities in education and vocational training.

Another recommendation encouraged schools to increase student enrollment and shorten the span of educational programs by improving the quality of teaching. Although it seemed likely that additional new schools would be established, another approach to the production of more physicians was available. Strong liberal-arts colleges and major universities were offering alternative pathways to clinical studies for those interested in careers in medicine. Many students were coming to medical school with excellent preparation in biochemistry, physiology, and microbiology, and it was unnecessary for them to take the standard medical school courses. With comparatively little additional expense, undergraduate schools with good biology and chemistry departments could provide the other requisite preclinical courses, making it possible for more young graduates to enter clinical studies at the start of medical school. The exact pattern was still vague, but some institutions had the potential to establish excellent preclinical programs: the California Institute of Technology, the Massachusetts Institute of Technology in collaboration with Harvard, and other universities with strong natural-science departments. The Fund could encourage this kind of effort by supporting the development of more effective teaching methods, and grants could be given to modernize the teaching of such subjects as anatomy. Community hospitals could also be put to greater educational use, and Newton and Glaser's report suggested pilot programs encouraging physicians to teach in the hospitals with which they were affiliated. Efforts to shorten the span of years consumed by undergraduate medical education and residency training would have to be viewed as experimental and subject to careful assessment; methods of evaluation were still being developed, and measuring the success of new curricula and educational formats was difficult. Projects to develop criteria for evaluation of medical students and internists were then being sponsored by the Fund under the direction of the National Board of Medical Examiners and the American Board of Internal Medicine.

Newton and Glaser also advocated grants for the training of paramedical personnel. The Fund was prepared to continue support for efforts to define new categories of personnel; organize training programs for individuals at several educational levels, including those with relatively limited formal education; study the role of paramedical personnel and its relation to the role of physicians; and examine the function of paramedical personnel with respect to sophisticated technological aid.[97] In addition, by underwriting the study of the National Commission on Accrediting, the Fund hoped to avoid the chaos that could result from a lack of nationwide standards for licensing the multitude of paramedical individuals.

Paramedical personnel and physicians were not adequately exposed to new information, even though medical centers and professional societies recognized the rapid advances taking place in scientific and medical knowledge. Continuing education had to be related to the physician's daily life—something that could not be accomplished by attending occasional brief courses. Newton and Glaser suggested that a closer relationship between community hospitals, ambulatory care units, and urban teaching centers would lead to more effective educational programs.

Their report suggested that the Fund continue to support projects concerned with psychosocial behavior, including human sexuality. In complex times it was urgent to acquire a greater understanding of normal and aberrant human behavior. Although the Fund's part in the necessarily massive effort would be small, careful selection of projects and recognition of innovative approaches could make its role an important one.

Violence, although always a characteristic of the animal species, was thought to have become even more prevalent in American society over the past seven years. Newton and Glaser believed that well-planned studies might lead to a better conception of the mechanisms of violence—a necessary prerequisite to lessening violence on a personal as well as a political level. Concern with the effects of violence in early childhood motivated the report's interest in studies of child abuse—a far greater menace than had earlier been thought. Increasing evidence pointed to the influence of early childhood in determining later behavior, and Newton and Glaser believed that more knowledge in this area might decrease the psychological trauma that manifests itself in later life.

By 1971 the growing use of marijuana and narcotics was creating far-reaching problems. The prevailing ignorance about drug abuse underlined the need for a massive, well-planned approach. Fundamental and clinical research and a better understanding of the sociological and psychological factors contributing to drug use would require the talents of an interdisciplinary force including physicians, basic scientists, political scientists, and law enforcement officials. An attack on drug abuse would also have to include consideration of alcoholism, and Newton and Glaser felt that here the Fund's role was vital.

They also advised the Fund to maintain its interest in the population problem through support for projects in medical research and to international medical education and health care through grants that would make textbooks in medical subjects available at low cost. In the past, grants had been made to medical schools around the country for collaborative work with developing medical schools in other parts of the world. The staff felt that these projects had distinct merit, although the schools often found it difficult to maintain the programs after the grants ended. The strengthening of medical education in Latin America through the collaboration of medical schools in various Latin American countries was encouraging, as was the Fund's support of the Pan American Federation of Associations of Medical Schools and the Regional Library of Medicine for Latin America. The Fund's resources and those of even larger foundations were clearly insufficient to underwrite the development of a significant number of medical schools worldwide, yet there were ways in which a small injection of support might lead to an important contribution. Newton and Glaser believed that first emphasis should be given to the production of high-quality physicians and the training of those who could use public health measures for treatment of water and sewage to reinforce rudiments of health care.

Decreasing federal support for medicine in universities and research institutes was providing more opportunities for the Fund. Newton and Glaser wanted to reestablish the Fund's Fellowship Program on a small scale: A few fellowships should be awarded annually on a competitive basis to senior individuals who wished to pursue important work in institutions other than their own, and junior fellowships should be awarded to especially promising young men and women. Newton and Glaser wanted to use the expertise of past fellowship recipients, distinguished scientists, and medical educators whose sabbatical year had been supported by the Fund. In retrospect, it was clear that the Fund had not taken advantage of the continuing relationship these individuals might offer as informal advisors.

Newton and Glaser believed that it was important for the Fund to maintain its current flexible policy regarding requests for projects outside the scope of its regular programs. This included participation in major, nonrecurring capital drives of New York City's leading civic institutions, as an expression of the Fund's responsibility for the well-being of its community. The Fund was also advised to respond on an ad hoc basis to other requests falling outside its primary areas of interest, when the request had particular promise "for the welfare of mankind."

For the future, Newton and Glaser advised the Fund to explore ethical problems in medicine, environmental quality and technology, and problems of aging. In the case of biomedical research projects on aging, support should be limited to unusually promising endeavors that as pioneering ventures were not apt to attract funds from the NIH or the National Science Foundation.

Newton and Glaser also addressed a variety of in-house considerations. Fitz's new program was a well-integrated response to their suggestion that the Fund provide more detailed follow-up for evaluating grants. They also addressed the question of collaboration with other foundations. In recent years the Fund had worked effectively with the Carnegie Corporation, and they felt that joint efforts should continue—but only if the Fund was always a full partner. The Fund's officers and staff were encouraged to accede to requests for consultation from universities and other established organizations, when the subject fell within their competence and when the time involved was not excessive. Finally, the format of Board meetings needed revision: Newton and Glaser believed that the present structure prevented members from exploring topics in depth. They wanted to devote a portion of each meeting to a detailed review of one area receiving, or scheduled to receive, Fund support, and to invite outside authorities to attend board meetings when major presentations were under consideration. Newton and Glaser also proposed convening board meetings at 9:30 A.M. instead of 4:30 P.M. and continuing the meetings through lunch. Social aspects of board meetings could be continued at an annual dinner, to which emeritus members of the board would be invited.

Grants during Glaser's Vice-Presidency

Awards in 1971 and 1972 continued the Fund's emphasis on medical education, the allied health professions, and health care (see app. J). One particularly prescient grant supported the increasing use of computers as instructional tools. The Fund joined the Carnegie Corporation in providing three-year support to the National Board of Medical Examiners and the American Board of Internal Medicine for an experiment in the application of the computer in teaching and testing "clinical competence"—a term embracing the complex skills of logic and judgment that underlie the physician's professional capabilities. This grant of $361,800 followed an award in 1970 to the National Board of Medical Examiners to explore the potential of the computer as an alternative to oral examinations and paper and pencil tests. The Board of Medical Examiners had designed and field-tested a computerized examination that gave precise and authoritative indices of individual clinical competence. Over the three-year span of the present grant, research staff hoped to make this computer-based system fully operational.[98]

The University of Rochester School of Medicine received a grant of $75,000 pooling the resources of schools to meet the health manpower requirements of a ten-county area in western New York. Incorporated as the Genesee Regional Educational Alliance for Health Personnel, the program was a consortium of all types of institutions engaged in education for the health occupations and professions, including school districts, colleges, community hospitals, and the University of Rochester's professional schools and teaching hospitals.[99]

Joining the Kaiser-Permanente Medical Care Program and the Association of American Medical Colleges, the Fund granted an award to an innovative three-day meeting in March 1971 on the organization and delivery of medical care. The meeting brought together a group of 288 executive, academic, and financial administrators from almost every medical school in the country and from a number of leading clinics. Participants considered the advantages of prepaid, group-practice medical care as a major means of health service. The symposium examined in detail the program's three component parts: the Kaiser Foundation Health Plan, which enrolled subscribers and their families; the Kaiser Foundation Hospitals, which built and equipped the facilities for the plan members and their physicians; and the Permanente Medical Groups, the six autonomous physicians' groups that provided complete care (including hospital care) for their members. The proceedings of the symposium were edited by Anne R. Somers, a medical economist, and published in book form through the Fund's publication program.[100]

A grant from the Fund that year also supported a program at the University of Colorado Medical Center illustrating the role of medical disciplines in helping society confront harmful forms of human behavior—in this case, the widespread problem of parental abuse and neglect of children.[101] The leader over the past decade in the study of child abuse was C. Henry Kempe, chairman of the Department of Pediatrics at the University of Colorado, whose book *The Battered Child* was published with support from the Fund. Its expanded third edition included discussion of all forms of abuse—physical, sexual, nonorganic failure to thrive, and neglect—with much emphasis on prevention and emergency evaluation.[102] Kempe had pioneered the idea of the child-abuse team as a means of medical and social intervention. A small hospital-based interdisciplinary unit (including pediatrics, psychiatry, social work, and public health nursing) offered a promising approach for advanced research into the causes of the problem and a means of rapidly translating the findings into programs of service and teaching. Kempe characterized child abuse as a transmitted pattern of child-rearing, frequently passed down through several generations. It appeared to be equally prevalent in every social class and ethnic group, and it almost always had its roots in the background of the abusing parent, which was characterized by punitive behavior and emotional deprivation. A three-year grant of $278,142 to Colorado's medical center enabled the child-abuse team to add three new dimensions to its role as a national model for research: an experiment in the training and use of family therapy aides to work with parents involved in child abuse; an experimental day-care nursery service to shelter children and help parents in times of family crisis; and follow-up research on the current status of the large population of abused children who had been cared for at the center.[103]

Other timely and productive grants made during Glaser's tenure at the Fund spanned the full range of the Fund's interest at the time: awards for the regionalization of medical education, through the WAMI program (whose name was an acronym for Washington, Alaska, Montana, and Idaho); for the modernization of the Departments of Medical Genetics and Anatomy at Yale; for the Beth Israel Ambulatory Care Center in Boston; for the Hospice in New Haven, Connecticut; for the study of violence, at Stanford's Laboratory of Stress and Conflict; and for a program linking medicine with public policy, at Harvard's John F. Kennedy School of Government.

THE WAMI PROGRAM

The decentralized program of medical education was an educational innovation developed between the late 1960s and early 1970s. Regionalization had two forms: networks of universities and hospitals within a state, as in a Fund-supported program in Illinois, and pooling of resources throughout an entire geographic region. From the viewpoint of medical educators, "successful programs depend increasingly on precise definitions of institutional educational objectives, effective student evaluation procedures, and skillful program administration by the college or the school. They also require the fullest engagement of new technologies in communication and learning resources."[104]

One of the most successful regional projects was the WAMI program, established in 1970 to meet the needs of the Pacific Northwest. The Commonwealth Fund supplied seed money for this program at its conceptual stage.[105]

The four participating states represented 22 percent of the nation's land mass in 1970 and contained approximately six million people. Only Washington supported a state medical school. Two-thirds of the physicians and other health professionals in the region lived in three areas: the Puget Sound region of Washington, the Anchorage area of Alaska, and the Treasure Valley of Idaho. The remaining third practiced in the towns and rural communities of a region stretching across five time zones—a mountainous, inaccessible, and sparsely populated land. In the previous twenty years, local and regional attempts by state and federal agencies to find solutions to the health problems of this area had been ineffective and at times even detrimental.

Impediments to the delivery of medical care in this region in the late 1960s included a dearth of family physicians, primary-care internists, and primary-care pediatricians. The majority of physicians were located in the cities and larger towns, so the deficiency was particularly severe in the more rural areas. Physicians in isolated communities also had restricted access to educational and health-care resources, as only a limited number of tertiary health-care centers existed in these four states. The number of practicing physicians would continue to be concentrated in Washington, since a progressively greater number of students was applying for admission to the University of Washington School of Medicine without corresponding increases in class size, and residents were favored over out-of-state applicants. Nor did the WAMI states have the resources to build and maintain additional medical schools, and a program designed to meet the requirements of the region could not look forward to any capital expenditures for new facilities.

The University of Washington Health Sciences Center had eighteen major health care units, including a neonatology complex and a burn and trauma center. It seemed desirable to develop a program that would bring these resources to all communities in the region. The idea for the program emerged in September 1969; while attending a meeting of the Washington State Medical Association, Thomas E. Morgan and August G. Swanson were challenged by a family practitioner to develop a way of subsidizing his four-man group practice so that it might provide a program for teaching family medicine in rural Washington.[106] Intensive discussion ensued within the dean's office at the University of Washington School of Medicine, and during the next two months the basic concepts of the WAMI program evolved.

Swanson was an experimentally oriented medical educator, and Morgan was working with Swanson on a major curriculum revision at the University of Washington. They were both creative in their approaches to improvement of the educational process. Also involved in the early stages of planning was John N. Lein, associate dean for continuing medical education at the University of Washington, whose experience gave him the ability to perceive the needs of practicing physicians, especially those in rural areas. Lein had his finger on the pulse of the region and was able to help shape the program to make it politically attractive. As assistant dean for admissions, M. Roy Schwarz was making yearly visits to twenty-eight Northwest schools supplying the University of Washington with medical school applicants, reviewing the applicants in the pool, meeting with premedical advisers and administrators, and giving seminars on the admissions process and the criteria used for selection. He recognized the enormous resource that existed at these feeder schools: faculty members who could teach first-year medical students at the University of Washington. While a few more faculty members would be required for the WAMI program, a large number of highly trained, sophisticated faculty members were already available.

By December 1969 the group was ready to present their ideas informally to potential sources of funding. They went to Washington and set forth their embryonic plans to Kenneth Endicott, who had just become director of the Federal Bureau of Health Manpower. The visit represented not an application but simply a step designed to inform Endicott of their thinking. Following that presentation, Swanson visited with Newton at the Fund's offices in New York, where he described these concepts of regionalized medical education in the Pacific Northwest. Newton was very interested and asked that he be kept informed as plans developed. In February 1970 Swanson stepped down from his position as acting dean of the medical school; early in March he prepared a proposal, which he sent to the Commonwealth Fund and several other foundations. Within a month Newton had telephoned him with the suggestion that he visit Swanson during a planned trip to the West Coast in late June. Newton spent a day with the group in Seattle, accompanied by Glaser and Terrance Keenan. Although the Seattle group had by that time developed a more sophisticated presentation of the program, they did not yet have a specific budget proposal. Swanson remembers the conversation in his car as he drove the group to the airport: Newton asked that Swanson prepare a brief proposal with a budget and submit it as soon as possible. Keenan simultaneously advised him on how much justification would be needed for the budget but was interrupted several times by Newton, who said, "We don't want too much, we don't want too much."

The Fund's advice to make haste caused the planners to realize that the proposal was known only to a small group in the dean's office. A meeting was quickly arranged with Charles E. Odegaard, the president of the University of Washington, and his staff, who were enthusiastic about the plan. Odegaard suggested that the university-based portion of the program first be introduced into Alaska, since it was the only state of the four with a single public university and thus would not involve the plan in competition between institutions.

By mid-July the group was in Alaska presenting their ideas to the staff in the governor's office, and by September preliminary plans were underway with the University of Alaska. The group was advised by the regional medical program coordinators in Alaska, Montana, and Idaho to consult with leaders in the practicing community about the plans. Meanwhile, at its meeting in November 1970, the Fund's board of directors had allocated a three-year grant of $996,678 to implement the program. As Schwarz pointed out, this source of flexible funds, provided through the efforts of Newton and Glaser, not only gave the planners enough leeway to cover unexpected problems but also covered essential needs that emerged during the early stages of planning and development. This Commonwealth Fund grant also supplied the seed money to obtain federal dollars for implementing the program in all four states.

The experimental plan opened at the University of Alaska during its first year, moving to Idaho during its second and Montana in its third. The responsibility for degree-granting and accreditation of the WAMI program resided with the University of Washington School of Medicine. Administration and evaluation of the program were centralized at the University of Washington, and the program's evaluation would demonstrate whether learning and behavior development occurred in the WAMI sites at a rate equal to that in a home base in Seattle. The planners hoped to phase out federal support if the program proved valuable, replacing it with state funding on a contractual basis.

If all this was to be achieved, the school of medicine at the University of Washington would become a regional medical school and assume responsibility for the entire continuum of medical education (undergraduate, graduate, and continuing education) for this four-state region. (It would not, however, have to modify its research orientation or expertise, nor its patient-care activities.) The school would be dependent upon four state legislatures, and would have to deal with four governors, four boards of regents, and four medical societies. These requirements made the program one of the most massive political undertakings ever attempted in the history of medical education in the United States. Its planners would be challenging existing dogma about medical education, confronting faculty members at each of the participating universities. The secret of making WAMI work, in Schwarz's view, was to create the belief in everyone involved that he was a full partner in this unique undertaking. Each person who played a role had to be made to feel that he owned a piece of the program and that if he did not perform the entire program would be jeopardized. Schwarz, who became the program's director shortly after it began, was largely responsible for its success.[107]

In the first, or university, phase of the program, three universities without medical schools provided the first year of the medical school curriculum to entering students. This arrangement permitted the first-year class to expand from 102 to 175 students, with appropriate allocations given to Alaska, Montana, and Idaho. Courses for the first phase were planned jointly by faculty from the five universities (including the University of Washington) so that a "single, region-wide course" was taught at five locations by a "region-wide" faculty. Medical faculty from Seattle traveled to the universities to cover those portions of the educational material requiring more than local faculty resources.

All students went to the University of Washington campus in Seattle for the second year of the curriculum and for the initial clerkships in the third year of the undergraduate program. A student at this stage had the opportunity to enroll in the second, or community, phase of the WAMI program; the student would spend six weeks in a community clinical unit (CCU) working with a private physician in a rural community in one of the four states. House staff in residency programs were also assigned to a CCU for up to six months. These experiences in family medicine, internal medicine, pediatrics, psychiatry, and obstetrics and gynecology were designed to provide a participant with an understanding of how the community functioned, what roles a physician must play, and what skills and knowledge were required to deliver high-quality health services. The planners hoped that this exposure would attract a larger number of students to careers in primary care in underserved areas. At least once every six weeks, faculty from the medical school in Seattle visited each unit.

By the late 1970s, the number of students admitted to the University of Washington School of Medicine since the start of the program had increased by 81 percent. The performance of these students was equivalent to that of their peers who were training in Seattle. The number of students entering pathways to training in primary care increased by 100 percent. In addition to the 45 to 50 percent of each medical-school class that chose careers in family medicine, another significant percentage chose the route to clinical specialties, opting for careers in primary care, internal medicine, and pediatrics.

Although data sufficient for firm conclusions were not available by the late 1970s there were indications that the maldistribution of physicians in the Pacific Northwest was being at least partially corrected. Only nine of the students participating in the university phase of the WAMI program had completed their undergraduate and graduate training in 1979, too small a sample to justify any solid conclusion. On the other hand, eighty participants in the community phase had rotated through the CCUs and entered practice. When the participants in the WAMI program were matched with a corresponding control group of 276 house officers who had not rotated through these units, the WAMI group showed a significant increase in the number choosing small towns for practice and a corresponding reduction in the number who chose towns with populations greater than 100,000.

Varied methods were used to bring the resources of Seattle's health science center to outlying communities. In 1974 the University of Washington School of Medicine began to use highly advanced communication satellites able to transmit two-way color television images and voices simultaneously. Experiments with this technology in the admissions process, minority recruitment, faculty sharing, consultations, and independent learning indicated that satellite communication appeared to have valuable applications for the region's health care and education. At the urging of Dean Robert L. Van Citters, the medical school established a regional consultation program, MEDCOM. This telephone network allowed a physician anywhere in the WAMI states to call the school, toll-free, for advice on patients' problems. All costs for this service were met by the medical school, and during the 1977–78 academic year 9,332 calls were received from physicians in the four states. The faculty also assisted the region's practicing physicians by acting as special consultants in routine visits to the program sites (326 visits in 1977–78), supplementing the teaching program in the university phase and the required review and consultation in the community phase. Members of the faculty also presented 162 continuing education programs attended by 3,412 health professionals.

Some remodeling was done at several campuses to accommodate special curricular needs, but because the WAMI program called for no construction of new buildings, no capital funds were needed. By the late 1970s, the program seemed to be an ongoing success. In 1977 it received the Richard and Hilda J. Rosenthal Award from the American College of Physicians for significant contributions to the improvement of health care.[108]

Seed moncy from the Commonwealth Fund helped the WAMI program's planners obtain other grants to implement their innovative endeavor, the cost of which was later assumed by other institutions. The Fund's support of the WAMI program also represented a continuation of its enthusiasm for the regionalization of hospitals, an effort that began in the 1930s. Although the purpose of this particular project was to distribute medical teaching and patient-care personnel throughout the Pacific Northwest, the process also facilitated the education of nurses and allied health personnel in areas where they were critically needed, through cooperative enterprises with community colleges, other four-year institutions, and hospitals. Talented teachers already available in the region and the clinical material available in private clinics and community hospitals allowed a considerable increase in the number of medical students, and students and house officers trained in a milieu of academic excellence away from the traditional medical center appeared to have a greater inclination to practice in smaller towns and cities. Through the WAMI program, health care in remote areas was distinctly improved.[109]

Revitalization of Medical School Departments

MEDICAL GENETICS AT YALE

A Commonwealth Fund grant to Yale University in 1967 enabled the university's president, Kingman E. Brewster, to initiate a two-year study of the overall potential of the school and its associated institution, the Yale–New Haven Medical Center. Brewster wanted a comprehensive assessment of Yale's capabilities and opportunities in medical education, research, and service in light of rapidly changing conditions in medicine and society. Directing the study, Brewster and the university's provost, Charles H. Taylor, were assisted by a committee of ranking staff members at the medical center, including representatives of the hospital and the nursing school. Also collaborating were outside consultants in medical education and its administration; in hospital development, organization, and management; in community health care systems; and in health-care personnel.[110]

Among the possibilities identified for development by this committee was the field of genetics. In 1970 Brewster decided to set up a Genetics Advisory Committee to make recommendations about the future of this area at Yale. A year of study led to the conclusion that the field was exciting, Yale was strong, and the time was right to establish a department of genetics in the medical school. The plan to draw the new department's staff from existing departments required that these departments find the venture worth the risk of parting with their resources, since they would be sacrificing faculty members and space for the good of the university.

No discrete faculty grouping or course in human genetics existed at Yale until 1965, when a Section of Medical Genetics, staffed by two junior faculty members, was established in the Department of Medicine to present an eight-hour block of lectures on "Human Development" to first-year medical students. By 1968 the faculty of the medical genetics section had grown to four, the organization had become an interdepartmental division sponsored jointly by the departments of pediatrics and medicine, and the lecture hours in the course devoted to human genetics had increased to twelve.

When the Department of Human Genetics was established in 1972, its members were scattered over the campus. Brewster placed first priority on raising money for facilities to bring this group together. His efforts to obtain support from Newton resulted in a grant of $2.5 million. This grant was critical: As the department's first major donation, it served as seed money for the grants to follow, including smaller gifts from the Kresge Foundation and the National Institutes of Health (NIH). The Commonwealth Fund money permitted the renovation of some fifteen thousand square feet of space; consolidation of the basic science portion of the department; and provision of office space, a conference room, and laboratory facilities.

Leon E. Rosenberg, chairman of the new department, could not overemphasize the significance of the Fund's contribution. He viewed this grant as catalytic, the key to the developments of the next ten years. Even with this grant, the human genetics portion of the department remained scattered, but later gifts from other foundations allowed Yale to build the structure bridging Cedar Street that would house the entire department. Grants from other foundations also established a Cancer Center and developed a program in molecular genetics. In Rosenberg's words, "Kingman [was] 'playing a chip' at an absolutely key time. He could have played it in a number of directions with the Commonwealth Fund and other foundations but he chose to put it on the square labeled 'genetics.' The results breathed vitality into what was previously a paper organization."[111]

The new department was based on the idea that the application of fundamental genetic principles to the hereditary diseases of man can best be carried out in an atmosphere in which basic and clinical scientists are appointed to a single faculty. As planned, the faculty was initially established by reappointment: Ten faculty positions were created by transfering individuals from medical-school departments (medicine, pediatrics, and microbiology), and five joint appointees were named from the medical- and graduate-school departments (biology, molecular biophysics and biochemistry, and therapeutic radiology). All were committed to research across the entire range of genetic phenomena from the molecular to the clinical levels. By 1973 Rosenberg, a research scientist and clinician with a national reputation who had spent almost ten years at Yale, had assembled nineteen full-time faculty, six of them at the level of full professor, and was offering a comprehensive, integrated program in three main areas:

1. *Research.* Activities were underway in medical genetics, molecular genetics, somatic cell genetics, population genetics, cytogenetics, and developmental genetics, with the help of a five-year grant from the NIH and additional support from the university and other sources.
2. *Service.* In cooperation with the Departments of Medicine and Pediatrics, the Department of Human Genetics was providing health-care services in genetic counseling, antenatal diagnosis, nutritional management of inherited metabolic disorders, and early detection of metabolic diseases.
3. *Education.* Faculty in the medical school, the graduate school and Yale College cooperated to provide training in human genetics for medical students, Ph.D. candidates in the graduate school, postdoctoral students preparing for an academic career, and physicians obtaining a Ph.D. degree under the medical scientist training program.[112]

Several outstanding clinical scholars trained in the medical genetics program achieved important academic positions. Louis J. Elsas took charge of medical genetics at Emory; Morris Mahoney became full professor at

Yale and head of the prenatal diagnostic activity; Margretta R. Seashore was to become director of the genetics clinic at Yale; Robert Fineman, director of pediatric genetics at the University of Utah; Richard E. Hillman, director of the metabolic division at the Washington University School of Medicine in St. Louis; Seymour Packman, associate professor of pediatrics and genetics at the University of California at San Francisco; Barry Wolf, assistant professor at the Medical College of Virginia; and William Rhead, assistant professor in the pediatrics-genetic unit at the University of Iowa.[113]

The department contributed significantly to the academic mission of Yale's medical school and the rest of the university by housing creative investigators who asked interesting and important questions, attracting new faculty to the fields of eukaryotic and human genetics, introducing students and practicing physicians to genetic principles, and providing health services to patients and families suffering from heritable diseases. Rosenberg believed that by choosing the status of a department, rather than some other academic structure such as a free-standing center or interdepartmental division, Yale created a stronger and more creative program in medical genetics that fortified the university in the process.

THE DEPARTMENT OF ANATOMY AT YALE

A large grant from the Commonwealth Fund in 1972 permitted Yale to bring the distinguished cell biologist George E. Palade and key members of his outstanding research group to the School of Medicine.[114] The sum of $750,000 was appropriated, payable on the condition that Yale provide $350,000 from other sources.

The Yale University School of Medicine intended to achieve a strong, unified capability for work at the frontiers of the basic life processes and their disease-causing impairments. Palade was a pioneer in the field of electronmicroscopy and in the relation of biochemical function to morphologic structure. His elucidation of the properties of cell membranes— their role as gateways in the transport of molecular materials within the cell, and to and from the cellular environment—was a landmark in the progress of biological science and had earned him a reputation as a world leader in the field. His group's move to Yale not only made possible the establishment of an outstanding Department of Cell Biology but was a key element in the transformation of the Department of Anatomy.

The seeds for this modernization were sown in 1959, when Russell J. Barrnett left Harvard to join the Yale faculty. In 1968 Barrnett became chairman of Yale's Department of Anatomy. The department at that time was cast in the traditional mold and except for Barrnett's appointment had made no move to update its biomedical facilities.[115] Barrnett's objective was to create competent groups in cell biology and developmental biology, and to strengthen neurobiology. His dowry as the new chairman included five new positions (one professor, one associate professor, and three assistant professors), which he was able to match with five positions supported by NIH grants. There were no funds for renovation, but the dean, Frederick C. Redlich, had promised a response to individual needs as appointments were made.

As Palade's close friend, Barrnett talked with him about these plans and ideas. Although they explored the possibility that Palade and his group would move to Yale, no formal discussions were held at this stage. Barrnett did, however, notify Yale's Biological Sciences Advisory Committee of his contact with Palade when he gave the committee his plans for developing the department.

In 1968, on Barrnett's nomination, Palade received an honorary degree from Yale. The following year Palade expressed an interest in moving to New Haven. Financial matters at Yale by then had become more pressing: It appeared that funds for renovation might soon be more difficult to obtain from medical-school sources; furthermore, unfilled positions, rather than remaining on departmental budgets, would go before the Planning and Priorities Committee, to which chairmen could apply for these resources. Although the freeze on positions did occur, the dean acknowledged the steps that Barrnett had taken earlier and agreed that further negotiations with Palade should proceed.

When it became clear that Yale would need to obtain outside funds to bring Palade's group to New Haven, the Commonwealth Fund was contacted, and in March 1970 a group from Yale conversed with Glaser.[116] Glaser was familiar with the work of Palade and his group and appeared receptive to the notion of providing money for departmental renovations that would allow Palade to come to Yale. Negotiations between the dean and Palade waxed and waned practically to a stalemate. But with urging from a strong faculty group, the dean made his first offer to Palade by letter on February 2, 1971. Palade and the Dean met on February 23, and an amended offer was sent to Palade on March 2. In none of these communications was the Commonwealth Fund mentioned. Charles H. Taylor was now acting president of Yale, and he negotiated with the Fund over the next few months, convincing its staff of Yale's strong support for Palade and his group and persuading them that the Fund's $750,000 would allow the move to be made. Yale's situation had become urgent, as considerable pressure was on Palade to remain in New York. Toward the end of November 1971, the Commonwealth Fund's grant was assured, and on November 24 Palade accepted Yale's offer.

On April 22, 1972, Barrnett delivered the necessary documents to the Appointment and Promotions Committee. Although Palade was appointed as of July 1, 1972, his move was not completed until two more years had passed—the time required for the renovations.

Two years after Palade arrived at Yale, Gross Anatomy became the Section of Human Anatomy in the Department of Surgery. Barrnett became chairman of the Section of Cytology, which along with Palade's Section of Cell Biology had a partnership in a common graduate training program. The section of cellular neurobiology was subsequently formed with Pashko Rakic from Harvard as chairman. In 1978 the two sections merged, establishing a strong group that has made great progress under Palade in both research and teaching at Yale.

Palade left the Rockefeller University, where he had spent most of his career, because he was convinced that his basic research in cell biology could be systematically applied to larger biological systems—and that this work could be accomplished best at a university medical center with a strong tradition of interdisciplinary collaboration between the basic and clinical sciences of medicine. Yale's commitment to the new department in faculty support, equipment, and space gave this group the best possible start. The renovation made possible by the Commonwealth Fund created some 7,300 square feet of laboratory and office space. Yale itself purchased the very expensive scientific equipment required by Palade and his group.

A special problem arose in 1972 during the completion of the renovation—money was needed for installation of an electronmicroscope. Since the medical school had used university sources to the utmost to bring the move to that point, the Commonwealth Fund made an additional small grant of $23,700 to bring matters to a happy conclusion.[117]

THE BETH ISRAEL AMBULATORY CARE CENTER

The Commonwealth Fund's participation in programs for the care of ambulatory patients illustrates the long life of an idea in the history of a foundation. The Fund's interest began in 1945, in conversations between Lester J. Evans and Joseph T. Wearn, chairman of the Department of Medicine at Western Reserve University, whose ideas for curriculum reform included a university-based community health center to train medical students in the care of ambulatory patients.[118]

As specialization increased and the practice of medicine became more fragmented, teaching concentrated on inpatients, and general clinics in hospitals declined in quality. University teaching hospitals traditionally focused on inpatient care and paid little attention to their outpatient departments, which generally offered a less-than-optimal level of continuity and efficiency. Yet services to outpatients provided the bulk of doctors' practices, and these patients were becoming an increasingly large part of the hospital population.

Howard H. Hiatt and his colleagues at the Beth Israel Hospital were convinced that university teaching institutions must assume responsibility for the improvement of ambulatory care, and proposed to develop teaching, research and service in this area. The result was the Beth Israel Ambulatory Care Center (BIAC)—a semi-autonomous unit with its own administration, staff and budget, designed to serve the large population of patients from a cross-section of the community who depended on the hospital for their general medical care. The Beth Israel Hospital was chosen because of its considerable experience in community health care—as an essential part of the Harvard Community Health Plan (itself founded with grants from the Fund) and as a collaborator with neighborhood health centers in the Boston ghetto of Roxbury.

In 1971, the Fund gave the Beth Israel Hospital $7,500 as partial support for the planning of both an ambulatory care center and a program uniting community leaders and physicians to strengthen community-based ambulatory care. In May 1972 the Fund appropriated $300,000 for two-year support toward the BIAC's teaching and research program; this grant was matched by the Carnegie Corporation, with the encouragement of Carnegie staff member Margaret E. Mahoney.

When the center opened its doors in October 1972, with thoroughly renovated clinic, screening, and patient reception areas, all existing primary care units and service at Beth Israel were closed. The facilities of the center and its closely integrated specialty clinics were designed to provide maximum operating efficiency while preserving the atmosphere of the private physician's office. Its physical and administrative autonomy (including, for example, an allocation for the cost of hospital space occupied by the program) made possible the precise measurement and monitoring of the costs of service, teaching, and research in the ambulatory setting. The center operated as a hospital-based group practice with front-line care delivered by primary health-care teams in internal medicine, obstetrics and gynecology, and pediatrics. These teams, composed of a physician, nurse, and health aide, provided continuity in care that had hitherto been lacking. A carefully defined division of labor among physicians and allied health workers on each team allowed patients to receive comprehensive care at a controlled cost per unit, maximizing the center's revenue. Backup services were provided by the hospital's specialty clinics, including dermatology and hematology units. To integrate mental-health care with more traditional medical care, the program began with a full-time psychiatrist and seven social workers.

Several projects were started by the center during its first two years of operation:

1. An "Ambulatory Care Project," in cooperation with MIT's Lincoln Laboratory and with funding from the Department of Health,

Education, and Welfare, to develop a system of protocols permitting allied health workers to assume a wider role in the diagnosis and management of frequent minor health problems and chronic diseases
2. A "cost-revenue center" to establish the cost-finding and accounting procedures needed to document and evaluate the financial impact of the experiment's various components
3. A system of computerized medical records that would also help integrate the center's records of outpatient care with those of the hospital's inpatient services
4. Streamlined laboratory reporting procedures, community outreach, and extensive family planning services

Under the direction of Thomas L. Delbanco, the Beth Israel's new enterprise was also a laboratory for teaching, research and experimentation in the delivery of cost-effective ambulatory care—a modern version of Wearn's ambulatorium. It introduced and tested several innovations, working closely with community physicians, health centers, and other hospitals to transfer its experience into the mainstream of medical practice. Cost-finding and accounting procedures were established to separate teaching and research expenditures from service cost.

These experimental services were, in turn, the basis of BIAC's work in teaching and research—the special object of the grants from the Fund and the Carnegie Corporation. Harvard's medical students and Beth Israel's house staff were trained, for example, in the team approach to health care and in methods of monitoring the quality and cost of ambulatory practice. In research BIAC concentrated on evaluating the effectiveness and efficiency of an ambulatory-care service, through the analysis of data such as utilization rates of costly laboratory procedures. The methods applied to evaluating the BIAC service were also offered as a resource to community practice, health centers, and hospital outpatient departments.[119] From the outset, data on the center had been collected systematically and its operations evaluated independently by the Harvard University Center for Community Health and Medical Care.

During 1974 the center intended to expand its activities over the next three years in several areas:

1. *Service:* Substantial enlargement of the center's clinical facilities to permit expansion of its core medical staff. Special attention was to be given to obstetrics and gynecology, as the center was establishing a comprehensive program to meet the special health needs of women. The center was also to assume full responsibility for Beth Israel's Home Care Program.
2. *Teaching:* A program of residency training stressing organization

and delivery of primary care was made possible by a grant from the Robert Wood Johnson Foundation in 1974. In cooperation with the Harvard Medical School, the center was also starting a program that would include medical students and residents on all center health-care teams. Under a grant from the Hyams Trust, the center developed a plan for the health education of the patients themselves, based upon individual health education "prescriptions" drawn up by the patient's primary-care team. Implementing this plan and systematically evaluating its medical and financial results would be a major goal of the center.

3. *Evaluation:* The center would continue to direct its work toward establishing reliable measures of the quality of ambulatory care by refining its computerized medical records, disease-specific protocols, and cost-revenue accounting. Responsibility for evaluating the center's work would be shifted to an in-house unit.

The estimated total cost of the existing center programs from 1975 to 1977 was $3,269,000; the cost of instituting new programs and expanding existing ones was estimated at $716,500 for the same period. The Beth Israel Hospital itself was committed to providing $2,776,900 toward these costs, leaving a shortfall of more than $1 million over the next three years. The Fund's staff thought that the center was well worth supporting as a model ambulatory care system within the hospital setting: Its staff participated in national conferences on primary care and published studies of its problems and achievements, and in 1974 the center was selected as one of eight subjects of a major report to the Department of Health, Education and Welfare on experiments in ambulatory care. In November of that year, the Fund renewed its grant to BIAC, providing $300,000 over the next three years.[120]

BIAC's next decade has been marked by consolidation and expansion of its efforts. One-third of all house officers in internal medicine at Beth Israel are now in a special BIAC program that prepares them for careers in general medicine and primary care. Originally supported by the Robert Wood Johnson Foundation, this program has been federally funded since 1977 and has served as a model for other programs nationally. BIAC is also the "control" in the Johnson Foundation's evaluation of its fifteen new programs in general medicine based at university hospitals.

National attention has focused on BIAC's studies evaluating the optimal management of common respiratory and urinary infections. These studies represent the more clinically oriented path taken by the center's research, which has included investigations of the nature and extent of functional disabilities in patients seeking hospital care, techniques of breast examination for patients, the content and frequency of periodic health examinations, and the utility of exercise for elderly patients. A grant to

BIAC in 1981 for a program educating general physicians about the early diagnosis of alcoholism has marked the Commonwealth Fund's continuing interest in this organization and in the special health problems of ambulatory patients.[121]

THE HOSPICE IN NEW HAVEN

In the early 1970s, more than 60 percent of all the deaths in the United States were caused by chronic diseases such as cancer, heart ailments, and central nervous system disorders. Terminal illness frequently confronted the patient with an extended period of fear and anxiety, which was shared by his family and friends. Often the high cost of treatment in acute-care hospitals added a financial crisis. Yet despite the magnitude of the problem, there were few special facilities for patients who were beyond recovery and needed special medical management to relieve their discomfort and careful attention to prepare them emotionally to face death. The acute-care hospital, while effective in fighting the illnesses and medical crises of dying patients, had not developed an approach to their special needs. Nor did acute-care hospitals incorporate help for the patient's family, either during his illness or after his death. Nursing homes were reluctant to accept patients facing a prolonged period of severe pain and usually lacked both expertise in pain control and adequate staff to care for patients incapacitated by terminal illnesses. Home care was also difficult because doctors rarely made home visits.

The inspiration for a hospice in New Haven—a place where terminally ill patients might live in comfort and dignity—came from Cicely Saunders, an English physician who worked with patients suffering chronic pain, especially from advanced cancer. While she was planning the Saint Christopher Hospice in London in 1953, she made the first of many visits to the Yale–New Haven Medical Center. There she inspired Florence S. Wald, dean of the nursing school, to relinquish her post and develop the concept of palliative care of the terminally ill in the New Haven community. With Ira Goldenberg, Morris A. Wessel, and the Reverend Edward F. Dobihal, Jr., Wald conducted a two-year study of existing facilities—medical centers, community hospitals, nursing homes, and patients' homes—that were caring for dying patients. Wessel, a pediatrician in practice in New Haven, was active in a wide range of community projects; Dobihal was director of Religious Ministries in the Yale–New Haven Hospital and associate professor in the Divinity School; and Goldenberg was professor of clinical surgery at Yale's medical school.

The study was sponsored by the School of Nursing with grants from the United States Public Health Service's Department of Nursing Resources and the American Nurses Foundation. The information emerged from diaries which the four kept (with the consent of the patients and their families) in the course of their care to those with terminal illnesses, wherever they were—at home, in a hospital, or in a nursing home. The group found that continuity of care was difficult to achieve throughout a patient's terminal illness and that collaboration between disciplines and agencies was difficult to sustain. To occupy a hospital bed, patients had to be receiving curative treatment—but for terminally ill patients such treatment often did more harm than good. Symptoms were difficult to manage because doctors and nurses were unaccustomed to preventing pain and were afraid to prescribe a regular schedule of drugs such as morphine, benadryl, Dilaudid, and codeine. They worried about addiction and increased tolerance, and they believed that such drugs would make patients obtunded. Often patients were told in the last few weeks or months of their illness to find a place for themselves, as nothing more could be done for them in a hospital. Families were not considered part of the care-giving team, nor was their physical and psychologic well-being considered the responsibility of care-giving agencies either during the illness or when they were working through their bereavement. A feeling of helplessness was common and distressing to both patients and families.

Care-givers in community health agencies and many physicians in practice welcomed the help of the research team, and patients' families were particularly grateful. The group felt that a solution to the problem of care for the terminally ill was an inpatient facility modeled after the Saint Christopher Hospice, and the four met with heads of community agencies and with whichever hospital chiefs of service were sympathetic to the need for a hospice when "our job is done." The group soon realized that the medical community was not in a position to offer comfort: Tertiary hospitals had their own unique roles in society, which did not include participation in the terminal care of patients.

The deans of the medical, divinity, and nursing schools were very supportive of the project, as indeed was Yale's president, Kingman E. Brewster; all agreed that in a community the size of New Haven an autonomous institution with links to all health agencies would be best. In the search for money to support their work, Dobihal, Goldenberg, Wald, and Wessel went to New York to see Robert J. Glaser of the Commonwealth Fund. (Some years later, Glaser confessed that what drew his attention most was a confrontation with an ensemble consisting of a nurse, a doctor, and a chaplain.) In early 1973 the Fund gave the group a small grant to study the feasibility of establishing a hospice.[122]

The staff at the Saint Christopher Hospice had discovered that patients going home after a stay in the hospice needed additional special care. Between 60 and 70 percent of the patients chose to die at home, but they feared that the doctor or nurse would not come when needed and that they would be left all alone. The New Haven group's five-year plan for full development of the program provided for home care—back-up care along with help from the family physician.

In May 1971 work began in earnest with a feasibility study prepared by Henry J. Wald, who was finishing his master's degree in health-facility architecture.[123] A functional flow chart was prepared to project the sequence of the many facets in planning, and the decision was made to provide home care while plans for the inpatient facility were still in progress.

A private foundation and the Connecticut Regional Medical Program together supplied $33,000, but the work moved forward more rapidly when the Commonwealth Fund, the Van Ameringen Foundation, and the Ittleson Family Fund gave the hospice substantial grants (of $100,000, $100,000, and $25,000, respectively). These funds enabled a complete planning staff and home-care staff to be assembled.[124] A British physician, Sylvia A. Lack, and a nurse from the Mayo Clinic, Sister Mary Kaye Dunn, were hired to establish a home-care service. The hospice was planned to care for 100 terminally ill patients in their homes and in a building with forty-four beds. The planning was in the hands of five coordinators, each responsible for a facet of the work (home care, finances, community relations, etc.), and the coordinators had task forces to help and critique their efforts. Members of the board of directors also shared the work of these task forces, which included physicians, nurses, hospital administrators, and businessmen. Yale's medical and nursing schools and the New Haven Visiting Nurse Association offered its generous cooperation in establishing the unique services to be offered by the hospice. In 1974, after the dean of the nursing school, Donna Diers, made Lack aware that the National Cancer Institute could provide money for the demonstration of home care for cancer patients, the group received a grant of $1,500,000 to keep the home-care service going for two to three more years.[125]

That same year two major hurdles to introduction of the hospice system were overcome: Blue Cross and the Connecticut Medical Service approved the program as eligible for regular reimbursement of patient cost, and the Connecticut Commission on Hospitals and Health Care approved plans for the hospice to be designated a chronic disease hospital. Now the way was clear for construction of the hospice building, which was financed by grants of $1 million from the NIH and another $1 million from the state of Connecticut. This funding arrangement required the hospice to accept patients from the entire state. The working drawings of the inpatient facility presented to the board of directors by the architect Lo-Yi Chan were accepted in late 1974. A major capital campaign committee was then formed in the greater New Haven area. From 1973 on the

Commonwealth Fund's grant provided the staff with support for general planning and fund-raising efforts and for development of other aspects crucial to the facility's successful start:

1. The internal organization and administrative systems of the hospice facility
2. Services that would create a therapeutic milieu for hospice patients and their families;
3. Relationships with home health agencies and medical personnel to enable the hospice to operate as an integrated part of the health-care system
4. A volunteer program to link the hospice's home-care program with community groups
5. A forum for education about the needs of terminally ill patients and their families

Continued support from the Ittleson Foundation met the costs of staff salaries, legal fees, office expenses, consultants, research planning, and fund raising. The task forces were now studying issues of research, professional relations, patient care, building and site, finances, and community relations; among the more than 100 task-force volunteers were members of Yale's faculty in economics, medicine, hospital administration, nursing, and religion.

When patients insisted on use of the hospice, many of their physicians would tag along, but others still resisted. Yet many of the physicians who were at first against the idea of the hospice later became its enthusiastic supporters. Individuals from all over the country continue to visit this model program, and training courses are available for those interested in hospice work. The pioneering New Haven Hospice Program is still considered a model for the inpatient and home care of terminally ill patients.[126] On December 1, 1982, the home care portion of the program celebrated its tenth birthday.

Florence S. Wald recently offered her interpretation of the events leading to the founding of the first hospice in the United States:[127]

> [Along with the Commonwealth Fund] the Van Ameringen Foundation simultaneously gave its support as did the Ittleson Family Fund. Once these solid and prestigious foundations lent their support other ones felt more comfortable in following suit. Dr. Albert J. Solnit of the Child Study Center at Yale played an important role in the very beginning. He knew of our plans and without asking us or telling us beforehand he mentioned our work to Dr. Robert Glaser and urged his support. . . .
>
> The role that the Commonwealth Fund took was unusual and in a way daring because by the time we asked for its help we had separated ourselves from

Yale.... From our point of view we avoided the high indirect costs and the stumbling blocks that town-gown relationships present. From Yale's point of view, it has difficulty in taking under its wing an endeavour of any service except in the very beginning phase. However, the then Deans of Divinity, Medicine and Nursing were in agreement with this decision and were supportive—but it did take the trust of Commonwealth!

THE STANFORD UNIVERSITY LABORATORY OF STRESS AND CONFLICT

One of the Commonwealth Fund's strengths was its refusal to be deflected by external events. Through a world war and the Great Depression the Fund's programs in health continued straight on course. Harkness House was nevertheless not an ivory tower; the Fund's charter was flexible enough to accommodate programs concerned with new and immediate problems of American society.

The staff summed up the temper of the times in 1971: "Recent years have recorded unprecedented waves of riot and insurrection in our cities and campuses, increasing racial militance and tensions, and profound alienation among youth manifested by life styles of hostility, distrust, and drug-taking. Finally, the extent and degree of violent crime have made fear and disquiet a widespread feature of American community life."[128]

The Stanford University School of Medicine proposed to become the first medical school to examine the problems of aggression and violence in an academic setting. A committee of Stanford faculty members had already published the results of a two-year study of the subject, *Violence and the Struggle for Existence*. A Laboratory of Stress and Conflict, based in the Department of Psychiatry, would invite participation of the best minds from throughout the university and from the nearby Center for Advanced Study in the Behavioral Sciences. In addition to generating and conducting collaborative research, the laboratory would be a facility for teaching medical students and undergraduates.

The school's leader in planning was David A. Hamburg, chief of the Department of Psychiatry, who believed that although ignorance about the causes of violence was substantial, the existing base of knowledge left "little doubt" that this inquiry could yield important results. Although a characteristic of aggression was the multiplicity of its dimensions—evolutionary genetic origins, endocrine and other biochemical mechanisms, family and cultural factors, and social factors—most of these lines of inquiry had been pursued separately; the unique feature of the Stanford program was its plan for an interdisciplinary study of the underlying causes of the problem.

Specifically, Stanford planned to concentrate on four topics:

1. *The evolutionary bases of human behavior.* These studies would involve field investigations on primate species in their natural habitat, building particularly on Stanford's collaboration with the Gombe Stream Reserve in Tanzania; investigations would be primarily concerned with the intricate threat-and-attack behavioral patterns of the chimpanzee, man's closest living biological relative. The aim was to identify the fundamental modes of aggression—how they are learned and how and when they occur—that comprise man's ancient instinctive legacy.
2. *The role of the early years of life in the formation of human aggression.* This research would concentrate on recent findings that the events of infancy and childhood have profound consequences for subsequent behavior. It had been ascertained, for example, that adolescent and adult disturbance—especially violence—is highly correlated with abuse or neglect during childhood.
3. *Problems of stress and conflict in early adolescence.* These transitional years seem to be a crucible for the formation of attitudes of alienation and hostility and for experimentation with psychoactive drugs. Although this is the age at which preventive measures could be most useful, virtually no research had been done to improve understanding of early adolescence as a crucial period in human development.
4. *The impact of environmental stress on human behavior.* Animal research had indicated that the combination of crowding, forced contact with strangers, and competition for shelter has powerful effects on levels of aggression and conflict. The laboratory would explore the parallels for human society.

These studies would entail basic and clinical research on the biochemical and physiological phenomena associated with dominant, assertive, and violent behavior. Each subject area would thus involve the integration of biological, psychological, and social determinants of aggression.

Stanford's request for start-up funds covered the cost of personnel, travel, and bricks-and-mortar. A grant would pay for three faculty members to work with Hamburg in directing the program; research associates, laboratory assistants, and secretaries; collaboration with the Gombe Stream Reserve, including visits to Stanford by Jane van Lawick-Goodall, director of the research in Tanzania; and renovation of a facility on campus to house the laboratory.

The Fund's staff was enthusiastic about supporting work on a problem that it termed "of vital significance to the stability of American life."[129] The program seemed intellectually strong: Not only would it call upon faculty from throughout the university, but its leader was seen as a "scientist and educator of national and international standing, who has made the search for solutions to aggression and violence in modern society the central goal of his scholarly work."[130]

The staff therefore recommended to the board of directors that $505,686 be appropriated for a three-year period beginning in 1970. Half of the grant would be designated for the first year, and one quarter for each of the remaining two years.[131]

From 1970 through 1973, the research at the laboratory focused on the problems of adolescence, both in chimpanzees and in humans. Some projects were continuations of efforts instituted before the Commonwealth Fund's grant (e.g., Goodall's study, begun in 1961, of the aggressive behavior of chimpanzees in their natural habitat); others could not have started without the Fund's support. A project funded through a grant from the National Institute of Mental Health (NIMH) and the object of special enthusiasm at the laboratory was a "peer counseling" program, which by 1973 had trained several hundred students ages twelve to eighteen in a twelve-week course. Graduates of the course who were assigned to elementary schools tutored younger students; worked to improve students' physical skills, peer relations, and social skills; helped physically handicapped students; and assisted with behavioral research. At the secondary school level, peer counselors offered support to students making the transition from elementary to junior high school; participated in group projects and work with foreign students, students with personal problems, and minimally mentally retarded students; offered tutoring; performed structured interviews for special guidance projects; and assisted the leaders in the peer counselor training program. The program's effectiveness was judged chiefly by "remarkably positive" reports from teachers.[132]

The laboratory's staff was also conducting a drug counseling program; research on drug use in adolescents; peer counseling with disadvantaged youth; a Clinic on Alcohol and Violence; and studies of sex hormones and aggressive behavior, the expectations of black students and white university administrators, the use of mental health services by black students at Stanford, conflict resolution in psychotherapy, vicarious reinforcement and "pro-social" behavior in young children, therapeutic alternatives to incarceration for adolescent offenders, and the present knowledge of human hatred and violence.[133]

In fulfilling its educational commitments, the laboratory offered a required course for undergraduates in Stanford's Human Biology Program, a course concerned with the evolution of human behavior. At the advanced level of the Human Biology Program, the laboratory's staff established several new courses: one on the psychobiology of aggression; one on human aggression, which surveyed biological, psychological and social approaches to the topic; and one on primate behavior. Altogether, these courses reached about five hundred undergraduates a year.

Psychiatric residents participated in the work of the Alcohol and Violence Clinic, and medical students were exposed to new material on drug-related hostility and violence, adolescent problems, paranoid attitudes and paranoid psychosis (relating particularly to schizophrenia in young adults and depression in the middle years), and the treatment of violent offenders in institutions.

The Peer Counselor program represented the laboratory's reach into the high schools of Palo Alto, and the program's staff was also involved in international education through UNESCO and the World Health Organization.[134]

The Fund's support was crucial for the establishment of the laboratory, which had, as its leaders said, "come at a difficult time. . . . Most important is the present climate in respect to Federal funding. In addition, we are part of a private university that became seriously overcommitted during the 1960s when it underwent a dramatic period of growth including the creation of what was virtually a new medical school. Further, the Laboratory of Stress and Conflict does not fit the usual categories of granting agencies."[135] In requesting a renewal of the Fund's grant for three more years, Hamburg said, "it will take several more years before the Laboratory is fully effective at that level of quality to which we aspire."[136] The continuing decline in the availability of federal funds had resulted in the phasing out of some of the laboratory's activities, and the soaring construction cost of creating the laboratory facility had depleted the Fund's 1971 grant earlier than planned. Hamburg was hoping that the Fund would not only renew the grant but would allow the renewal to begin on January 1, 1974, about five months earlier than the originally scheduled termination of the first grant.

Hamburg asked for a total of $319,731 for 1974 through 1976 to cover partial salaries of seven faculty staff members, as well as the services of a secretary, supplies, and travel. No additional money was requested for facilities: "Core faculty support is the essential need of the laboratory in the next three years."[137]

Before committing the Fund to a renewal of the grant, Carleton B. Chapman, the Fund's president, put two questions to Hamburg in an August 1973 site visit: Are you able to give adequate time to this, an expansive project that would suffer if your input of time were inadequate? And in so complex a project, how can we be sure that our funds are being spent on the project itself and not on some of its numerous ramifications?[138] Since he had relinquished his position as chairman of the Department of Psychiatry, Hamburg replied, the laboratory was now his prime professional activity, and he believed he would be spending at least 50 percent of his time on the laboratory's work. All of the Commonwealth Fund's money was going to the core project; the ramifications, some of which he termed "very elegant and promising," were pure dividend.[139]

Examples of these dividends were a study of paranoia in patients at the Palo Alto Veterans Administration Hospital—an investigation run by the staff of the laboratory but not funded by the laboratory itself; and the expansion of the peer counseling programs to minority-group community centers in San Francisco. Chapman found Hamburg's replies convincing and recommended that the Fund renew the grant for the requested amount, but he specified that this should be the final renewal and that any future requests for funding should be considered as an application for an entirely new grant.[140]

With the renewal of the grant, the Fund's staff foresaw expansion of the laboratory's research, teaching, and service.[141] During the next three years, the work of the laboratory centered around clinical studies of human male behavior and hormone interaction, studies of human adolescence in a natural setting, and studies of chimpanzee development and behavior with particular emphasis on hormone-behavior interactions.

In the first category, the staff had studied the differential dose-response curve of normal young human males injected with gonadotropin-releasing hormone. A wide range of behaviors and moods was monitored. The results indicated that there was no change in sexual arousal or aggression, as had been hypothesized, but that there was an indication of a decrease in fatigue and an increase in activity level with increased testosterone levels. In addition, a longitudinal study of the relation of testosterone to orgasmic frequency in young adult males had revealed that the techniques of isolating individual and ecological correlations could be generalized to the problem of studying component interactions within any dynamic system.

The group working with human adolescents completed its study of drug use in the adolescents of Palo Alto, and funding for the peer counseling program was assumed by the Palo Alto School District when the grant from the NIMH expired.

Commonwealth Fund support in the final period of the grant was primarily to complete the data accumulation, storage, and processing in the chimpanzee studies.[142] Since the opening of the Stanford Outdoor Primate Facility in 1974, the laboratory had performed daily observations of behavior as well as periodic anthropometric measurements, dental examinations, and hormone determinations. The behavioral data were gathered under strict sampling procedures, using trained observers who were required to pass proficiency qualification tests and whose observations met quality control standards. The laboratory termed both the quality of the behavioral data and the combination of behavioral data and physiological data "unprecedented" since they were longitudinal data from chimpanzees living in a free social structure within a partly free environment. Studies concentrated on the adolescence of the chimpanzee as a model for man. By the close of the program, preliminary analyses of the developmental changes were completed.[143]

A counterpoint to the success of the laboratory at Stanford was the closing of the research facility in Tanzania in June 1975, in the wake of the kidnapping of four Stanford students working at the Gombe Stream Reserve.[144] (Hamburg went to Africa to negotiate, and they were released several months later.) The following year he left the laboratory to become president of the Institute of Medicine at the National Academy of Sciences, and his successor, Seymour Levine, was overseeing the continuation of the laboratory and the winding down of the Fund's grant.

In November 1976 Stanford asked for an extension of its grant through June 1977, to allow the completion of the project's current publications.[145] Uncommitted funds of $15,500 would be used for salaries of laboratory personnel, but no new funds would be requested.

At a site visit that same month to assess the gains of the program to date, Reginald H. Fitz and Walter Donway agreed that all of the laboratory facilities built by the Fund seemed to be heavily used and that the projects underway appeared to be related to the Fund-supported project on stress and conflict.[146] A key aspect of the program had been the identification of correlations between hormones and behavior changes in early adolescence. The human study had been pursued in particular by Betty Hamburg, but the work was shelved when she left the laboratory with her husband. The chimpanzee study continued, and one of the laboratory's early achievements in biochemistry was the accurate measurement of testosterone levels in animals. Staff members were now turning their attention to the study of catecholamines: Once these substances had been accurately measured, the project planned to move to a study of their psychological concomitants.

This was one grant that the Fund staff had found "fascinating and fun."[147] Watching the chimps' activities—including bouncing rocks off the outside of the observation screen and showing their "fiendish cleverness" at putting together sticks and whatever else was handy to build ladders for scaling the high concrete walls of the facility—made site visits exciting, and a presentation by Goodall and Hamburg to the board in 1974 was greeted with enormous enthusiasm. Newton wrote to the two after their appearance: "I am especially pleased because we have never tried anything like this before. The members of our Board who were present were obviously delighted. They read about the grants we make, but we have found no way to make our grants come alive. For the first time, they have heard one of our grant recipients describe a project in vivid terms. In other words, you have started a precedent, but I am afraid it will be hard for anyone else to follow you."[148]

The Fund's staff concluded that many of the activities initiated under Hamburg's direction should continue, although "the payoff in terms of results would obviously and almost by definition be in the distant and indefinite future."[149]

After a decade of distance from the program, Hamburg has concluded that parts of the payoff may already be in hand:[150]

> The laboratory was deeply concerned not only with non-human primates, but also with the distinctive problems and opportunities of human primates. The interplay between the two was certainly stimulating for us and there is reason to believe that both lines of inquiry are continuing to be useful. . . .
>
> I do feel very good about the close link we established between the field studies and laboratory work. . . . This was a novel and attractive model which stimulated a lot of interest in the field. We were also involved in a "now or never" situation. Given the rate of attrition of tropical forests in Africa, the opportunity to study chimps in nature will probably not be with us much longer. Even now, the serious political problems of the kind we encountered in the 1975 hostage episode provide a powerful inhibitor. Still, efforts are being made by some people in the field to follow up on the kind of precedent we established in the work of the Laboratory of Stress and Conflict.
>
> The semi-natural facility we built for the chimps at Stanford was a considerable improvement upon existing laboratory facilities. . . . I understand that this has had some useful effect in the field. There is more attention being paid now to taking good care of the animals along the lines that we established in order to achieve more effective breeding colonies as well as for research purposes. Also, the methodological sophistication in systematic observational techniques, reliability analyses and qualitative measures, has had a useful effect. . . .
>
> The work on chimpanzee adolescence showed something of the relation between anatomical, hormonal and behavioral changes in early adolescence. This work discovered an unanticipated and sex-differentiated change in behavior of wild chimpanzees associated with puberty. This discovery challenged the conventional wisdom of the time that adolescence is a human invention at least in its behavioral aspects. . . .
>
> The work of the laboratory helped to focus attention on early adolescence which had until then been a seriously neglected phase of the life cycle. The work led by Dr. Betty Hamburg on human adolescence did much to clarify the distinctive biological, psychological, and social factors bearing upon the 10–15 age period. This work differentiated between earlier and later phases of adolescence in ways that have now become widely accepted and clinically useful. . . . The work on stress and conflict in adolescence contributed directly to Betty's peer-mediated approaches for coping with these problems. These approaches have now been incorporated into many school systems. To my knowledge, Palo Alto was the first one. Moreover, the peer-mediated approaches have now usefully extended to a number of other contexts—e.g., the prevention of cigarette smoking in adolescence. . . .
>
> There is a natural tendency in considering the work of this laboratory to focus on the chimpanzee research because it was so very unusual, vivid, even dramatic. Other aspects of the work were less fundamental and less vivid, more applied, yet perhaps no less significant.

THE JOHN F. KENNEDY SCHOOL OF GOVERNMENT

The Fund's intent to engage the full range of university scholarship to solve the nation's health-related problems was reflected in a three-year grant to Harvard University's John F. Kennedy School of Government in 1971. The grant assisted the school's Public Policy Program, a new curriculum launched in 1969, which was preparing students in medicine, law, and other professions for leadership roles in the governmental aspects of health care.[151]

The inadequate return the nation was receiving from its health expenditures—then approaching $70 billion annually—was partly attributable to a lack of skill in policy-making. The scale and complexity of America's health service arrangements required solutions to such difficult questions as financing mechanisms; resource allocation; and organizational structure, function, and control.

In response to this need the Kennedy School's program was intended to equip superior students from professional schools for careers at the policy-making levels of public service. A two-year curriculum led to the master of public policy (M.P.P.) degree, which could be followed by an additional year of study and a dissertation for the doctorate. The first year provided both a grounding and a practicum in the essentials of public policy formation and evaluation. Actual problems currently confronting government agencies were used in conjunction with the latest methods of analysis from mathematics, economics, statistics, and the political sciences. The second year was devoted to individual research and related course work in a major area of policy or of government operations.

The two-year curriculum had been organized to enable students to arrange a joint degree program toward a medical or other professional degree and a master's degree in public policy. This arrangement extended the students' total period of study by only one year, since the second-year studies for the M.P.P. were counted as electives toward the professional degree. Students were also admitted to the Public Policy Program following graduation from professional school, or after a period of professional experience or government service. All joint-degree students were pursuing their first degrees at a Harvard graduate school.

The Fund's grant of $300,000 provided interim support toward the basic teaching and administrative costs of the program, while the school sought permanent funding through an endowment drive. At the same time, the program was also receiving support from the Ford Foundation.

Twenty-five students entered the Public Policy Program each year; medical students were in the minority, and law students were the most prevalent. By 1974, six had completed the combined M.D.–M.P.P. degree program and six more were in progress. In addition to the combined-degree candidates, four physicians had returned to the Kennedy School to work toward an M.P.P. degree. The Commonwealth Fund's grant enabled the school not only to offer fellowships to these four but to recruit faculty members with a special interest in the health field. Of the students these faculty members turned toward the health field, several went on to positions in the public sector.

The Fund's grant also allowed the program to work closely with the Harvard School of Public Health. Three junior faculty members held joint appointments in the two schools. One was helping to develop a new degree program at the School of Public Health in health policy administration; the second was spending part of his time as a research associate in the school's Center for the Analysis of Health Practices; the third was termed "one of the outstanding degree candidates" in the joint degree program. Finally, the Fund's grant enabled the Public Policy Program to participate in an interdisciplinary seminar on medical experimentation.[152]

By the time the Fund's grant terminated in 1974, Don K. Price, the school's dean, could report that "this experiment has already succeeded in the eyes of the two faculties concerned and the students who have participated."[153]

In the ensuing years the school's program has included two or three medical students each year. Graduates of the program include Harvey Feinberg, now dean of the Harvard School of Public Health; David Calkins, special assistant to the Secretary of the Department of Health and Human Services and now director of the primary care residency program at the Beth Israel Hospital in Boston; David Blumenthal, who served on Senator Edward Kennedy's staff and is currently the acting executive director of the Center for Health Policy and Management at the Kennedy School; Al Mulley, director of the Division of General Internal Medicine at the Massachusetts General Hospital; Mark Rosenberg, head of a section on the epidemiology of violence at the Centers for Disease Control; and Earl P. Steinberg, assistant professor of medicine at the Johns Hopkins University School of Medicine.

Steinberg applied for admission to the Master of Public Policy Program as a third-year medical student. "Having completed almost three years of medical school," he wrote, "I have come to two realizations. First, the practice of medicine alone does not permit me to utilize many of my analytical skills in problem-solving situations to their fullest extent. Secondly, through direct involvement in patient care and a closer consideration of the evolving public issues in the area of health care that that exposure has fostered, I have become aware of both the tremendous need for an imminency of change in this field. . . . I have been concerned about the discrepancies I foresee between the background of those that should play a role in formulating policy in these areas and those who most likely will do so."[154] Steinberg wanted not only the skills to deal with policy issues and an understanding of the political process—he wanted access to public officials. During his first year in the program, he was a research assistant to Richard Zeckhauser, whose work related to food safety regulation; this project led to Steinberg's summer job as a special assistant to Donald Kennedy, commissioner of the Food and Drug Administration (FDA).

This experience served as the basis of Steinberg's thesis, written during his second year in the program. Kennedy School theses, at that time, had two parts: a general overview of a policy area and an in-depth analysis of a particular policy issue within that policy area. Steinberg's thesis dealt with federal regulation of cosmetics, particularly the health hazards associated with these substances. The policy issue he chose to analyze dealt with whether or not the FDA should continue to allow lead acetate to be used as a color additive in hair dyes.

Since completing the Kennedy School's program, Steinberg has pursued a career that he terms "predictable." A three-year residency in internal medicine was followed by joint faculty appointments at Johns Hopkins, in both the Department of Medicine at the School of Medicine and the Department of Health Policy and Management at the School of Public Health. Steinberg's two main areas of research have been technology assessment and health-care finance. He has completed a major assessment of nuclear magnetic resonance technology for the congressional Office of Technology Assessment and has written two papers dealing with physicians' use of liver-spleen scans in the diagnosis of metastases. He is also nearing completion of three years of work studying physicians' use of exercise thallium testing. In the field of finance, Steinberg has been studying the ramifications of the prospective payment system that is based on Diagnostic Related Groups (DRG) and has been implemented by the federal government for the Medicare program, and he is working under contract with the American Society of Parenteral and Enteral Nutrition to analyze the impact of prospective payment on the future use of parenteral nutrition. In addition, he will devote the next year and a half to working with colleagues at the School of Public Health on a possible successor to DRG-based payment: capitation methodologies.

"As you can see, my research is highly collaborative, and benefits directly from my training in both medicine and public policy. . . . The Public Policy Program has proven to be a tremendously beneficial experience for me."[155]

The Vice-Presidency of Carleton Burke Chapman (February 1, 1973–January 31, 1975)

In 1972 Robert J. Glaser returned to Palo Alto as president and chief executive officer of the Kaiser Family Foundation. It was an unhappy time for Newton, who had leaned heavily on Glaser in conducting the Fund's affairs, but their programs were already in place and Newton could take his time in selecting Glaser's replacement. Since Newton would soon be reaching retirement age, the board decided to choose a vice-president who would eventually become the Fund's next president. Carleton B. Chapman came to the Fund's vice-presidency with the understanding that if all went well, he would be Newton's successor.

Carleton Burke Chapman (fig. 30, see p. 462) was born in 1915 in Sycamore, Alabama. He attended the local public schools and then entered Davidson College, where he majored in English and the classics. After graduation he became a Rhodes Scholar at Oxford, where he took an A.B. degree in physiology. In 1939 he entered the third year of the Harvard Medical School, receiving the M.D. degree in 1941. His internship and residency training in medicine were spent on the Harvard Medical Service at Boston City Hospital. After a brief period at the Harvard School of Public Health, he served in the Army Medical Corps in the Balkans, the Middle East, and the Far East.

His academic career really began when he joined the faculty at the University of Minnesota School of Medicine, working first in internal medicine and then with Ancel Keys in stress physiology. He also collaborated with Richard V. Ebert in opening the Heart Hospital and was active in the medical school's educational programs. In 1953 Chapman went to Southwestern Medical School at the University of Texas in Dallas. During his nineteen years there as professor of medicine, he specialized in cardiology, and his research produced important studies in exercise physiology.

Increasingly dissatisfied with the shape of medical education, Chapman became convinced that the standard pathway to the medical degree was not the best one possible. During the early 1960s, he became interested in the conferences on this subject sponsored by the Association of American Medical Colleges. He was given the opportunity to put some of his ideas into practice when in 1966 he accepted the deanship at the Dartmouth Medical School. His first assignment was to convert a two-year school into one granting the medical degree, and this endeavor received support from the Commonwealth Fund. In the process Chapman realized that the standard educational process was missing great opportunities by failing to stimulate even minimal cooperation between the faculty of arts and sciences and the faculty of medicine. By the time Dartmouth's first class graduated in 1973, an entirely new program had been put in place for the clinical years without relinquishing the standard Flexnerian preclinical requirements.

When Chapman left Dartmouth, he stepped into a newly created post at the Fund, "Executive Vice President." He devoted his time to several specific projects, including a reassessment of the Fund's publications; a follow-up study of the advanced fellowships; and the preparation of a new program for the support of medical education, which he had been planning before his arrival in New York. To form a sound base for decision making, Chapman studied the Fund's previous programs in detail.

During Chapman's vice-presidency, the general direction of the Fund's efforts remained the same as it had been under Glaser (see app. K). The Fund continued its support for medical schools that were modifying their curricula, and for studies of those socially important behavioral problems with roots in medicine: drug and alcohol abuse, the causes of violence and aggression, the social effects of the population explosion, the nature and treatment of learning disabilities, and the ethnic beliefs and traditions that inhibit the access of some groups to modern medical care. An effort that continued to command an appreciable part of the Fund's resources was the education of medical students in human sexuality and problems of sexual dysfunction.

The largest single grant ever awarded by the Fund was given during Chapman's vice-presidency, in September 1973—to the Columbia–Presbyterian Medical Center. This gift supported the construction of a "Library–Health Sciences Center," as well as renovation and expansion of the Vanderbilt Clinic. The Fund's donation was a major contribution to the center's recently announced ten-year, $133-million capital campaign to modernize the center's facilities and increase its endowment. Board members of the Fund who were also associated with the center advanced the idea that by making a large grant early in the campaign, the Fund could provide a crucial precedent—an endorsement that would multiply the value of its gift. Conversely, if the Fund, with its widely known relationship and continuing investment in the Columbia–Presbyterian Medical Center, did not show its unequivocal determination to do its share in moving the center to a new level of excellence, there was real danger that others would demonstrate less enthusiasm for this effort. The Fund's staff concluded that "it is entirely appropriate to view the Columbia–Presbyterian Medical Center's capital campaign as a special exception, *not* in terms of the Fund's program interests—which the projects described fit very well, but in the importance and magnitude of the investment that should be considered."[156]

The center had requested a total contribution of $10 million, half for the Library–Health Sciences Center and half for the Vanderbilt Clinic. The staff believed that the Fund's appropriate share was $5 million and agreed that this support should be earmarked for these two crucial projects, which fell directly within the Fund's priorities. The report of the Fund's president and staff to the board of directors reveals between its lines the degree of controversy that had preceded the final decision: "There are two factors involved in this recommendation. First, the medical center has developed a very loyal constituency during its four and a half decades of operation; this constituency should be expected to provide exceptional support for the center's capital needs. Second, the Fund has worked hard, through many years, to develop strong relationships with many other leading medical institutions, which look to the Fund for support; even now, the urgently needed basic program support sought by these institutions far exceeds the Fund's limited resources."[157]

While Chapman was vice-president, the Fund also continued to support links between medicine and other fields (the Yale Law School Program), and it maintained its interest in controlling the cost of medical care, through programs at the Harvard School of Public Health and Boston's Affiliated Hospitals Center, Inc.

THE YALE LAW SCHOOL PROGRAM IN LAW, SCIENCE, AND MEDICINE

As science and technology became more complex through the 1960s, problems spanning law, science, and medicine called for expertise and breadth that few scholars commanded. Yet law schools had not revised their curricula to reflect the legal complications of interdisciplinary problems. In 1973 the Commonwealth Fund gave $530,265 to the Yale Law School, which had been a leader in linking law with the physical, behavioral, and social sciences.[158] Among the school's influential projects had been a sociological jurisprudence program introduced in the 1930s; a program bringing together law and psychiatry in the 1940s; and projects joining law and urban studies, and law and social sciences in the 1960s. In each instance the law school identified a domain where law had broad implications, and where interdisciplinary work was required to define legal principles. Now, with the Fund's support, the law school set out to provide new opportunities in education and research for graduate students from a wide variety of backgrounds. This new, integrated program was to add a full-scale teaching component to the faculty's substantial research in law, science, and medicine.

The grant made possible curriculum development and research examining three general questions about the relationship between law and new scientific knowledge: What systems and guidelines can a society command to deal with the effects of new scientific and medical knowledge? What are the philosophical underpinnings of scientific and medical progress? What is the effect of advances in science and medicine upon the medical order and upon society as a whole? Additional research projects would be integrated with the larger inquiry to address the problems posed by medical experimentation, organ transplantation, and technological advances such as genetic manipulation, medical and technical aspects of pollution control, population control, regulation of energy sources, and the delivery of medical services.

The new program would bring four to six graduate fellows to the law school for a year or more of interdisciplinary study and research. Fellows would be either recent law graduates or young law teachers; instructors preparing to teach, supervise research, or enter public administration; or advanced science or medical students who wished to spend a year in the law-school setting to complete dissertation work in law, science and medicine, to do advanced work in preparation for teaching, or to pursue a particular research interest. All graduate fellows would be able to participate in law-school courses, undertake research, and, in the case of nonlawyers, familiarize themselves with legal thought and methods. In addition to Yale's intellectual resources, the program would include visiting faculty from other universities, private legal practice, and government and business. A steering committee composed of faculty from the law school, medical school, and graduate schools was to select candidates, recommend visiting and permanent faculty, monitor curriculum development, and coordinate research.

When the grant request was submitted in April 1972, some of the law-school faculty were offering sporadic interdisciplinary courses, but their efforts had never been coordinated. To structure these courses was the first major objective under the grant. The second was to invite young, promising persons from various disciplines to the law school for a year, where they would explore the substantive areas in the program and prepare themselves for teaching and research. With Robert A. Bert as program director, courses in law and medicine became an integral part of the curriculum, and the law school became a magnet for graduate and undergraduate students.

Soon seventeen physicians had applied for admission to the law school. The faculty also attracted others interested in this interdisciplinary area, and the fellowship program was successful as well. Of the twenty fellows who spent a year at the law school, many returned to their own institutions as teachers and researchers in law and medicine. Richard Delgado, for example, became professor of law at the University of California at Los Angeles, in its Program in Medicine, Law, and Human Values. Arnold Arluke, Paul Starr, and Michael Waitzkin—all sociologists—taught and wrote many reports integrating the discipline of law, medicine, and sociology. Lance Tibbles became professor of law at Capital University, where he offered seminars in law and medicine; Angela Holder became an associate professor of pediatrics and legal counsel at Yale Medical School; and Sally Sharp taught courses in medicolegal issues at the University of North Carolina School of Law.

After four years Yale wanted to extend its program to discover whether more structured, integrated courses could be used to establish closer ties between the law and the medical schools. In 1977 the Fund renewed its grant for $300,000.[159] The only change in the program was its new plan to attract medical educators in midcareer. The program would offer them joint teaching opportunities with law-school faculty members, develop seminars and materials suitable for both law and medical students, and, most important, establish an interest in law within the medical school itself.

One of these educators in midcareer was Howard M. Spiro, professor of medicine and chief of gastroenterology at the Yale University School of Medicine, who had worked closely with Bert since the program's inception. In addition to teaching at the law school, Spiro developed an independent program at the medical school. Few law schools had established interdisciplinary ventures, but no medical school had a program to educate future physicians about the social and political forces affecting medical practice. To strengthen the medical school's program, a new core curriculum for first- and second-year medical students was designed to supplement the courses offered at the law school. The new courses would analyze medicine's ethical framework by exploring the problems of physicians, lawyers, social scientists, legislators, and judges in four major hospital services: surgery, pediatrics, cardiology, and medicine. Courses would be supplemented by clinically oriented seminars designed for third- and fourth-year medical students, as well as interns and residents on these services.

This curriculum represented the logical continuation of the work already completed under the two Commonwealth Fund grants. Through the help of the Fund, Yale had progressed in examining problems on the border of law and medicine and in establishing permanent bridges between the two fields.

THE CENTER FOR THE ANALYSIS OF HEALTH PRACTICES

The proliferation of new diagnostic and therapeutic procedures since World War II had resulted in both unequivocal benefits and serious problems. Often-controversial procedures were introduced and tested under varying conditions and degrees of control. Medical science's astonishing armamentarium included many techniques too expensive for universal application and raised questions about cost effectiveness and equitable distribution. An additional concern was that controversial new and established procedures continued to be widely used in large segments of the health-care system. Not only technical procedures were at issue but the validity of clinical decisions made by physicians, including the need for surgery and the economical use of well-established laboratory tests. Among many such concerns, these were of pressing importance:

—Hysterectomy, the operation that accounted for a higher total of

hospital days than any other surgical procedure performed in this country, was done far less frequently in other nations with comparable medical-care systems.
— Little was known about the relative effectiveness of various medical and surgical techniques for treating peptic ulcers, which accounted for five million days of hospitalization a year.
— Many clinicians believed that coronary artery bypass should undergo further clinical trials. Others felt that the procedure was too widely accepted to make such trials relevant; furthermore, if such surgery were offered to all who could benefit from it, the cost would be staggering.
— The medical value of prolonged hospital stays after such common procedures as gallbladder surgery was being questioned; millions of hospital days were at stake.
— Dramatic developments in diagnostic laboratory testing, resulting in wide application of hundreds of tests that could add hundreds of dollars to the patient's bill, had led clinicians to scrutinize the cost-effectiveness of routine use of these tests.

There was little doubt that the cost of medical practice could be greatly reduced if a qualified institution conducted a systematic investigation and used its prestige to evoke a significant response to its recommendations throughout the nation's system of health care.

Harvard University had established a Center for the Evaluation of Clinical Procedures to explore such problems. Leading the center was Howard A. Hiatt, dean of the School of Public Health. Hiatt was well-qualified for this role: Before assuming the deanship in 1972, he was a successful investigator in the field of cancer research and physician-in-chief at one of Harvard's major affiliated teaching hospitals, the Beth Israel. Supervising the new center was a steering committee of representatives from different Harvard schools and health-care experts from outside the university. The core staff could call upon Harvard's numerous experts in medicine, health-care research, law, public policy, the basic sciences, and the humanities; for clinical studies, the center could turn to the outstanding resources of the Greater Boston medical community.

The center asked the Fund to support four major activities during its early years:

1. *Inventory and analysis of crucial clinical procedures.* Each year, the center planned to study five clinical procedures with controversial effects on the nation's health-care system. Each study would relate costs and benefits of alternative approaches to certain medical problems. The center's staff hoped that clearer criteria would emerge

for judging clinical procedures in medical, ethical, economic, legal, and social contexts.
2. *Analysis of procedures used in clinical trials and other human experimentation.* The center intended to examine critically conditions obtaining in human experimentation. Participants in a regularly scheduled seminar would discuss guidelines for human experimentation and more effective ways to collect essential clinical data.
3. *Study of the spread, acceptance, and, later, replacement of new clinical procedures.* This program would involve preparation of in-depth case histories of new procedures and implementation of effective methods of disseminating the center's recommendations.
4. *Education.* The center planned to establish a limited program to educate medical students and practicing clinicians in the statistical and analytic techniques essential to proper evaluation of clinical procedures.

These programs were estimated to cost $693,385 a year to operate, but $250,000 would be defrayed each year by a grant from the Robert Wood Johnson Foundation. The Commonwealth Fund's board of directors approved an appropriation of $225,000, to be paid at the rate of $75,000 for each of three years.[160]

The program did not realize its full potential during its first two years of operation,[161] but Hiatt had recently recruited a new program director, Howard Frazier, who brought to the project a rich background in clinical and investigative medicine. A detailed report to the Commonwealth Fund four months later was much more sanguine.[162] The renamed Center for the Analysis of Health Practices was drawing the interest of promising young faculty members from a variety of departments within the university, and the volume and quality of its research activities was improving. In the wider community, faculty seminars on the analysis of health and medical practices and the program's public health rounds attracted individuals representing a spectrum of responsibilities and disciplines. Three monographs had been completed and seventeen articles had appeared in the primary literature, contributions ranging from highly theoretical studies to solutions for specific contemporary problems.

The center was becoming known as a source of guidance for specific problems of evaluation and policy analysis, and its staff was frequently approached for advice by directors of operating programs. Constructive relationships had been established with the Centers for Disease Control, the National Institute of Mental Health, the Massachusetts Eye and Ear Infirmary, and with innovative programs of ambulatory care at the Massachusetts General and Beth Israel hospitals in Boston (see p. 423).

From 1976 to 1977, the center produced almost four dozen articles for the technical periodical literature, along with three monographs and four technical reports. Equally significant were the center's investigations of the most important problems in contemporary health care: cost inflation, the effect of innovation, and ambulatory care. Its programs attracted the participation of individuals from insurance companies and government agencies, as well as the financial support of the agencies themselves.[163]

The center continued to be enriched by the quality of its visiting investigators. In 1976 these included the chairman of the Department of Statistics from the University of Chicago, the director of research in medical education at Michigan State University (recipient of a Commonwealth Fund grant), and the chairman of the management science and information systems group at the University of Massachusetts. Among the projects completed or well advanced during this third year were: *Hypertension: A Policy Perspective* (a book published simultaneously with the report of the study itself); three monographs (*Risks, Costs and Benefits of Surgery; Medical Inquiry: Theory and Practice;* and *Hypercholesterolemia in Children: Detection, Treatment and Policy Implications*); and *Policy Studies*, a shorter series on a wide range of topics such as the problems of diagnosing disorders of the fetus early in pregnancy; the use of tangible rewards to improve patient adherence to medical programs; the assessment of programs to prolong life, including intervention directed at the complications of atherosclerosis; the control of hypertension in certain populations; the diffusion and regulation of medical innovations; the management of blood resources in the United States; improving performance in the diagnosis of acute appendicitis; programs to reduce motor vehicle deaths; recommendations regarding goals and guidelines for health planning; and health maintenance organizations as a resource for teaching primary care to medical students. (These last three items were the subjects of unpublished studies; the remainder generated articles or parts of monographs.)

Many new activities were underway, including studies on the economic behavior of the physician, the cost-effectiveness of medical care under Medicaid, patient adherence to anti-hypertensive programs, the psychosocial effects of breast cancer, fetal monitoring, the value of medical data, the diffusion of medical technology, and analysis of clinical decisions.

The center became the research arm of the Harvard Community Health Plan in 1983 and changed its name to the Center for Health Research.[164]

THE AFFILIATED HOSPITALS CENTER, INC.

The merger of three renowned Harvard teaching hospitals created an unusual new tertiary-care institution in Boston: the Affiliated Hospitals Center, Inc. (AHC). AHC combined the staffs, boards of directors, and medical services of the Peter Bent Brigham Hospital, the Robert B.

Brigham Hospital, and the Boston Hospital for Women. Its move into a $76 million facility on Francis Street in October 1979 was the result of years of frustrating effort and negotiation.

AHC was a model institution, implementing ideas then being advocated for the nation's entire hospital system. The total number of beds for the three hospitals was not increased but reallocated according to realistic service requirements; expensive equipment and facilities were employed more intensively; economies were sought in inventory and purchasing, demonstration, insurance, financial and legal services, security, and service contracts; manpower was gradually redistributed among departments and specialties; and the management of all information, including computer-assisted record keeping, was consolidated.

There was wide speculation about the financial aspect of these changes and of hospital mergers in general. But economists and hospital administrators agreed that very little reliable documentation existed on the means of achieving economies through hospital mergers. In this context, the Affiliated Hospitals Center was not to be allowed to develop as an "uncontrolled experiment." AHC trustees, administrators, and senior medical officers believed that it presented an opportunity even more significant than an experiment in merger economics. In the early and necessarily experimental years of the new institution, when policy of all kinds would be defined, AHC had the chance to design, test, and implement changes in the way doctors approached the relationship between the cost of care and its clinical effectiveness.

AHC's proposal to the Fund in 1979 requested money to establish a "Center for Cost-Effective Care" (CCC), a separate unit within the highest management and policy committees of its parent organization. The CCC would coordinate all research related to merger economies and cost-effective care and would translate the research results into AHC policy and daily operations. The proposal was the special interest of several active AHC trustees, a group of influential AHC senior physicians, and Robert G. Petersdorf, AHC president and a medical educator and administrator with a national reputation.

Even before occupying its new facility, AHC had initiated several money-saving measures. The evaluation of these experimental initiatives would be the responsibility of the CCC. Mergers between hospitals were increasing, with and without physical consolidation, and it was important that some group evaluate the short- and long-term financial and healthcare effects of this new corporate venture.

Whatever economies might be achieved by hospital reorganization, it was the hospital's individual physicians who decided what medical resources would be used, how often, and for what purposes. These decisions determined charges to a hospital's patients and, ultimately, the hospital's overall costs. AHC believed that the early years of the merger offered a promising opportunity to develop and implement the appropriate use of health resources and that the new center should make an enduring commitment to this effort.

During a site visit in early December 1979, the Fund's staff and a consultant, Howard H. Newman, president of the Dartmouth–Hitchcock Medical Center, heard reports about research already underway, including studies of the use of radiological facilities. Costly radiologic diagnostic and treatment procedures were then at the center of the national debate about "over-utilization" of costly medical services. Computerized tomographic scanning—the computer-assisted procedure for producing a more revealing x-ray photograph—was only the most recent and controversial example. The issue, of course, was cost-effectiveness of such procedures compared with alternative uses of medical-care dollars. Six major interrelated projects at the AHC were demonstrating the cost versus the results of the use of a given piece of hardware. Under investigation was the statistical likelihood of a "positive" finding from a specific type of test, given certain preliminary indications. Another question concerned the efficacy of routinely ordered larger versus smaller numbers of x-ray photographs in increasing the chances of a "positive" finding. A grant from the National Library of Medicine was enabling two AHC investigators to study clinical decision making. One aspect of their work was the development of a computer-assisted consultation system that would give physicians a preliminary reading on the appropriateness of ordering a particular expensive procedure. AHC was also collaborating with the well-established Center for the Analysis of Health Practices, which concentrated upon models of cost-effective clinical care for illnesses frequently encountered by primary care doctors and was particularly interested in the AHC's extensive ambulatory care services.

To extend the AHC's research, the Center for Cost-Effective Care enticed the best young investigators. The galaxy of clinical research talent brought together in the AHC (for example, Eugene Braunwald, CCC's chairman of medicine) and talent available in the Harvard Medical School orbit would be difficult to match anywhere in the country and gave AHC a unique potential for success. The entire AHC was to be a clinical laboratory for CCC research and demonstration projects, so that CCC recommendations would be put into practice throughout inpatient, intensive care, acute care, and outpatient services. Strengthening this marriage of research results with hospital policy, the director of the CCC was to be part of the highest AHC management. CCC advisory and steering committees and a visiting committee from outside AHC would be composed of administrators, hospital trustees, clinical department heads, and scholars of sufficient stature to give CCC recommendations weight. Ultimately, the CCC would try to bring residents, attending physicians, and other hospital staff to greater awareness of the need to weigh the cost-effectiveness of procedures.

The CCC's substantial start-up costs could not be met from AHC revenue during the period of financial pressure and uncertainty attendant upon the merger. But the establishment of the CCC could not be postponed if the unit was to become an accepted, integral part of the new venture. The total recommended by the Fund's staff in 1979 for three years was $956,000, $458,000 less than the amount requested by the AHC.[165]

Petersdorf and AHC administrators agreed that the CCC could make excellent progress with this support. Under the direction of Barbara J. McNeil (professor of clinical epidemiology and radiology) and Deputy Director Anthony L. Komaroff (AHC vice-president for management systems and chief of the Division of General Medicine and Primary Care), the CCC was developing effective management tools, including sophisticated systems that surveyed hospital costs in new ways. (One, for example, revealed the costs for which each individual physician was responsible.) Komaroff's responsibilities were mainly on the clinical side, but he was also responsible for integrating the most successful analytical tools of the center into the daily workings of the hospital.[166]

The CCC's conference, "Relating Clinical Practice and Hospital Administration," in October 1982 was attended by over two hundred hospital administrators from all sections of the country. The CCC also conducted a monthly seminar series featuring speakers from widely divergent parts of the biomedical complex. Since termination of the Commonwealth Fund grant, the center has been funded by the Blue Cross/Massachusetts Hospital Association Fund for Cooperative Innovation.[167]

To encourage more cost-effective care in teaching hospitals and to influence physicians and other personnel to use hospital resources effectively, the CCC needed to identify a hospital's resources and compare their use to a predetermined goal. In feeding back information to hospitals, it hoped to create a system of accountability that would provide an incentive for physicians to act cost-effectively. The CCC's Management Control System determines the cost of care provided by a clinical center through an internal "pricing system," in which the cost of services provided by other hospital departments becomes a cost for the clinical center. These "transfer prices" initially reflect the budgeted direct cost for each unit of service, and the total cost of such services is based on the volume and type used by the center. Transfer prices are also calculated for the components of a "bed-day" for patient-care units. The CCC's current projects include the creation of centers of groups of physicians with efficient patterns of practice; developing standards of productivity for ancillary (e.g., laboratory) and support (e.g., housekeeping) centers;

setting up an incentive system to reward or penalize managers based on their staff's performance; and structuring systems transferable to other acute-care institutions.[168]

Other Experimental Health Services

Although the Fund sponsored no formal program in medical ethics, several grants, including an award to the Hastings Center (the Institute of Society, Ethics, and the Life Sciences in Hastings-on-Hudson, New York), addressed this and other currently important social issues and helped create useful arrangements for the scholarly pursuit of solutions. Grants to the Maternity Center encouraged the professionalization of midwifery in the United States, and the Fund's support of the Community Blood Council helped to eliminate the waste, confusion, and shortages resulting from the uncoordinated activities of more than 150 institutions that were attempting to meet New York City's need for blood. A grant from the Fund allowed Yale University's Program on Non-Profit Organizations to make, in the words of its director, "a promising start . . . in our rather ambitious effort to develop a substantial body of knowledge and understanding about this profuse and unruly world of nonprofit organizations.[169] In all its efforts, the Fund's staff believed that its responsibilities included informing all members of the health professions about controversial issues and encouraging debate about the problems and their possible remedies.

In awarding these grants, the Fund followed its usual route of seeking the most qualified recipients in the highest-quality institutions to carry out the programs. Beginning with Edward S. Harkness and Barry C. Smith, and continuing through the tenures of Malcolm P. Aldrich and J. Quigg Newton, Jr., the leaders of the Fund preserved the Fund's "trickle-down" concept of philanthropy. As in the support of programs in medical education and medical research, the Fund's policy assured the education of excellent students who could migrate to other universities to seed programs that would train additional individuals in their fields.

Although programs classified by the Fund as Experimental Health Services enjoyed varying degrees of success, some served as prototypes for later efforts by other organizations, and a larger number made an important imprint on the course of development of effective medical care in the United States.

Newton's Administration of the Fund

Newton brought to his position at the Fund many of the personal traits necessary for success as a foundation president. He was, first of all, a good listener, able to inform himself about significant problems and advantageous approaches through conversation with leaders in medicine. Lester J. Evans's contacts with universities and hospitals had made the Fund well known as an organization receptive to new ideas, and Newton was able to choose intelligently among the varied proposals coming his way. While Newton respected the opinions of experts in planning the Fund's programs, he also evaluated their ideas. He had a good sense of people, knowing whom to trust and whom to disqualify.

Newton also had a good political sense, an ability to develop strategies for handling sensitive areas. He could identify worthwhile projects even when they existed outside an organized framework or special program. When Evans was organizing the experiments in medical education, the Fund followed a general plan that guided its contributions. No such umbrella existed during Newton's tenure, but he turned this problem into an advantage, using the resulting flexibility to move the Fund into new programs. In collaborating with the Carnegie Corporation, Newton accommodated easily to that organization's point of view. The collaboration allowed the two foundations to undergird each other: Carnegie supplied staff assistance, and Newton and the Commonwealth Fund offered the strengths of a long tradition in the health field and a sensible, sensitive president. Newton was a skilled opportunist in the best sense of the word, at a time when opportunism could help the Fund move discreetly but effectively into important areas.

As a good public servant, Newton also supported proposals that benefited the Fund's surrounding community. Using his law degree specifically, he was active in the New York Arbitration Society, and his participation in other public functions enhanced the Fund's image.

Newton was described as "an explorer of where the frontiers of knowledge needed to be expanded."[170] He welcomed innovation, believing that foundations were generally not as creative as they should be. This characteristic, he felt, might be related to the dynamics of policy decisions, which were often made in an adversarial atmosphere: the board versus the director. The affairs of most foundations were managed by a board composed of individuals who did not want to change society in quite the same way as did their staffs. At the Commonwealth Fund a good balance existed between the staff's innovative leanings and the more leavening attitudes of the board members. Regarding environmental health, for example, the staff pushed for an attack on pollution, but proposals to involve the Fund did not receive enthusiastic support from the board. As staff members were aware, such problems were sensitive issues in the business community. On the other hand, to the board almost anything proposed by a medical school was within bounds—including programs in sex education and prevention of child abuse. (Programs dealing with drug abuse, however, were never very popular with the board.) The Fund's directors necessarily placed a great deal of importance on public opinion, and in general, trustees were not as daring in matters of Fund policy as they would have been in their own businesses. From their platform, they had to be conservators of tradition, but it was sometimes difficult for them to appreciate that had Edward S. Harkness still been alive, he would have kept pace with the times. It was through Harkness's sense of innovation, exhibited strikingly during his presidency, that the Fund was able to advance so many pioneering projects. Harkness, of course, did not have to struggle with the countervailing influence of his board, as he was dealing with his own family money and the board was composed of friends who followed his leadership implicitly.

Newton was nevertheless able to bring the Fund into a pattern of grants compatible with the innovative spirit so evident in its early years. Although Newton's staff was the smallest in the Fund's history, it had the talent to recognize important ideas. Plans were crystallized after talks with the staff and with Aldrich, so that what Newton brought to the board for discussion were specific programs in final form. After presentation to the board, the idea for a program would go back to the staff for final development, returning to the board as a specific project for a decision on funding.

The President's Discretionary Fund

A mechanism for increasing the Fund's flexibility, the President's Revolving Fund, as it was first known, was established during the presidency of Malcolm P. Aldrich. Aldrich had suggested to the board of directors that a small sum would allow him to make minor disbursements between board meetings without having to obtain the specific approval of the board's executive committee. It was Newton, however, who used the Discretionary Fund most creatively, financing projects as diverse as collaborative ventures with the Carnegie Foundation, the printing costs of the proceedings of a conference sponsored by the New York Academy of Sciences, and summer fellowships at Emory University for medical students interested in population control. The approval of the board of directors for Newton's use of the money can be inferred from their willingness to raise the stakes. When the Discretionary Fund was set up in 1953, it contained $5000; nine years later, as Aldrich began to use it more extensively, the amount was doubled. In 1965, during Newton's presidency, the board allocated $25,000 annually; in 1967, $50,000; and in 1972 the board gave Newton a practically unlimited amount to dispense as he saw fit—a single appropriation of $225,000, of which any balance remaining at the end of the year would revert to the General Fund.[171]

The first $5000 sat untouched for five years, until $1,300 of it was used to cover the travel expenses of a physician at the Mary Imogene

Bassett Hospital.[172] During Newton's presidency, however, the Discretionary Fund became an administrative mechanism that touched many of the Commonwealth Fund's major program interests, as well as its distinguished investigators and consultants. The Institute for Policy Studies received $4,165 from the Discretionary Fund in 1965 for a series of seminars on "Dimensions and Determinants of Health Policy";[173] an international conference on schizophrenia at the University of Rochester, led by John Romano, received a $6000 award in 1967; and the New York Academy of Medicine was given $1000 for a preliminary study of the affiliation between voluntary and municipal hospitals in New York City. The Group for the Advancement of Psychiatry received help from the Discretionary Fund in its early years, as did the University of Toronto, which was using computer simulation techniques to plan model medical curricula.

Joint programs with the Carnegie Corporation received much of the contents of the Discretionary Fund during Newton's tenure, and the Board's enthusiasm for these projects in particular led to its decision to double the Fund in 1967.[174] Half the operating costs of collaborating with the Carnegie Corporation that year were met by a $7000 disbursement from the Discretionary Fund. The Fort Lauderdale Conference of 1966— that seminal meeting between federal administrators and medical educators—was supported in part through a disbursement from the Discretionary Fund, as was an ensuing study by Robert A. Aldrich, professor of pediatrics at the University of Washington School of Medicine.[175] The Discretionary Fund supported another joint Carnegie-Commonwealth meeting the same year in Swampscott, Massachusetts, on the role of the behavioral sciences in medical education.[176] The Commonwealth Fund's share of the operating expenses of the National Conference on Medical Costs totaled $3000 in 1967, and, matched by the Carnegie Corporation, provided for lunch and dinner sessions for a panel of three hundred participants, led by Secretary of Health, Education and Welfare John Gardner, who were considering the problem of soaring medical costs against the background of a federal report, *Medical Care Prices*.

One recipient of a Carnegie-Commonwealth grant wrote jubilantly to A. McGehee Harvey about the timeliness of the Fund's response to his request:[177]

> In July 1968 I moved . . . to Gainesville, Florida. For the previous nine years I had been immersed in private practice of internal medicine in a community of 20,000 people. Dr. Leighton E. Cluff, who had been my mentor for several years during residency and fellowship training at Johns Hopkins, had two years earlier become professor and chairman of the Department of Medicine at the University of Florida College of Medicine. It was he who had encouraged me to join him at Gainesville to assist in the then-beginning emphasis on ambulatory care in training medical students and residents.

I admit to perplexity during my first few weeks in Gainesville. The teaching hospital patient constituency, as a result of earlier negotiations with community physicians, was limited to referral patients. My ambition to develop ambulatory and general medicine experiences for medical students and residents was thwarted by this arrangement.

During the summer and early fall of 1968 I began to explore the rural counties of Northern Florida. Specifically, I was looking for a county with few or no physicians and with a population that was not so large that it would overwhelm the resources of a medical school-sponsored clinic. There were several counties west of Gainesville that met these specifications. By the fall of 1968, I had met with and gained approval of the county commissioners of Lafayette County to develop a university-sponsored rural health clinic to serve the 3,000 residents who were then without the services of a physician and had been for ten years. . . .

The health center opened the first week of January and 16 patients requested services. From the outset the citizens of the county, the commissioners, and medical school representatives had agreed to a fee-for-service medical practice, but all understood that no one would ever be refused medical attention. The county commissioners provided the facility rent free and made a contribution of $8,000 to the clinic. (Of some interest is the fact that they underwrote their county veterinary services with $13,000.) The services of medical and nursing students, residents in internal medicine, and faculty were given without charge. In fashion typical of resident behavior in the late sixties, considerable supplies from the teaching hospital would appear in the rural health center.

In spite of these contributions by the university and community, it was clear by the end of the second month that the patient fee revenue would not cover the operating costs. Sometime near the end of February or March 1969, Lee Cluff wrote a letter to Colin MacLeod describing the education and patient services of the Lafayette County Health Center, and requesting some financial help. Dr. MacLeod responded with a check for $19,000, which he stated was the remainder of the President's Revolving or Discretionary Fund for the year.

This $19,000 was probably the most important grant money I ever received. It made possible the survival of this newly started program, and in some part, vindicated the controversial educational efforts of a then-young and naive faculty member. With this money we were able to guarantee the salaries of local people working in the clinic and purchase the supplies needed for patient care until patient revenue was generated and a contract negotiated successfully with the Florida Department of Health to reimburse the county health center for public health services. The recognition by the Commonwealth Fund of this education and patient service venture was critically important and timely.

Late in the first year of operation, Dr. Emanuel Suter, then dean of the University of Florida College of Medicine, and I visited the Commonwealth Fund at the Harkness House in New York. I well remember the meeting. We were hosted by Terrance Keenan of the Commonwealth Fund. He received us in his office on the second floor. Coffee was served in china cups and saucers with linen napkins. Mr. Keenan indicated that he was interested in our rural health clinic with its amalgam of students and residents and faculty working together with community members to provide around-the-clock health services to the residents of Lafayette County while broadening the educational mission of the medical school. He suggested that he would discuss our proposal with the Carnegie Corporation as they sometimes shared in the support of similar requests.

In subsequent months, we were visited by Margaret Mahoney and Bob Glaser and in time were awarded $300,000 jointly by Commonwealth and Carnegie. I cannot tell you what this meant to me and the University of Florida College of Medicine. The state had recently passed legislation mandating state medical schools to establish departments of community medicine. Overnight I was appointed chairman of this department with its only program, the Lafayette County Health Center.

The $300,000 was a two-year grant which I carefully nurtured for three and a half years. We were by then contemplating expanding our rural health services into two additional counties and were developing a physician's assistant program partly on the theory that trained paramedical personnel would be helpful to physicians practicing in rural areas.

Although not directly intended, the Commonwealth–Carnegie grant was responsible in part for the development of the department of community health and family medicine The department, spurred by the rural health ventures, had broadened its activities to include units dedicated to social science and humanities, computer science, and a family medicine residency program that assumed care for all the indigents in Gainesville, Florida.

In 1974 or 1975, the department was successful in a $900,000 grant application to the Robert Wood Johnson Foundation that was based on the now-interdisciplinary rural health care project that embraced three counties and included a retirement village and a one hundred bed nursing home. At one time or another, in varying combinations that differed in each county, residents in medicine, family medicine, and pediatrics, faculty from all three disciplines, nursing students and their faculty, occupational therapists, clinical psychologists, physicians' assistants, and social workers all participated in the patient care, teaching and research activities in the rural counties.

In the middle seventies, Lee Cluff and I, representing the departments of medicine and of community health and family medicine, jointly applied to the Veterans Administration for a grant to enrich the training of medical students and residents in ambulatory health care. This grant was not limited to describing and developing further the already existing rural health ventures. In my mind there is no question that these activities were most helpful in our successful application which over a seven-year period brought 1.7 million dollars to the two departments. I never missed an opportunity to take visiting professors to the Lafayette County Health Center in Mayo, Florida, so they could experience first hand our version of the "Mayo Clinic." You were one of the first. Every site visit somehow concluded in Mayo, Florida, where dinner was served by a club of retired folks. At times I wondered if the citizens of Mayo were not becoming too sophisticated in responding to these visitors, invariably from urban, and usually Northeastern, cities.

Let me be more personal. I staked a lot of myself on the development of these clinics. I received considerable support from many, but particularly Lee

> Cluff. These projects still function after 15 years. Last week my son told me he had received a letter from one of his high school classmates who now attends the University of Florida College of Medicine. His friend remarked that his recent weeks at the "Mayo Clinic" had been his best experience in medical school.
>
> The Commonwealth Fund should be proud that at one critical time in the history of a community health project being developed by a totally unknown medical school professor in an eight-year-old medical school, it was able to contribute $19,000—and what a significant $19,000!

Newton also used the Discretionary Fund to support local causes. He gave $3000 to Columbia University for a conference aimed at stepping up efforts to expand careers in health services for persons from poverty-level backgrounds. The conference built on the work of neighborhood health centers sponsored by the federal Office of Economic Opportunity and on another Fund-supported project at Lincoln Hospital, which had demonstrated that under appropriate conditions people with relatively little formal education could become highly proficient in a wide range of health-service occupations. The Better Business Association, Inc., of New York City received $10,000 to study the creation of a Health Science Hospital Authority, which would give Bellevue Hospital autonomy by altering its status as a public hospital. A model demonstration facility sponsored by Friendly Homes, Inc., for children in mental hospitals who could not be discharged to their own homes was given $5000. Here the Fund's contribution was relatively minor, as the program had received more than $75,000 from the City of New York and $42,000 from private sources.

Today the President's Discretionary Fund is still used for a limited number of smaller grants, usually given one time only, and its amount has not increased substantially since Newton's presidency.

Newton and the Fund's Traditions

Despite his enthusiasm for new approaches, Newton was sensitive to the Fund's traditional ways. In assessing new proposals, Newton built on the legacy of the annual reports, which he used as a textbook outlining the basic problems in medicine and health over a long span of years. The reports outlined the progress of regionalization and integration in the Fund's programs—traditions that had stemmed from projects generated by the Fund's staff. Programs during Newton's tenure also reflected the Fund's bias toward support of the great private institutions rather than state schools. This attitude reflected in part the Fund's traditional special relationship with certain schools, including Yale, the Columbia–Presbyterian Medical Center, Johns Hopkins, Tulane, the University of

Rochester, and Harvard. These ties may also have demonstrated the Fund's traditional dependence upon the quality of the recipient institution. Often the reputation of the institution would carry more weight than the proposed program. When Thomas B. Turner, dean of the Johns Hopkins University School of Medicine, met with Newton in 1967, he offered no specific proposals at all, telling Newton only of plans under consideration by the faculty. The Fund's decision was to provide the dean with a sizable grant that would permit faster progress toward implementation of the programs under study.

The belief that safety lies in grants to institutions and investigators of proven quality presents certain problems. Does the competitive advantage given to institutions having such an "inside track" tend to work against a less well-known institution that may have an unusually innovative proposal but not "blue ribbon" credentials to bolster its chances of grant support? And if, for example, the presidents and the deans of two outstanding schools visited the Fund with a proposal to put the resources of their prestigious institutions together, even though the nature of the project, while sound and constructive, was not world-shaking—would it be foreordained that the Fund would respond positively? Without Lester J. Evans, the Fund would have been more likely to answer affirmatively. Evans was very good at recognizing the potential of small, little-known institutions that could be more innovative than more prestigious schools steeped in tradition. Underlying Evans's ability was the realization that good ideas are not confined to renowned universities. The roster of grants awarded during Newton's tenure as president of the Fund reveals that he, too, had a similar appreciation for outstanding talent in the less famous schools of medicine—for example, support of the state universities of Utah, Florida, and Nevada—even though it might be more difficult to uncover. Newton's tendency to rely on institutions and investigators of proven worth appears to reveal a conservative attitude toward philanthropy, one weighted heavily toward broadly acceptable programs, but the impression is belied by his willingness to support the fields of population control, sex education, midwifery, the allied health professions, and international medical health.

Of obvious importance for medicine was Newton's concern with public policy, and grants during his tenure supported the Institute of Medicine of the National Academy of Sciences, Duke University's center for education and research in the formulation and analysis of health policy, and Harvard's new interdisciplinary effort to improve public understanding of the role of science.

In all the Fund's endeavors, Newton wanted to give the universities a primary and the Fund an adjunctive role in decision making. He said: "Our limited staff did not have the experience and perspective to cook up the ideas themselves, but they did have the background to respond appropriately to good ideas that came to the surface and knew where to get independent expert advice. We did not want, however, in any way, to attempt to tell potential grantees what they should do."[178] The role of the staff was to listen, sort out the university professionals' best ideas, and then help the universities to implement them. The Commonwealth Fund's philosophy according to Newton was that the medical schools had been the source of much of the new medical knowledge; they would be the most likely source of new ideas along the path to improving medical care.

When Newton turned the Commonwealth Fund's presidency over to Carleton B. Chapman on February 13, 1975, he did not leave the Fund entirely; he served as vice-chairman of the board of directors from 1975 to 1976.

9

Integrating Medical Education into the University

Let us labor to place the teaching of medicine in its true position. Let us emancipate the student and give him time and opportunity for the cultivation of his mind, so that in his pupillage he shall not be a puppet in the hands of others, but rather a self-relying and reflecting being. Let us ever foster the general education in preference to the special training, not ignoring the latter, but seeing that it is not thrust upon a mind uncultivated or degraded. Let us strive to encourage every means of large liberal education in the true sense of the term, and so help to place and sustain our noble profession in the position which it ought to occupy.

—William Stokes, 1861

The Fourth President: Carleton Burke Chapman (1975–1980)

Carleton B. Chapman's first task as president was to give the board of directors a complete assessment of the Fund's programs at their meeting in February 1975. He found his assignment both fascinating and difficult; to obtain the board's guidance, he offered a preliminary statement at the meeting of November 1974. Although it was mid-February before he assumed the presidency officially, Chapman had spent the last year of his vice-presidency preparing his recommendations.

Chapman's tactic was to comment on Newton's presentation to the board of directors three years earlier.[1] In general, Chapman believed that Newton's priorities were sound. All Newton's recommendations would need updating, of course, but Chapman believed in the Fund's focus on projects designed to resolve the population problem and eliminate socially destructive psychosocial behavior. He also wanted to continue the Fund's fellowship and publication programs and believed that the Fund should continue to respond to individual requests outside its primary areas of interest.

Chapman and Newton differed on one major point, however: Newton

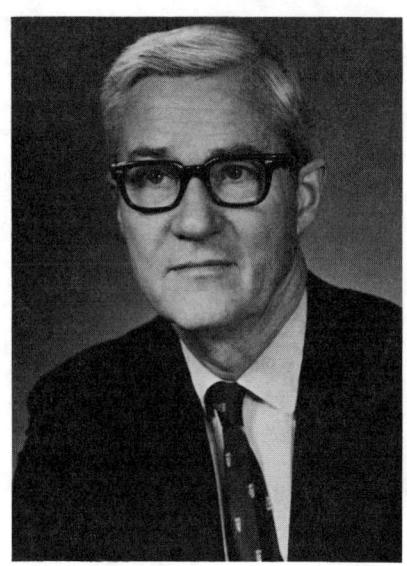

Figure 30. Carleton Burke Chapman

thought the Fund should maintain its programs to improve the health-care system, but Chapman now proposed that it think seriously about withdrawing from this field. Since Newton's appraisal, the Robert Wood Johnson Foundation had moved its newly increased resources into the medical area, focusing on the problem of health-care delivery in the United States. (The Johnson Foundation's annual expenditures were at least six times those of the Commonwealth Fund.) In addition, the Johnson Foundation's programs in its first few years were mainly transplanted Fund programs. For example, when Margaret E. Mahoney moved from the Carnegie Corporation to a vice-presidency of the Johnson Foundation, she took with her the Clinical Scholars Program and other joint Carnegie–Commonwealth activities.

The Fund would be outspent, but more important, Chapman doubted the value of most of these "experiments" in health care delivery—whether funded by the Commonwealth Fund or by other foundations. Foundations cannot determine the main shape of the system, Chapman believed—it is the product of legislative planners in Washington. Although some experimental results can influence legislation, especially if the men who carry out the experiments are allowed to write the laws, most programs are not designed to yield clearcut results. The extreme difficulty of evaluating these "experiments" while they are in progress was another reason for the Fund to divert its interests.

Chapman advocated other shifts in the Fund's policies as well. Newton had supported awards for international medical education and health care, but Chapman felt that this emphasis was no longer pertinent to the Fund.

He also felt that a small in-house program for visiting fellows was not practicable: The Fund was not in any sense an educational research institution within its own walls, and major universities were more suitable hosts for visiting fellows and distinguished scholars. Instead, the Fund should regard the university, and especially the private university, as its most logical instrument and client.

At the time of Newton's appraisal, the Fund's focus was mainly on education in the health professions. Three and one-half years later, the Fund was spread too thin. The programs of 1971 were admirable, but they were designed to fit a particular era—which even then was coming to an end. What the Fund now needed was not a rejection of the board's actions but a shift of emphasis among Newton's recommendations that would yield an even sharper focus on education for the entire sweep of the health professions.

The Interface Program

The Development of the Program

The crux of Chapman's presentation to the board was a variation on one of Newton's recommendations.[2] Newton had suggested that the Fund continue to support the production of more physicians, train more paramedical personnel, and offer continuing education programs for both types of professionals, but Chapman believed that the emphasis on increasing the number of physicians produced each year was rapidly becoming irrelevant. Instead, the Fund should broaden its interest in refining the process of education for medicine, especially at its juncture with prebaccalaureate education.

Chapman saw medical education separated from its natural ties of liberal education as an unmanageable, incomprehensible monster intimately and disturbingly analogous to those Mesozoic giants of the group Dinosauria which, unable to adapt to a changing environment, became extinct a hundred million years or so ago.[3] His impression was that faculties the country over were masters at the art of presenting a tiny change designed to preserve the status quo as something enormously innovative and valuable. Tinkering would not solve the problem, however: Any attempt to repair the grotesque structure that was medical education solely by tampering with the so-called basic sciences was a task exceedingly difficult, if not altogether hopeless. Substantial improvement required the participation of many different individuals, faculties, and university departments.

Practically all factions paid lip service to the proposition that doctors should be liberally educated. But in the same breath, those academicians who did not belong to the medical faculties claimed that the major enemy of the liberal education process at the college level was, collectively, the premedical requirements in the natural sciences: a year of elementary biology, a year of elementary physics, a year of general chemistry, a year of advanced biology of some sort, exposure to organic chemistry, and often courses in elementary calculus and in what used to be called analytical and physical chemistry. Chapman chose Elizabeth Kennan's statement to represent the university's standard lament: "The graduate, and particularly the professional, schools have encouraged and, in some cases, required a pinpointing of undergraduate preparation. Medical schools, of course, are a prime case in point. So comprehensive are their requirements . . . [in the natural sciences] that they virtually blanket three years of an undergraduate experience."[4] In other words, if those excessive and intellectually repressive premedical science requirements could somehow be shoved out of the way, all students opting for medicine would find liberal education within easy reach.

Chapman also wanted to stimulate the elimination of barriers between the basic sciences in the medical schools and the natural and behavioral sciences elsewhere in the parent institution. He hoped to improve the quality of the exposure to learning in the natural, behavioral, and biomedical sciences.

Specifically, the Fund should give substantial awards for innovative programs at a relatively small number of universities. Grants would be made to the university and not specifically to the medical school; they would contain no provision for endowment, although they might contain matching requirements. The focus would be on meticulously planned changes with far-reaching effects, not on programs susceptible to ill-considered "add-ons."

In disclaiming credit for his proposal's originality, Chapman pointed out that the Fund's staff (particularly Lester J. Evans) and the board had supported related programs since at least 1950, the year that marked the start of Case Western Reserve's curriculum revision. Chapman's own ideas had only recently been developing in parallel. As dean of the Dartmouth Medical School he had become aware of a kind of academic, intellectual, and political barrier between the faculty of arts and sciences and that of medicine. About five years earlier, he had started to consider ways to turn the barrier into a connection. By the time Chapman arrived at the Fund, his plans had begun to assume a coherent shape. He found Newton receptive, and bit by bit specific designs were presented to Newton and the board.

Chapman's program would begin where the Fund had left off in its experiments in medical education. During the 1950s and 1960s, the Fund's staff had scrutinized the preclinical phase of medical education; Chapman envisioned an "interface program" designed to deal specifically with the premedical and preclinical phases. The eight years of premedical and medical education were traditionally divided into four years of college and four years of medical school. Premedical requirements were met haphazardly during the four years of college as a prelude to the preclinical education of the first two years of medical school. Across the gulf between them passed only minimal faculty interaction, sporadic cooperation and coordination of curricula, and little discussion of the real needs of students preparing to study medicine. The object of the Fund's efforts would be the years from college through the first two years of medical school (fig. 31).

The barrier between the so-called basic biological sciences in the medical school and the natural and behavioral sciences in the arts and sciences division of the parent university had been neglected, both in general and by private foundations. At what Chapman called the "interface" existed the greatest opportunity for evolution of education, especially for the health professions. In particular, the premedical and preclinical portions of the educational sequence leading to the M.D. degree (usually the four years of college and the first two years of medical school) needed detailed analysis. Scarcely anyone in the university world seemed content with this sequence, but most faculty members appeared to hold solidly to the belief that significant change was difficult or even impossible. Chapman wanted to design a program that would encourage faculties to consider the possibility that the quality of the students' intellectual development was not optimal during these years, and that both sequence and content were ready for change.

Chapman identified the early stages of medical education as the source of the sequence's main defect. For a time he believed one of the academic

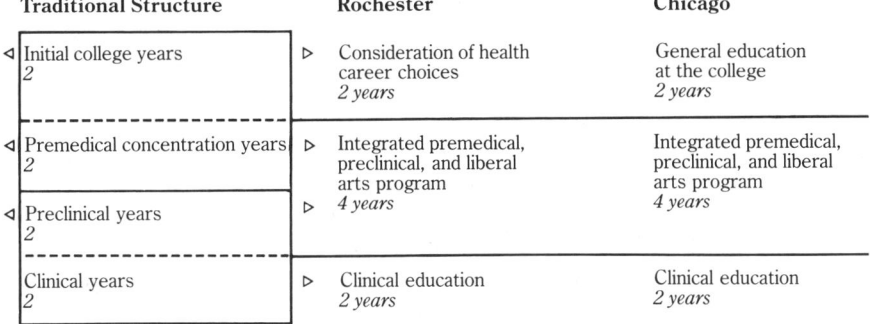

Figure 31. Comparison of the traditional structure of college and medical school education with Interface Programs at the universities of Rochester and Chicago Adapted from the Annual Report of the Commonwealth Fund, 1976.

Integrating Medical Education into the University

myths perpetuated especially by college arts and science faculties: Premedical requirements were detrimental to the whole concept of a liberal education. Later, he recognized that responsibility for the problems rested with both sides, especially with the natural sciences faculty, but also with the faculties responsible for teaching the preclinical sciences.

Chapman explained the isolation of the basic sciences from the rest of the university as a paradoxical consequence of the Flexner Report. A collection of strong basic science departments had been established within each medical school, each entirely separate from its analogue in the parent university.[5] These biomedical science departments exerted a profound influence on educational activities at the college level, and by imposing their own standards on the entry process into clinical medicine, they were in a position to control the end educational product. The final step was the formal recognition of the pattern through state licensure laws, most of which were enacted between the two world wars. The paradox was that Flexner had not intended this particular result—in fact, he had recognized it as grossly undesirable. Indeed, some argued that the preclinical sciences were not really "medical" at all, and that faculty working in basic science departments in medical schools risked cutting themselves off from intellectual currents generated in other parts of the university.

The Flexner report had produced other strange and deleterious effects, not the least of which was a considerable waste of university resources in the process of bringing a student from his first years of college to the M.D. degree. Just as serious, in Chapman's view, was the effect of this rigid and extraordinarily durable system on scientific, as well as linguistic, literacy. The problems growing out of the juncture between the basic and natural sciences were not confined to the medical school but spanned the university. To date, the university itself had been unable to view its activities critically, and with few exceptions had had little success in introducing constructive revision. But money was becoming scarce, and it is much more difficult to induce a university to examine itself critically when resources are abundant. Chapman hoped that the Fund's approach would provide considerable leverage in encouraging universities and their medical schools to confront some of their basic difficulties.

Chapman hoped that the Fund could restore Flexner's emphasis on the broad education of the physician, but nowhere could Chapman find anyone fervently espousing the philosophy that a student should acquire a liberal education before going on to deal with patients.[6] He felt that attacking the barrier between the basic and natural sciences would lead to rapid change in the university's intellectual mainstream, to the benefit of students at all levels, whether they were headed for medicine or not. "Liberal education" would regain some of its lost meaning.

Flexner was not the only outspoken proponent of a liberal education at the time. Thomas H. Huxley delivered a warning in 1876 that is still pertinent: "There is no position so ignoble as that of the so-called 'liberally-educated practitioner,' who may be able to read Galen in the original; who knows all the plants from the cedars of Lebanon to the hyssop upon the wall; but who finds himself with the issues of life and death in his hands, ignorant, blundering, and bewildered, because of his ignorance of the essential and fundamental truths upon which practice must be based."[7] But what in the light of present-day knowledge are those essential and fundamental truths? At what educational stage and in what academic setting should they be taught, and does the premedical option really make it impossible for students to obtain a sound liberal education? If so, can ways be found to correct the defect without impairing the student's education in those truths? It was these critical questions that Chapman wanted the Commonwealth Fund to address.

Despite the negative aspects of the Flexner report, its net effect was undeniably positive and its intent worth preserving. It was also an example of the best use of money from private foundations. The Carnegie Foundation funded the Flexner report itself, and Flexner's recommendations were implemented mostly through money from the Rockefeller Foundation, supplemented by donations from private individuals. Until about 1940 the Rockefeller Foundation and the General Education Board (also a Rockefeller creation) spent more than $100 million on the intricate business of restructuring American medical education, mostly under Flexner's personal direction. To Chapman it seemed not unreasonable to conclude that since private foundations produced the Flexner report and brought about its implementation in the first half of the century, these foundations should be concerned with correcting the report's defects and the undesirable consequences emerging in the last half of the century.

In developing this program, Chapman planned to deal with the entire university and not with its medical school alone. A Fund-supported survey in 1974 examined educational experiments at Brown University, the University of Chicago, Columbia University, Duke University, the Universities of California at San Diego and at San Francisco, and Washington University in St. Louis, to discover potential recipients of grants through this new approach.[8] This survey revealed that the climate for converting barriers to working relationships was gradually becoming more favorable and advised the Fund to support medical schools associated with universities, with the assumption that institutions already related could be led to work together more closely. The ideal programmatic structure was far from clear, however, and there was certain to be plenty of objection, mostly from powerful (and in Chapman's opinion, hide-bound) departmental chairmen. In discussing the Fund's concerns, Chapman routinely tried to assuage their fears by emphasizing the Fund's primary interest in improving the quality of the student's entire university education, and he would refer them to an article by Michael Simpson: "To devise a system which will consistently and significantly enhance the student's learning and create the sort of doctors our community really needs—that is the real challenge we are only beginning to meet. Our system of values will need to change. For example, we still consistently overvalue poor research and semi-literate publication; again, partly because quantity, in number of publications, is easier to measure than quality."[9]

At the board of directors' meeting in February 1975, Chapman proposed assembling a group of the nation's most able experts in higher education, including medical education, who would be aware of major defects and the urgency of correcting them. Over the next few months, a concrete program would be developed for presentation to the board. Chapman specified what he believed to be the program's important features:

1. The primary grantee would probably be the private university with a medical school.
2. A consortium of five to ten institutions of high quality or potential should be established as grantees. In selecting the recipients, Chapman did not propose to stage an open competition. Instead, consultants would help the Fund to identify those institutions most likely to participate successfully.
3. An institution's progress would be monitored and evaluated from the beginning.
4. Over several years, the program would have the effect of committing the Fund to the support of a relatively small number of major projects in higher education.
5. While the program's unifying theme would be some version of what Chapman called the Interface Program, its ultimate design must mobilize analytic talent within the best universities. Although it should not be part of the Fund's purpose to tell each institution what to do in detail, there must be agreement on realizable educational goals.

In closing his presentation to the board, Chapman pointed out that this approach was being developed within a few outstanding institutions. It was capable of producing a profound improvement in education for medicine in all of its premedical phases. It was also capable of undoing some of the negative effects of the Flexner report without eliminating its positive influence. And, finally, an Interface Program could exert constructive influences within higher education that would go far beyond matters pertaining to medicine or health. What Chapman was proposing was not total withdrawal from all the activities the Fund had considered worthwhile in the past but commitment of a large proportion of the Fund's annual income to a new program. Although all prior commitments would be honored, supporting the Interface Program would necessitate temporary or permanent withdrawal from some projects, including excursions into health-care delivery and behavioral problems in society.

The Board of Directors' Response

Most of the board members approved of Chapman's recommendations, but his proposal opened the way for lively discussion.[10] Lewis M. Branscomb felt that the time was right for an approach to the problems of medical education. The federal budget for the current year had reduced research funds, both for the activities of the National Institutes of Health and for the educational component of the National Science Foundation. To him, it seemed that the federal government was turning away from medical programs, pursuing the policy in effect since the beginning of the Nixon administration. Branscomb felt that this paucity of federal funds gave the activities of foundations even greater importance, and Chapman's proposal offered considerable leverage in bringing about institutional change—unlike many projects that, although worthwhile in themselves, did not have any fundamental effect on a system or an institution. Enough progress had already occurred to indicate that the system could permit knowledge to move freely between scientists in university and medical school science departments. Branscomb felt that the system's real problem was its definition of a "medical doctor." What are the appropriate credentials for a physician? Is the process of acquiring these credentials one way in which the training of doctors contributes to the welfare of society? And what about other types of medical professionals? In the mid-1970s, the choice of medical careers was limited, and the university structure implied that the student in the biomedical sciences was going to become either a basic scientist, a medical doctor, a nurse, or one of a very few other medical professionals. Branscomb felt that students in the biomedical sciences should have a far wider variety of choices and very different kinds of backgrounds, including, in some cases, financial and business training.

All these factors made the barrier between the medical school and the university—and, by implication, a complete perspective on these institutions—the appropriate target for the Fund's efforts. Since credentials are an educational institution's essential output, and the prime concern of students, the Fund should be examining the credentials necessary for both institutions to produce people with a variety of skills in the biomedical sciences. Branscomb characterized Chapman's proposal as considerably broader than any program the Fund had ever tackled—no less than an attempt to redefine medical education.

Calvin H. Plimpton advised the rest of the board to give Chapman every encouragement, and additional support came from board member

Robert J. Glaser. It was crucial that medicine emphasize human biology, Plimpton thought, so that education in biology and the other sciences could be brought within the sphere of the humanities. Chapman's enthusiasm for the plan was the vital element for its undertaking; practical proposals needed to implement it would follow. Others asked probing questions, but any dissent was gentle, limited to the observation that university faculties were notorious for their ability to impede innovation.

Chapman replied that he recognized the problems ahead. He was well aware that programs to reform medical education tend, sooner or later, to revert to dead center. Even worse, concepts are distorted, plans go awry. Flexner himself was disappointed at the perversion of his ideas, but his angry denunciations came too late; many aspects of the Western Reserve experiment ultimately disappointed even its chief supporter, Thomas Hale Ham. Chapman wanted to persevere, nevertheless, with a program that would repair the damage to the student's education at the premedical and preclinical levels and diversify the "standard product" of preclinical medical education.

The Interface Program Underway

This new endeavor represented a fundamental alteration in the structure of the Fund's overall program. Chapman understated the extent of the change in June 1975, when his introduction to the Annual Report alerted Fund-watchers to a "modest focusing and redirection of the program now in progress."[11] He did not specify the nature of the shift, partly because the program was still in its formative stages, but mainly because a unique feature of the program was the Fund's refusal to dictate the precise direction of revision. Its intention to allow each school to develop a unique pattern was entirely characteristic of the Fund's past dealings with universities.[12]

The Fund's staff had approached several universities that were planning or actually executing changes at the juncture of premedical and medical education. The result was two proposals to the Fund, one from the University of Rochester and the other from University of Chicago. In November 1975 Rochester was awarded the first grant under the Interface Program, and Chicago's program was approved when the board met the following May.

These programs both proposed to unify the educational experience of the two final years of the baccalaureate period and the first two years of medical school instruction without reducing the time between graduation from high school and the awarding of the medical degree. Both allowed students to switch easily to nonmedical graduate programs at various points in the sequence, and both intended to provide abundant exposure to the humanities and behavioral sciences. To emphasize the integrity of the educational process, the Fund broke tradition by designating as beneficiary the institution as a whole rather than its medical school and by giving responsibility for each program's success to the university's chief executive officer.

Eventually, seven institutions received support under the Interface Program: the University of Chicago, the University of Rochester, Boston University, Brown University, Duke University, Dartmouth College and Medical School, and the Johns Hopkins University. The awards were all substantial, spanning at least three years; an additional two years of support would be possible if the program was progressing satisfactorily. Two other institutions not considered an official part of the Interface Program—the City College of the City University of New York and the University of California at San Diego—also made Fund-supported contributions to integrated premedical and preclinical education.

The Interface Universities

THE UNIVERSITY OF ROCHESTER

The Commonwealth Fund had already made a substantial long-term investment in medical education at Rochester, which it considered a well-managed institution.[13] Institutional strength was a sine qua non for the Interface project, since far-reaching changes would inevitably bring problems, including opposition from some quarters. The Fund's staff believed that Rochester's record of cooperation between administration and faculty, its dedication to rigorous education, and its sound financial planning made it an excellent candidate for the first commitment under the Interface Program.

The key problems identified by Rochester's faculty were common throughout the nation's institutions: The college and the medical school operated separate and, to some extent, overlapping departments and faculties in the biomedical sciences, and these strong, independent departments interacted only sporadically in the total educational process. Students admitted to the School of Medicine faced two years of preclinical science so intensive and tightly scheduled that they were forced to abandon most earlier interests abruptly, especially in the humanities and social sciences. In the College of Arts and Sciences, students heading for medical school tended to pursue a highly standardized curriculum in the premedical sciences, dictated largely by medical-school admissions requirements. Many faculty members also agreed that the first six years of education for medicine were poorly sequenced and redundant. They focused upon many aspects of science unrelated to the needs of future physicians and lacked integration with other university offerings. In addition, although a large percentage of undergraduates declared themselves "premedical," only a small proportion of those qualified for medical school were admitted. Facing a highly competitive period of undergraduate study, premedical students tended to avoid challenging courses in the humanities that might endanger the high grades needed for admission to medical school. The heavy concentration in the natural sciences characteristic of the most commonly pursued premedical curriculum left many students at an academic disadvantage if they failed to gain admission to medical school, but counseling to increase an appreciation of alternative health careers and encourage a more flexible pattern of study was inadequate at most institutions. Ironically, the intensive science courses that medical schools demanded left too many students disillusioned with the entire scientific enterprise—whether they won or lost the medical school admissions contest.

To lead premedical students to the broader goal of a "liberal education," a committee of sixty faculty members at the University of Rochester proposed changes that would completely reorder the sequence of education for medicine. The first step was a pilot program, which envisioned the eight years of preparation for the medical degree as a two-four-two sequence (see fig. 31).

The first two years would be spent in the college, where students would be counseled about the many careers available in the health field and the way in which they might be pursued at Rochester. Four subsequent years would include what was then called "premedical and preclinical education," but which in the Rochester plan would be an individually planned but unified program in the biomedical sciences, with additional concentration on the behavioral sciences, humanities, and social sciences; and, as in the traditional model, the two final years would be devoted to study of the clinical disciplines.

Rather than grafting new programs onto present ones, the Rochester plan proposed a transition to a different pattern of education for medicine. Students interested in health careers would be given a broad range of choices and intensive counseling; all university schools, including nursing and engineering, would cooperate in developing courses, coordinating schedules, and planning career options. The faculty was also considering the idea of revising the current qualifications for admission to the School of Medicine.

A pilot group of sixteen students would enter the middle four years of this experimental curriculum in September 1976, at the end of their sophomore year at the college. Their admission to the University of Rochester School of Medicine would obviate the anxiety and competitive pressure that was the traditional lot of premedical students. Each student could elect to qualify for a M.A. or M.S. degree, which would be awarded at the end of the four-year sequence (six years after matriculation). Others would simply take a B.S. or B.A. degree. The crucial point was that the longer, integrated sequence of education for medicine—with admission to medical school out of the way—would permit a more flexible education and leave students at no academic disadvantage if, at the bachelor's or master's degree level, they chose another career.

From the outset the Fund's concept of improvement in medical education focused on quality, not length or even cost. Yet the Fund's staff could not imagine that the new plan should be any more expensive than the existing one, once the costs of the transition had been met. The staff recommended a total grant of $2,058,000 to the University of Rochester for the first thirty-month period.

A major portion of these funds would pay for the time of faculty in developing and implementing the plan. Other large budget items included summer support for College of Arts and Sciences faculty involved in the plan; participation of faculty in the new counseling effort; central administration, including large parts of the time of various deans; instructional materials, travel, and consultations; and evaluation.

All parties agreed that this last item was crucial to the plan's development and its potential effect. An objective evaluation was the most difficult task facing both the university and the Fund, requiring vigilance during the entire transition period to ensure that problems and shortcomings would be identified quickly and the plan revised accordingly. Rochester's request to the Fund included a substantial sum for the university's own evaluation, but the Fund's staff also provided for independent assessment at all stages to complement as well as to verify the university's efforts. The success of the experiment would ultimately be judged by the peer review of the medical-education community itself, and the Fund's staff selected respected national figures in the fields of medical and science education who were willing to provide a continuing evaluation of the Fund's entire Interface Program.

A particularly thorough scrutiny of all aspects of the plan would take place toward the end of the thirty-month grant period. Final support of the plan's development was contingent upon evidence of genuine progress. If Rochester seemed unable to continue the plan, the school would not request renewal and would return any balance of the Fund's initial grant. If the plan was successful, at the end of the five-year developmental phase the university would be prepared to continue its support from university resources, which were being budgeted for the purpose.

By 1977, 31 college sophomores from the University of Rochester had been admitted to the School of Medicine through the Rochester Early Selection (or so-called 2–4–2) Program. Irving Spar, the administrator at Rochester in charge of the program, discussed the selection process: "We tried not to accept the anxious student who just wanted an early acceptance into medical school. We selected the students on the basis of their ability to take advantage of the medical school courses earlier and interdigitate them with an undergraduate degree or a master's degree. The student who wants an early acceptance in his back pocket is often not imaginative enough to work out an interesting 2–4–2 program."[14]

The faculty developed and taught fifty new interdepartmental courses related to education for medicine and considered thirty-five of them good enough to keep. These courses were open to all students in the university. Cooperation between the basic sciences department at the School of Medicine and the biology department at the College of Arts and Sciences also led to a program allowing students to obtain an undergraduate bachelor's degree in the biological sciences while emphasizing a biological subspecialty. While some of the subspecialties were conventional within the biology department—molecular genetics and population genetics, for example—others were more traditionally associated with the medical school—such as biochemistry, microbiology, and the neurosciences.

From this increased cooperation between medical school and undergraduate college came the Bridge Fellowship Program, which developed a group of faculty with skills in more than one discipline. The long-term hope was for a network of faculty members who could act as conduits of information, values, and concerns across departments and colleges, throughout the entire university. Spar believed that this program was an even more important use of Commonwealth Fund money than the Early Selection Program: "Bridging started only because of the new courses that made it possible for the faculty to get to know each other. It's something you can't mandate; it's something that has to evolve."[15]

Similarly, a new university format, dubbed the "cluster system," had begun informally, with Commonwealth Fund seed money paying for a few dinners for faculty members and outside speakers. The success of these meetings of groups of faculty with common research and teaching interests eventually made their standing more formal. Departments still had primary administrative power, and responsibilities were divided among departments and deans, but the clusters helped to determine which new degree programs and courses were needed, which departments and colleges should teach them and to which students, and which departments should recruit new faculty to handle the added load. Clusters were consulted in actual recruitment of new faculty as well. Their interdisciplinary, interdepartmental character was intended to allow the university to plan programs that spanned several colleges; examine the entire six years of education for medicine as a continuum, eliminating duplication and overlap; and in other ways influence use of the university's resources as a whole. Clusters in genetics and aging were already operating at the university, and other clusters were planned in behavioral sciences in medicine (important for students in medicine, engineering, education, and management);

bioethics (which had received a strong expression of interest from about three dozen faculty members throughout the university); and bioengineering. Spar was part of a committee of four or five that met every week, eleven months of the year, to develop new ideas and participants for clusters. Some clusters died, others were able to obtain outside funding, and some developed degree programs that were incorporated into the University's system.

Two years after receiving its initial grant from the Commonwealth Fund, the university obtained a renewal of $1,500,000, which extended from June 1977 through June 1980.[16]

The university's request for continuation of the grant argued that several new clusters, then in the talking and planning stage, could broaden the Interface Program at Rochester before it was consolidated. The most important new cluster, the one for which the university sought most of the support, would reform the university's entire approach to teaching biology. The proposal stated the problem succinctly:[17]

> Traditionally, human biology has been the province of physicians and surgeons in training. . . . Preclinical faculty in the Medical School have concentrated on teaching medical and graduate students with almost no involvement in teaching undergraduates. Most faculty in the biology department, who are primarily modern molecular, cellular and developmental biologists, have not been interested in offering . . . courses in human and mammalian biology. . . . Premedical undergraduates need the opportunity to acquire knowledge concerning the function of the human body. Nursing undergraduates should have more comprehensive courses in this area. . . . This phenomenon is not confined to the University of Rochester. Biology majors from other leading schools also have the same narrow background. . . . [Human biology] should be available to those bound for careers in social sciences, management, chemistry, engineering and health professions.

The university had set up a committee to devise the best possible programs in human and mammalian biology that the university's resources could provide for undergraduate and graduate students. The committee's chairman was the new provost of the university; the committee comprised the heads of the departments of biology, biochemistry, physiology, microbiology, radiation biology and biophysics, and psychology, and the head of the Center for Brain Research. The curriculum they designed called upon all resources of the university, especially those of the medical-school departments, which had not been available for teaching undergraduate biology. More than 160 faculty members throughout the university were teaching some aspect of the biological sciences—to undergraduates, graduate students, medical students, nursing students, graduate physicians, engineers, and so forth. A cluster in this area was intended to use faculty talent coherently and economically.

The Fund was receptive to the university's request for a final one-year grant of $402,240. The Fund's staff was pleased to see the university promoting the Interface Program's strong supporters. Key administrative appointments showed the university's commitment to the Interface Program and presaged progress in the next few years. From July 1980 through June 1981, the university would complete the difficult task of eliminating activities and courses superseded by the Rochester Plan. Much of the Fund's support would compensate the university for released time of faculty developing the clusters. In addition, the grant would help faculty members requiring technical assistance for courses in the sciences and engineering. To complete the Fund's support of Rochester's program, the board of directors approved a grant of $350,000 for a final year.

The program succeeded, according to Spar, because its administrators were always aware of the Damoclean sword that hung over them: the end of the Fund's grant.[18]

> Everything was set up so that when the Commonwealth money was gone, they could continue with a small amount of university money. . . . Miriam Rock, associate dean of the college of art and sciences, and I, being administrators, were always aware of budgets—college budgets and university budgets—and therefore, as we planned things, planned for the future. . . . I think our attitude was much different from that of a faculty member in this position. . . . Uppermost in our minds was the idea that "some day, somebody's going to have to eat this." None of us wanted to commit ourselves to the idea that other medical schools with similar programs would accept our Early Selection students. All this took place in the days of the mandated increase in third-year students by the federal government, students from the Caribbean medical schools. Many medical schools are limited in the number of clinical students they can train, and if the government mandated a 5 percent increase there was no way we could guarantee another school that we could accept a few more of their students. We had to protect our capitation money at the expense of the Interface Program.

The Early Selection Program itself did not require a large outlay of university money, and the end of the Commonwealth Fund's grant did not jeopardize the program. The admissions committee agreed to accept sophomores from the undergraduate campus, who could devise their own programs and take advantage of the educational opportunities between the two campuses. Unlike programs at other universities, this plan did not mean a loss of students (and student revenue) to the home school, as the only students accepted into the program were already at the university. When new courses were devised, departments did not have to hire biochemists or microbiologists but could "buy" a little of the time of medical-school faculty. The program also spilled over into the university's nonmedical segments: When students destined for a career in law, for example, felt that they were not getting the full benefit of advisory services, Rochester was forced to build up the counseling program for students in other parts of the university.

Spar said, "I think the program is continuing not only because of our planning, but because the university is putting some of its resources into it. . . . The university saw it had a good thing. Furthermore, the program will help in the university's competitiveness for undergraduate students in the future."[19] The program's final report in February 1982 expressed continued satisfaction with its accomplishments.[20]

THE UNIVERSITY OF CHICAGO

The plan developed by the University of Chicago's Pritzker School of Medicine and presented to the Fund's board in May 1976 extended a program already underway.[21] The three issues it addressed were the same ones that had concerned the faculty at the University of Rochester: the content and sequence of the basic sciences as they were taught at most colleges and medical schools, the role of the humanities and social sciences in the education of physicians and other health professionals, and the imbalance between the number of students pursuing premedical studies in college and the number admitted to medical school.

Responsible for organizing the proposal presented to the Fund was the University of Chicago Program Supervisory Committee, which included representatives of the basic natural sciences, clinical sciences, social sciences, and humanities. This committee's responsibilities also included recommending policy regarding admission of students and evaluation of the program, and initiating course development and implementation. The proposal had the support of a large cross-section of faculty and was approved in principle by groups in both the college and the medical school. Daniel C. Tosteson, head of the Division of the Biological Sciences, a university-wide unit responsible for teaching at both college and medical school, would be chief administrator of the proposed program. As a relatively new dean at the university and one with wide experience in medical education, Tosteson would have a large stake in the program's success.

The University of Chicago proposed to deal with the problem of coherence in traditional medical education by melding the final two years of college and the first two years of medical school into an integrated sequence (see fig. 31). Students interested in medicine and human biology would share their first two years in the college with other undergraduates in a sequence of general education; they could enter the program at the beginning of their third year and pursue a four-year sequence that integrated premedical, preclinical, and liberal arts studies. In this way the program would use the resources of the university rather than a highly specialized curriculum to combine the scientific and humanistic development of the student interested in human health.

The student's first two years in the program would meet the college's requirements for a B.A. degree, as well as introducing the substantial preclinical study usually provided in medical school. During these years students might decide to apply to a medical school other than the University of Chicago, leaving the program at the baccalaureate level. Others might simply terminate their formal education at this point. The faculty expected, however, that most students would apply for admission to Pritzker and continue in the program for an additional two years. They would then be ready for the two clinical years leading to the M.D. degree, either at Pritzker or at some other medical school. Others who completed the four-year program might elect to receive an M.S. degree in human biology and enter another branch of the health professions, or pursue the Ph.D. degree in one of the biological sciences. The variety of tracks open to students in the Chicago program would reduce the academic disadvantage to premedical students not admitted to medical school.

Unlike most universities, where the college of arts and sciences and the medical school maintained separate, often isolated, faculties in the biological sciences, the University of Chicago included all such faculty in its Division of the Biological Sciences, which was responsible for teaching at both the college and the Pritzker School of Medicine. The approach proposed by the University of Chicago was in many respects similar to that already being implemented at the University of Rochester. But the Fund's staff believed that combining Chicago's biological sciences into a single division would improve all science education at the university, including the sciences most relevant to medicine.

Faculty of this division had developed an array of new courses for the science component of the four-year program. The basic, or premedical, sciences were linked with the preclinical sciences in a sequence that eliminated redundancy. Because the science component of the four-year program served students preparing for careers in human biology and other health professions as well as those preparing for medicine, new courses stressed science in itself, not some conception of the basic sciences as an adjunct to medical education. Human Genetics, Evolution, Human Morphology, Pharmacology-Physiology, and the Biology of Diseases were among the new courses that constituted the science core of the four-year program. Some replaced courses, such as Gross Anatomy, that were traditionally taught at the medical school; others replaced courses taught at the college.

The roster of new courses was designated the Liberal Arts of Biology and Medicine (LABM). Each student in the four-year program, whether headed for medical school or for some other health-related or scientific career, was required to take eight of these courses, fulfilling certain requirements for the college's B.A. degree and obtaining a broader view of the nature, opportunities, and obligations of a career in the health field. Because the medical school's clinical faculty had been involved in developing these courses and would cooperate in teaching them, students could grasp at an early stage the relevance of other disciplines to clinical medicine.

Other LABM courses included Philosophy and Medicine, Nature and Culture, and Ethical and Biological Aspects of the Control of Human Reproduction; and new courses planned included Human Behavior, Human Ecology, Socioeconomics of Medicine, and Ethical Issues in Biology and Medicine. LABM courses were to be opened to all University of Chicago students, not just those formally enrolled in the four-year program.

The program would begin as an optional track for students interested in human biology and medicine. At first, it would be conducted in parallel with the university's regular premedical and preclinical sequences. Although this approach was conservative, it reflected the justifiable desire of faculty to test and evaluate the ambitious group of new courses that must be developed, taught for the first time, and modified as a result of initial experience. Thirty students would be admitted to the program in the first year, forty-five in the second, and sixty in the third. Sixty students would be admitted each succeeding year, until the program's four years contained a total of 240 students. The Pritzker School was committed to accepting a minimum of twenty of these students into each of its classes. If the program was successful, the university would begin to replace its regular premedical-preclinical sequence with the new courses. The objective was to implement the new program fully in no more than six years.

While the program was being developed and evaluated for a limited cohort of students, the university would need additional faculty to teach the new courses that would run temporarily in parallel with existing ones. As the experimental program expanded to replace the existing premedical-preclinical sequence at both the medical school and the college, the faculty time required would subside to approximately previous levels. The number of faculty would eventually be reduced through attrition, returning to a level not higher than would have been reached by ordinary increments in the existing program. This expansion and reduction was a sine qua non of the Fund's involvement, and would be one requirement for renewal of Fund support.

The Fund's staff recommended a grant to the University of Chicago ASHUM (Program for Education in the Arts and Sciences Basic to Human Biology and Medicine) of $1,130,000 for the first year (July 1976 through June 1977) and $730,000 for the second (July 1977 through June 1978).

Less than six months into the program, Tosteson resigned to become dean of the Harvard Medical School. His successor at the University of Chicago, Robert B. Uretz, also supported the ASHUM program, but the change in leadership and the university's receipt of the award late in the academic year caused a year's delay in implementing the program, and expenditure of the grant was extended over three years instead of two.

ASHUM's class entered the program in September 1977 and finished its second year in May 1979. These students received their M.S. degrees in June 1981; some entered the clinical years of medical school in September 1981—an important benchmark, since clinical faculty were then in a position to pass judgment on ASHUM as preparation for this segment of medical school. Approximately half of the ASHUM students were not seeking the M.D. degree but wanted an integrated high-quality education in human biology, including access to courses—in such subjects as pathology, anatomy, physiology, and pharmacology—usually reserved for medical students but relevant to other career interests such as human ecology, public health and epidemiology, nutritional sciences, behavioral sciences, administration of health care, human genetics and genetic counseling, medical ethics, and public policy in health.

In 1979 the University of Chicago requested an additional three years of support: $800,000 for the first year, $650,000 for the second, and $500,000 for the third.[22] The renewal would support the released time of faculty who were developing and teaching new courses; the cost of replacing the old track with the new courses; the cost of recruiting new faculty; and the expense of minor laboratory renovations and equipment. This use of the grant would continue only during the first year of the renewal period. Other major expenses were administration, which included costs of ASHUM planning committees and time devoted to ASHUM by deans of the college and the biological sciences division; equipment and supplies required for the new courses, especially those that entailed extensive laboratory work; salaries of course assistants, who partially assumed the duties of faculty released for ASHUM work; and support for summer students.

The Fund's staff decided to recommend the ASHUM program for two years of support at the level requested, and a final year of support at a lower level.[23]

DUKE UNIVERSITY

Duke University opened its hospital and admitted its first medical students in 1930.[24] Forty-five years later its School of Medicine was accepting about 115 students each year and had a reputation for strength in the biomedical sciences. Also on the university campus was a school of nursing, a program for physicians' assistants, and a school of engineering that concentrated on biomedical engineering and the biosciences. Trinity College, Duke's division of arts and sciences, was a nationally important site for premedical education, the only institution in the southeastern United States that provided more than 100 entrants each year to American medical schools. The physical proximity of Trinity College to the School of Medicine and the traditional interest of both schools in curricular innovation made Duke a prime candidate for a program to improve the continuum of education for medicine.

Departure from the standard medical school curriculum began at Duke in 1966, supported by a $750,000 grant from the Fund. Instead of following the usual two years of basic medical-science courses with two years of clinical science and electives, the Duke University School of Medicine offered the following sequence:

Year I: Required courses in all of the basic medical sciences, including gross anatomy, microscopic anatomy, biochemistry, genetics, human behavior, microbiology, neuroanatomy, neurophysiology, pathology, pharmacology, and physiology.
Year II: Clinical training in medicine, surgery, obstetrics-gynecology, psychiatry, and pediatrics spanning five terms, each eight weeks long.
Year III: Electives in the basic sciences, including options for special study in interdisciplinary areas such as endocrinology and virology.
Year IV: Electives in the clinical sciences.

The faculties of the school of medicine and Trinity College had initiated discussions about improving the early years of medical education even before the Fund became involved. Their concerns paralleled the problems identified at Rochester and Chicago. Duke's proposal to the Fund outlined further deficiencies of the existing system:

—Premedical faculty at Trinity College in such subjects as chemistry and biology worked in isolation from basic biomedical scientists in the School of Medicine; collaboration and communication were limited.
—Alternative career opportunities related to medicine often were not well-developed and were not presented to premedical students as reasonable, attractive alternatives.
—The university offered other students—for example, those preparing for law, business, and engineering—too few opportunities to learn about the biomedical sciences.

Duke University proposed to treat the entire sequence leading to education in the clinical sciences as a university responsibility, a cooperative effort between faculties in the medical school and the college. Key faculty members and administrators seemed ready to make the concessions in departmental prerogatives needed for success. The proposal was approved overwhelmingly by Trinity College's Undergraduate Faculty Council and by the medical school's Advisory Board; it had the enthusiastic sponsorship of Duke's vice-president for health affairs, William G. Anlyan; and Duke's president, Terry Sanford, assured the Fund's staff and consultants that the university's senior administration was behind the plan. Duke asked the Fund to contribute support for starting costs and for the expenses of the transitional years.

First, the faculties of the medical school and of Trinity College planned to examine the content and sequence of science courses offered to students during the traditional four premedical and two preclinical years. Some of the courses might no longer be necessary, but, more important, some might be restructured so that students could take them in different sequences. Duplication in course content could be eliminated; certain physical sciences and mathematics courses could be oriented to the needs of students preparing for medicine; new courses could be developed to reflect advances in neurobiology, genetics, and other fields of central importance to the biomedical sciences.

The medical school's Department of Biochemistry was already cooperating with Trinity College departments to offer a shorter chemistry sequence for premedical students. Greater emphasis on biochemistry and increased laboratory work would open up the crowded preclinical years of medical school by enabling students to satisfy the medical school's requirement in biochemistry while they were still undergraduates. Similar streamlining and reorganization of premedical and preclinical sequences were planned in mathematics, physics, biology, and cell biology, but crucial to these developments was the willingness of departmental chairmen in the medical school to augment their programs at the college level.

New courses and sequences of courses in the biological and basic medical sciences were also being planned or were actually in progress— particularly in molecular biology, cell and developmental biology, and the neurosciences. All these courses would be available to premedical students, permitting a flexible and more relaxed six-year sequence of medical education. Cooperation between the Department of Zoology at Trinity College and the departments of anatomy, physiology, and pathology in the School of Medicine, for instance, had produced a course entitled "Structure and Function of Tissues and Organs." Traditionally, Duke's Department of Zoology had taught cell biology to undergraduates; this new course would meet the needs of advanced students in cell biology but would also satisfy the medical school's preclinical requirement in microanatomy.

Another part of the plan enabled faculty to use the increased flexibility of the premedical-preclinical sequence to introduce courses in humanities, social sciences, and behavioral sciences for students headed for medical careers. Restoration of the "liberal arts" to the years of medical education would ultimately depend on new attitudes signaled by the medical school's admissions committee and by Duke's premedical student advisors. New courses in the liberal arts at Duke would focus on the role of professionals and the professions in society, and on the institutional settings in which health-care professionals practice.

Trinity College had traditionally stressed independent study for undergraduates under the guidance of faculty advisors. Duke's new plan would extend independent study for premedical students. Like the Interface programs at Rochester and Chicago, the Duke plan allowed certain students to be admitted provisionally to the medical school while they were still sophomores or juniors at the university's college of arts and sciences. At Duke, however, the early admission option would proceed as part of the independent study program. At any point in their undergraduate careers, premedical students at Trinity College might propose individualized plans of study spanning their premedical and preclinical years. If a plan was approved by the undergraduate faculty, it would be reviewed by the medical school's admissions committee. Each year, the committee would guarantee fifteen students admission to Duke's medical school— pending satisfactory completion of the premedical phase of the student's study plans. The students accepted in this way might pursue premedical and preclinical study as a continuous integrated sequence, with the increased flexibility and relaxation attendant upon long-range planning. Curricular plans devised and carried out by these students were expected to provide insight into the variety and potential of many new premedical-preclinical sequences.

This increased flexibility would place increased demands on the university's system of counseling students, but career planning was already well-developed at Duke. As part of the proposed plan, the Office of Advisors for the Health Professions would be strengthened by permanent advisors from the physical and biological sciences who could call upon a network of faculty advisors from Trinity College and the School of Medicine.

A portion of the grant requested by Duke released the time of faculty involved in implementation of the plan. Other support would permit the university to hire faculty in the humanities and social sciences to develop and teach new courses integral to the plan. As with the earlier Fund grants to the Universities of Rochester and Chicago, some overlap of new courses with existing courses was necessary while the new curriculum was being developed. In addition, support would be given to departments asked to begin extensive teaching outside their usual duties. The Fund clearly designated such support for the transition, and not for the continuing costs of the program.

Overall administration of the plan would be the responsibility of Anlyan and Frederic N. Cleaveland, provost of the university, who would report directly to the president and chancellor. An advisory committee of twelve faculty and three senior administrators would monitor the plan, directing all program activities related to health education and the health sciences, identifying and developing new projects, and recommending certain budget allocations. A subcommittee appointed by the university's administration would nominate the program's day-to-day director or directors, and the Committee for Health Science Education would conduct all the program's services concerned with advising students. This committee would represent Trinity College and the engineering, medical, and nursing schools.

Full implementation of the plan, including the phase-out of some existing courses and material, was expected to require about five years. New courses and faculty would be fully established by that time, and a reasonable initial evaluation of the plan completed. Duke administrators assured the Fund that the university would then be prepared to continue the program under its regular budget. In accordance with policy, the Fund's staff recommended a three-year appropriation representing the maximum available to Duke during that period: $2,800,000.

Duke's proposal included plans to evaluate the new program at each step. The Fund would select its own consultants as well,[25] and it was made clear to university officials that the opinion of these consultants would weigh heavily in the Fund's decision about renewal of the grant.

Duke's expenditure of its initial grant began July 1, 1977; the three-year grant would end on June 30, 1980. In October 1979, the University requested an additional two years of support.

On the positive side, Duke had organized a concentration in Science, Society and Human Values that was expected to attract many premedical students who did not want to major in the sciences. Another new major, in biology, brought together the offerings of Duke's departments of zoology and botany. Most universities had instituted this type of a major long ago, but at Duke the change was important because it could not be accomplished easily. Duke had also instituted a useful program enabling about sixty students to work in hospital wards and emergency rooms as "Health Careers Volunteers." Its system of independent study had progressed, and it offered greater opportunities for undergraduates to work with medical school faculty.

Yet these developments could not be considered a substitute for essential curricular reform. Although Duke had developed several entirely new courses in the basic medical sciences during the past two and one-half years, disagreements between the college's Department of Chemistry and the medical school's Department of Biochemistry about granting medical school credit for courses in college biochemistry seemed to Fund staff and consultants a symbol of the problems impeding Duke's progress. Duke's program of guaranteed admission to medical school—and the programs of other universities participating in the Interface Program—also started and remained small, and the highly qualified Committee on Health Science Education was not permitted to identify the early-selection candidates without a second screening by the medical school's admissions committee.

The Fund's staff nevertheless found evidence of sustained, vigorous, and still-increasing faculty attention to the themes and objectives of the Interface Program. Every facet of the premedical and preclinical educational sequence had been analyzed by faculty groups. Faculty cooperation between Trinity College and other university components was everywhere evident. Many younger faculty members were enthusiastic about possible changes, and two of Duke's top administrative positions were taken by new appointees with long-standing commitment to the success of the Interface Program. Opposition to parts of the Duke plan—significant three years ago—was far less. In short, the Fund found in Duke's Interface Program a mixture of achievement and disappointed expectations, of intense concern and lack of concrete accomplishment.[26]

The Fund's staff approved the renewal of support to Duke University, and the board of directors awarded a one-year grant of $750,000 (for July 1980 through June 1981).

BOSTON UNIVERSITY

The sum requested by Boston University was modest compared with the grants to Rochester, Chicago, and Duke, as Boston University's Interface Program represented a carefully negotiated reduction in scope and budget.[27] Boston University's Modular Curriculum emphasized improvement in the quality and flexibility of the education offered to students preparing for health careers. It also addressed directly the need for cooperation between liberal arts and preclinical faculty in dealing with the final two years of college and the first two years of medical school.

The plan would continue the direction taken in 1961, when the University inaugurated its Six-Year Combined Liberal Arts-Medical Education Program, a Fund-supported, nationally recognized prototype that generated a series of fourteen variations at other institutions.[28] About fifty students were admitted to the entire B.A.–M.D. sequence directly out of high school each year; this admission entailed acceptance to the medical school. Students spent two years, including two summers, in the College of Liberal Arts, followed by four years in the School of Medicine. Their achievements in both segments of the accelerated program had been consistently excellent, and the attrition rate was extremely low. Summer study by six-year students reduced the length of the program by about one-tenth, from seventy-three to sixty-six months.

The university's early statements about the program indicated its intent both to accelerate the college–medical school sequence and to integrate its liberal arts and biomedical sciences components. In practice, however, the acceleration had been achieved by compression of the college years, while the medical school years had continued, for the most part, in the classic four-year pattern. The plan was an "accelerated" program with overlapping components, rather than a "shortened" or "integrated" one. Its most important achievement had been the convincing demonstration that able students could be selected after high school and educated to the medical-degree level in six years. Boston University's success in choosing these students raised serious questions about the assumptions and procedures of standard medical school admissions committees.

The current proposal would enable Boston University to take the next step, by turning to genuine integration of the liberal arts and preclinical components of medical education. John I. Sandson, dean of the medical school, proposed that the medical school and liberal arts faculties cooperate in developing teaching units of what was then segregated as either "premedical" or "preclinical" education. These "modules" would be offered to students in a flexible four-year sequence, spanning the last two college and the first two medical school years.

This approach was intended to lessen the current sharp division between college and medical school courses, between the years designated for the natural and social sciences and those designated for the "biomedical" sciences. It would lead to a reexamination of the quality and sequence of all the educational components offered to students working toward the M.D. degree or other health careers. Students who chose to study one of the preclinical sciences during the college years would open up the congested first and second years of medical school. They would benefit from a longer, less pressured period in which to develop understanding of the sciences related to their future medical careers and be exposed to medical school faculty before making a final decision about whether or not to seek the M.D. degree. By completing one-fourth of medical school's first-year courses before entering medical school itself, students would also have eased their transition. Finally, the "premedical syndrome" of competition for high grades, approval of instructors, and superiority over other premedical students would be relieved.

"Modules," defined units of instruction being developed jointly by liberal arts and medical school faculties, included Biochemistry, Cell Biology, Psychology, Microbiology, Histology, the Socio-Medical Sciences, Humanities, and Epidemiology. At the start, 100 students would be admitted to the Modular Curriculum track each year. These students, identified during the sophomore year in the college, would for the next four years pursue a combined premedical-preclinical sequence of great flexibility, based upon their individual selection of modules. Modules would be offered repeatedly during each year, allowing for reduced class size, more intensive laboratory work, and adaptability in sequence of study.

A substantial number of such students were to be admitted to the Boston University School of Medicine at the same time they were admitted to the four-year Modular Curriculum. Although the premedical students were the obvious beneficiaries, the new program was intended to improve the quality of science education for all students, regardless of whether they continued through the medical school years at Boston University or continued their education elsewhere.[29] Students who entered the new curriculum, starting with their third college year, might elect to take a B.A. degree at the end of two years and apply to another medical school, or they might choose to pursue another health-related or scientific career.

The proposed Modular Curriculum was intended not as a replacement for the university's six-year program, but as a complement. Most students admitted to the new program would earn the B.A. and M.D. degrees in either seven or eight years, but the modules would be open to students in the six-year track as well.

One possibility was to open basic medical science courses to the program's college juniors and seniors. Medical school faculty would not, however, take the risk of examining the entire content and organization of the basic medical science courses unless the proposed new courses were first conducted as an "experiment," in parallel with the regular ones—a conservative approach that the Fund recognized as simply a fact of life in medical education. Boston University therefore proposed entirely new courses for college juniors and seniors in most of the basic medical sciences, social sciences, and humanities related to medical education. Yet if the integration sought by the Modular Curriculum was achieved, as had been the acceleration sought by the six-year program, the university had to face the problem of combining the best features of the two tracks. Willingness to act upon the implications of success in both programs was a condition of the Fund's support beyond its initial grant.

The Fund had invested $2,007,500 in Boston University's six-year program between 1955 and 1971. The university now requested $1,034,621 for development and operation of the Modular Curriculum during the twenty-eight months beginning March 1, 1977. The chief requirement was support for released time of faculty who would develop the new modules. The Fund's board approved Boston University's proposal at the requested levels of support.[30]

In February 1978 Boston University requested a second grant for support of its Modular Medical Integrated Curriculum (MMEDIC), as the program was then known. The request covered an additional three years of diminishing support for a total of $1,420,025.

By the time the Fund's board of directors met, the MMEDIC program had admitted two classes. In September 1978 a third class would be admitted and at the same time, the first class would enter the Boston University School of Medicine. Courses needed for the program had been restructured to reflect both modern knowledge of subject matter and the interests of future physicians, and most had been taught once, some twice. For example, in the regular curriculum of the medical school, all aspects of biochemistry were covered in a 110-hour course, squeezed into the first year along with about six other extremely difficult courses in the basic medical sciences.

Boston University's renewal request covered five main activities. First, the new courses, or modules, had to be evaluated. An executive committee and a Modular Academic Program Advisory Committee would oversee this effort. Next, because the first class of MMEDIC students would be entering medical school in September with many of their first-year requirements out of the way, a decision would have to be made about use of the resulting free time. Among the possibilities were advanced study of the basic medical sciences, early exposure to clinical work, research, continued study of the liberal arts, or simply unscheduled time. The important element in any final arrangement was some release from the overwork and unnecessary rigidity of the first-year curriculum. Third, several more modules were needed, especially in advanced physiology, gross anatomy, and the neurosciences. Additional modules were planned in the social sciences and humanities as they related to medicine. Fourth, "premedical" courses, especially biology and chemistry, would be evaluated in view of changes being made in the Modular Curriculum. Finally, continued support of the evaluation built into the MMEDIC program was requested for the medical school's Department of Socio-medical Sciences, which had a creditable record in its longitudinal studies of the six-year program.

In considering Boston University's initial proposal in 1976, the Fund's staff had been concerned with the university's refusal to enlarge the population of the demonstrably successful six-year program. With the development of the MMEDIC program, however, there were three "tracks" into the Boston University School of Medicine. Students might make a formal commitment to medical school after high school, after the sophomore year of college, or at the end of college. Boston University also allowed its six-year students the option of an additional year, so that programs of six, seven, or eight years were available. The variety of entry points and program lengths might be valuable features, but the university understood that three substantially independent tracks could not be operated permanently. The special courses developed for students in the MMEDIC program might prove superior to courses in the basic medical sciences then taught in the School of Medicine, and social sciences and humanities "modules" related to medicine might replace some courses in the College of Liberal Arts. Whatever the decisions about individual courses, eventually the relationship between the two special programs would have to be clarified.

The university requested a three-year grant from the Fund, but questions about the university's intentions remained unanswered, and the Fund's staff believed that university officials had to consider some bold possibilities:

1. Making the new modules in the basic medical sciences the standard courses in these disciplines for all premedical students and medical students who needed them.
2. Enlarging the MMEDIC program, with its early identification for medical school and flexible sequence of courses in the basic medical sciences, beyond the existing restriction to 15 students.
3. Raising the admittedly arbitrary limit on the number of students permitted to enter the School of Medicine through the six-year program.
4. Cooperating with other universities in the Interface Program to give students standard credits for medical school work completed in other colleges.
5. Adopting a common academic calendar for the College of Liberal Arts and the Medical School, at least for the overlapping years, as a tangible indication that faculties were prepared to make real concessions to achieve integration.

The Fund's staff recommended a renewal grant of $900,000, covering the two years from July 1979 through June 1981. A third and final grant might be considered if Boston University signified its willingness to make other difficult choices.[31]

BROWN UNIVERSITY

The Fund's support for Brown University began in 1960 during the University's earliest consideration of a medical sciences program and continued through 1972, when the school established a program granting the medical degree.[32] Its awards to Brown during that time totaled $2,030,000. The Interface Program at Brown capped a dozen years of university interest in integrating premedical with medical education, liberal arts in the college with professional education for medicine.

Brown was a college and graduate school with a single unified faculty and no professional schools. Education for medicine at Brown was a university program, run by a division of the biological and medical sciences that also included faculty from the departments of biology and zoology.

The Master of Medical Sciences (M.M.S.) Program, started at Brown in 1963, admitted students as college freshmen and directed them through an integrated, six-year curriculum that prepared them for the clinical or final two years of study for the M.D. degree. Brown did not offer the medical degree, but the quality of its M.M.S. program enabled graduates to transfer to medical schools with advanced standing. Candidates pursued a sequence of courses that stressed the humanities and social sciences, presentation of preclinical subjects over a longer period, and continuous student involvement with a single university faculty rather than with "premedical" and later "preclinical" faculties having different demands, standards, and attitudes.

When Brown added a year to the M.M.S. program, creating a full sequence leading to the M.D. degree, its affiliation with five hospitals (having on their staffs clinical faculty appointed by the university) made transition to the extended program essentially trouble-free.

Approximately 40 of the physicians graduated from Brown each year had pursued the seven-year B.A.–M.D. sequence (a total of 118 by 1977); another 20 had followed a regular premedical course at Brown or elsewhere and had entered Brown as freshman medical students. From this perspective, Brown's program could be called a 3–2–2 sequence, admitting two-thirds of its students as college freshmen and one-third as first-year medical students.

About 160 students applied to a medical school after their four years at Brown, and about 130 were admitted—an extremely high "success rate." Brown offered these regular premedical students a large variety of courses in the biological and other sciences. The multiplicity of courses resulted partly from the demands of the seven-year program, but partly from Brown's structure, which treated all medical teachers as university faculty, expected to concern themselves with all students.

Brown's Interface proposal differed substantially from the others already funded, as early admission of students to medical school had been an integral part of Brown's medical program for fifteen years. Brown's proposal dealt primarily with premedical education, the portion of the university that required modification and strengthening. It also addressed the familiar problems of premedical competitition, disjunctive courses, and narrow opportunities for students who were not accepted into medical school. Increased flexibility in the premedical sequence was part of the solution, but the key was improvement in the quality of university science education offered to all students, whether they were admitted to medical school or not. Brown's faculty agreed upon several new approaches:

1. A jointly taught, integrated sequence to replace the unstructured sequence of six courses in mathematics, applied mathematics, physics, biophysics, and physiology

2. A similar coordination of course work in organic chemistry, biochemistry, and molecular biology
3. A new premedical concentration in the neural sciences, integrating offerings in mathematics, psychology, applied mathematics, physics, and linguistics
4. Involvement of medical and other faculty in a sustained attempt to make effective communication part of the students' education from entry to college through the end of professional study
5. Cooperation of faculty from philosophy, religion, biology, and medicine in developing and extending Brown's program in biomedical ethics
6. A systematic course of study dealing with health-related behavior and organization of health care, bringing social sciences to the clinical setting

The faculty was obviously willing to examine the quality of education in the sciences. Members of the liberal arts faculty would reassert some control over premedical education and feel that they had some stake in it, and medical faculty would assume some responsibility for the serious issues and difficulties of premedical education: "This effort . . . should not result in a dilution of the scientific preparation for medical students, but in its strengthening. Meeting premedical requirements outside of the current ritualistic formula should . . . mean building an intellectual capital, instead of the exercise in futility it has too often become."[33]

Finally, Brown's proposal stated: "Brown can and should experiment with dismantling the traditional course requirements for admission to medical school, and restructuring them in an intellectually more effective manner; and Brown can give credence to this effort by liberalizing the admissions requirements for its own medical students, and allowing for experimentation in the college component of the seven-year continuum leading to the M.D. degree."[34]

Brown's vice-president for biology and medicine, Pierre M. Galletti, seemed prepared to extend the school in attacking the "premedical syndrome"—even to the point of simply dropping most of the standard requirements for admission to Brown's medical-education program. Operation of the program was to be the joint responsibility of Brown's vice president for biology and medicine and the dean of academic affairs; a full-time academic director would coordinate activities among university departments, organize an evaluation of the program, and pay special attention to teaching materials and other "exportable" elements of the experiment.

The university estimated that new activity during the initial years of the plan would require the equivalent of twelve full-time faculty the first year, eleven the second, and nine the third. The Fund's staff was willing to support 6.5 "full-time equivalent" faculty in the first year of the program, the same in the second, and 4.5 faculty in the third. Brown also required support for laboratory renovation, equipment and supplies to be used primarily in the proposed organic chemistry-biochemistry-physiology sequence. The Fund's staff recommended total three-year support of $1,200,000.

By 1983 Brown was convinced of the superiority of the "continuum approach" to medical education, in which "the challenges of scholarship—synthesis, creativity and discovery—are expected to supplement the more mundane demands associated with the survey course/test-passing mode which characterizes medical education today."[35] Almost 90 percent of the students admitted to Brown's program out of high school were graduating with a medical degree seven to eight years later. Brown planned to continue its program by dismantling standard medical school admissions requirements entirely, replacing them with an equally demanding set of individualized expectations.[36]

DARTMOUTH COLLEGE AND MEDICAL SCHOOL

A key proposition of the Fund's Interface Program was that science education, including education for medicine, could be improved if it was conducted as an integrated activity of the entire university. The advantages of this integration would be particularly evident at Dartmouth, where separate basic medical science departments were maintained on a shared campus by an amply funded college with strong departments in the natural and behavioral sciences and a small medical school having a total enrollment of less than 170.[37]

Until 1967 Dartmouth had a two-year medical program, which sent all students on to other medical schools for the M.D. degree. In May 1958 the Fund appropriated $1 million to strengthen this program and encourage its integration of three years of college (premedical education) with two years of medical school (preclinical education). Over the next eight years, Dartmouth moved toward the development of a full medical school; the Fund helped in February 1965 with $300,000 for establishment of a department of medicine. By 1966 Dartmouth's program was in the advanced stages of planning, and the university had decided to organize a "three-year" medical school, which would enable students to earn the M.D. degree and complete an internship within seven years after high school. In November 1968 the Fund awarded $750,000 for five-year support of the new school, which admitted its first students in 1970.

The "refounding" of the medical school at Dartmouth, which had not awarded a medical degree since 1914, was considered a major achievement by the Fund's staff, and they thought the money for its support (a total of $2,050,000 between 1958 and 1974) had been well spent. Yet Dartmouth had found it difficult to force the integration of the premedical and preclinical programs. After extended discussion among faculty (and an earlier proposal that did not satisfy the Fund's consultants), Dartmouth presented a workable plan. Dartmouth's proposal to the Fund in 1977 stated its problems and objectives: "Faculty members of the medical school and of the natural and behavioral science departments elsewhere in the university, despite their closely related scientific interests and activities, commonly interact with one another little more than they did in 1950 . . . a lack of close working relationships is likely to represent opportunities lost. . . . Through the concerted use of the total resources of the university, programs in instruction at all levels—undergraduate, graduate and professional school—can potentially be enriched and rendered more effective."[38]

The proposed approach had already been applied to Dartmouth's teaching program in biochemistry. Support from the Fund would enable refinement of this plan and its extension to other basic and preclinical science departments—a step rapidly becoming a necessity for the medical school.

Most universities in recent decades had increased the number of faculty members teaching biochemistry. Some universities maintained biochemistry departments both in the medical school and in the arts and sciences division; biochemists were also located in other basic science and clinical departments. Coordination of course offerings in biochemistry was usually informal, and the resulting courses were often of poor quality. At Dartmouth, resources had not been available to maintain an overlap; study of biochemistry beyond the introductory level was a medical school "preclinical" subject, unavailable to undergraduate students. In 1975 the medical school and the college developed an integrated, institution-wide "Program in Biochemistry," taught by all biochemists at Dartmouth and available equally to undergraduates, graduate students, and medical students. The program had four novel features:

—An undergraduate major in biochemistry. A Dartmouth College student who completed his work in this new major was automatically exempt from biochemistry work in the medical school and could use the released time in any other academic pursuit.
—A combined Ph.D.–M.D. program for medical students wanting to specialize in biochemistry.
—A program of graduate study leading to the Ph.D. degree in biochemistry.
—Advanced medical school courses for students who wished to go further in biochemistry.

In addition, a new basic course in biochemistry for all students replaced two introductory courses offered separately by the Department of Biochemistry and the Department of Biological Sciences, providing a foundation for a new series of intermediate and advanced courses. The school was able to alter the premedical-preclinical sequence substantially, as graduates of Dartmouth College represented about 40 percent of each medical-school class. Opening biochemistry to undergraduates was important, also, for those preparing for careers in the basic sciences, and in other health-related areas.

Relying heavily upon its experience with biochemistry, Dartmouth proposed further integrating college and medical-school efforts in environmental health, the neurosciences, genetics, and the social sciences and humanities. In addition to these major cooperative efforts, the Dartmouth program included an "internship" program for undergraduates, with opportunities outside the classroom for dealing with health-related problems; counseling of undergraduates interested in health careers by medical school faculty (a continuation of "experience-oriented" career counseling began in 1974 with a small grant from the Fund); and planning for an early admissions program.

Although site visits were standard procedure for evaluating requests under the Fund's Interface Program, the opinion of consultants was unusually important in this case: Carleton B. Chapman had left his position as dean of Dartmouth's medical school to become president of the Commonwealth Fund, and this close connection precluded his considering the proposal until the opinion of the consultants had been delivered.

The consultants agreed that if medical education at Dartmouth was to continue, it must draw upon the institution's full, unified strength in the sciences—an "interface" effort was mandatory. Walsh McDermott, a biomedical scientist, medical educator of national stature, and at the time Special Advisor to the president of the Robert Wood Johnson Foundation, wrote: "Dartmouth, unlike almost any other school, has a built-in motivation to make an interface-like activity go . . . a non-state-supported school in today's world cannot possibly hope to compete on an equal basis with the other quality medical schools. . . . It must become in some way unique . . . to have the spine and major structure of the science base of a medical school such an intimate part of the university as would be the case with a Commonwealth-supported interface program, would indeed make Dartmouth unique."[39] Consultants acknowledged the importance of Dartmouth's proposed activities in genetics, neurosciences, and environmental health, but stressed that like biochemistry, these activities would require strengthening. Fund support for Dartmouth should be focused on fortifying the basic sciences, and the university should incorporate at least the premedical-preclinical portions of medical education into the university at large.

John G. Kemeny, Dartmouth's president, and James C. Strickler, the dean of the medical school, were responsible for implementation of the overall plan. Like other institutions involved with the Fund's Interface Program, Dartmouth created a Council on Health Studies to represent the college and medical-school faculties in making major academic decisions about the plan. The council would review plans and accomplishments of the program, allocate resources according to program priorities, and recommend staffing consistent with college and medical-school personnel policies. Day-to-day operation of the plan was assigned to a program director.

Requested support was intended chiefly for released time of college and medical-school faculty involved in planning, implementing, and evaluating integrated courses and programs in the basic sciences. Approximately half the budget would support extension and consolidation of the coordinating developments underway in biochemistry. The staff believed that the remaining support should be available for released time of faculty involved in other aspects of the development of Dartmouth's basic sciences—including but not limited to genetics, neurosciences, and environmental health. Finally, about one-tenth of the budget would be set aside for undergraduate internships, career counseling, procedures for early admission of students to medical school, and related activities.

At its meeting in May 1977, the board awarded $1,040,000 to Dartmouth College and Medical School for three-year support of "an integrated, institution-wide approach to the basic sciences."

Dartmouth's request for renewal of its grant occasioned a two-day visit by the Fund's staff and consultants in December 1979.[40] The site visitors concluded, unanimously, that Dartmouth had carried out the promises of its initial proposal.[41] They found that in at least five key areas, Dartmouth's faculty was cooperating to improve teaching in the biomedical sciences, humanities, and social sciences. The most significant change had occurred in the field of biochemistry. In May 1979 seventy-four Dartmouth College students were majoring in biochemistry and from 30 to 40 percent of the twenty-five Dartmouth students admitted each year to the medical school had satisfied its biochemistry requirement. Without enlarging its faculty, Dartmouth had created a broad, flexible institution-wide science program in this area. The other four areas, representing less advanced cooperative efforts, were based upon the biochemistry model:

Neurosciences: Faculty from eleven departments had come together to teach and conduct research in the neurosciences. An unusual freshman-level college course, Introduction to the Neurosciences, was made possible by support under the Interface Program, and was taught by faculty of the departments of psychology, the biological sciences, biochemistry, and medicine. Also jointly taught was an upper-level college course, The

Synapse, with faculty from the departments of biochemistry, pharmacology, and psychiatry. Advanced college students were able to enroll in a medical school neuroanatomy course, Nerve, Muscle and Synapse, and in the planning stage were two new advanced courses in the medical school, Nerve and Muscle Pathology and Functions of the Cerebral Hemispheres, both to be taught by the Department of Medicine.

Environmental Health: The college's Environmental Studies Program, already well established, was cooperating with the Departments of Microbiology and Community and Family Medicine to teach a new medical school elective, Environmental Health, which was also open to college students. The same cooperation had produced an intermediate-level course, Topics in Environmental Health, lodged in the college but open to medical students.[42]

Genetics and Immunology: In 1978 and 1979, Dartmouth's Departments of Biological Sciences, Maternal and Child Health, Microbiology, and Pathology developed and taught two new courses in the college, Population Genetics and Evolution and Genetics and Society. Dartmouth was also planning new offerings in virology and immunology to replace an existing course that combined the two. The need for two separate courses grew out of the new policy of opening medical school immunology courses to college students wanting to satisfy a medical school requirement. An advanced course in immunology was being developed for students who elected advanced study in medical school.

Health-related Courses: Faculty of six college and three medical-school departments had cooperated to develop courses in the humanities and social sciences as they devolved upon medical and health issues. These and related courses actually constituted a new health-care studies program at Dartmouth. Among the new courses were International Health: Cross-cultural Perspective (Anthropology 12), Philosophy of Medicine (Philosophy 29), and Introduction to Medical Care Organization and Health Policy (Policy Studies 80). During the next phase, the same faculty groups would develop two required courses in the medical school: Health and the Physician and Therapeutics.

Most new courses developed in the college were open to medical students and depended on the assistance of the medical faculty. Fewer new courses had been set in the medical school because Dartmouth's three-year medical curriculum left little time for electives. Later Dartmouth decided to add a year to this curriculum, moving to the conventional pattern of a four-year medical school. Renewal of the Fund's grant would allow faculty groups to turn their attention to new courses for this expanded curriculum, so that equally valuable changes might be undertaken in the education of physicians.

Like all the universities participating in the Fund's Interface Program,

Dartmouth was conducting supporting services and extracurricular programs. The Dartmouth undergraduate internships involved college students in health care service or medical research, but with strong academic as well as field experience. Dartmouth also established a counseling program for students interested in medical education and other careers in the health field. Finally, it offered certain college sophomores early assurance of admission to the medical school.

The university requested $1,086,280 for all Interface activities during the three years from July 1980 through June 1983. Each of the five areas of significant faculty cooperation required continued support, including that for released time of faculty developing new courses and faculty seminars and colloquia, which often initiated new projects among departments. Supporting programs, such as the undergraduate internships, health careers counseling, early assurance of admission, and program evaluation, required additional support as well. In 1979, the Fund awarded Dartmouth College and Medical School a two-year grant of $755,000.[43]

THE JOHNS HOPKINS UNIVERSITY

The Johns Hopkins University became the seventh and final institution to receive major support from the Commonwealth Fund for reexamination of the premedical and preclinical years of education for medicine.[44] The university's proposal to the Fund stated its fundamental purpose as "reintegrat[ing] to the best of our ability work in basic science *throughout* the university. . . ."[45] Although discussion of this type of reform had begun at least twenty years earlier at Johns Hopkins, specific plans had been formulated only recently.

In May 1956 a committee at the School of Medicine under John C. Whitehorn recommended a "Year I Program" to integrate premedical and medical study and eliminate a year from the conventional eight years of the B.A.–M.D. sequence. After two years at college, some students would be admitted to the Johns Hopkins medical school. They would first spend one heavily scheduled year (called "Year I") studying the basic sciences at the medical school and liberal arts at the Homewood (arts and sciences) campus, and would then enter the medical school for the conventional four years of study. Since 1958 Hopkins had admitted 310 students into this program.

In May 1971 a Faculty Committee on Medicine and Human Biology recommended a six-year B.A.–M.D. sequence. A student's four years at the Homewood campus would include the first two years of medical school; his undergraduate degree would be in Human Biology and Medicine. Liberal arts, human biology, and some clinical work would be combined during these first four years. The student could earn the M.D. degree by completing two years of clinical clerkships in the medical school. At the college level, courses in the physical sciences, mathematics, and biology would be revised to suit the requirements of future medical study. Several academic governing boards at Johns Hopkins approved this proposal in principle, but nothing was done to implement it.

Two years later a report of the Joint Committee on Human Biology and Medicine rejected the key recommendations of the May 1971 report, but suggested six-, seven-, and eight-year "options" for the B.A.–M.D. sequence. It proposed a review of premedical courses (and some preclinical ones) and added that "the liberal education ideal in premedical studies is most strongly endorsed."[46]

In November 1976 a report of the Biological Sciences Task Force became the basis of the Johns Hopkins University's proposal to the Fund.[47] A Human Biology Program would use a 2–2–3 sequence to eliminate one year from the conventional eight-year program. After the sophomore year of college, at Johns Hopkins or elsewhere, a student could choose to begin a major in human biology, which the college of arts and sciences had added to its other tracks in biology. At that time, the student could be admitted to the Johns Hopkins University School of Medicine. The student's junior and senior years at the college of arts and sciences would combine study of human biology, liberal arts, and some preclinical subjects usually taught in the first year of medical school. During these final college years, the student would not be competing for admission to medical school and would be more free to sample courses in the humanities and social sciences. The difficult first year of medical school would also be spread over two years. Upon graduation from the college, with a B.A. in human biology, the student would enter the second year of medical school at Johns Hopkins.

Structuring the Human Biology Program involved the faculties in a new look at the content and order of college and medical school subjects. Anatomy, physiology, and other courses normally reserved for first-year medical students would be available to college juniors and seniors. Since first-year medical school courses would now be available regularly to college students, cooperation between basic scientists in the university's college and medical school was expected to increase. The two faculties were developing joint courses in biochemistry, genetics, physiology, neurobiology, and cell and developmental biology. Neuroanatomy and neurophysiology, for example, were being integrated into a single, interdivisional course, and parts of anatomy and physiology were being taught together as systems physiology. Biochemistry, long needed at the undergraduate level, was to be offered at both the college and the medical school, with an advanced medical school course for those who had completed the undergraduate course. Microbiology had been moved from the second year of the medical school to the first, and a new course in epidemiology was added to the second year, which in turn had been redesigned.

The college planned new offerings in the departments of biology, biophysics, and physiology. In addition, these departments would participate in the interdivisional courses already described. Many other college departments were developing or modifying courses to offer education of substantially higher quality for all students interested in the biological sciences, including those preparing for careers in other health-related fields.

Before submitting the proposal, Johns Hopkins faculty met over several months to synchronize the academic calendars of all university divisions, a step most universities find extraordinarily difficult. The new calendar, which took effect in September 1978, cleared the way for participation of all faculty and students in interdivisional courses.

The university's president, Steven Muller, was to be responsible for overall implementation of the program. Richard S. Ross, vice president for health divisions and dean of the medical school, would direct the crucial involvement of medical-school faculty. The continuing responsibility for the program would be in the hands of Simeon Margolis, who had a joint appointment in the departments of medicine and physiological chemistry.

The Fund's board of directors gave Johns Hopkins a grant of $1,736,000, covering the period July 1978 through June 1981. The university was able to raise the money needed to fulfill the requirements of a related "challenge" grant the following year; this money was used toward the construction of a new preclinical teaching building, which brought together classroom and laboratory activities previously conducted at five different sites on the two Johns Hopkins campuses. This final two-year grant from the Fund in 1981 completed its support of the Johns Hopkins Interface Program.

Additional Grants in the Interface Program

THE CITY COLLEGE OF NEW YORK

In 1976 the Fund renewed its support, begun in 1974 with a three-year grant, for the Program in Biomedical Education of the City College of the City University of New York.[48] A cooperative arrangement with eight medical schools had enabled City College to offer students interested in the problems of medical practice in needy urban areas an integrated education leading to the M.D. degree six years after graduation from high school.

The Program in Biomedical Education operated within City College's new Center for Biomedical Education, which included the college's Health, Medicine, and Society Program, its graduate programs in biomedical engineering and biomedical physics, and its new programs in public health and the allied health professions. The center's director, Alfred Gellhorn, was an experienced medical educator, a dean of the college, and vice-president for health sciences.

High-school graduates admitted to the Program in Biomedical Education pursued a four-year curriculum that integrated college education with the equivalent of the first two, preclinical, years of medical school. Students who completed the program were awarded a B.S. degree by City College and could enter the third year of medical school. Under an agreement with seven medical schools—Howard, Meharry, Mount Sinai, New York University, University of Puerto Rico, University of Rochester, and the State University of New York at Stony Brook—students in the program were interviewed at the end of the undergraduate sophomore year, and almost all were then given assurance of advanced standing in a specific medical school. Students not guaranteed a place at that time could continue in the program and reapply for the same advanced standing during their senior year at City College. Under the same arrangement, a smaller group of students was granted early admission to the University of Pennsylvania School of Dentistry.

The four-year sequence at City College itself was organized to offer students integrated education in the basic sciences, with a consistently realistic orientation to the needs of medical practice; training in such preclinical sciences as anatomy, pharmacology, and social medicine; exposure to clinical work in hospitals and health agencies throughout the city; and an emphasis upon instruction in the social and behavioral science components of medicine and health-care delivery. The student's early commitment to medical education allowed this thorough preparation for medical school to be combined with an exposure to the humanities and social sciences comparable to that available to City College undergraduates in other fields.

The course in community health may have been the most innovative in the program. Designed to educate and motivate the future physician to practice medicine in underserved urban neighborhoods, it was different from any other taught in medical school. A required course spanning the four years at City College, it integrated rigorous academic work with learning and service in the field. In its first year, the course covered sociology, demography, history, educational and recreational resources, employment, political structure, economics, transportation, and medical-care services. This year included preparation of a report on a broad, health-related problem and field placement in one of forty city day-care centers, senior-citizen facilities, or alcohol treatment centers, where the student provided health education, preventive disease screening, or antenatal care. There the student devoted at least twenty hours a week to serving as the associate of a physician, visiting nurse, medical social worker, or home-care technician. Through this experience the students learned about health problems of people in the urban community, the difficulties of access to the health-care system, and the impact of the social and physical environment on individuals. In the second year, course work emphasized occupational health and disease, environmental health programs, epidemiology, and preventive medicine. Students continued their field work and began to write individual reports that identified social health-care problems and proposed solutions.

The course in behavioral sciences was closely correlated with work in community mental-health centers. Excellent field placements had been arranged in cooperation with more than twenty health-care centers and agencies in Manhattan and the Bronx. Here the students were exposed to the myriad functional and organizational mental-health problems that were such frequent concomitants of urban life. Students learned how to interview patients with empathy and to participate with psychiatrists in the psychological management of patients' problems.

The basic medical sciences, traditionally taught during the first two years of medical school, were spread out over four years at City College and were closely correlated with their clinical applications. Courses in the natural sciences, such as chemistry, physics, and mathematics, were redesigned to meld college and early medical-school education.

In the Program in Biomedical Education at City College, basic and preclinical science courses had been designed to produce a broadly educated physician. Integration of premedical and preclinical education, a key goal of the Fund's Interface Program, was a reality. The program's early guarantee of admission to medical school with advanced standing was unprecedented, since the medical schools were not affiliated with the college's premedical program. The program also appeared to be exportable to other universities, at less cost than starting a new medical school.

The Program in Biomedical Education admitted its fourth class in September 1976. Its 180 students had been selected from a large and increasingly qualified pool of applicants who expressed interest in providing primary care to medically underserved communities. The next year the Fund's grant was unexpectedly complemented by support from the state and the city of New York. The New York State Board of Regents unanimously recommended—eighteen months earlier than initially planned—that City College's Center for Biomedical Education become a permanent unit. At about the same time, the city and state doubled their subvention to the center for the 1977–78 academic year. These two grants were the first step toward full government support for operation of the center.

By 1978, the year of the Fund's final grant to the program, students had been recruited from all public, parochial, and private high schools in metropolitan New York. Composition of the student body was as diverse racially and ethnically as the city itself; by any academic standards the students were among the very best graduated from city high schools. Measurable evidence of their excellence came from scores on the anatomy and biochemistry sections of the National Board examinations, which students in the City College program took at the end of the sophomore year. Their average score fell among the top third of scores attained by the nation's medical-school sophomores.

The program at City College demonstrated that some high-school seniors could make the transition to college work and postgraduate studies in a single step. Yet the education of future primary care physicians should be different from—but not inferior to—that of future biomedical investigators. The Fund's staff believed that it was possible for medical schools to identify the best students for M.D.–Ph.D. training, but that one could not use the same criteria without quantitative distinctions in selecting other medical students.

THE UNIVERSITY OF CALIFORNIA AT SAN DIEGO

The University of California at San Diego (UCSD) and its relatively new school of medicine epitomized many of the ideals of the Fund's Interface Program.[49] The well-established pattern at UCSD represented a goal toward which most other universities were moving only gradually. The university's five colleges, including the medical school, occupied the same campus under a comprehensive administration. Each discipline was the responsibility of a single, university-wide department, to which faculty were jointly appointed by all the colleges. The medical school itself maintained no independent basic science departments, but paid for nine faculty members of the university-wide biology department and six of the chemistry department. Departments such as medicine, although chiefly oriented to medical instruction, took part in teaching basic biology, pharmacology, anthropology, and sociology. This structure encouraged integration of teaching in medical and related sciences with instruction in the natural sciences and with courses in disciplines centering on man and society. Administrative complexities and intellectual distances did not divide the medical school from the parent university, so the university offered ideal opportunities for contact among undergraduate, graduate, and medical students.

Despite its ideal structure, UCSD was still having difficulties in coping with the "premedical syndrome" that plagued the country's liberal arts institutions. Warren College, newest of the university's institutions, was a liberal arts college emphasizing preprofessional education. About half of its freshmen had stated that they planned to enter medical school after graduation; almost certainly many more were "closet" premedical students. In liberal arts programs all across the country, such students tended to major in biology or chemistry, because they knew many medical schools preferred such a background. Enrollment in these science departments was huge, even when contrasted to the early 1970s, and despite the predominance of premedical students, these courses were usually organized to suit the needs of future graduate students in biology and chemistry.

To address the problem of the "premedical syndrome," the Fund in 1978 made a grant to Warren College and the School of Medicine to develop a new undergraduate major in the biological sciences, intended to provide "a demanding intellectual experience for students interested in man's well-being in its broadest definition."[50] Human biology and related studies of man would begin in this program much earlier than usual in undergraduate curricula, and by defining and stressing material actually needed in preparation for medical school, the program intended to forestall the premedical student's pointless compilation of natural science credits. Instead, some courses traditionally limited to medical students would be available to undergraduates, making possible advanced placement in the many medical schools that had such arrangements. The university's unusual organization allowed undergraduates to receive instruction from the same departments and faculty that taught preclinical courses in the medical school. Many students in the program could do extensive medical-school work in their senior college year and would have time later for additional work in humanities and social sciences. These studies would be encouraged in depth by two required "minors" that would complement the new major by relating the social and behavioral sciences and humanities to problems of man's well-being. The program would also include experience in clinical settings during the freshman and sophomore years, when students would work under the direction of the university's already functioning "life/career planning" program. Systematic counseling stressing varied opportunities in the health field would also be part of the program.

Because UCSD was a publicly supported institution, it had to operate on a "steady-state" budget. Innovations would require redirection of faculty time, and without additional support, existing activities would have to be abandoned. The Fund's grant would support the university's permanent faculty in developing and teaching the new program, while regular university funds would support visiting faculty and graduate students hired to teach the current program. In this way permanent faculty would build commitment to the new program; if it was successful, current programs could be phased out without affecting entrenched interests, since visiting faculty would be returning to their home universities. The few faculty hired permanently for the new program would replace faculty lost through attrition.

In 1978 the Fund made a two-year planning grant of $150,000 to UCSD. The program that evolved from this grant was known as the "Health Professions Honors Program" (HPHP).[51] Although it was based upon cooperation of college and medical school faculty, it was not an "interface" program per se, since it concentrated solely on the premedical phase of medical education.

Students were considered for admission to the program during their freshman year at Warren College and began the HPHP work as sophomores. Students might major in any subject, but the core of their work as sophomores was a year-long course in human biology. Most college biology departments emphasized molecular biology, while medical school courses, where the best human biology was taught, were generally not open to undergraduates. The course taught for the HPHP by Gregory Erickson of the medical school's Department of Reproductive Medicine concentrated upon aspects of human biology most relevant to future medical or other health-professional education: developmental biology, cell structure and function, and organ systems physiology. The course was open to other undergraduates as well, and provided an excellent introduction to human biology as part of a liberal education.

Students were also required to work in a health-care setting where they could evaluate their interest in varied aspects of the health professions, and a Communication Seminar helped them to interpret their experience. Students also spent two quarters in field work in a clinic, hospital, or research laboratory, and wrote an honors thesis.

The curriculum made work in the humanities an important part of college education, not simply an afterthought of preprofessional preparation. Students could select courses in the economics of health care, the philosophy of science, the behavioral sciences and anthropology, and political science and policy studies. Special courses and seminars for students in the HPHP program included Biomedical Writing, which used guest lectures by medical school faculty and two detailed writing projects to introduce students to collection, organization, and written communication of biomedical information. Overview of the Health-Care System, a seminar reserved for HPHP students, analyzed current health-care delivery systems in the United States. The Health Professions dealt with concerns about the current state of health manpower in this country's health-care system, and Health Communications explored the interaction between health care, profession, and patient.

HPHP students were not given an early guarantee of admission to the school of medicine, as were some students in programs at the Interface universities. They were nevertheless identified within the university as students receiving unusually rigorous preparation for medical-school studies, and in their junior and senior college years could take certain medical-school courses. Students who completed HPHP requirements would have worked with faculty from the medical school, and HPHP work was noted in their transcripts. This, it was hoped, would allay the fears and pressures that tended to undercut effective premedical study. In fact, the initial plans for the HPHP program had recognized the possibility that students would be skittish about committing themselves to a program that did not have proven acceptability to other medical schools. In an effort to lessen this concern, plans from the start had included the full participation of faculty from UCSD's medical school. If it seemed advisable as the program developed, the School of Medicine was prepared to guarantee early admission to students in the HPHP program.

The Fund's staff found that the university had completed its planning for the HPHP program on schedule under its initial two-year grant. On January 1, 1979, Allen Lein of UCSD's medical school became director of the HPHP, and, in May of that year, a first class of students was accepted. The Fund's staff believed that three years of support at approximately the same level would permit essential features of the program to continue until the university could incorporate them. In 1979 the Fund's board of directors awarded $225,000 to Warren College and the University of California at San Diego, School of Medicine for final support of the Health Professions Honors Program.

The Diversity of the Interface Programs

In viewing the process of medical education in the 1970s as one of "bewildering ferment,"[52] the Fund was loath to impose rigid strictures on the universities participating in its Interface Program. The Fund's position was that "Where education for medicine is concerned, no one since Flexner has been so bold as to present a precisely worked-out model to be imposed nationwide."[53] The resulting freedom produced programs that appeared to reflect each school's unique virtues and frailties, and in the aggregate may have tipped the balance in favor of a better model for premedical, preclinical education.[54]

The integration of the final years of college and the initial years of medical school into a coherent unit was emphasized at Brown University, the University of Rochester, the University of Chicago, Boston University, and the Johns Hopkins University. The achievements of these schools seemed to rest not only on the merit of their programs, but on the power of their leaders: A strong administration could overcome the scheduling problems, the bruised egos, the philosophical differences, whereas under a weak administration even a putatively successful program might flounder.

Brown University could be considered the standard bearer of virtually every major principle of the Interface Program. With integration of premedical and preclinical education already accomplished, Brown's initial application for support concentrated on problems of premedical education in the natural and behavioral sciences, humanities, and social sciences that future medical students study in college. Brown did not have to win its considerable accomplishments in the teeth of the kind of established, contrary patterns that prevailed at some of the other Interface universities, as the changes in its curriculum continued a line of development begun more than a decade earlier.

Brown's administrative structure allowed its Interface Program to offer an individualized course of study to students bound for medical school, since medical education was conducted by a division of biological and medical sciences that was simply one unit of the university, rather than a separate "medical school." Duke, Johns Hopkins, and Rochester were also able to give their students this type of flexibility. At Rochester, for example, during the middle four years of its program, a student might pursue B.A. and M.A. degrees in English—with integration of humanities, premedical, and preclinical courses—followed by two clinical years leading to the M.D. degree. Another student might pursue a B.A. in biology and an M.S. in genetics, again combining premedical, preclinical and liberal arts education throughout the four years, and then finish with two years of clinical work for the M.D. degree. Related to individualized choice of courses was the selection of paths to the medical degree. Boston University offered the most flexibility, with a choice of three tracks, but this number of choices for the student worked to the financial disadvantage of the school, which could not support so many programs indefinitely.

Flexibility in choosing courses permitted students to rediscover the liberal arts; the restoration of this segment of the curriculum was a particular strength of the programs at Duke, Boston University, and Brown. Similarly, as premedical students were investigating knowledge outside the natural sciences, courses in the Interface programs at Duke, Brown, and Johns Hopkins were open to nonmedical students. This exchange affirmed the idea that the medical school, too, was part of the university and a potential resource for all students.

The two ends of the continuum—early admission to medical school and help for students not entering medical school—were respected to varying degrees by all seven Interface universities. Early admission was offered by all schools except Chicago, and students at Chicago were unhappy about the absence of this feature. Counseling about other career choices related to medicine was a strong part of the programs at Duke, Dartmouth, and Rochester.

Final Recommendations

At its meeting in September 1980, the Commonwealth Fund's board of directors approved in principle an amount not to exceed $2 million for final grants to universities supported under the premedical-preclinical Interface Program.[55] The board promised to consider the staff's recommendations for final grants at its regular meetings during 1981, but the Fund would make no commitment to the universities beyond agreement to review their renewal requests. Any appropriations would come from allocations for 1980–81.

President Margaret E. Mahoney informed executive officers of the five eligible universities—Boston University, Brown University, the University of Chicago, Duke University, and the Johns Hopkins University—of the Fund's plan, and invited their submission of final proposals.[56] (The two other Interface schools, Rochester and Dartmouth, had already received final grants.)

All five eligible universities submitted requests, amounting to $2,973,400, and their proposals were reviewed by a committee of outside consultants and Fund staff.[57]

One condition of support for schools in the Interface program was that each develop a plan for evaluation; each Fund grant included a modest amount for this facet of the program. By 1981 each university's program was undergoing a systematic evaluation, conducted by faculty not directly involved, and some data were already available. Those evaluating the programs in the seven universities met several times to compare notes and to share plans.

The Fund's own evaluation committee, headed by Robert H. Ebert, recognized the limits of present techniques for assessing educational experiments, as did medical educators themselves. Neither the programs nor the evaluations of their results resembled laboratory experiments. What was needed was one final evaluation of the entire Interface Program by an outside, independent group. The appropriate time for this comprehensive evaluation would be determined by Ebert's committee. The final evaluation would include the seven core universities and other universities that had adopted aspects of the core universities' experiments, and it would examine the process of implementing the programs and the resulting changes. The cost of an excellent professional evaluation was estimated in 1981 to be $250,000, just over 1 percent of the total then invested in the Interface Program.

An interim evaluation had been conducted for the Fund by Alfred Gellhorn, former dean of the University of Pennsylvania School of Medicine and emeritus director of City College's Center for Biomedical Education. His assignment began in January 1979, and for the next sixteen months Gellhorn was a constant presence at the decision-making meetings of the

Fund's staff and consultants. He reported his findings and his personal evaluation to the board of directors at its meeting in May 1980.[58]

Gellhorn found that in each Interface Program the medical school was drawn closer to the parent institution. Faculty members gained a new sense of being a part of a university rather than of a medical school or college. Those with common interests and complementary skills revised existing courses and developed new ones; the number of joint appointments of faculty in medical school and college increased. Interdisciplinary curricular developments joining faculty from departments of history, philosophy, literature, sociology, religious studies, economics, law, and medicine were expanded in all participating institutions, to the benefit of all students.

The "premedical syndrome," with its competitiveness among students for grades, its overemphasis on the natural sciences, and its demoralizing instances of cheating and "dirty tricks," was affecting not only the premedical student population but all undergraduates and faculty members. At the seven institutions with Interface Programs and at City College, the severity of this syndrome was reduced, principally by early selection of students for admission to medical school. Students in the Fund-supported programs were practically unanimous in their sense of release from anxiety, their increased pleasure in the educational process, and the almost complete disappearance of destructive interpersonal competitiveness. The conventional wisdom that four years of college were necessary in order to assess the applicant's "maturity" and "commitment" was convincingly destroyed. The experience at City College and at Brown indicated that high-school seniors could proceed through college and into medical school (and, in the case of City College, through medical school and internship) with performance equal to that of students who were accepted in their last years of college.[59]

Improvements in student counseling probably decreased the number of students frustrated because their aspiration toward medicine was so unlikely to be realized. At the same time, the availability of broader information on other health-related careers appeared to encourage students to retain their commitment to the health professions.[60]

But despite the general evidence of salutary change, all did not go well in some institutions. Gellhorn and the Fund's staff agreed: More time would be needed before the real value of the Interface Program could be determined.

By 1981 the seven universities had received $18,933,621 in grants from the Commonwealth Fund. In addition, support for programs at the City College of the City University of New York and the University of California at San Diego, amounting to $1,675,000, raised the total expended to $20,608,621. The three grants recommended by the evaluation committee as final support amounted to $1,500,000, bringing the total of the Commonwealth Fund's support of Interface Programs to $22,108,621.

Chapman's Retrospective Look at the Interface Program

As the father of the Fund's Interface Program, Carleton B. Chapman related most of his career at the Fund to the outcome of this project.[61] It was the culmination of three decades of Chapman's fascination, hope, frustration, and despair in working with first medical education and, for at least twenty of those thirty years, with "that amorphous process usually referred to as liberal education."[62]

Just before his retirement in 1980, Chapman wrote briefly about the problems of medical education and the solutions that his Interface Program had attempted.[63] The subject was too vast, he felt, to be encompassed in a retiring foundation president's final words. Instead, he framed three questions that hinted at possible solutions. The first concerned the position of beginners in the vast intellectual kingdom of the natural sciences: How could students be fitted with the intellectual equipment required for more advanced work without driving them to loathe the whole business, without creating a virulently negative attitude from which many (including some who go into medicine) never recover? Chapman thought the first priority was to redesign the teaching of elementary natural science, a need that should be apparent to anyone even casually familiar with the problem. The fact that the very names of the disciplines and courses had long ceased to convey precise or accurate information ought by itself to have suggested that redesign was in order. There was other evidence as well: at Yale about 40 percent of students who opted for majors in the natural sciences in the 1970s rejected their chosen field before they graduated. In contrast, less than 20 percent of those who chose to major in the humanities switched to other fields before graduation.[64] Nor was this an isolated example; other schools had noted the same unpopularity. Chapman's explanation lay in the way the individual courses were planned and taught to beginners. He believed that the elementary offerings of the departments of chemistry, biology and physics at the college level were simply unsatisfactory—even though this proposition was regarded by many faculties as a consideration of no merit whatsoever. Whatever else students should have acquired at the hands of the natural scientist, they should have learned something of how science works. Their failure to comprehend even this basic point led Chapman to conclude that the natural scientists that students encountered early in their careers failed to comprehend the basic needs of the beginner and perhaps the simplest rudiments of pedagogy. Our universities housed natural scientists of sufficient talent and inspiration who, lifted out of the standard constraints imposed by departmental structure, might readily design a new approach to natural science for beginners, one that would require little more time than the past offerings and might appropriately be entitled "the basic concepts of natural science." Properly planned and ably taught, such a course could almost certainly meet the requirements of the student opting for medicine better than did the battery of courses then required.

Chapman's second question—What precisely are the medical sciences?—was one of the most basic queries in medical education. University faculty tended to look on the scientific underpinnings of medicine as something of a piece. They could not, for example, devise an effective course in immunology and microbiology for medical students without referring to what had been covered earlier in college-level courses in elementary and not-so-elementary biology. Investigation of this question might also contribute to more streamlined and effective courses.

His third question—What is a liberal education—encompassed an urgent topic, one that was at once familiar, obscure, and ill-defined. Chapman felt that the Interface Program's most valuable service was to force the reexamination of liberal education. A liberal education was not only worth having in itself, but courses in the humanities could be directly valuable to premedical students: "[medical] students generally do not understand science. They have little grasp of how it works, of what its genius consists, what theories are, how they are tested, and what defeats them. . . . Science for them is a catalogue of facts—complete and beyond question. Philosophy could lead them to new understanding and appreciation of science which would be far more crucial than their catalogues of facts in making them creative researchers and perceptive diagnosticians."[65]

Early review of the Interface Programs had shown the pace of change to be painfully slow, Chapman acknowledged, and the ultimate effect of the program would not be known for years or perhaps decades. If the Interface Program did no more than to bring these three topics under honest and conscientious scrutiny, however, he felt that it would have been worth far more than its total cost in dollars. By the year 2000, Chapman believed, we would be able to identify specific turning points in medical education. The first would be the Flexner report in 1910; the next would be the Fund-supported experiment in medical education at Case Western Reserve University in the 1950s; and a third might be the Interface Program.

As for the future, medical educators believed that we were on the threshold of another big change in medical education. Although most looked apprehensively at what the future might hold, Chapman thought it might be possible to make the next step of the educational process more rational. He hoped that the Interface Program would influence faculties themselves to produce the next curricular design.

Chapman's Stewardship of the Fund's Traditions

The Interface Program represented the Fund's willingness to examine long-range problems of major importance, a tradition transmitted from each chief executive officer of the Fund to his successor.[66] Chapman could not explain this coherence in the Commonwealth Fund's planning and performance, but he sensed it from the beginning of his association with the foundation. He found himself caught up in the Fund's traditions, a subtle and powerful influence whose origins he was never able to ascertain.

The Fund's traditions were concrete as well as philosophical, recent as well as long-standing. The President's Discretionary Fund, for example, Chapman found extremely valuable in emergencies, for causes needing a relatively small amount of money immediately (see p. 454). Although the upper limit of a single grant was fixed at $25,000, Chapman instituted an additional safeguard: He always involved other members of the staff when deciding to use this resource.

Another tradition was the Fund's special consideration of projects related to New York City institutions, even those outside any particular interest of the Fund. As a New York organization, it felt a responsibility to support worthwhile programs in the city—for example, projects at Columbia and Cornell universities. Most of these grants were one-year allocations.

Despite the addition of the Interface Program, the other grants allocated by Chapman and his staff reflected the Fund's traditional priorities: The Fund continued to support projects concerned with medical education, medical centers in the community, social medicine, health policy, and medical problems in human behavior.

Yet another tradition concerned the recruiting of staff. In some foundations this was traditionally carried out through "a kind of old-boys network," which Chapman felt had worked satisfactorily most of the time. He himself would probably not have entered foundation work otherwise, and he thought that the system had worked better than one had any right to expect. At the Commonwealth Fund, however, staff recruitment had not been carried out only through this network. Barry C. Smith, Lester J. Evans, and Mildred C. Scoville were altogether an outstanding group, and in Chapman's opinion, the concentration of these talented individuals at the Fund was not just pure luck; someone had been very perceptive in choosing them for the Fund's staff. (Evans was, in his view, the model of an effective foundation officer.) Formal search committees can be useful, but in a small organization like the Commonwealth Fund, with a small staff that works intimately together, success finally depends on the compatibility as well as the excellence of the staff. One reason for the Fund's ability to move in some strikingly innovative ways was its small size and consequent lack of bureaucracy.

The Fund's board of directors had also become an excellent group, one that Chapman found very supportive. Hulbert S. Aldrich was chairman of the board when Chapman arrived at the Fund, and the Aldrich brothers were walking archives, providing answers that could not be found in the records. As custodians of so much early information, they helped preserve the Fund's traditions. The current excellence of the board also reflected a new method of identifying prospective new members, who were now chosen for their professional backgrounds, talent, intelligence, interest, and ability to contribute to the Fund's programmatic development. Previously there had been no women on the Board, but in 1979 Harriet Bundy Belin, chairman of the Century Fund at Radcliffe College, was appointed. Discussions at board meetings reflected the wisdom of these changes. Meetings were longer and much more interesting, and their structure now allowed ample time and a receptive environment for intelligent discussion of issues.

Chapman did not use the board's executive committee to any great extent. For proposals that involved important administrative units such as the Interface Program and the Book Program, he preferred to inform the board of the direction of any proposed change well before asking them to vote. His strategy was to report informally at one meeting and present a proposal for action at the next meeting, several months later. Chapman talked to various board members between meetings when he thought it necessary to enlist their support or to inform them more fully than was possible during a meeting. He relied on certain board members for certain types of proposals, depending on their particular interests. Two or three times a year a member would tell him, "So-and-so approached me at lunch with this proposal. I am transmitting it to you and you handle it as you see fit." None ever said that he was particularly interested in a proposal and wanted Chapman to support it. Malcolm P. Aldrich offered the Fund's traditional viewpoints, but he put no pressure on Chapman and did not try to influence the outcome of any proposal beyond the normal discussion process.

By the time Chapman arrived at the Fund, it had accumulated over twenty years of experience in influencing the process known as medical education. Most important were the concrete "do's and dont's" handed down by the staff, but what the Fund's experience dictated was the creation of incentive programs not necessarily requiring huge sums of money. In framing the Interface Program, Chapman benefited from Lester J. Evans's advice: Don't be too rigid in your definition of the ground rules or you will hamper the project. It would have been wrong, in Chapman's opinion, to say that the Fund's staff encouraged the development of six-year programs. He felt that to specify any given number of years would have been so divisive as to defeat the whole effort. At first the only ground rule for the Interface Program was that the money not be spent on bricks and mortar, but the staff's experience and their observations in the field soon led them to realize that even this limit was inappropriate; physical alterations were sometimes necessary to give a program a reasonable chance of success.

The Fund's staff felt that grants should enable an institution to continue the original program when the grant was over, or, alternatively, to improve the program without further investment. Although it was not necessary for a program's endpoint to be clear, the staff wanted to be certain before making a grant that the institution would not be worse off financially when the grant ended, for an institution could not usually assume the continuing cost of a program without additional financial resources. It would be irresponsible to induce an institution to undertake an expensive program with Commonwealth Fund support and then without any further specific consideration expect it to be carried on in the absence of that support. Universities were already spending a great deal of money on medical education without achieving optimal results, and the Fund's Interface Program added money for planning in the expectation that a university would eventually be able to do a better job for the same amount it was already spending.

The Fund had been fearless in plunging into some extremely complicated and long-range projects over its several decades of activity. Chapman wanted to extend his predecessors' traditional rejection of the thesis that one designs only programs that can provide quick, definitive results. Although a foundation could sponsor projects offering fast answers, any effects of the foundation's work might soon disappear. The Interface Program was described by one critic as "irrelevant and passé," but its specific emphases would have to be viewed as fundamental unless one relegates the entire process of medical education to the status of vocational training. In all its years of involvement with medical education, the Fund's leaders regularly resisted such a doctrinaire inclination. That, in Chapman's view, had been one of the Fund's most significant achievements.

The Selection of Chapman's Successor

One tradition Chapman questioned: the method of selecting the Fund's president. "One can look down the list of major foundations and find that the tradition of selecting broken-down deans or retired college presidents to head the operation was widespread—sort of a pre-retirement process."[67] When Chapman reached the retirement age of sixty-five, the choice of his successor was complicated by his dual role at the Fund: As president he was also a member of the board. Some other board members did not want him involved in the selection process at all. Chapman disagreed—not because he wanted to select his own replacement, but because he felt that he had an obligation to help the Fund with this most important problem.

Chapman saw the president of a foundation as a "listening post." Foundation executives were in a position to take in all sorts of information, and they should not only permit but actively encourage the process. Success depended also upon the chief executive officer's willingness to spend much time traveling away from home base. When foundations proliferated between the 1930s and the years after World War II, there was no cadre of individuals specifically trained for this type of work. Foundations had to turn to people in academic life still capable of taking on a new assignment. In the next thirty years, however, a group of what might be called "foundation professionals" had grown up, including some very impressive individuals. Although Chapman wanted to use what influence he had to persuade the board to look at these professionals, he felt that to "bureaucratize" the process would be dangerous. To limit the field of candidates to these professionals would prevent the Fund from breaking out of such a mold when some obviously "grand opportunity" presented itself. Yet accountability had become so important in this country that it was not going to be easy for a private foundation to choose a major officer without being able to offer the public definitive justification for its choice.

The board's solution was to appoint a search committee in the manner of academic institutions. Under the chairmanship of Robert J. Glaser, this group selected two candidates from the group of "professionals," and one of them—Margaret E. Mahoney—captured the job.

Part IV:
The 1980s

10

Programs for the 1980s

Our grand business in life is not to see what lies dimly, at a distance, but what is clearly before us close at hand.
—*Thomas Carlyle*

The Fifth President: Margaret Ellerbe Mahoney (1980–)

Margaret E. Mahoney was born in Nashville, Tennessee, and received the B.A. degree from Vanderbilt University, magna cum laude, in 1946 (fig. 32). Early in her career, Mahoney was a foreign affairs officer in the United States Department of State. As a staff member of the Carnegie Corporation, she directed a program to mesh health manpower policy with the national need for health service. Mahoney came to the Fund on July 1, 1980, after eight years as vice-president of the Robert Wood Johnson Foundation, where as one of its first senior officers she developed and managed major programs to improve health services. Her many professional affiliations include membership on the President's Task Force on Medicaid and Medicare; on the Medical Assistance Advisory Council of the Department of Health, Education and Welfare; on the Health Advisory Committee of the Office of Technology Assessment, United States Congress; and in the Institute of Medicine. To the presidency of the Commonwealth Fund she brought deep experience in policy planning and institutional development, and a particular interest in encouraging opportunities for new careers.

The Environment for Health Programs in the 1980s

The late 1970s witnessed the end of a twenty-five year era of public willingness to pursue health goals almost without reference to cost. The

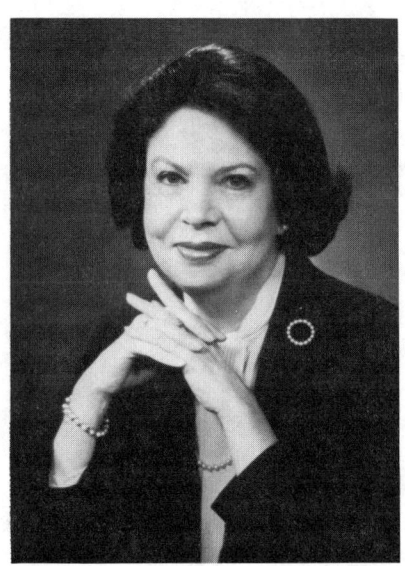

Figure 32. Margaret Ellerbe Mahoney
Photograph by Bachrach

substantial slowing of the American economy had affected the availability of health care: Federal support for health programs diminished, and levels of economic well-being that varied from region to region put an even greater burden on some local areas. To remain effective yet solvent, health-care institutions in the early 1980s could be forced to change their objectives, their specific programs, and their day-to-day operations.

The best predictor of the rate of spending for medical care in most nations, including the United States, had been the rate of growth in real income.[1] Some economists predicted that the pace of the nation's real economic growth would be substantially slower between 1980 and 1985 than it had been since World War II, with growth rates expected to be one-third less than those of the 1960s. In response, real growth in governmental spending was expected to be far less than in the previous two decades.[2] This was particularly important to the field of health, in which, for example, 54 percent of hospital expenditures, 50 percent of medical-school expenditures, and 55 percent of nursing-home expenditures came from government funds.[3]

Circumstantial evidence supported the conclusion that as public spending slowed, the rate at which health expenditures grew would also diminish. National health expenditures had rapidly outpaced the overall national growth, increasing from 5.3 percent to 9.5 percent of the gross national product since 1960 and possibly surpassing 23 percent by the end of the 1980s if allowed to grow unabated.[4] Defense and energy programs were likely to claim a larger proportion of federal funds between 1980 and 1985 than in the past. The United States could spend more on these programs without spending less on health care by raising taxes or by running even larger national deficits, but since increasing deficits were inflationary and tax increases were certainly unpopular, neither solution seemed likely.[5] In addition, the public in general and physicians in particular were worried about the rising cost of medical care. When both groups were polled each year from 1977 through 1979, cost was named as the most important problem facing the health-care system.[6] Cost was the problem mentioned first by the public, more often than problems with the distribution or quality of services and dissatisfaction with the extent of governmental involvement in health affairs combined.

When a society attempts to advance rapidly in a relatively short period, not every effort can be expected to succeed. In 1980 the economic downturn and the awareness that not all sociomedical investments had been equally successful reduced the public's willingness to pursue health goals without weighing the cost. Professionals and the public alike were asking for tangible evidence that what they were paying for then and recommending for the future actually worked. It was the practical value of the current programs in relation to tomorrow's health that was likely to emerge as the major theme in health affairs over the next five years. As the nation faced health issues in the 1980s, the Fund's staff believed that without the resources to address all aspects of this challenge, the Fund would have to react selectively.

The Fund's Program for the 1980s

In July 1981 the Fund's new directions were announced. Its first and most important mission, intended to further the Fund's basic goal of enhancing the common good, would be to stimulate opportunities for Americans to live in good health. This first mission would be carried out by providing grants to nonprofit institutions throughout the United States for individuals who would develop services, educational programs, or research programs focusing on elderly persons, alcohol abusers, or single mothers and children, or concentrating on the capacity of academic health centers—the nation's teaching hospitals—to carry out their multiple responsibilities in education, research, and service. Some support would also be given to programs for minority-group members seeking careers in the health professions and for ways of using medical technology more discerningly. Special consideration would be given to programs to improve the quality of life in the Fund's hometown, New York City.

What all programs require is more effective coordination through collaboration among leaders of voluntary and city health agencies, voluntary and municipal hospitals, medical schools, private and public employers, and insurers. The Commonwealth Fund would support planning efforts, particularly proposals offering specific ways of keeping crucial health services available for large groups of people who risk losing them, of combining programs of health-care agencies, and of achieving solutions replicable by other institutions.

Emphasis on complex national problems in the delivery of health care began at the Fund during the presidency of J. Quigg Newton, Jr. Again in the 1980s, the Fund is in no position to explore all of society's urgent difficulties; yet by careful selection, it can support research and demonstration that may lead to new approaches to eliminating the deleterious influences on medical care made by changes in society at large. Addressing the fundamental problems is not easy. Principles of scientific investigation are far more difficult to apply outside the laboratory than inside, and studies of actual environments often provide only partial answers. The Fund's position is that practical proposals for the future can be built only on a realistic understanding of how things have worked.

The Fund's emphasis in the 1980s on research and demonstration continues its commitment to encouraging advances in the general well-being of Americans and thus the institutions that serve them. The Fund's basic goal remains, although the groups of people receiving attention change; as America's resources have been mobilized on behalf of some groups, the Fund has been able to shift its attention to problems facing others. Although it began by establishing child guidance clinics and building hospitals, its annual grant-making resources are too limited today to build facilities or maintain ongoing programs. (For comparison, the Commonwealth Fund's annual appropriations in 1985 are less than the operating cost of the average New York City teaching hospital for one month.) Accordingly, the Fund's policy in the 1980s is to help develop and test new approaches, to bring results to public attention, and to help mobilize resources for the beneficiaries of the programs it supports.

To further this policy, the Fund is continuing its longstanding interest in a publications program. Its new program, directed by Lewis Thomas, encourages the creation of authoritative, exciting books written primarily by working scientists for a literate lay audience—especially books about the biomedical sciences, and about the behavioral and social sciences as they relate to human health. The program's premise is that science needs the public's support, which, as Lewis Thomas points out, depends in turn on widespread understanding of the problems, methods, and objectives of scientific research.

To achieve concrete results today requires more than an imaginative program to advance knowledge, or mechanisms such as a book program to improve public understanding. The basic structure of the Fund's management, particularly its investment policy, has been substantially altered under President Mahoney to provide the Fund with both a range of expertise and financial viability. The tradition set in motion by Edward S.

Harkness seems to continue with a staff that is competent but not complacent, one that is enhanced by a group of experienced consultants and led by a dedicated and informed board of directors. It is too soon to measure the success of the Fund's current work; that is a task best left to others. What is clear is the path of continuity at the Commonwealth Fund, in both purpose and spirit.

Part V: Educating the Public and the Physician

11

The Book Program

> *If sufficiently good reporting is done, the Fund's publications may carry some hint of the imponderables which play so large a part in all cooperative social enterprises—matters of relationship between voluntary and public agencies, of balance between subsidy and self-help, of tactics in program building and diplomacy in community leadership.*
>
> —Annual Report,
> The Commonwealth Fund, 1931

The Commonwealth Fund's book-publishing program has always been predicated on a negative answer to the philosophical question, "If a tree falls in the forest and no one is present, does it make a sound?" Before there was a formal program, before there was even a structure within the organization to accommodate a program, the Fund made certain that the results of its grants did not go unnoticed. As an annual report flatly stated, "Research without publication may be rewarding to the individual, but it is socially unimportant."[1] In spreading the word, the Fund has used its flexibility as a philanthropy to pursue a policy that in a commercial publishing house would be considered at best eccentric, at worst financially ruinous. That policy has been to publish what it believes merits publication, no matter how small the audience, how lengthy the book, how expensive the production. The result is a list of more than three hundred books—some of them classics in their fields—that illuminate social and medical thinking in the United States over the past sixty years.

At first, in 1922, the Fund saw the printed word as just one of its various educational efforts to extend the knowledge and use of "the sound methods of treatment developed by the program." The program in question was the Program for the Prevention of Juvenile Delinquency, and the Fund's first publication, aside from its annual reports, was Barry C. Smith's description of the program, first included in the 1922 annual report and reprinted the same year as a pamphlet.[2] By the next year, ten manuscripts were in progress, a series of case studies of "problem children." These were educational but not propagandistic and were intended for lay groups, avoiding technical language while at the same time adhering to high scientific standards. Not all ten came to fruition, but those that were published met with a "gratifying" reception: For example, *Three Problem Children,* which came out in 1924, received "exceptionally favorable comments" in magazine reviews and letters and sold 2,329 copies, with orders for 352 copies received from universities and high schools. Another 1,170 copies were distributed free of charge, and the success of the early publications encouraged the Fund to expand this kind of effort: The child health demonstrations were attracting wide attention, and the Fund's staff believed that these demonstrations would not attain their full educational value unless descriptions of the work and its results were disseminated to a wide audience.

What the Fund gained by becoming a publisher was not only the dissemination of results but control over the product. Participants in the Fund's delinquency-prevention program were already publishing a dozen articles and monographs a year; the articles appeared in such standard journals as the *American Journal of Psychiatry* and *Proceedings of the American Sociological Society,* and the books were published by organizations such as the National Committee for Mental Hygiene. The Divisions of Educational Research and Legal Research had been producing such publications as *The Story of Human Progress, Part I* (a junior-high-school textbook), an overview of the financing of education in the United States in thirteen volumes, and an intensive study of the Federal Trade Commission—all published by either university presses, commercial publishers, or organizations besides the Commonwealth Fund. But when the Fund hired Dr. Emma Winslow in 1924 to prepare material about the child health demonstrations for publication, it was beginning to take responsibility not only for the selection of the material published but also for its presentation: its clarity of language and its appearance. The Fund's editorial services were always more extensive than those of a commercial publishing house, often amounting to virtual rewriting of a book. As an annual report lamented, "Scientific writing in the United States is not distinguished for simplicity or grace, and much of the work in which the Fund is interested has been done in fields where concepts are still shadowy and terminology undisciplined."[3]

By 1926 the Joint Committee on Methods of Preventing Delinquency had distributed almost 80,000 copies of eleven publications; circulation of a number of miscellaneous pamphlets brought the total distribution close to 100,000. In fact, supervision of publications was becoming the most important facet of the committee's work. The following year the committee was dissolved, but its staff was retained as the nucleus of a new, autonomous administrative unit, the Division of Publications. This division comprised four sections: publications, distribution, statistical services, and library and information services. The director of the committee, Graham Romeyn Taylor, was made director of the new division, housed at 578 Madison Avenue, which was to oversee the publication of all the Fund's departments. Curtis E. Lakeman was assistant director; Geddes Smith, Mary B. Sayles, and Mary A. Clark were writers and editors; and the division had its own statistician.

After graduating from Harvard University in 1903, Taylor spent a brief time as a newspaper reporter. He then joined the Chicago staff of the *Common*, a periodical that later merged into *Survey*. As Western correspondent for the *Common*, Taylor wrote a series of articles on planned industrial communities that were published in book form in 1915 under the title *Satellite Cities: A Study of Industrial Suburbs*. In 1916 he was appointed special assistant to the American ambassador to Russia and was on the staff of the American Consulate General in Moscow during the revolution. Returning to the United States, in 1919 he became secretary of the Chicago Commission on Race Relations.

Until 1951 the Fund was officially a publisher, identifying, editing, advertising, and distributing its own books.[4] Taylor presided over the division's expansion and diversification until his death in 1943. His determined eclecticism kept the division from concentrating too narrowly on one subject or one type of book. The largest category of books published by the Fund were handbooks—working tools that "precipitate[d] in usable form many years of field experience mulled over by many workers. The manual on public health record-keeping, for instance, draws its authority from the toil of a small army of executives and clerks in many health departments. Fund books offer help in classifying and recording medical diagnoses, administering serum treatment in pneumonia, identifying intestinal infections, standardizing small hospital routines, running a rural health department, training health officers, organizing and running child guidance clinics and visiting teacher service, caring for patients suffering from encephalitis and brain injury."[5] Another group of books was based on field observation in the form of surveys and special inquiries. Whereas the first category illuminated technique, this second group discussed policy and included studies of maternal mortality in New York City, teachers' attitudes toward children's behavior, and the predictive accuracy of vocational guidance. Most of the books in the third category, those aimed at the everyday reader, grew out of the Fund's programs in mental hygiene. Reports of research—medical and legal—included a five-volume analysis of the function and methods of the Interstate Commerce Commission; by 1930 this category included a book representing the results of research to which the Fund had given only limited assistance (*The Hospital Treatment of Post-Encephalitic Children*, by Earl D. Bond and Kenneth E. Appel of the University of Pennsylvania Hospital). A final category offered reprints and works of historical interest.

The winnowing process was meticulous. A Committee on Publications, experts in varied fields, advised the division's staff. This committee never met as a whole, but manuscripts being considered for publication were referred to the appropriate members for critical reading; this stage was frequently followed by a group conference, and manuscripts were often subjected to yet additional criticism through reading by persons outside the committee. The result of this painstaking and time-consuming effort was an emphasis on the quality rather than the quantity of production—an emphasis reinforced by the Fund's attitude toward distribution of its books. Although the number of copies sold provided one answer to the question "How are we doing?" the Fund always intended to distribute its publications selectively. It systematically developed lists of interested readers: "leaders in education, teachers and professors in schools, colleges and universities; physicians, psychologists, social workers, judges and probation officers; executives and technical workers in public health; writers, editors, and leaders of public opinion along many lines; and a wide range of organizations and institutions in the fields of education, public health, mental hygiene, and child welfare."[6] Free distribution of books was never allowed on a large scale because of the Fund's desire to make the material available only to those likely to give it real thought.

Distribution of books at no cost to recipients would also have wrecked the division's budget. Although the Publications program was not intended to be a profit-making wing of the Fund, it was intended to pay its own way, and, as budgets increased over the years, the income from the sale of books did cover publication costs. After five years of operation, the division could boast that the average cost of manufacture had been reduced, a higher standard of format was being maintained, and processes of distribution had been systematized. Moreover, the demand for the Fund's publications as measured in volume of sales was greater in 1932 than in any other year since the division was organized.[7] Particularly popular were Mary B. Sayles's three books, *Three Problem Children*, *The Problem Child in School*, and *The Problem Child at Home*: Nearly 28,000 copies of the books in this series were sold.

After ten years the Fund had published sixty books and pamphlets, some in several editions, representing 120,000 copies. The Division of Publications continued to perform a dual function: "widen[ing] the reach of the Fund by putting into circulation, in print, experience and new knowledge gained in the activities which the Fund subsidizes; and . . . aid[ing] in the dissemination of useful facts and sound ideas originating elsewhere but pertinent to the Fund's major objectives."[8] In many cases direct grants to workers in the field were followed by provision of editorial services, distribution facilities, and payment of overhead costs, without reference to the selling price of the resulting book. In no case, however, was a Fund activity undertaken for the purpose of producing a publication. As early as 1929, the Fund's staff could say that "the policy adopted by the Fund has already demonstrated the usefulness of developing publications out of projects undertaken for their own sake and in themselves educational."[9]

On occasion books were commissioned by members of the Fund's staff. One example was a handbook, *Lobar Pneumonia and Serum Therapy*, by Frederick T. Lord and Roderick E. Heffron. The Fund's 1936 annual report tells the story:[10]

> Serum therapy was not, until recently, generally accepted and in use; its value had been recognized in medical centers, but by and large the general practitioner was not sufficiently sure of himself to employ it. In Massachusetts the state department of health (with financial support from the Fund) undertook to get serum into the hands of practitioners all over the state and to make it easy for them to learn how to use it. Other state health departments also became interested, notably those of New York, Michigan, Maine, and Connecticut. The time was ripe for a fresh presentation of the essentials of current medical knowledge about pneumonia, with specific instructions for the use of serum, and the encouraging success in Massachusetts lent weight to the story. Accordingly, the Fund asked a young physician closely associated with the work in that state to write, in collaboration with an older colleague, a handbook addressed directly to practitioners of medicine.
>
> The result, a small volume modestly priced, has been offered for sale generally and appears to be fulfilling the purpose for which it was designed. In the opinion of the *New England Journal of Medicine*, it "should prove of incalculable value to practicing physicians, particularly those with remote connections with the larger medical centers." A study of the first 1,000 sales to individual purchasers showed that physicians of all ages were buying it, with the largest percentage in the group from 36 to 45 years old, and that nearly one-half the sales were made to physicians practicing in towns of less than 25,000.

Another seminal book published in the division's first decade was *Aphasia*, a 656-page treatise by Theodore H. Weisenburg, M.D., and Katharine E. McBride, Ph.D., which presented the results of the first extensive controlled study of the disease. This book represented the culmination of five years of work and was regarded as the capstone of Weisenburg's career.[11] A report of the Fund's general director in 1935 characterized the book as the Fund's first major contribution to the literature of clinical research. Perhaps the most important book to emerge from this first decade was *A Standard Classified Nomenclature of Disease*, the preparation of which had been supported by the Fund. This compendium became widely accepted as the basis of case recording in hospitals, and went through several editions. Favorable reviews of *The Biology of Pneumococcus, Supervision in Public Health Nursing, Brucellosis in Man and Animals, Essentials of the Diagnostic Examination*, and *The Patient as a Person* appeared in such publications as the *British Medical Journal*, the *Journal of the American Medical Association,* and the *American Journal of Public Health.*

By 1943 orders for books were received from purchasers at more than seven hundred educational institutions. The audience for the Fund's books was also expanding as translations appeared: Four books of earlier years were transmitted to China on microfilm for use by that country's Ministry of Social Research, and three were translated into Portuguese by the Federal Office of the Coordinator of Inter-American Affairs.

Taylor's death gave the division a difficult year, however, and the next half-dozen years were equally turbulent. His successor was Porter R. Lee, Jr., son of the former director of the New York School of Social Work. Born in Buffalo, Lee received his A.B. degree from Cornell in 1928, taking honors in English. Before assuming his post with the Fund he had been a staff member of the publishing firms of Doubleday Doran and Company and Blue Ribbon Books. Upon his death in 1946, Lee was succeeded by Roger A. Crane, the division's distribution manager. Crane directed the Division of Publications until his retirement in 1966.

The division continued to publish about a dozen new books a year and maintained a back-list of over 100 publications. Among the new books that appeared in the 1940s were Helen B. Taussig's *Congenital Malformations of the Heart,* which was "almost lyrically praised by the medical journals and which, to the temporary confusion of the Division, went out of stock within four months of publication";[12] *Atlas of the Blood in Children,* by Kenneth D. Blackfan and Louis K. Diamond; *The American Hospital,* by E. H. L. Corwin; *Teaching Psychotherapeutic Medicine,* a transcript of the essential parts of the teaching done in a pilot course organized by the Fund and held at the University of Minnesota in the spring of 1946; and *Neural Mechanisms in Poliomyelitis,* by Howard A. Howe and David Bodian. The work described in this last-mentioned book won the Mead Johnson Award for Research in Pediatrics in 1942.

Of the 86 books newly published by the Fund between 1939 and 1949, 56 stemmed from Fund-sponsored activities or were written at the Fund's suggestion; 11 were published in response to the requests of other organizations; and the remaining 19 were submitted on the initiative of the authors. The Fund was moving away from operating programs of its own design, a trend reflected in the activities of the Division of Publications;[13] but in 1949, the Fund decided to "clear the decks"—to return to the policy of its earlier years, that of publishing only books and pamphlets that had grown directly out of work financed by the Fund, except in "special circumstances, where publication of other material, chosen according to rigorous standards, will help substantially in advancing the Fund's principal objectives."[14] The Fund's staff believed that this would "eliminate the publication of books, germane to the Fund's interests in a more general way, whose authors or sponsors have sought the Fund's imprint mainly for the sake of its prestige or for the advantages of the division's highly specialized editorial or distribution facilities. In the long run this policy may reduce output but should make it more purposeful."[15] Fifty-three titles were allowed to go out of print (eighty-three stayed available for purchase), and the division concentrated on completing its existing commitments and working more closely with the rest of the Fund's operations.

This substantial change in the division's program was the result of the impending passage of a tax law that would have penalized the Fund for receiving income from an enterprise that had the form, although not the essential quality, of a business.[16] It was this legislation, too, that led the Fund to link the division with the Harvard University Press in 1951. The collaboration would turn over the production and distribution of books to Harvard while retaining sponsorship and editorial functions in the division's offices, and the Fund would pay subsidies to the press as necessary. Books would bear a joint imprint and, consequently, each manuscript would be subject to the approval of the press's own editorial board. The volume of mailing and bookkeeping done at the Fund's offices would decline, and the staff of the division would be reduced by half. The press would retain 35 percent of proceeds from the sale of books, paying royalties and crediting the remainder to a manufacturing fund and a sales promotion fund. The Fund agreed to replenish these two accounts as necessary.[17]

During the next two years of transition, the collaboration produced only two or three books each year, but by the late 1950s, five to ten books were being published annually. These reflected the Fund's primary interest: the support of biomedical research. Such titles as *Atlas of Exfoliative Cytology*, by George N. Papanicolaou, and *Coronary Heart Disease in Young Adults: A Multidisciplinary Study*, by Menard M. Gertler and Paul D. White, developed from research long supported by the Fund.

The Division of Publications emerged from its relative dormancy in the mid-1960s, when it established a number of new liaisons with both publishing houses and nonprofit organizations. An affiliation with the Hoeber Medical Division of Harper and Row, similar to the Fund's arrangement with the Harvard University Press, began in 1962. Franklin Book Programs, Inc., received $25,000 in 1964 for the translation and publication of books for medical personnel in Latin America. In 1965 the Fund appropriated $41,181 to the National Commission on Community Health Services for an editorial unit to prepare reports for publication. A grant to the Harvard University Press in 1966 provided partial support toward the press's employment of a senior editor in the biomedical sciences. In 1967 the Child Research Council at the University of Colorado School of Medicine was given a grant toward the preparation of a three-volume series of monographs. The following year the Fund assisted with the publication of the proceedings of a workshop on interprofessional care of the ambulatory patient, of an international symposium on radiology, and of an annual meeting of the American Association of Planned Parenthood Physicians.

But the most important change in administrative policy occurred in 1964, after the Fund's staff recognized want in the midst of plenty: "Vast sums of money are now available for medical research from the National Institutes of Health and from various national societies concerned with specific diseases, but individuals who have had research grants from these sources often find that it is difficult to secure money for publication of their findings when subsidy is needed. It appears that a gap may exist here in which the Fund might meet a pressing need."[18] The first tentative step occurred the following year, when the division gave Harold I. Lief, professor of psychiatry at the Tulane University School of Medicine, a small grant for secretarial assistance in preparing for publication the report of a study of medical students and their adaptational problems.

This support turned out to be the first in a series of grants-in-aid that continued until 1982. By turning to the recipients of its Awards in Support of Creative Scholarship, the Fund's staff hoped to identify and help medical scholars interested in preparing books for publication. (In fact, the entire Creative Fellowship program was altered to reflect a specific orientation toward scholarly medical writing.) Beginning in 1967, between seven and twenty-one grants-in-aid were given annually. Support was intended to pay for scholars' released time for writing, related travel, and such other needs as secretarial assistance and the preparation of illustrations (but not for research that might lead to publication). A principal criterion for this type of assistance was commitment to a definite work program leading to a draft manuscript, but in contrast to the publication-subsidy program, these manuscripts did not need to appeal to either of the Fund's cooperating presses as a condition of support.

Meanwhile the Fund had decided to fortify that other half of the division's activities. Grants in the publication-subsidy program were made for manuscripts that because of a limited market or high production costs might not otherwise find an outlet for publication. To qualify for support, the manuscript had to be accepted by either the Harvard University Press or the Hoeber Medical Division. In addition to bearing the publisher's imprint, subsidized books were designated as Commonwealth Fund Books—an identification linking them with a series of titles that over the years has won recognition for scholarly merit. Between two and ten subsidized books were published each year. Among the most notable were *Venous Thrombosis and Pulmonary Embolism*, by Michael Hume; *Psychoanalytic and Psychophysiological Investigation in Gynecologic Disorders*, by Alfred O. Ludwig and Somers H. Sturgis; *The Red Cell*, by John W. Harris; and *Episodic Behavioral Disorders*, by Russell R. Monroe.

In the six years after Roger A. Crane's retirement, the Division of Publications had no official director. In 1972 Reginald Fitz took the position, remaining until his retirement in 1981. The program over which he presided had an annual budget of about $500,000. Its concerns had changed little over the years: Although the focus of the program was chiefly on biomedical research, books dealt with educational, social and economic aspects of medicine; biomedical ethics and philosophy; legal matters as they pertained to the biomedical field; and historical topics.

As the new vice-president of the Fund, Carleton B. Chapman made the Book Program one of his first targets of inspection:[19]

> Evaluation of the program has never been methodically carried out partly because it is so difficult to discern what items to scrutinize. There can be little doubt that in many parts of the English-speaking world of scholarship, the Fund is better known for its books than for its other activities. A very rough estimate of the success of its publications suggests that perhaps 20 percent have made an outstanding contribution in a particular field. Some—especially those having to do with the Fund's earlier programs—were extremely influential for a time but are now largely forgotten. Most have been important to some workers in some fields at some time. A few are long-time classics.
>
> A flattering estimate of the success of the book subsidy and the grant-in-aid segments of the Book Program comes from Dr. Martin Cummings of the National Library of Medicine, which operates the only comparable program in the country. Dr. Cummings and his associates say emphatically that our list of applicants (and awardees) is more prestigious than theirs and that the two programs, taken together, do not meet the need. Authorities in infectious disease, cardiology, and public health are equally emphatic, from their own points of view.
>
> Yet much of the testimony does not answer the basic question our Board must face: how, in comparison with other programs that we are supporting, or are considering supporting, does the Book Program stack up? . . . Is it serving the public optimally? And is its cost, when compared to the costs of other Fund programs, at an optimal level?

Chapman's own bias was that its long-term results were disproportionately small when compared with the cost of the program. Yet "as we ran it, it was relatively high risk, and I couldn't see how it could be otherwise."[20]

The Book Program changed in accordance with Chapman's ensuing recommendations. It continued to publish a few scholarly works that would not otherwise have found their way into print, along with books that complemented the Fund's other activities. Chapman had called for a conference of consultants: Biomedical scholars, representatives of university and commercial presses, as well as the director of the National Library of Medicine, met early in 1974 and advised the Fund to continue and strengthen this program. Although the program continued to work primarily through the Harvard University Press, the subsidy for a biomedical editor at the press was terminated upon negotiation of a new contract.

Fitz's retirement prompted another appraisal of the Book Program. In the fall of 1982, Lewis Thomas was appointed editor and director, and the program's purpose was redefined to encourage "the creation of authoritative yet engrossing books"[21] written primarily by working scientists for a literate lay audience. For science to obtain its rightful share of public funds, Thomas thought, the public must understand "what the scientists are up to, what research is really like, how it is done and where it seems to be heading."[22] Although all aspects of science will be considered, the program favors books in biomedicine and in the behavioral and social sciences related to human health. Publication subsidies have been replaced by grants-in-aid allowing authors to work full-time on a manuscript and covering editorial and related expenses. The program offers direction in writing as well as assistance in arranging contracts with publishers.

As in the 1920s, the Fund is emphasizing the dissemination of science to the public. In the sixty years since its inception, the Commonwealth Fund's Book Program has come full circle.

Epilogue

Progress occurs in crises, a crisis taking place when the science making most rapid progress turns its attention to the class of humanity most in need.
　　　　　　　　　　—Mary Everest Boole

Each generation of foundation officers in the United States has faced different problems as the societal setting shifts. Foundations have always needed the sensitivity to recognize changes and the flexibility to alter strategies of giving promptly and effectively. To cope with societal change, a philanthropic foundation must have both suitable form and purpose.[1] Its staff must have the means of accumulating knowledge about its areas of interest (the passive phase), and it must be in a position to evaluate and use its experience (the active phase). This two-step process allows a foundation to develop programmatic goals and creates the potential for innovative approaches. The result is a window through which the staff and board of directors can judiciously survey events, a view enabling the foundation to offer timely support.

As important as the choice of recipient is the timing of a grant in relation to scientific and social progress. The advance of medical science was characterized by George Rosen as a series of "explosion phenomena": A period of relative quiescence is followed by a crescendo to a critical, explosive level.[2] The quiet growth of knowledge and interest in bacteriology, for example, reached this critical level about 1880 and was followed by the explosive discovery, within little more than a decade, of the bacterial cause of many diseases. The gradual growth of knowledge about nutrition, which reached a critical level around 1910, was followed by the explosive discovery of vitamins. Arnold R. Rich used a similar concept—the alternation of "quiescence" and "flux"—to describe the history of medical education, and he expanded this idea to include almost all human endeavor.[3] The most important periods of flux, according to

Rich, originate in a widespread, spontaneous feeling that the existing form of any enterprise is inadequate to permit the best expression of its purposes. This feeling intensifies: Thought and energy are extensively applied to render the form of the endeavor more suitable to current demands or expectations. As participants experiment, changes—often unduly radical or reactionary—are tested freely. Finally, a modified form comes to be regarded as enough of an improvement to permit a temporary relaxation of activity. Another period of quiescence ensues, during which the outward form of the activity remains relatively static. Inactivity at these times is only apparent, however, since imperceptible changes may be occurring that will lead a new generation to find the outlines, laws, or dimensions of their social endeavor inadequate—after which a new period of flux will occur.

The Commonwealth Fund, founded in 1918, has met these peaks and swales in medicine. The evolution of its philosophy of giving; the decision-making process developed by its staff and board of directors; its relation to other institutions; and its innovative reactions to rapid changes in medicine and society over more than six decades reveal an organization successful in applying its limited resources at crucial points in the nation's systems of medical education, medical research, and health care.

Much of this success results from the Fund's traditions, attitudes toward the core problems of medicine that have persisted over the years. Tenure of officers and staff often overlapped, allowing a thread of continuity. Unlike many other foundations, the Fund has a small staff, its procedures are nonbureaucratic, and it relies heavily on outside consultants. Here again, the Fund's traditional use of consultants dates back to the days of Edward S. Harkness, the first president, and Max Farrand, the first general director; and early decisions about the organization of the staff and the process of awarding grants were made in the 1920s by Barry C. Smith, Farrand's successor.

Edward S. Harkness had a perceptive grasp of the fundamental precepts of effective institutional arrangements, including the affiliation among hospital, medical school, and parent university. He obviously understood quality, and he knew where to find it when he chose advisors in medicine and public health. Barry C. Smith, too, had a gift for selecting and placing staff members. He and his associate, Mildred C. Scoville, had backgrounds in social welfare; when the Fund's programmatic direction veered toward medicine and public health, Smith wisely brought Lester J. Evans to join the flagship staff. Evans's chance combination of experience in medical practice, public health, and education in a school dedicated to research in the basic sciences gave him the resources for his work over the next two decades. With his arrival, the Fund's central team was complete: Smith had acquired a staff member who could give him the day-to-day medical information necessary for effective decision making.

An important part of the Fund's form has been the staff members' special talents, background, and experience, along with their ability to work well together in a rare spirit of mutual respect. They have learned from each other, thought as a unit, and developed the capacity to react fluidly. Through their continuing contacts with medical schools and universities, they have used the view from their window to detect early stirrings in a field, the beginning of a period of flux. In quiescent periods the Fund has turned to the support of ancillary institutional arrangements and other services that would provide a base for advances during future times of flux. The development of a uniform medical nomenclature in the late 1920s, for example, attests to the alertness of Smith's staff to new opportunities for assistance and their ability to identify the broad, important problems in medicine. In this instance, their award cut across organizational lines, but they have also supported basic institutional needs through organizations such as the Association of American Medical Colleges and the National Academy of Sciences.

Research, education, and prevention have been the cornerstones of the Fund's programmatic structure, and over the years it has maintained a balanced program that has reached all aspects of health and all segments of society.

Concern for the Welfare of Children

From 1918 through 1920, the Fund directed its attention to the pressing problems of European relief work that followed World War I. The next programs, developed by Max Farrand, were long-range commitments in educational (1920–23) and legal (1920–43) research. These early endeavors served as only the prelude to the Fund's major work, begun in the early 1920s: projects intended to improve the nation's health.

"Child health" as a field of study was entering a period of flux in the 1920s. Clifford W. Beers had furnished the leadership to stimulate public interest in mental health and the proper treatment of the emotionally ill, and William Healy had begun his pioneering work in the juvenile courts, arousing widespread public concern about juvenile delinquency. This choice of a field of interest and the need for a broad attack on a broad problem could not have been more timely. Child health, a field with high public visibility, was ready for rapid progress, and it provided the ideal issue for shaping the form and purpose of a recently created private philanthropic foundation. Recognizing the beginning of a period of change, the Fund was able to mount an innovative program in child guidance, one with far-reaching implications for the development of child psychiatry. Again, the Fund made an excellent choice of consultants: Thomas W. Salmon, head of the new National Mental Health Association, which administered the Fund's Child Guidance Program; and Adolf Meyer, the father of dynamic psychiatry in this country, who conceived the Fund's training programs for psychiatrists.

This initial project in mental health led to educational programs in the 1920s for all levels of professionals. In the child guidance clinics, the activities of psychiatrists, psychologists, pediatricians, and psychiatric social workers were integrated, and teamwork was recognized as an important approach to both preventive and curative medical care.

At this time, too, the Fund's staff realized that even important accomplishments have no social significance unless the findings become widely known. Here was the start of the Fund's Publication Program—an endeavor that disseminated the results of outside as well as Fund-supported projects.

Once the Fund's interest in child development was established, the staff saw related fields to be plowed. Emerging concepts of public health were ripe for trial in a preventive program that would encompass immunization against communicable disease, provision of a potable water supply and a milk supply free from contamination, availability of dental care, and attention to the general health of the children of the community. Public interest had been fueled by the disclosures of the World War I Selective Service examinations: 35 percent of young men drafted were unfit for service, and a high percentage of their defects were traceable to neglect in childhood. Once again, the Fund recognized a field in flux, and it responded by creating child health demonstration units in four small communities.

A thread of continuity was developing—the experience gained in one program was leading the Fund's staff to perceive the need for the next. The welfare of the child was first addressed through the Program for the Prevention of Juvenile Delinquency, then through the child guidance clinics, and finally through the child health demonstration units. Now the Fund realized that children must be considered as part of their community and child welfare as a part of community health. The child guidance clinics and the child health demonstrations of the 1920s showed the staff one of the most important tools for progress in health: training individuals with unique capabilities, professionals who could develop new knowledge and apply it to important problems. In seizing upon this fundamental approach, the Fund's staff shaped a well-rounded program that attempted to fill gaps at several levels of expertise. The thread of continuity that extended from an emphasis on mental health to training for psychiatrists led directly to the Fund's focus on medical education. In the field of psychiatry and mental health, for example, the Fund provided support to train not only psychiatrists, but psychologists and psychiatric social workers, as well as internists and pediatricians who would integrate psychiatry with their specialties. Nor did the Fund neglect the need to support these professionals' guilds: notably, in the early days of the Fund, the Group for the Advancement of Psychiatry and the American Psychiatric Association. To establish standards, the Fund backed the American Board of Neurology and Psychiatry; to maintain these standards, it supported programs of continuing education. In all its endeavors, the Fund's staff was recognizing the need to integrate its various approaches to the problems of health.

Concern for the Welfare of the Community

Hermann M. Biggs, health commissioner for the state of New York and a consultant to the Fund, stressed the integration of practical medicine and public health. Greatly admired by Barry C. Smith, Biggs was a successful physician as well as a pioneer in uniting the institutional arrangements for maintaining health and curing disease. His plan for the first municipal diagnostic medical laboratory in the country is viewed as one of America's most important contributions to public health, and the country was soon populated with similar facilities. What made Biggs a statesman and innovator was his unique view of public health. He saw preventive medicine and curative medicine as part of a continuum—not as separate areas of activity but as integrated functions. As a consultant, Biggs helped to elucidate the purposes of the Fund, and its Rural Hospital Program was designed to fill a need that Biggs had identified.

In response to a growing nationwide interest in programs promoting good health, especially in rural areas, the Fund mounted a two-pronged attack in the late 1920s on rural public health problems, creating a Division of Public Health and a Division of Rural Hospitals. In public health as in child guidance, the Fund's organizational structure—its form—enabled its staff to recognize entry points for innovative programs.

The Division of Public Health concentrated on the development of rural health care in general, with two particular purposes: to provide field consultant service to the former child demonstration units; and to select states, communities, and institutions for new activities, establish necessary cooperative relationships, arrange evaluation of results and compilation of educational material, and furnish whatever technical and investigative services were required. This stimulus to collaboration between state and local governments was a new activity for a foundation. The Fund's general intent appears to have been to strengthen rural health service by setting up a cooperative relationship with state health departments in selected states; in several counties in Massachusetts, Mississippi, and Tennessee, public health efforts were designed to staff existing or new health departments adequately and plan local programs in accordance with standards developed collaboratively by the Fund and the American Public Health Association. Reinforced by traveling field units provided by the Fund as well as statistical, epidemiological, and other services, state health departments supervised these efforts and carried their lessons into other counties.

Traveling field units were found to be particularly valuable in fortifying local public health work. Originally a field unit consisted of a physician trained in public health work, a public health nurse, a sanitation officer, and a record clerk, but specialists in epidemiology, nutrition, and other areas were soon added. Field units were later established in other states, and the Fund's experience with these units led its staff to conclude that the best machinery available to improve the standards of rural health work had two aspects: a mobile unit teaching good public health practice as it circulated among the local health departments, and a specimen county in which to develop better-than-average standards. The field unit helped to build the demonstrations; the demonstration in turn gave the field unit teaching material. It was the formal liaison with the state health department that enabled towns to benefit from these mobile consultant services.

Other programs of the Division of Public Health also used the Fund's experience in its child health programs to offer an integrated approach to public health problems. Fund-sponsored programs produced better-trained rural physicians by combining public health with professional education. The division fortified courses in preventive medicine, strengthened facilities for postgraduate study, and offered scholarships for medical students who intended to enter rural practice and for rural physicians already in practice who wished to familiarize themselves with recent advances in medicine. An innovation was the Fund's Division of Health Studies, established in 1931 as a support service for the Division of Public Health, which enabled the Fund's staff to validate its impressions and document the results through statistical studies and research projects. The success of an integrative approach in the Child Health Program led the Fund's staff to use this same tactic in these more comprehensive public health efforts.

Under the rural-hospital construction program, the first modern hospital facilities for specific communities provided a center for combined public health and medical services. In what the Fund's staff perceived as a logical sequence, the Fund next implemented a plan for the regionalization of hospitals in order to encourage a degree of improvement in the quality of care that could not be attained by individual rural hospitals alone. A new demonstration to provide community health and hospital services at the Hunterdon Medical Center in New Jersey was the prototype for future efforts in primary care in both rural and urban areas. The Fund's grants to Hunterdon supported the services of consultants, planning and preparatory expenses, comprehensive health activities, building costs, a county-wide health inventory, and the center's mental health section. Its broad program enabled the Hunterdon Medical Center to exceed the usual community hospital's attainments in coordinating local, public efforts with private medical care.[4]

Later, the Fund expanded its support of health services to urban areas as well. Large grants given during the 1950s encouraged the development of the Home Care Program at Montefiore Hospital in the Bronx, New York, and a program of maternal and child health in Richmond, Virginia. Each of these ventures confirmed the idea that success in improving the nation's health depended on the availability of well-trained individuals.

Support of Medical Education and Medical Research

Medical schools and their parent universities became an important and logical constituency in the late 1940s. Fifteen years earlier the effects of the Flexner Report of 1910 had created a new flux in the structure and purposes of medicine. The Fund again recognized an opportunity, as it had in its child welfare and public health programs, and Edward S. Harkness's $5 million addition to the Fund's endowment in 1937 gave the staff the income to support projects in medical research. Staff and consultants used the proceeds of the gift wisely: Several investigators supported by the Fund later won Nobel Prizes for medicine or physiology. As a companion program, fellowships were awarded to young faculty members to develop their expertise in research.

Again, Harkness's "trickle-down" theory was vindicated as recipients of research grants attracted outstanding young medical scientists, who in turn trained the next generation of basic and clinical investigators. "Knowledge is power," Francis Bacon said some four hundred years ago, and the Fund's staff saw the fellowship as one of the recipient's most important tools for the acquisition of this power. The Fund's fellowships over time were intended to create leaders, not simply trained individuals, and the pathway to creative leadership was widened when young fellowship recipients were exposed to exceptional senior investigators. Awards for psychiatrists, for interdisciplinary training for young full-time faculty in schools of medicine and public health, for faculty members of professorial rank retooling their investigative skills, for nurses and members of minorities acquiring their academic qualifications—all have succeeded in supporting deserving individuals, many of whom have come into the forefront of their fields.

By the 1960s increased governmental support led the Fund to discontinue its program of fellowships. Similarly, medical research received a large proportion of the Fund's assets until the late 1950s, when the federal government began to increase its support in this area.

Awards for medical education were more controversial than awards for medical research. By 1949 the Fund's staff was scrutinizing the gap between the real and the ideal physician:[5]

The art of medicine is at once so difficult and so desperately needed that its most thoughtful practitioners, never satisfied with its attainments, are continually trying to better it. Always in flux, it moves in cycles. From time to time it shifts pace or direction. These periods of accelerated change are crucial, and we are in one today.

Sometimes the people who are trying to change medicine have a word for the quality they want to add to it. The last important shift of direction came early in the present century, when the medical schools began to take seriously the implications of what Pasteur, Claude Bernard, and Virchow had added to medicine in the preceding half century. Then the word was *scientific*. Scientific medicine was rooted in the laboratory. It was to tease out the physical components of disease and set them in order. It has given us superb microscopy, masterful biochemistry, precision in diagnosis, and—in some areas—brilliant therapy. It has led to the flowering of specialization.

Now that kind of medicine, for all its achievements, is seen to be not enough. Specialization has gained at the expense of something equally valuable—a sound general view of the patient. The parts have run away with the whole. The medical center has become a specialist's paradise, but not a good place to learn everyday medicine. There are too many people who undeniably are not helped by laboratory study and accomplished surgery. There are too many people who are allowed to develop ailments that medicine, either alone or in partnership with various kinds of social manipulation, could prevent. All this has become a commonplace criticism of medicine, and many medical educators and other leaders are trying to change the situation.

There is no one good word to describe what medicine ought to become. Those who believe doctors should be wiser than they are now deny the exclusive claim of the older medicine to the name *scientific*: they believe medicine should become more scientific, in the sense of admitting data now commonly left out of consideration. Medical progressives use the word *preventive* when they think of what medicine could do before pathology developed; *constructive* when they set "positive health" as their goal; *comprehensive* when they as doctors deal with people whole instead of in parts; *social* when they feel the pressure of the human environment on the individual and want the doctor to be at least aware of it. All these concepts are facets of good medicine; taken together they mean something different from the kind of medicine that now prevails. Specifically, without leaving out anything that is now essential to good medicine, they add new dimensions to it: breadth, to include more attention to the patient's environment; depth, to include some comprehension of his inner motivations; and duration, to relate the patient's present condition to his past and future.

The Commonwealth Fund . . . is sympathetic to these objectives and is doing what it can to foster them. They give point to its contributions to medical education and influence the choice of experimental projects in the field.

The Fund's definition of good medical practice as "comprehensive medicine" was widely misinterpreted as an attack on medical education based primarily on scientific principles. During the 1950s the medical literature contained scathing essays by defenders of the Flexnerian tradition who advocated the preservation of Flexner's scientific principles as the cornerstone of medical education.[6] The two viewpoints were nevertheless not polar opposites: Supporters of comprehensive medicine wanted to build upon the scientific aspects of medicine, which they too saw as the basis of good medical practice. Studies of the relations between patients and physicians were rare before World War II, and the Commonwealth Fund's interest in comprehensive medical care was important in bringing "patient-care research" to the public's attention. The time was right, the Fund's staff believed, to incorporate to the greatest degree possible the rapid advances in medical science into the day-to-day practice of medicine.

The reasoning was as follows. In the late 1940s the physician was becoming increasingly dependent upon a team of collaborating health professionals, each with his own technical expertise. Yet even in the face of these extensive changes in the form of medical practice, the patient still clung to the traditional image of the physician as the benevolent family doctor. At the same time public education had popularized the concepts of health as a pervasive human right and medicine as a social institution, and the universities were finding themselves the object of pressure to lead the search for better ways to distribute health care. The societal forces themselves were indistinct, however, as problems and demands were much less pressing than they later became. The universities' educational programs were also being challenged by the growing volume and complexity of medical investigation—all of which led to a perceived imbalance in the triad of teaching, service, and research.

These conflicting expectations created a new flux, which was recognized by the Fund's staff. Lester J. Evans saw the university as the agent of cultural synthesis, the guardian of medicine's future. In a series of perceptive memoranda to the staff, Evans promulgated the idea that medical schools were responsible for maintaining medicine as a profession, rather than a trade, and he generated enthusiasm among the staff for greatly increased support of medical education.[7] Evans preached the gospel of rediscovery: of the student as the primary reason for medical and professional education, and of the patient as the reason for medicine's existence. For the patient, the Fund would join forces with the medical schools to unite his life history, present environment, and social and personal needs.

Focus on Comprehensive Medicine

The Commonwealth Fund's emphasis on comprehensive medicine marked the start of its enduring partnership with the medical school. The Fund's staff agreed that many of the answers to the nation's problems of health services could be found in the university medical centers, and Evans was crusading for an approach to medicine that would make the patient's personal and emotional needs as important as his physical well-being. Change in the form of medical practice, he believed, must begin in the medical school, the ideal setting for collaboration between medical scholars and scholars in the social sciences. Education and research, rather than direct medical service, seemed to be the university's primary responsibility to society, yet concern with patient care could lead to improvements in the other two areas. No one of these three aspects of medicine could remain static when confronted with advances in another. Although progress in the biological sciences grew logarithmically after World War II, medicine was still using the organizational patterns and ideas that were appropriate when fifty years was the average life span in the United States. The Fund's staff believed that if medical schools were to educate physicians capable of meeting the demands of practice ten years in the future, universities would have to pay more attention to societal, technological, and economic changes beyond their control— factors that were dramatically altering the practice of medicine as well as the educational patterns of undergraduate and postgraduate training. The learning process and the quality of patient care in the teaching environment should be legitimate subjects of university-caliber research, and medical schools' interest in these two areas should be tackled with the knowledge and skills of the educational process itself. Medicine was not only failing to exploit the significant products of research in the social and behavioral sciences—it was virtually ignoring them.

In the first few decades of this century, medicine was a well-circumscribed field. Its activities were directed mainly toward the study of specific illnesses and their ramifications: the pathogenesis of a disease, a drug's mechanism of action, a new surgical procedure, more accurate diagnostic tests. Comprehensive medicine superimposed an attack on other problems, ones based in medicine but so broad that definition and practical solutions required trained individuals from many different fields. The Fund's staff believed that only this intellectual cross-fertilization could produce innovative yet practicable ways to improve health care.

The resulting programs in medical education in the 1950s, like the Fund's efforts in public health, were to emphasize "integration" of disciplines, so that medical education would relate to the "whole patient" and not just his disease. These programs in comprehensive medical care were the start of another thread of continuity in the Fund's programmatic development. Grants for curricular changes at Cornell University and the University of Colorado in the late 1940s and early 1950s were supported by research programs that studied the integration of all aspects of medical care. Fund-supported biomedical research also carried out the theme, focusing not on individual organs, but on the integration of organ systems for normal physiological function. Investigations concentrated on the endocrine system, emphasizing how hormones interact to control body function, and on the integrative role of the nervous system in health and disease.

In the 1960s the Fund supported expanded programs, which integrated the teaching of comprehensive medicine with community needs by founding departments of community medicine in medical schools and special units related to medical care in defined populations. In studying health care delivery in their own local areas, these programs presented a clearer picture of medical practice to the student, developed models of medical care that could be used elsewhere, and raised standards for day-to-day medical practice. As in the past, the Fund's programs linked the local practitioner and the university, to the benefit of both: The physician gained a resource for continuing education, and the university was helped to create a more effective training environment for the practice of general medicine.

As the Fund's involvement in medical education deepened, the staff extended its awareness of deficiencies to the entire system. Continuing through the late 1950s and into the next decade, grants from the Fund helped medical schools to restructure their curricula, develop closer ties to parent universities, shorten the period of premedical and medical education, offer personal counseling to premedical students, and foster research in problems of medical education. All these projects focused on the responsibility of medical educators toward the preparation of future teachers, investigators, community leaders, and medical practitioners.

The scope of the Fund's programs continued to spread through the 1960s: Next, medical schools used the needs of their local communities for comprehensive care as a laboratory for the study of both health-care delivery and research in patient care. The nature of these laboratories changed over the years. From the ambulatory clinics of university hospitals, programs in comprehensive care moved first into rural and then into urban settings. The target of these programs changed too, from individual outpatients to a group of patients considered as a unit, as in the Harvard Community Health Plan.

Of the Fund's total appropriation of $48 million between 1947 and 1956, 51 percent was allocated to medical education. Unrestricted grants to nineteen universities accounted for slightly more than half of these awards. From 1947 to 1962, fifty-five institutions received grants for such projects as recasting medical curricula, teaching comprehensive medicine, integrating medical schools with their parent universities, streamlining and shortening medical and premedical education, and undertaking research in problems of medical education. In financial terms alone, the stakes were enormous. By the academic year 1958–59, these institutions had combined operating budgets of over $319 million, which did not include construction costs, support for students, or operation of affiliated hospitals. Between 1949 and 1977, twenty-eight institutions each received $1 million or more from the Fund for medical education (see app. L). These were large sums, but the Fund's staff felt that this leverage from the private sector offered real potential for improving the nation's health.

As the Fund's staff became active partners with medical school faculties in directing change, Evans's emphasis on people over proposals was again justified. One of the most profitable of these symbiotic relationships was the collaboration between Evans and Joseph T. Wearn, which culminated in Western Reserve University's experiment in curriculum reform in the 1950s. They agreed that the quality of teachers and students with a capacity and drive for self-education far outweighed the importance of other factors. Medical education should be planned not for the exceptional, highly gifted student, nor for those at the bottom of the ladder of talent; the most effective medical curriculum would be targeted at the average good student—in other words, the majority.

In his approach to decision making, Evans relied on his numerous contacts with young and seasoned faculty members; in the 1950s most stayed at home, and Evans had no trouble capturing their time for a thorough discussion of varied ideas. His train rides to and from universities provided ample time for him to ruminate and disseminate his thoughts in memoranda to the Fund's staff. In the 1960s, however, the advent of the National Institutes of Health and their study sections and, most of all, the airplane changed the form of information gathering and development of programmatic ideas by the Fund's staff.

All aspects of medicine changed dramatically during the 1960s. By the early 1970s, more flexible medical curricula became widespread, more physicians were being graduated each year, and new medical specialties proliferated. Medical centers nationwide involved themselves increasingly in community health services, including prepaid group plans. Until the 1960s medical schools had looked inward at their own problems of education and research, but society now demanded that they look outward at social needs—a new responsibility for most universities.

The Fund still relied on the university as its major constituency. Under President Newton, it continued its emphasis on the critical problems in medical education—how the medical curriculum could come to terms with the expanding body of biomedical knowledge, how to improve coordination between premedical and professional studies, and how to strengthen postgraduate training. Related problems such as the seemingly inadequate financial base of medical education (particularly of private medical schools), the need for more effective means of keeping practicing physicians in stride with accelerating advances in medicine, and the beginning of a never-ending rise in medical costs also received attention. But now the Fund added another dimension to its support of educational institutions: It placed a high priority on encouraging universities to devise model programs addressing the management and distribution of health care.

In the 1960s and early 1970s, the Fund's staff saw the need for change throughout the entire system. Medical care must be more efficiently organized; new types of paramedical personnel must be educated to extend the capacities of physicians; new patterns of medical practice and new methods of paying for health services must be developed. Good health care would not result simply from training more physicians. Society could not afford the cost of their education nor the cost of delivering medical care on the traditional fee-for-service basis of physicians in private practice. High-quality, low-cost medical care for all would also require more nurses, technicians, and medical assistants; their functions would have to be carefully delineated, and they would have to be deployed efficiently. The Fund's support of programs creating and training new types of professionals—such as physicians' assistants and nurse practitioners—was intended to diffuse the burden of medical care, which had rested mainly with the physician. The staff believed that medical institutions should be modified to include new patterns of working in the community and should not be restricted to education centered on patients admitted to hospitals.

Like the assumptions of earlier directors and staff members toward comprehensive care, the attitude of the Fund's present board and staff toward a new system of health-care delivery echoed the belief that it would be most likely to come from universities because of their perception that medicine was no longer a circumscribed field. The design of an efficient health-care system would require the participation of economists, systems analysts, political scientists, architects, engineers, and legal scholars. Indeed, an interdisciplinary effort was mandatory if the country was to extricate itself from what appeared to be a health-care crisis.

During the early 1960s, the Fund supported a broad investigation of health and its maintenance, awarding grants to universities with an interest in the health of their surrounding communities. These studies took into account the diminishing role of the general practitioner and the expansion of group practice and hospital services. Several major issues were then selected for study, and grants were awarded to institutions with innovative, "experimental" solutions.

By 1974 a significant number of medical schools had a department of community medicine or its equivalent, and the advent of the larger Robert Wood Johnson Foundation had necessarily altered the direction and scope of the Fund's programs. Applications to the Fund for programs in comprehensive medical care had become relatively inconsequential, and the staff felt that support of an idea that had received great attention in the preceding years no longer represented the optimal use of its resources. A perceived problem in the premedical and preclinical curricula and educational trends within the medical schools themselves led the Fund in a different direction. Its plan under a new president was to tackle some of the basic problems of medical education, particularly the interface between the medical school and the university. The Fund's Premedical-Preclinical Interface Program in the mid-1970s was a continuation of its traditional interest in higher education, now no longer directed specifically at medical education per se. During the 1970s private funding of higher education in general had fallen off drastically in favor of other urgent projects concerned with community needs and the public interest. By its change in direction, the Fund was sending an important message: Higher education was an indispensable resource to any nation, the more so when the rate of social and political change was rapid.

The Interface Program was the endpoint of Lester J. Evans's prediction in the 1960s that there would be no slowing of the continuing development of the biological and physical sciences and advanced medical technologies. Ever sharper and more sophisticated diagnostic tools were to be developed over the next decade, with advances in preventive medicine keeping pace and the basic sciences seen as demanding unified presentation. Evans anticipated that new knowledge of the fundamental aspects of the mechanisms of disease and the process of life itself would force medicine to examine "the circumstances under which disease and illness occur in the human who is a social thinking and feeling being";[8] centrally important to this examination would be the integration of teaching in the basic scientific disciplines. Of all the curricular changes of the 1950s and 1960s, integrated teaching in the basic sciences was the most successful. The Interface Program incorporated all the experience that the Fund had gained with the educational process through its grants for new schools, for the reorganization of schools, for curriculum change, and for integrated teaching.

Yet the results of the Interface Program are not clear; the problems it addressed are long-standing and complex. Medical education in the United States over the past century—the effort to produce "technically competent and compassionate physicians"[9]—has elicited from medical educators attitudes running the gamut from despair to dissatisfaction. Some have said the process of education cannot be improved: in the words of one medical-school professor, changing the medical-school curriculum is like rearranging the lifeboats on the Titanic. The most prevalent response, however, has been a sort of reinvention of the wheel, as individuals and committees separated by a generation rediscover familiar problems and propose similar solutions.

Recurrent Problems in Medical Education

Even before graduation from college, the premedical student is subject to a skewed education, and it has been that way for a long time. He is a "crammer and a grinder," said Thomas H. Huxley in 1876.[10] According to a report in 1985 by the Association of American Medical Colleges (AAMC), "Physicians for the Twenty-First Century," he is a test-passer not interested in obtaining a liberal education in his undergraduate years but only in gaining admission to medical school.[11] Once he arrives at medical school, his inclinations are perpetuated. As educators have noted since the 1840s, hours of lectures supplant independent work and laboratory research, subjecting him to too many facts at the expense of understanding.[12] As a report by the AAMC charged in 1932, lectures are delivered by a parade of physicians,[13] most of whom are inadequate teachers who encourage the student to memorize rather than think.[14] The courses themselves (as Abraham Flexner and Derek Bok, the current president of Harvard University, pointed out a half-century apart) largely ignore the social, psychological, and preventive aspects of medicine.[15] In particular, introductory classes in the natural sciences reflect the "narrowness that is an inevitable part of academic departmentalization."[16]

As for the remedies, some seem unarguably worthy yet difficult to implement in many schools: Help students to become aware of the social aspects of medicine by instructing them in such subjects as medical ethics and the cost of medical care. Teach them to recognize their patients' feelings so that they can converse empathetically and ensure patients' compliance with their recommendations. Make medical schools less competitive and more generally pleasant.[17] Use an interdisciplinary approach to the teaching of the natural sciences to beginners to obviate the narrowness of those introductory courses—an idea integral to Columbia University's Program in General Education in 1919, Robert Hutchins's innovations at the University of Chicago in the 1930s, Harvard's 1945 plan for General Education in a Free Society, President Bok's 1983 Report to Harvard's Board of Overseers, the recent report of the Association of American Medical Colleges, and, in the fall of 1985, Harvard's Oliver Wendell Holmes Society, "an experimental medical curriculum, intended to enhance teaching of the 'caring' aspects of medicine."[18]

Other proposed solutions to the problems of medical education have been more controversial: The Commonwealth Fund was an early supporter of physicians' participation in health-care teams including paraprofessionals—a solution that President Bok resists, as it would diffuse responsibility for medical care.[19] Brown University has recently merged its premedical and M.D.-degree programs into a single 7- or 8-year course of study and is admitting most of its medical students directly from high school;[20] and two professors of psychiatry have recently suggested that physicians embrace the increasing impersonality of medicine rather than trying to circumvent it: "A public that has accepted fast-food chains, automatic bank tellers, and shopping mall emergicenters is unlikely to balk at health care delivered by an institution in a fast and convenient manner."[21]

The reforms suggested by President Bok and the AAMC's "Physicians for the Twenty-First Century," provide a shopping list of all the important needs in medical education visualized by Lester J. Evans and the Commonwealth Fund's staff.[22] What President Bok has termed Harvard's "most impressive innovation of the 1980s," its "entirely new curriculum" featuring "sweeping innovations," replicates many of the Fund's attempts over the past forty years to solve the problems of medical education. Bok believes that the medical school curriculum should give more attention to neglected areas of knowledge, such as medical ethics, patient psychology, and computer applications—all incorporated some years before into Fund-sponsored curricula at Western Reserve, Duke, and Boston universities. By introducing preclinical students to patients, the innovative curriculum at Western Reserve University in particular emphasized the psychological and behavioral factors that influence health.

Reform of the curriculum at the college level was a feature of all seven Fund-supported Interface Programs, in line with Bok's belief that faculty need to agree on the minimum of knowledge needed to enter medical school and then devise courses that cover the necessary material; and Bok's idea that college faculties should develop more medically oriented courses in the humanities and social sciences was carried out at the medical schools of Stanford University and the State University of New York at Stony Brook with Fund support.

President Bok's emphasis on new methods of pedagogy also echoed the Fund-supported work at the University of Buffalo. Many professors think that they can teach by the discussion method, but it is no simple matter to prepare a faculty to use new forms of instruction, especially when they have few good models to remember from their own student days. Progress in training teachers has been enhanced by the use of videotapes, which enable instructors, with the help of an experienced critic, to observe themselves in the act of teaching.

The new medical school at the University of Kentucky stressed principles of public health and the prevention of disease; this aspect of medical care was also emphasized by Bok and, before him, by John R. Paul, president of the Association of American Physicians, who advised that[23]

> there should be numbered among us, groups of physicians or perhaps individual physicians intent upon the study, not only of the patient by himself, but also of the circumstances under which the patient got ill and may remain ill. . . . It calls for the measurement by physicians of factors which concern the ecology of disease, be they extrinsic or intrinsic, and their integration. It calls for

liaison officers between intramural and extramural points of view who, besides using spectroscopes and microscopes, may even feel as if they could use telescopes now and again. It is their task to build their ecological findings into the clinical picture which is incomplete today, whether the disease in question be infectious or non-infectious, without a word or two about ecology, endemiology, or even epidemiology. Perhaps this approach to extrinsic factors can be developed by techniques which are brought to bear largely upon sick patients in bed, stripped as it were of their environment, stripped of their clothes, isolated, put into a theoretical test tube, crystallized there—like a virus perhaps. But there are other techniques which we should not shun because they are time consuming and require us to go outdoors now and again. . . .

I could mention a host of cases, some of which belong in the field of psychosomatic medicine, some in geriatrics, but all in medicine, and all of which call loudly for a doctor in the house—not necessarily as an amateur psychiatrist, and not wholly as a dispenser of "home care," but as a clinician, a pathologist, or a clinical investigator, a detective, if you will, intent upon factors which are related to the pathogenesis of disease, which some day can be measured and perhaps interpreted far better than we can measure them today.

Research in patient care, an integral part of the Fund's programs in comprehensive medicine, is singled out by Bok as deserving of more attention by physicians who "cling tenaciously to estimates based on poor information and exaggerate the informational value derived from small samples. As problems grow more complicated, such weaknesses become more costly; to avoid them, doctors will need to be proficient in the uses of statistics, computer analysis and decision theory."[24]

The Harvard Planning Group has put at the top of its list for a new curriculum "an understanding of the central physical, chemical and biological principles and mechanisms that underlie human health and disease, including awareness of the natural history and manifestation of diseases."[25] This recognition of the basic importance of traditional science in training the physician was also well-recognized by the Commonwealth Fund's staff in the 1950s.[26]

Yet such insights do not necessarily lead to desired change. Even when faculty resistance was overcome and changes were carried out, the history of efforts to reform medical education has not been one of complete success. In the late 1960s and early 1970s, student demands led to rearrangements in the curriculum that were not preceded by careful study. The focus in those years was the content of the curriculum—what everyone agreed the student should know when he graduated from medical school. Today's issues concern the goals of medical education, and specifically the role of the physician in the health-care system. The issues thus seem to recycle.

But "if there is little new in what the [AAMC] report finds and recommends," asks Steven Muller, president of the Johns Hopkins University and chairman of the AAMC panel responsible for the report, "if in fact we all have heard almost all of it before—what reason is there to expect that anything will change? Well, for whatever it is worth, my personal opinion is that this time much *will* change; indeed, that major changes are already under way. This process and prospect of change may in the end have only marginal relationships to the . . . report; it relates more directly to external circumstances. . . . The great driving forces for change are being generated largely outside the immediate context of academic medicine."[27] These forces include the need for teaching hospitals to survive in an environment of stringent cost control and intense competition, which enforce redefinition of the clinical faculties' organization and mission. The medical school and teaching hospital will continue to depend on each other, but both will pursue alternative settings for health-care delivery, the medical school in order to diversify clinical instruction, and the hospital for the sake of economic survival. The cost of health-care delivery will continue to press on the cost of medical education, and the power of economic determinism will require medical education to adjust to new constraints. Finally, increasing regulation of physicians' fees will affect both students' choice of career and professional compensation.[28]

Why is it so difficult to change medical education when, over the past fifty years, specific glaring needs have been repeatedly identified by intelligent and devoted educators?

One answer lies in the importance accorded the responsibilities of those in academic positions, whose duties have been likened to the three legs of a stool: teaching, research, and patient care. Most individuals cannot be equally adept in each. In the prestigious schools, academic advancement and better facilities go to those who are making the most evident advances in research, and less acclaim is accorded those principally concerned with undergraduate teaching and patient care. In both the preclinical and clinical departments, postgraduate scholars in the basic sciences, and resident and research fellows in the clinical departments, receive the most attention.

In choosing departmental chairmen, committees give the greatest weight to the research accomplishments of the candidates. Less value is placed on a candidate's competence as an effective clinician and teacher, and those in charge of the choice may appear to have given insufficient thought to the difference between a research institute and a medical school. This bias can be damaging to the undergraduate teaching program, particularly in the clinical departments. In a perversion of the trickle-down theory, the example commended by the committees in their choice of departmental chairmen is reemphasized by the chairmen themselves and filters through their departments.

The system is a downward spiral, and as a result, in each major flux in medical education, the same needs are reexpressed. This is the case at present. The key question is how to implement the needed changes and make them stick—a question that has not been answered by all the impressive efforts mounted in the past. The schools with the greatest influence, those that set the standards, must make these needs in medical education a major priority, mustering the resolve and faculty support for necessary changes. The particularly turbulent societal shifts affecting medical education today make it mandatory for recent appraisals and recommendations to succeed.

Directions for the 1980s

There is no shortage of questions engendered by rapid societal change and other outside influences on medical education: Have technological advances made it undesirable to use the tertiary hospital for the major portion of medical education in the clinical years? And, to quote the title of a recent article by Arnold S. Relman, "Who will pay for medical education in our teaching hospitals?"[29] With the public's demand for more adequate primary health care and better integration of health care with other social services, medical schools will be pressed to reassess their institutional goals and objectives. Alterations will not be limited to adjustments in the curriculum but will involve the mix of patient-care resources and the connection between the community and the medical school. New technology, in the form of data storage and retrieval techniques and other applications of computer technology, will also have an important effect on medical education, as medical schools address the need to integrate the increase in technological capacity with improvement of patient care systems through educational arrangements essential for productive solutions. Medical schools must also continue to face the problem of the relationship of undergraduate to graduate medical education and their responsibilities in the field of continuing education. What is the best setting for undergraduate education? How can the present system be altered to meet the changing environment for the practice of medicine? Should the educational setting be different for different purposes—for example, training generalists and training specialists?

The present multiplicity of questions now makes the Commonwealth Fund's hypothesis of the 1950s and 1960s seem rather simplistic. Its "experiments in medical education" were based on the assumption that reform in the practice of medicine would follow changes in the pattern of medical education. In the intervening years, a variety of outside forces have had a greater impact than reform of the medical curriculum on patterns of practice. Among these factors are the organization of medical practice in terms of payment, the continuing emergence of many new technologies, and the development of increasing areas of specialization. One of the most striking changes in the past twenty-five years has been the blurring of the sharp division between practicing physicians and academic physicians. Another is the increase in the number of the nation's medical schools. Nearly fifty new medical schools have come into being, the number of medical students graduated each year has more than doubled (from 7,500 to 16,000), and the size of medical school faculties has increased even more. This growth was encouraged partly by the increasing population of the country at large and the corresponding demand for medical care; it thus reflected the conclusion of the early 1960s that there was not a sufficient number of physicians, particularly primary-care physicians, to meet the needs of the nation's entire population.

This was in sharp contrast to the perception of the late 1940s that the most direct pathway to improvement in medical care was an enormous program in biomedical research. That belief led to massive grants from the federal government, particularly the National Institutes of Health. These grants in turn made it possible to train increasing numbers of individuals for faculty positions, particularly in the various subspecialties of medicine and surgery. The addition of new full-time units in the subspecialties influenced a majority of medical school graduates during the 1960s to choose specialty training and abandon general pathways. A leveling-off in grant money for research in the 1970s, however, made medical schools more dependent on income from practice. To balance the budget, more faculty time would have to be given to patient care and less to teaching and research.

The resulting accountability and restriction led to other changes as well. More than one-half of all active physicians in the United States have a defined relationship with a medical school. When medical school faculties contained only a small percentage of the total number of physicians, it was easier to separate academic physicians from those in practice. In 1979 there were some 45,000 full-time faculty members, not including interns and residents in training; twenty-five years earlier there were only 8,000 full-time faculty members. Medical students, some 60,000 in number, increased the academic total to over 165,000, to which one could add the 86,000 physicians who served as part-time or voluntary faculty in the nation's 124 medical schools.[30] Requirements in the 1970s for specialty recertification and incentives for membership in state medical societies have also brought about a strong increase in continuing medical education. When Commonwealth Fund programs in medical education began, continuing medical education represented only an occasional visit to a county medical society meeting or, through the Fund's encouragement in its Rural Hospital and Public Health programs, the return of a practitioner to a medical center for a brief course of reorientation. Now continuing education includes a continual series of meetings, using highly technical educational devices, all over the country, in locales convenient to physicians.

Financially, the disparity between full-time academic physicians and those in private practice has lessened dramatically. In the 1950s salaries of full-time academic physicians were much lower than those of practicing physicians performing similar activities. By the late 1970s, if one includes fringe benefits and retirement plans, the income of full-time medical school faculty had come much closer to that of the average income earned by successful private practitioners. Financial considerations have also brought about a marked change in the type of patients looked after by academic health centers. Medical schools are now providing more continuous and comprehensive care to population groups in reorganized outpatient clinics, health maintenance organizations, and ambulatory health centers. Complex problems formerly sent to the large university centers are now often handled locally by medical specialists going into private practice and becoming associated with their community hospitals.

Many medical schools have become increasingly dependent on income from private patients, and more full-time clinical faculty are engaged in the private practice of medicine. In this respect the wheel has made a full turn. The development of full-time professorships in clinical departments in the early 1900s made it possible for those of professorial rank to devote their time to teaching and research without the need to support themselves by private practice. Now the teachers are once more the practitioners, setting in relief again the problem that William H. Welch and others sought to alleviate. The major difference is that the practice of medicine by "full-time" teachers is now conducted within the hospital and not in outside individual private offices.

How medical education is to be paid for and carried on in these circumstances is a matter of great importance. Academic physicians and those in private practice face similar problems in dealing with social and political forces relating to the practice of medicine. Their solutions will greatly influence the educational programs as well as the practice of medicine. When Medicare and Medicaid legislation was passed in 1965, for example, the federal government in the individual states became the largest purchaser of health care, and both types of physicians had to cope with the scrutiny that accompanies the use of tax money for a given service.

The ever-changing social and political influences on medical education and practice must be taken into account in structuring the whole system of medical education, from the premedical to the postgraduate years. Although the simpler situation of the 1950s has changed greatly, in some respects the state of medicine has come full cycle as the Fund's efforts over time to integrate the science and the art of medicine are once again a center of attention. Promotion of the teaching of comprehensive medical care is a vision of the desirable that became submerged when the emphasis on specialty training increased. It is a goal now being revived at all levels.

The Commonwealth Fund's program for the 1980s emphasizes the public responsibilities of the academic medical center. The connection between the medical school and the community has been a constant theme throughout the history of the Fund's programs in medicine and health care—in the context of the 1980s, it is a prime emphasis, rather than a new idea. Now the link between education in preventive and in curative medicine is control of the cost of medical care. And as Edmund D. Pellegrino foretold fifteen years ago, "Effective evaluation research, if it is to produce change, must do so on the basis of observations directed to the suitability of a curricular mode in producing physicians adapted to the major social uses of medicine."[31]

The current efforts to modify medical instruction and medical practice have as their antecedent the Fund's Experimental Health Services. In the 1960s the Fund's staff and directors saw the most serious problem of American medicine as the lack of uniform quality in medical care: The health needs of a large segment of the nation's population were unmet. Despite its inclusive name, the Commonwealth Fund's Experimental Health Services Program was confined in the 1960s to investigating two main aspects of the nation's health services: integrative efforts to improve the delivery of medical care, and special problems related to critical events in American medicine. These problems either had not previously received careful attention from academic health centers or were beyond their defined scope of responsibility. They covered a wide range of needs, from better care for dying patients to emergency care for trauma cases and the needs of young families in relation to childbirth. The Fund's programs for health-care delivery took advantage of a variety of institutional arrangements and, in some instances, such as the Hospice Program, created new arrangements. As in the Yale Trauma Program, an innovative approach often opened up a new field which in turn generated wide national support from civilian as well as governmental sources. Indeed, many of these Fund-supported experiments soon evolved into practical components of the nation's systems of medical education and care.

The illustrative programs grouped together under the title "Experimental Health Services" appear to be a varied assortment, with little connection among them. Actually, they represent a deliberate effort by the Fund to build a programmatic structure in which peripheral as well as central endeavors are properly nourished. As in the past, the Fund supported interdisciplinary approaches. In trying to improve the delivery of health care, the Fund's programs relied not only on physicians but on nurses, technicians, physicians' assistants, and other aides. Awards to national organizations helped to maintain or set standards of medical practice and provided forums for discussion of social problems related to medicine. The assumption was that the design of a better system should also address the ethical and social questions raised by the increasing technological complexity of medicine. Here, programs would need the help of economists, systems analysts, political scientists, architects, engineers, legal scholars, and anthropologists. Another aspect, sound financing, would depend upon the cooperation of fiscal experts. (Had the federal government given enough weight to the application of financial expertise, the gross underestimation of the potential costs of Medicare and Medicaid might have been prevented.) The best possible medical care at the least possible cost required an exchange of ideas and a common understanding of purpose. The Fund's board and staff felt that its integrative approach would lead to symbiosis and not just a quantitative addition of divergent resources.

Today the direction of the Fund's programs continues to reflect the background of its leaders, beginning with the general directors who worked with Edward S. Harkness—Max Farrand and Barry C. Smith—and extending through the tenures of combined chief executive officers and presidents—Donal Sheehan, Malcolm P. Aldrich, J. Quigg Newton, Jr., Carleton B. Chapman, and Margaret E. Mahoney. In each succcessive era, the basic goal of improving American medicine remained intact, but the means changed, and the qualifications of the Fund's leaders changed accordingly (see app. M). Barry C. Smith and Mildred C. Scoville's background in the social sciences was supplemented by Lester J. Evans's experience in public health, community relations, and, later, medical research and education. After Evans's retirement, presidents without medical training obtained the necessary expertise by selecting as vice-presidents men with the requisite medical and scientific backgrounds. In the 1970s the fourth president of the Fund, Carleton B. Chapman, combined medical training with administrative experience. In the administration of Margaret E. Mahoney, the advice and involvement of a distinguished group of men and women in medicine undergirds a staff experienced in addressing public issues from a foundation's point of view.

The Capabilities of Foundations

The Commonwealth Fund's relationship with the recipients of its grants exemplifies the special power of the foundation. As one fellowship recipient wrote, "Catalysis is what I felt from The Commonwealth Fund. . . . By this process, you [the Fund] increase your influence by a factor of more than ten because there is a kindling of enthusiasm of the participants in the program. Therefore, your support can bring greatness to the project that is asking you for help. This is the power of strategic rather than tactical (full) funding. It is the role of the private foundation and I know its importance."

Foundations have a unique place in American society—one far different from that of government. They can:

—Exert influence at the cutting edge during the early period of a flux. A foundation's independence allows it to act quickly to support proposals in their embryonic stage.
—Be partners with their grant recipients, offering broad knowledge of a field and access to expert consultants.
—Support visionary projects.
—Sustain projects that have not yet acquired peer recognition.
—Respond to proposals promising only future benefits, while public funds must be allocated for ongoing support of established and politically pressing needs.
—Formulate new projects, since a foundation's flexibility in the early phases of a program is greater than that of the federal government.
—Exceed privately or governmentally imposed limits, as did the Fund in supporting training for physicians' assistants and health maintenance organizations.
—Give grants for independent and unbiased studies documenting health needs, monitoring activities in the public sector, and evaluating progress.

The physician in society has been an enduring theme of the Commonwealth Fund's efforts, and its leaders have tried to make others aware of its history of support for "courageous moves"[32] toward change. "I am not concerned with massaging the Fund's institutional ego," wrote Margaret E. Mahoney, "but in stressing to the public and the world of philanthropy that foundations have an important role in helping educational reform. The Commonwealth story is but one of several, but I see it as one of the best examples."[33] Over the years the Fund has documented the unique role of the private foundation in American society, a role undiminished by the inroads of government or by economic inflation. Seemingly intractable problems encompassing urgent needs and challenges will make the dedication of private philanthropic organizations vital in the fields of medicine and public health. The history of the Commonwealth Fund vividly displays the ways in which this foundation has exercised its mandate to "do something for the welfare of mankind."

Appendixes

Appendix A

Recipients of Psychiatric Fellowships

Henry Phipps Psychiatric Clinic

Name	Last Known Position*
Betz, Barbara J.	Adjunct Professor of Psychiatry, Cornell University
Bigelow, Rena M.	Member, Department of Mental Health, New York State
Billings, Edward G.	Professor of Psychiatry, University of Colorado
Cameron, Norman A.	Professor of Psychiatry, Yale University
Challman, S. Allen	Clinical Professor of Psychiatry, University of Minnesota
Clarke, Dean A.	Medical Director, Massachusetts General Hospital
Cohen, Robert A.	Director of Clinical Investigation (1953–68), Director, Division of Clinical and Behavioral Research (1968–), National Institute of Mental Health
Conn, Jacob H.	Emeritus Professor of Psychiatry, Johns Hopkins University
Fox, Henry M.	Director, Psychiatric Liaison Service, Peter Bent Brigham Hospital; Clinical Professor of Psychiatry, Harvard Medical School
Frank, Jerome D.	Professor of Psychiatry, Johns Hopkins University
Harms, Herbert E.	Director, Colorado Springs Child Guidance Clinic
Hartz, Jerome	Associate Professor of Psychiatry, University of Maryland

*The tables in this appendix represent a partial list of recipients. In some cases, it has also not been possible to determine the recipient's most recent academic position.

Name	Last Known Position*
Hutchens, Wendell H.	Psychiatrist, Oregon State Child Guidance Clinic; Clinical Associate in Psychiatry, University of Oregon
Johnson, Adelaide M.	Associate, Institute for Juvenile Research, Chicago
Kanner, Leo	Psychiatrist-in-charge, Children's Psychiatric Clinic, Johns Hopkins Hospital; Professor of Psychiatry, Johns Hopkins University
Keller, William Carl	Professor of Psychiatry, University of Louisville
Klein, Elmer	Associate Clinical Professor of Psychiatry, George Washington University
Klein, Henrietta R.	Clinical Professor of Psychiatry, Columbia University College of Physicians and Surgeons
Lambert, John P.	Professor of Psychiatry, Columbia University College of Physicians and Surgeons
Lambert, Richard H.	Director, Santa Barbara Mental Health Clinic
Leighton, Alexander H.	Professor of Social Psychology and Head, Department of Behavioral Sciences, Harvard School of Public Health
Leighton, Dorothea C.	Professor of Psychiatry, School of Medicine; Professor of Anthropology, School of Arts and Sciences, University of North Carolina
Lemkau, Paul V.	Professor of Mental Hygiene, Johns Hopkins University School of Hygiene and Public Health. First full-time faculty member in the field of mental hygiene in a school of public health, and first commissioner of mental hygiene of New York City
Levine, Maurice	Professor and Chairman, Department of Psychiatry, University of Cincinnati
Levy, Norman A.	Clinical Professor of Psychiatry, University of Southern California
Lidz, Theodore	Professor of Psychiatry, Yale University
Matte-Blancho, Ignacio	Professor and Chairman, Department of Psychiatry, University of Chile
Miller, Wilbur R.	Associate Professor of Psychiatry, Iowa State University
Pappenheim, Else	Clinical Associate Professor of Psychiatry, State University of New York, Downstate Medical Center
Pavenstedt, Eleanor	Director of Psychiatry Liaison Service, Colorado General Hospital; Professor of Psychiatry, Boston University
Rennie, Thomas A. C.	Professor of Psychiatry, Cornell University; Director, Payne Whitney Clinic

Name	Last Known Position*
Reynolds, Chester L.	Psychiatrist, Rochester Guidance Center; Associate, Department of Psychiatry, University of Rochester Medical School
Rodger, T. Ferguson	Professor and Chairman, Department of Psychiatry, University of Glasgow
Rosenberg, Seymour J.	Clinical Professor of Psychiatry, Georgetown University
Sharp, Lewis I.	Associate Professor of Clinical Psychiatry, New York University
Trawick, John D., Jr.	Clinical Professor of Psychiatry, University of Louisville
Watters, Theodore A.	Associate Professor of Psychiatry and Head of the Division of Psychiatry, Tulane University
Welsch, Exie E.	Staff Member, Child Guidance Clinic, Rochester, New York; Associate in Psychiatry, Columbia University College of Physicians and Surgeons
White, Paul L.	Psychiatrist for the student body, University of Texas, Austin
Wortis, Joseph	Professor of Psychiatry, Health Science Center, State University of New York at Stony Brook
Wortis, S. Bernard	Littauer Professor of Psychiatry and Director, Laboratory of Experimental Neuropsychiatry, New York University
Young, Richard H.	Assistant Professor of Psychiatry, University of Nebraska

Boston Psychopathic Hospital

Name	Last Known Position*
Coon, Gaylord P.	Clinical Associate in Psychiatry, Harvard Medical School
English, O. S.	Professor of Psychiatry, Temple University
Finesinger, Jacob E.	Professor and Chairman, Department of Psychiatry, University of Maryland
Kaufman, M. R.	Professor and Chairman of Psychiatry, Columbia University College of Physicians and Surgeons
Michaels, Joseph J.	Director, Worcester Child Guidance Clinic
Roth, William F.	Professor of Psychiatry, University of Nebraska
Saul, Leon J.	Professor of Psychiatry, University of Pennsylvania
Scott, William C. M.	Associate Professor of Psychiatry, McGill University

Colorado Psychopathic Hospital

Name	Last Known Position*
Barnacle, Clarke	Assistant Professor of Clinical Psychiatry, University of Colorado
Brady, E. James	Medical Director, Brady Hospital, Colorado Springs Institute of Psychiatry; Clinical Instructor in Psychiatry, University of Colorado
Brosin, Henry	Professor and Chairman, Department of Psychiatry, University of Pittsburgh; President, American Psychiatric Association (1967–68)
Burnett, Richard	Instructor in Psychiatry, Columbia University College of Physicians and Surgeons
Bush, Stuart K.	Associate Professor of Psychiatry, University of Colorado; Assistant Director, Psychiatric Service, Colorado Psychopathic Hospital
Carnahan, Robert	Clinical Professor of Psychiatry, University of Arkansas
Challman, Allen	Clinical Professor of Psychiatry, University of Minnesota
Dixon, Henry	Professor of Psychiatry, University of Oregon
Durfee, Marion	Pasadena Child Guidance Clinic, Pasadena, CA
Evans, John	Assistant Professor of Psychiatry, University of Oregon
Ewalt, Jack	Professor of Psychiatry, Harvard University; Chief, Massachusetts Mental Health Center, Boston, Massachusetts; President, American Psychiatric Association (1963–64)
Felix, Robert H.	First Director, National Institute of Mental Health (1949–64); Dean, St. Louis University Medical School (1965); Professor of Psychiatry, St. Louis University Medical School
Finney, R. M.	Associate Professor of Neuropsychiatry, Baylor University
Gilbert, Howard	Assistant Professor of Clinical Psychiatry, University of Colorado
Heersema, Philip	Associate Clinical Professor of Psychiatry, Stanford University; Emeritus Clinical Professor of Psychiatry, Stanford University
Hirschberg, Cotter	Professor of Psychiatry, University of Colorado; Assistant Director, Mental Health Clinic, Colorado Psychopathic Hospital; W. E. Menninger Distinguished Professor of Psychiatry, Topeka Institute of Psychoanalysis
Hunter, Herriot	Associate Professor of Psychiatry, University of Colorado

Name	Last Known Position*
Jefferson, Roland	Assistant Professor of Psychiatry, Marquette University
Kiene, Hugh	Private practice, Providence, RI
Lemere, Frederick	Clinical Professor of Psychiatry, University of Washington
Lyon, John M.	Professor of Psychiatry, University of Colorado; Director, Division of Psychosomatic Medicine, Colorado Psychopathic Hospital
Messenheimer, Myron	Assistant Professor of Psychiatry, University of Minnesota
Murdock, Harry	Medical Director, Sheppard and Enoch Pratt Hospital, Baltimore, MD
Perry, Herbert	Chief of Psychiatry and Neurology, VA Hospital, San Francisco, CA
Reynolds, Chester	Psychiatrist, Child Guidance Center, Rochester, NY
Romano, John	Professor and Chairman, Department of Psychiatry, University of Rochester
Rymer, Charles	Associate Professor of Psychiatry, University of Colorado
Schiele, Burtrum	Professor of Psychiatry, University of Minnesota
Schube, Purcell	Director of Psychiatry, Pasadena Sanitarium, Pasadena, CA
Shanahan, William	Associate Clinical Professor of Psychiatry, University of Colorado
Wallner, Julius	Chief of Psychiatry, VA Hospital, Palo Alto, CA; Associate Professor of Psychiatry, University of Michigan
Young, Stephanie	Instructor in Psychiatry, University of Colorado

Appendix B

Advanced Medical Fellows, 1938–1956

Recipient*	School (Field)	Training	Ultimate Position
Adams, Raymond D.	Medical College of Virginia (neurology)	Massachusetts General Hospital	Prof. of Neurology, Harvard U.; Chief of Neurology, Massachusetts General Hospital
Armstrong, Wallace D.	U. Minnesota (physiology, biochemistry)	Prof. Krogh, Copenhagen	Prof. and Chairman, Dept. of Biochemistry, U. Minnesota Medical School
Blake, John B.	Harvard U. (history)	Yale U.	Director, Hist. of Medicine, Nat'l. Lib. Med.
Brooks, Frank P.	U. Pennsylvania (physiology)	U. Edinburgh	Prof. of Medicine and Physiology, U. Pennsylvania
Buddingh, G. John	Vanderbilt U. (bacteriology)	European and Canadian laboratories	Prof. of Microbiology, Louisiana State U.
Bunting, Henry	Yale U. (pathology)	Harvard–MIT	Prof. of Pathology, Yale Medical School
Burch, George E.	Tulane U. (medicine)	Sir Thomas Lewis, University College, London	Prof. of Medicine, Tulane U.
Childs, Barton	Johns Hopkins U. (genetics, biostatistics)	Galton Laboratories, London	Prof. of Pediatrics, Johns Hopkins U.

*Partial list

Recipient*	School (Field)	Training	Ultimate Position
Clark, Duncan W.	Long Island U. (medicine)	Yale U.	Prof. of Preventive Med., SUNY, Downstate
Comroe, Julius H.	U. Pennsylvania (pharmacology)	National Institute for Medical Research, London	Prof. of Physiology and Director, Cardiovascular Research Institute, U. California, San Francisco
Dawson, James R., Jr.	Vanderbilt U. (pathology)	Boston City Hospital	Prof. of Pathology, U. Minnesota
Dickes, Robert, Jr.	Long Island U. (medicine)	Western Reserve U.	Prof. of Psychiatry and Training and Supervising Analyst, SUNY, Downstate
Dripps, Robert D., Jr.	U. Pennsylvania (pharmacology)	U. Wisconsin	Prof. of Anesthesiology, U. Pennsylvania
Ferrebee, Joseph W.	Bassett Hosp, Cooperstown, NY (immunology)	Europe	Director of Research, Bassett Hospital
Flink, Edmund B.	U. Minnesota (medicine, biological chemistry)	George Thorn and A. Baird Hastings, Harvard U.	Prof. of Medicine, U. West Virginia
Frye, William W.	Vanderbilt U. (preventive medicine)	Vanderbilt U. (pediatrics)	Prof. of Preventive Medicine, Vanderbilt U.
Gammon, George D.	U. Pennsylvania (neurology)	National Hospital, London	Prof. of Neurology, U. Pennsylvania
Gaskill, Herbert S.	U. Pennsylvania (psychiatry)	several schools	Prof. and Chairman, Dept. of Psychiatry, U. Colorado
Genest, Jacques	U. Montreal (medicine)	Johns Hopkins U.	Prof. of Experimental Medicine, Scientific Director, Clinical Research Institute, Montreal
Gersh, Isidore	U. Chicago (anatomy)	U. of Chicago	Prof. of Anatomy, U. Chicago
Gordan, Gilbert S.	U. California (medicine)	Massachusetts General Hospital	Prof. of Medicine, U. California, San Francisco
Green, Harold D.	Western Reserve U. (physiology)	MIT	Prof. of Physiology, Bowman Gray School of Medicine
Ham, George C.	U. Pennsylvania (medicine)	U. Virginia	Prof. of Psychiatry, U. North Carolina

Recipient*	School (Field)	Training	Ultimate Position
Horstmann, Dorothy M.	U. California (rheumatic fever)	Yale U.	Prof. of Epidemiology and Pediatrics, Yale U.
Kaplan, Henry S.	Rush Medical College (biochemistry)	NIH	Professor of Radiology, Stanford U.
Kitay, Julian I.	Beth Israel Hospital, Boston	Columbia U. (endocrinology)	Prof. of Internal Medicine and Physiology, U. Virginia
Kretchmer, Norman	SUNY, Downstate (physiological chemistry)	Montefiore Hospital, NY	Director, NICHHD; Professor, Dept. of Nutritional Sciences, U. California, Berkeley
Leavell, Hugh R.	U. Louisville (public health)	Yale U.	Director, Harvard U. School of Public Health
Lewis, George T.	Emory U. (chemistry)	Columbia U.	Professor Emeritus, Biochemistry, U. Miami
Lindzey, Gardner	Harvard U. (psychology)	Boston Psychoanalytic Institute	Director, Center for Advanced Study in Behavioral Sciences, Stanford U.
Lowry, Oliver H.	Harvard U. (biochemistry)	Dr. Linderstrom-Lang, Copenhagen	Prof. of Pharmacology, Washington U., St. Louis
Machella, Thomas E.	U. Pennsylvania (medicine)	Dr. F. C. Mann, Rochester, Minnesota (liver disease)	Prof. of Medicine, U. Pennsylvania
MacLean, Basil C.	U. Rochester (public health)	Johns Hopkins U.	Director, Strong Memorial Hospital, Rochester, NY
Mandel, H. George	George Washington U. (organic chemistry)	Dr. Roy Markham, Cambridge U.	Prof. of Pharmacology, George Washington U.
May, Charles D.	Harvard U. (pediatrics)	Harvard U. (biochemistry)	Prof. and Chairman, Dept. of Pediatrics, U. Iowa
Milstone, Jacob H.	NYU (bacteriology)	Rockefeller Institute	Prof. of Pathology, Yale U.
Most, Harry	NYU (preventive medicine)	field study in Mexico, Guatemala	Prof. of Tropical Medicine, NYU
Mulholland, John M.	NYU (surgery)	various medical schools	Prof. of Surgery, NYU
Odell, Gerard B.	Yale U. (pediatrics)	Cambridge U.	Prof. of Pediatrics, Director, Division of Pediatric Endocrinology, U. Wisconsin, Madison

Recipient*	School (Field)	Training	Ultimate Position
Pappenheimer, A. M., Jr.	Harvard U. (bacteriology)	Pasteur Institute	Prof. of Microbiology, NYU
Recant, Lillian	Columbia U. (medicine)	Harvard U. (endocrinology)	Prof. of Medicine, Georgetown U.
Reichlin, Seymour	Washington U. (neuroendocrinology)	Maudsley Hospital	Prof. of Medicine, Tufts U.
Reiser, Morton	U. of Cincinnati	U. of Cincinnati	Chairman, Dept. of Psychiatry, Yale U.
Richards, Victor	Stanford U. (physiology)	Harvard U.	Chairman, Dept. of Surgery, Stanford U.
Richmond, Jonas E.	U. Rochester (biochemistry)	Oxford U.	Prof. of Preventive and Social Medicine, Harvard U.
Rothman, Stephen	U. Chicago (dermatology)	U. Chicago (pharmacology)	Prof. of Dermatology, U. Chicago
Runyan, John W.	Johns Hopkins U. (metabolic and endocrine studies)	Thorndike Laboratory, Harvard U.	Chairman, Dept. of Community Medicine; Director, Div. of Health Care Sciences, U. Tenn. School of Medicine
Senn, Milton J. E.	Wisconsin U. (pediatrics and psychiatry)	England and France	Prof. of Pediatrics, Yale U.
Shull, Harrison J.	Vanderbilt U. (medicine)	Harvard U.	Prof. of Clinical Medicine, Vanderbilt U.
Sodeman, William A.	Tulane U. (cardiac physiology)	U. Michigan	Dept. of Comp. Medicine, U. South Florida
Spellman, Mitchell	Howard U. (clinical and research training)	U. Minnesota	Prof. of Surgery, Harvard U.
Sprague, Charles C.	U. Texas (hematology)	Washington U. School of Med.	President, U. Texas Health Science Center, Dallas
Strominger, Jack L.	Yale U. (biochemistry)	Washington U.	Prof. of Biochemistry and Molecular Biology, Harvard U.
Swank, Roy L.	Harvard U. (neurology)	National Hospital, London	Emeritus Professor of Neurology, U. Oregon
Towery, Beverly T.	Long Island U. (medicine)	Thorndike Laboratory, Boston	Prof. of Medicine, University of Louisville
Turner, Joseph C.	Presbyterian Hospital (medicine)	Dr. A. R. Dochez, Columbia U.	Prof. of Medicine, Columbia U. College of Physicians and Surgeons

Recipient*	School (Field)	Training	Ultimate Position
Venable, John H.	Emory U. (anatomy)	Harvard U.	Prof. of Anatomy, Emory U.
Watson, R. Janet	Long Island U. (medicine)	Thorndike Laboratory, Boston	Prof. of Medicine, Long Island U.
Weens, H. Stephen	Emory U. (roentgenology)	three teaching hospitals	Prof. and Chairman, Dept. of Radiology, Emory U.

Appendix C Recipients of Fellowships in Support of Creative Scholarship, 1956–1966

Recipient*	Program	Chief Place of Study	Ultimate Position
Alexander, Benjamin, M.D.	To learn new methods for purification and analysis of special blood-clotting agents	Weizmann Institute, Israel	Director, Coagulation Laboratory; Clinical Prof. of Medicine, Cornell Medical College
Allison, Fred, Jr., M.D.	For cell studies and development of electron microscopy study of fate of white blood cells in damaged tissues	Rockefeller Institute, NY	Prof. and Head, Dept. of Medicine, Louisiana State U. Med. Center
Alway, Robert H., M.D.	To prepare for appointment as professor of pediatrics at Stanford, through review of new developments in the field	Guy's Hospital, London School of Hygiene and Medicine	Dean, Stanford U.
Anderson, Donald G., M.D.	New developments in medicine and medical education	U. Virginia Med. School and Great Britain	Dean and Prof. of Medicine, U. Rochester
Anderson, John A., M.D.	Rhythmical changes in physiological and biological variables occurring in the body in a daily cycle, and their interrelations in health and disease	Karolinska Institute, Stockholm	Prof. and Chairman, Dept. of Pediatrics, U. Minnesota

*Partial list

Recipient*	Program	Chief Place of Study	Ultimate Position
Anderson, Richard W., M.D.	To confer with experts in psychiatry	Dept. of Child and Family Psychiatry, Ipswich and Suffolk Hospitals, England	Prof. of Psychiatry, U. Minnesota
Atkins, Elisha, M.D.	Mechanism of fever production	Radcliffe Infirmary, Oxford U.	Prof. of Medicine, Yale U.
Austin, James H., M.D.	To act as Visiting Prof. of neurology and integrated basic sciences at a new, pace-setting medical school	All-India Institute, New Delhi	Prof. and Chairman, U. Colorado Health Sciences Center
Austrian, Robert, M.D.	Microbiology, emphasizing genetics	Pasteur Institute, Paris	Musser Prof. of Research Medicine, Chairman, Dept. of Research Medicine, U. Pennsylvania Medical Center
Ball, Eric G., Ph.D.	Integration of basic science teaching; to deliver paper on subject at ASME Conference, London	Medical schools in Great Britain	Prof. and Acting Chairman, Dept. of Biochemistry, Harvard U.
Barger, A. Clifford, M.D.	Medical education and coronary artery disease	Medical centers in Europe, U.S.S.R.	Assoc. Prof. of Physiology, Harvard U.
Barnett, Henry L., M.D.	To learn medical statistics and epidemiology, related to kidney disease	London School of Hygiene and Tropical Medicine	Prof. and Chairman, Dept. of Pediatrics, Albert Einstein Medical College
Barnett, Thomas B., M.D.	Investigations of physiology of breathing and muscle activity	Laboratory for the Theory of Gymnastics, U. Copenhagen	Prof. of Respiratory Diseases, Div. of Pulmonary Diseases, Dept. of Med., U. North Carolina School of Medicine
Beeson, Paul B., M.D.	To act as consultant on planning new med. school	U. of Nottingham, England	Prof. of Medicine, Oxford U.
Beierwaltes, William H., M.D.	Thyroid disorders; lead in tumor localization of radionuclide labeled compounds in malignant melanomas	Own laboratory, U. Michigan	Prof. of Medicine, Physician-in-Charge, Section of Nuclear Medicine, U. Michigan

Recipient*	Program	Chief Place of Study	Ultimate Position
Benditt, Earl P., M.D.	To prepare manuscripts for two books; to observe current teaching in pathology	Sir William Dunn, School of Pathology, Oxford U.	Prof. and Chairman, Dept. of Pathology, U. Washington
Bernheimer, Alan W., Ph.D.	To explore new techniques for studying bacterial proteins and review of related problems	Dept. of Pathology, Oxford U.	Prof. of Microbiology, NYU; Chairman, Basic Medical Sciences, Graduate School of Arts and Sciences, NYU
Berryhill, W. Reece, M.D.	To restudy medical undergraduate and graduate curricula in clinical medicine	Medical centers in U.S., Europe	Dean and Prof. of Medicine, U. North Carolina
Bland, John H., M.D.	Connective tissue research and survey of medical education	Rheumatism Research Center, Manchester, England	U. Vermont, Director, Rheumatism Research Unit
Blankenhorn, David H., M.D.	Research on vascular pathology, emphasizing atherosclerosis	Dept. of Medicine and Pathology, Rigshospitalet, Copenhagen	Prof. of Medicine and Director, Atherosclerosis Research, USC
Bogdonoff, Morton D., M.D.	To explore relationship between clinical medicine and social sciences	Duke U.; U. North Carolina	Prof. of Medicine, New York Hosp.– Cornell Med. Ctr.
Brown, Kenneth T., Ph.D.	Visual neurophysiological problems	Australian National U., Canberra	Prof. of Physiology, U. California, San Francisco
Bruce, Robert A., M.D.	Cardiovascular physiology and pathology	Royal Infirmary, Edinburgh	Prof. of Medicine, U. Washington
Burnett, Charles H., M.D.	Medical genetics	U. London; Galton Lab.	Prof. of Medicine, U. North Carolina
Buxton, C. Lee, M.D.	To review experience of foreign teaching centers with prepared childbirth techniques	Centers in U.S., Great Britain, Europe	Prof. of Ob./Gyn., Yale U.
Carnes, William H., M.D.	To review teaching programs and conduct virus research	Bland-Sutton Institute, Middlesex Hospital, London	Prof. of Pathology, UCLA
Chargaff, Erwin, Ph.D.	To teach and write on nucleic acid chemistry	Institute for the Study of Macromolecules, Strasbourg, France	Prof. and Chairman, Dept. of Biochemistry, Columbia U., College of Physicians and Surgeons

Appendix C

Recipient*	Program	Chief Place of Study	Ultimate Position
Clark, Duncan, M.D.	Social medicine	U. Birmingham, England	Prof. of Environmental Medicine and Community Health, SUNY Downstate Medical Center
Cohen, Philip P., M.D., Ph.D.	Physiological chemistry	Oxford U.	Prof. and Chairman, Dept. of Physiological Chemistry, U. Wisconsin
Cohen, Seymour S., Ph.D.	Action of nucleic acids	Pasteur Institute, Paris	Prof. of Microbiology, Hebrew U. Hadassah Medical School, Jerusalem
Cohn, Roy B., M.D.	Research on blood flow	St. Bartholomew's Hospital Medical School, London	Prof. of Surgery, Stanford U.
Craddock, William E., M.D.	Study and teaching of neuroradiology	Ulleval Hospital, Oslo	Prof. of Radiology, U. Virginia
Craig, Albert B., Jr., M.D.	To serve as Senior Lecturer at new medical school	U. Lagos Medical School, Nigeria	Prof. of Physiology, U. Rochester Medical Center
Craige, Ernest, M.D.	To confer with eminent cardiologists abroad	Laboratory of Dr. Aubrey Leatham, St. George's Hospital, London	Prof. of Medicine; Chief, Cardiology Division, U. North Carolina
Creger, William P., M.D.	Hematology and curriculum studies	Centers in Great Britain, Europe	Prof. of Medicine, Associate Dean for Student Affairs, Stanford U. Medical Center
Curtin, James A., M.D.	To continue study of bacteriology, infectious diseases	Dept. of Medicine, Johns Hopkins	Chairman, Dept. of Medicine, Washington Hospital Center, Washington, D.C.
Davie, Earl W., Ph.D.	Investigations of microbial genetics	Institute of Molecular Biology, U. Geneva	Prof. of Biochemistry, U. Washington, Seattle

Recipient*	Program	Chief Place of Study	Ultimate Position
Deuschle, Kurt W., M.D.	To review developments in social medicine, programs in community medicine for undergraduate, postgraduate physician education	WHO in Copenhagen and Geneva	Prof. and Chairman, Dept. of Community Medicine, Mt. Sinai School of Medicine
Dingle, John H., M.D.	To write on acute respiratory disease and on the role of influenza bacillus as a cause of disease	Geneva, Switzerland	Prof. and Chairman, Dept. of Preventive Medicine, Western Reserve U.
Duff, Ivan F., M.D.	Rheumatic disease studies in different populations	Centers in Far East	Prof. of Internal Medicine, Physician-in-Charge, Arthritis Division, University Hospital, U. Michigan School of Medicine
Eckenhoff, James E., M.D.	Study of new anesthesia procedures; exploration of teaching methods in his field	Special Hospital for Plastic Surgery, East Grimstead, England	Dean, Northwestern U. School of Medicine
Edelman, I. S., M.D.	Cellular and subcellular events in various disease states	Polymer Dept., Weizmann Institute, Israel	Prof. of Medicine, Cardiovascular Research Institute, U. California, San Francisco
Eder, Howard A., M.D.	Blood protein studies in animals and man; teaching of clinical medicine	Dept. of Chemical Pathology, St. Mary's Hospital, London	Prof. of Medicine, Div. of Arteriosclerosis Research and Human Nutrition, Albert Einstein Medical College
Epstein, Franklin H., M.D.	To review new techniques for extending his research on kidney function	Oxford U.	Prof. of Medicine, Harvard Medical School; Physician-in-Chief, Beth Israel Hospital
Featherstone, Robert M., Ph.D.	Use of x-ray diffraction techniques	Birbeck College, London	Prof. and Chairman, Dept. of Pharmacology and Experimental Therapeutics, U. California, San Francisco

Recipient*	Program	Chief Place of Study	Ultimate Position
Fischer, Harry W., M.D.	To review teaching, new diagnostic techniques and research in his field	Centers in Scandinavia, Great Britain	Prof. and Chairman, Dept. of Radiology, U. Rochester
Fishman, Alfred P., M.D.	Problems of pulmonary physiology	Nuffield Inst. for Medical Research, Oxford U.	Director, Cardiovascular-Pulmonary Division, Dept. of Medicine, U. Pennsylvania School of Medicine
Fitch, Frank W., M.D.	Studies of action of antibodies	Institute of Biochemistry, Lausanne	Prof. of Pathology, U. Chicago
Fitzpatrick, Thomas B., M.D.	To conduct research, write book on melanin pigment	Oxford U.	Prof. and Chairman, Dept. of Dermatology, Harvard Medical School
Fruton, Joseph S., Ph.D.	Protein research	Chemical Laboratory, Cambridge U.	Prof. and Chairman, Dept. of Biochemistry, Yale U.
Fulmer, Hugh S., M.D.	Training in biostatistics and epidemiology	Harvard School of Publ. Hlth.	Prof. of Medicine and Director, Div. of General Medicine and Primary Care, U. Massachusetts Medical School, Worcester
Furchgott, Robert F., Ph.D.	To learn new experimental techniques and concepts	Dept. of Physiology, U. Geneva, Switzerland	Prof. and Chairman, Dept. of Pharmacology, SUNY, Downstate
Gellhorn, Alfred, M.D.	To take stock, read, review research and new techniques; study chemically induced cancer formation at molecular level	Chester Beatty Research Institute, London	Vice-Pres. for Health Affairs, Director, Center for Biomedical Education, CCNY
Gellis, Sydney S., M.D.	Liver disease in the newborn	Centers in Great Britain, Europe	Prof. of Pediatrics, Tufts U.
Gemmill, Chalmers L., M.D.	To trace ancient history of medicine in Africa and Greece and the value of the ancient plant "silphium"	Great Britain, Libya, Greece	Prof. of Physiology, U. Virginia

Recipient*	Program	Chief Place of Study	Ultimate Position
Ginsberg, Harold S., M.D.	To engage in protein chemistry and virus research, and to review teaching on this subject	Institute of Biochemistry, Lausanne	Chairman, Dept. of Microbiology, Columbia U., College of Physicians and Surgeons
Glaser, Gilbert H., M.D.	To study new techniques of clinical and experimental neurophysiology and electroencephalography	Hospital for Sick Children, London	Prof. of Neurology, Yale U.
Glick, David, Ph.D.	To analyze research, prepare a book on histo- and cytochemistry	Centers in Europe	Director, Center for Histochemical Research, Stanford U. Medical Center
Gordan, Gilbert S., M.D.	Tissue culture studies	Strangeways Laboratories, Cambridge U.	Prof. of Endocrinology, U. California, San Francisco
Green, Robert H., M.D.	Air pollution research	British Medical Research Unit, London	Prof. of Pathology and Medicine, Yale U. School of Medicine, Associate Chief of Staff for Research, West Haven VA Hospital
Greep, Roy O., Ph.D.	Endocrinology studies	U. Sheffield, England	Director, Lab. of Human Reproduction and Reproductive Biology, Harvard U.
Grigsby, Margaret E., M.D.	To study for degree in tropical medicine	London School of Hygiene and Tropical Medicine	Prof. of Medicine, Howard U. College of Medicine
Grossman, Lawrence, Ph.D.	Mechanisms useful for genetic investigation	Institute of Molecular Biology, U. Geneva	Prof. of Biochemistry, Brandeis U.
Ham, George C., M.D.	Genetic factors and psychological and sociological adaptation	Genetic centers in U.S., Great Britain, Europe	Prof. and Chairman, Dept. of Psychiatry, U. North Carolina
Ham, T. Hale, M.D.	Research and writing on the program of medical education at Western Reserve	Western Reserve	Director, Div. of Research in Medical Education, Case Western Reserve U.

Recipient*	Program	Chief Place of Study	Ultimate Position
Hammon, William M., M.D.	To write up much unpublished research and clarify general principles in field of virology	U.S.	Prof. and Head, Dept. of Epidemiology and Microbiology, U. Pittsburgh Grad. School of Public Health
Hamolsky, Milton W., M.D.	To investigate new techniques for thyroid research	Collège de France, Paris	Physician-in-Chief, Dept. of Medicine, and Prof. of Medical Science, Brown U.
Harmel, Merel H., M.D.	To study the basic principles and techniques of cell biology	Laboratory of Biochemistry, Oxford U.	Prof. and Chairman, Dept. of Anesthesiology, Duke U. Medical Center
Harrison, Saul I., M.D.	To study techniques for analyzing psychiatric data, known as "Hampstead Index"	Hampstead Clinic, London	Prof. of Psychiatry, U. Michigan
Haugaard, Niels, Ph.D.	To investigate pharmacological problems and rhythmical biochemical reactions in cell-free systems	Dept. of Physiological Chemistry, U. Amsterdam	Prof. of Pharmacology, U. Pennsylvania School of Medicine
Hawkins, David, M.D.	To study the psycho-physiological influences of emotions	Institute of Psychiatry, Maudsley Hospital, London	Prof. and Chairman, Dept. of Psychiatry, U. Va. School of Medicine
Heald, Felix P., M.D.	Research on nutritional problems in children	Division of Nutritional Sciences, U. California, Berkeley	Prof. of Pediatrics and Director, Div. of Adolescent Medicine, U. Maryland School of Medicine
Hechter, Oscar, Ph.D	To review biomedical research literature and prepare manuscripts for three books	Worcester Foundation for Experimental Biology	Prof. of Physiology, Northwestern U. School of Medicine
Hiatt, Howard H., M.D.	Biochemical studies of cell growth	Pasteur Institute, Paris	Dean, Harvard School of Public Health
Howe, Calderon, M.D.	To study new techniques for investigating immuno-chemical and virus infections	Pasteur Institute, Paris	Prof. and Head, Dept. of Microbiology, Louisiana State U. Medical Center

Recipient*	Program	Chief Place of Study	Ultimate Position
Hudson, Robert P., M.D.	To study and obtain master's degree in History of Medicine	Johns Hopkins U.	Chairman, Dept. of the History and Philosophy of Medicine, U. Kansas Medical Center
Hurst, J. Willis, M.D.	To learn new vector ECG techniques related to electrocardiographic studies	Institute of Cardiology, Mexico City	Prof. and Chairman, Dept. of Medicine, Emory U.
Ingram, Walter R., Ph.D.	To review research in neurophysiology	Centers in U.S., Canada, Europe	Prof. and Head, Dept. of Anatomy, Iowa State U.
Jensen, Wallace N., M.D.	To review new methods of hematology research	School for Advanced Study, National Transfusion Center, Paris	Prof. and Chairman, Dept. of Medicine, George Washington U. Medical Center
Kaplan, Nathan O., Ph.D.	For biochemical studies of enzyme structure and action	Weizmann Institute, Israel	Prof. of Chemistry, U. California, San Diego
Kappas, Attallah, M.D.	To review problems relating to immunology and auto-immune mechanisms	Courtauld Institute of Biochemistry, Middlesex Hospital Medical School, London	Physician-in-Chief and Prof. of Medicine, Rockefeller U. Hospital, NY
Kern, Fred, Jr., M.D.	To review new techniques in gastroenterology	Dept. of Physiological Chem., U. of Lund, Sweden	Prof. of Medicine, Div. of Gastroenterology, U. Colorado Health Science Center
Kitay, Julian I., M.D.	To continue training in endocrinology; to engage in research in neuroanatomy and neurophysiology (2nd award)	Columbia U., College of Physicians and Surgeons; Cambridge U., with Dr. Barry Cross	Dean, School of Medicine, U. Texas Med. Branch., Galveston
Klatskin, Gerald, M.D.	To broaden his knowledge of metabolic and liver disorders and review new research techniques	Inst. of Pathological Anatomy, U. Copenhagen	Prof. of Medicine, Yale U.

Recipient*	Program	Chief Place of Study	Ultimate Position
Kolb, Lawrence C., M.D.	To review developments in social psychiatry, to write	Centers in Great Britain, Europe, U.S.S.R.	Prof. and Chairman, Dept. of Psychiatry, Columbia U., College of Physicians and Surgeons
Kretchmer, Norman, M.D.	To review pediatric research and special techniques; to carry on research related to developmental biochemistry and genetics, pediatric education, and international child health (2nd award)	Galton Laboratory, London, with Drs. Dent and Harris; Latin America, Europe, U.S.S.R.	Prof. of Nutrition, Obstetrics and Pediatrics, College of Natural Resources, U. California, Berkeley
Kruse, Cornelius W., M.S.	Further study in environmental health	U. Pittsburgh School of Public Health	Prof. and Chairman, Dept. of Environmental Health, Johns Hopkins U. School of Hygiene and Public Health
Landau, Bernard R., M.D., Ph.D.	To learn new enzyme techniques	Dept. of Biochemistry, Western Reserve	Prof. of Medicine and Pharmacology, Case Western Reserve U.
Landau, Richard L., M.D.	To learn new developments in the physiology of adrenals and gonads	Centers in Great Britain, Europe	Head, Section of Endocrinology, Dept. of Medicine, U. Chicago
Lawrence, H. Sherwood, M.D.	To participate in research on tissue sensitivity problems	University College, London	Prof. of Medicine, NYU
Lembcke, Paul A., M.D., M.P.H.	Investigation of the organization and operation of a Swedish hospital	Karlskoga Hospital, Sweden	Prof. of Public Health Admin., Johns Hopkins School of Hygiene
Lerner, Aaron B., M.D.	To investigate mechanisms of hormone function	Dept. of Biochemistry, Cambridge U.	Prof. of Dermatology, Yale U. School of Medicine
Lidz, Theodore, M.D.	To restudy teaching of psychoanalytic concepts, to prepare a textbook for medical students	Italy	Prof. of Psychiatry, Yale U.
Lief, Harold I., M.D.	To prepare a monograph, "The Making of a Physician"	Tulane U.	Center for Study of Sex Education in Medicine, U. Pennsylvania

Recipient*	Program	Chief Place of Study	Ultimate Position
Lippard, Vernon, M.D.	To review medical curriculum and relations between schools and hospitals, with special reference to preventive and social medicine	England and Scandinavia	Dean and Prof. of Pediatrics, Yale U.
London, Irving M., M.D.	Further studies of genetic control of proteins (enzymes)	Pasteur Institute, Paris, with Prof. Jacques Monod	Director, Harvard–MIT Division of Health Sciences and Technology
Long, Cyril N. H., D.Sc.	To review research, prepare a book on adrenal hormones	U. Hawaii	Prof. and Chairman, Dept. of Physiology, Yale U.
McManus, Joseph F. A., M.D.	To review recent work in histochemistry and biology and to write	Dept. of Zoology, Oxford U.	Dean, College of Medicine, Medical U. of South Carolina
Madden, Sidney C., M.D.	To participate in research in cell mitosis	Oxford U. with Sir Hans Krebs	Prof. and Chairman, Dept. of Pathology, UCLA
Mandel, H. George, Ph.D.	To participate in research on drug action on nucleoprotein synthesis	New Zealand	Prof. and Chairman, Dept. of Pharmacology, George Washington U.
Markham, Charles H., M.D.	To review research in neurology and neurophysiology	Max Planck Institute for Brain Research, Frankfurt	Prof. of Neurology, UCLA School of Medicine
Marks, Paul A., M.D.	To participate in studies of problems relating to genetics and cellular biology	Laboratory of Cellular Biochemistry, Pasteur Institute	Vice-President for Health Sciences, Columbia U.
Milstone, J. Haskell, M.D.	To do research on blood clotting factor	His own laboratory at Yale U.	Prof. of Pathology, Yale U. School of Medicine
Mirsky, I. Arthur, M.D.	To lecture and conduct seminars for medical students, graduates, on medical and psychiatric subjects	Hebrew U., Israel	Prof. of Medicine, Prof. of Psychiatry, UCLA
Mommaerts, Wilfried, Ph.D.	To review research and literature relating to physical chemistry and thermodynamics	Institute for the Study of Macromolecules, Strasbourg, France	Prof. and Chairman, Dept. of Physiology, UCLA

Recipient*	Program	Chief Place of Study	Ultimate Position
Monroe, Russell R., M.D.	To review the literature and write on episodic behavior disorder	Centers in Great Britain, Europe	Dir. of Research, Dept. of Psychiatry, U. Maryland School of Medicine
Moore, John W., Ph.D.	To review research on the physiology of interactions between a few neurons, and the characteristics of model neuron networks; to write	Centers in U.S.	Prof., Dept. of Physiology and Pharmacology, Duke U.
Morgan, Herbert R., M.D.	To engage in tissue culture studies	Institute of Cancer, Villejuif, France	Director, Independent Studies Program, U. Rochester School of Medicine and Dentistry
Moritz, Alan R., M.D.	To review the work and thinking of academic pathologists abroad	Centers in Great Britain, Scandinavia	Prof. of Pathology, Western Reserve
Parks, John, M.D.	To review patient care and teaching procedures in ob/gyn	Centers in Great Britain, Europe	Dean and Prof. of Ob./Gyn., George Washington U.
Parmelee, Arthur H., Jr., M.D.	To review research and examination techniques in maturation of central nervous system	Neonatal Research Institute, Paris	Head, Div. of Child Development, and Prof. of Pediatrics, UCLA School of Medicine
Richards, Dickinson W., M.D.	To gather new material for a book, *The Fabric of Cardiovascular Concepts*	Centers in Egypt, Europe	Prof. of Medicine, Columbia U., College of Physicians and Surgeons
Richmond, Julius B., M.D.	To review psychological literature, write, visit colleagues in connection with his interests in pediatrics and medical education	Centers in U.S., Europe, U.S.S.R.	Director, Judge Baker Guidance Center, Boston, Mass.
Romano, John, M.D.	To review educational activities, research in his field; possibly prepare textbook for medical students	Centers in Great Britain, Europe	Distinguished University Prof. of Psychiatry, U. of Rochester School of Medicine
Rose, Augustus S., M.D.	To review teaching in neurology, to write	Centers in U.S., Canada	Prof. and Chairman, Dept. of Neurology, UCLA School of Medicine

Recipient*	Program	Chief Place of Study	Ultimate Position
Rose, Noel R., M.D., Ph.D.	Advanced study of immunology Inst. of Biochemistry, U. of Lausanne (2nd award)	Pasteur Institute, Paris	Prof. of Immunology and Infectious Disease, Johns Hopkins U.
Samuels, Leo T., Ph.D.	To participate in research on problems of steroid hormones	Cambridge U., England	Prof. of Biochemistry, U. of Utah
Scheinberg, I. Herbert, M.D.	To study new biophysical techniques	Scripps Institute, La Jolla, CA	Division of Genetic Medicine, Dept. of Medicine, Einstein
Schilling, Robert F., M.D.	To review literature, learn new immunological techniques	U. London	Prof. of Medicine, U. Wisconsin
Seegers, Walter, Ph.D.	To prepare monograph on blood clotting	U.S., South America, Europe	Chairman, Dept. of Physiology, Prof. of Hematology, Dir., Thrombosis Specialized Center of Research, Wayne State U. School of Medicine
Senn, Milton J. E., M.D.	To review literature, write, reflect	Centers in U.S., Great Britain, Europe	Prof. and Chairman, Dept. of Pediatrics, Yale U.
Sims, Ethan A. H., M.D.	For studies relating to problems of the adrenal gland, electrolyte metabolism, renal function, diabetes mellitus	Western Reserve U.	Prof. of Medicine, Metabolic Unit, Dept. of Medicine, U. Vermont
Smith, Richard T., M.D.	Research relating to interactions between cells and chemical compounds	Tumor Biology Institute, Karolinska Institute, Stockholm	Prof. and Chairman, Dept. of Pathology, U. Florida Coll. of Medicine, Gainesville
Sprague, Charles C., M.D.	To review recent developments in medical administration	Centers in U.S., Great Britain, Europe	President, University of Texas Health Science Center at Dallas
Stetten, DeWitt, Jr., M.D., Ph.D.	To review medical education	Centers in U.S.	Deputy Director for Science, NIH
Stevenson, Ian, M.D.	To prepare a book on psychopathology	Zürich, Switzerland	Prof. of Psychiatry and Director, Div. of Parapsychology, U. Va. School of Medicine

Appendix C

Recipient*	Program	Chief Place of Study	Ultimate Position
Stotz, Elmer H., Ph.D.	To review new developments in general chemistry; to write	Cambridge U.	Prof. and Chairman, Dept. of Biochemistry, Yale U.
Swank, Roy L., M.D.	To participate in studies of vascular disease problems and fat metabolism	Biochemical and Physiological Institute, U. Cologne, Germany	Prof. and Head, Div. of Neurology, U. Oregon Medical School
Syverton, Jerome T., M.D.	To review research on host-cell-virus relationships and cancer; to write	Centers in Great Britain, Europe	Prof. and Head, Dept. of Bacteriology and Immunology, U. Minnesota
Taussig, Helen, M.D.	To complete manuscript of revised edition of book on congenital heart disease	Baltimore, MD	Prof. of Pediatric Cardiology, Johns Hopkins U.
Thorup, Oscar A., M.D.	To review medical education	Centers in Great Britain, Europe	Prof. and Head, Dept. of Bacteriology and Immunology, U. Virginia
Uhr, Jonathan, M.D.	To review research on the relation of delayed tissue sensitivity to virus immunity	Hall Institute of Medical Research, Melbourne, Australia, with Sir MacFarlane Burnet	Prof. and Chairman, Dept. of Microbiology, U. Texas Health Science Center at Dallas
Walker, James E. C., M.D.	To review systems, problems of health care and education, in preparation for new post as Prof. of Medicine and Society, U. of Connecticut	Centers in U.S., Europe, Africa, South America	Prof. and Chairman, Community Medicine and Health Care, U. Conn. Health Center
Watson, Cecil J., M.D.	To complete manuscripts for monograph on bile pigments and porphyrins in medicine	U. Minnesota; laboratories in Europe	Prof. of Medicine and Director of Unit for Teaching and Research, U. Minnesota
Weinerman, E. Richard, M.P.H.	To observe individual and group medical practice in its community setting; to write	Centers in Great Britain, Europe (primarily Eastern Europe)	Prof. of Medicine and Public Health, Yale U.

Recipient*	Program	Chief Place of Study	Ultimate Position
Welch, Arnold D., M.D., Ph.D.	To participate in research on drug effects on a certain type of virus	Inst. for Biochemical Therapeutics, U. Frankfurt am Main, Germany	President, Squibb Inst. for Med. Research, Vice President, E. R. Squibb & Sons, Inc.
White, Abraham, Ph.D.	To review new developments in biochemistry, medical education, social medicine	Centers in Great Britain, Europe	Distinguished Scientist, Inst. of Biological Sciences, Syntex (U.S.A.), Inc.
White, Kerr L., M.D.	To review research, teaching in epidemiology and social medicine; to write	Social Medicine Research Unit, London Hospital	Prof., Dept. of Medical Care and Hospitals, Johns Hopkins U. School of Hygiene and Public Health
Whitehorn, John C., M.D.	To write on influence of social and emotional factors on reactions to life situations	Johns Hopkins U.	Prof. and Director, Dept. of Psychiatry, Johns Hopkins U.
Wilkins, Lawson, M.D.	To revise textbook on pediatric endocrinology	Baltimore, MD	Prof. of Pediatrics, Johns Hopkins U.
Wissler, Robert W., Ph.D	To review nutritional problems and disease-linked protein factors in blood	Theodor Kocher Institute, Berne, Switzerland, with Dr. Ernst F. Luscher	Prof. of Pathology, U. Chicago
Wolf, George A., Jr., M.D.	To observe the organization and programs of medical centers, in preparation for new post as Vice-Pres. for Medical and Dental Affairs, Tufts U.	Centers in Great Britain, Europe, Canada	Dean and Prof. of Clinical Medicine, U. Vermont
Wolf, Stewart, M.D.	To complete a book, review neurophysiology developments	Centers in Europe	Director, Totts Gap Institute, Bangor, Pa.
Wood, Earl H., M.D., Ph.D.	Cardiovascular research; to review literature, write	U. Berne, Switzerland, with Prof. Weidmann, Dept. of Physiology	Prof. of Physiology, U. Minnesota, Mayo Clinic
Wood, Harland G., Ph.D.	Biological research on problems relating to carbon-dioxide fixation by the body	Max Planck Institute, Munich, with Prof. Lynen	Prof. and Director, Dept. of Biochemistry, Western Reserve U.

Recipient*	Program	Chief Place of Study	Ultimate Position
Wortis, Samuel B., M.D.	Intensive biologic studies of acute psychotic reactions in patients; to write a monograph	Centers in U.S., Canada, Europe	Prof. and Chairman, Dept. of Psychiatry and Neurology, NYU
Wyngaarden, James B., M.D.	Studies of genetic control of metabolic and related disorders	Curie Institute Paris, with Dr. François Gros	Prof. and Chairman, Dept. of Medicine, Duke U. Medical Center; Director, NIH
Zamecnik, Paul C., M.D.	Further investigations of protein synthesis problems	Cambridge U., with Prof. Alexander Todd	Director, Warren Labs., Harvard Medical School, Massachusetts General Hospital

Appendix D

Grants for Medical Research, 1919–1984

(*arranged chronologically by date of first grant*)

Columbia University, College of Physicians and Surgeons
James W. Jobling. Study of rickets. 1920–23

Columbia University, Neurological Institute
Charles A. Elsberg. Study of epilepsy. 1920–32

Columbia University, Neurological Institute
Charles A. Elsberg. Study of multiple sclerosis. 1920–35

New York University
William H. Park. Diphtheria immunization. 1921–23

National Tuberculosis Association
Occupations suitable to arrested tuberculosis cases. 1922

Presbyterian Hospital, Constitution Clinic
Walter W. Palmer, George Draper. Susceptibility of certain types to gall bladder disease, and support of the clinic. 1925–29

New York University, New York City Department of Health
William H. Park. Scarlet fever immunization. 1925–26

Pennsylvania Hospital
Earl D. Bond. Study and treatment of postencephalitic girls. 1927–33

Johns Hopkins Hospital, Cardiac Clinic
Edwards A. Park. Data on children recovering from chorea and rheumatic fever, and autopsy study. 1928–29

University of Michigan
R. L. Kahn. Blood serum test for diagnosis of tuberculosis. 1928–29

Saranac Laboratory
Hugh M. Kinghorn. Study of silicosis and pneumonoconiosis. 1928–31

New York University
William H. Park. Serum treatment for bronchial pneumonia. 1928–33

New York Hospital
May G. Wilson. Research in rheumatic fever. 1929–62

University of Pennsylvania School of Medicine
Theodore H. Weisenburg. Study of normals: speech, nature of aphasia. 1930–33

Michigan State College
I. Forrest Huddleston. Study of *Brucella* organism. 1930–33

Columbia University
Alfred Owre. Causes of dental caries. 1930–35

Child Research Council of Denver
Alfred H. Washburn. Study of growth and development. 1930–63

New York Academy of Medicine
Ransom S. Hooker. Study of puerperal mortality. 1930–33

Washington University
Harvey J. Howard. Trachoma research; virus disease. 1930–37

New York University College of Medicine
Charles Hendee Smith. Clinical pediatric research in pneumonia. 1931–32

Columbia University, Neurological Institute
Frederick Tilney. Motor development from birth to school age. 1931–33

Massachusetts Department of Public Health
George H. Bigelow, Henry D. Chadwick. Pneumonia study. 1931–36

New York University, New York City Department of Health
William H. Park. Research in rheumatic fever and allied diseases. 1931–32

University of Missouri, National Research Council
W. C. Curtis. Biological study of effect of radiation on organisms. 1931–32

University of Pennsylvania School of Medicine
A. Newton Richards. Research in function of kidney. 1931–44

House of the Good Samaritan
T. Duckett Jones. Research in rheumatic fever. 1931–41

Johns Hopkins University School of Medicine
John J. Abel. Chemistry of insulin. 1933–37

Columbia University, Neurological Institute
Frederick Tilney. Structure and development of the brain. 1933–38

Johns Hopkins University School of Medicine
Miriam Brailey, Janet Hardy. Study of tuberculosis in childhood. 1933–51

Harvard Medical School
Charles F. McKhann. Placental extract in prevention of measles; serum, proteins. 1934–41

Bellevue Hospital
James Alexander Miller. Tuberculosis teaching and research. 1934–38

New York State
Edward S. Rogers. Pneumonia program. 1935–37

Johns Hopkins University School of Medicine
Warfield T. Longcope. Study of essential hypertension. 1936–46

Michigan Department of Health
C. C. Young. Pneumonia study. 1936–42

Johns Hopkins University
Lowell J. Reed, Wade Hampton Frost. Study of chronic disease. 1937–42

Irvington House, New York
Ann G. Kuttner. Research in rheumatic fever. 1937–43

New York University College of Medicine
W. E. Studdiford, Howard C. Taylor. Obstetrics and gynecology study; toxemia of pregnancy. 1937–46

Johns Hopkins University School of Medicine
Howard A. Howe. Research in poliomyelitis. 1937–41

Harvard Medical School
W. Lloyd Aycock. Research in poliomyelitis. 1937–44

Washington University School of Medicine
Louis A. Julianelle. Studies in immunology. 1937–40

Harvard Medical School
Hans Zinsser. Typhus serum. 1937–39

University of Pennsylvania School of Medicine
William F. Wells. Prevention and control of airborne infection. 1937–47

Harvard Medical School
Walter Bauer. Study of arthritis. 1937–58

Western Reserve University School of Medicine
J. M. Hayman, Jr. Kidney disease; chronic nephritis. 1937-42

Salmonella Culture Center, Copenhagen, Denmark
Thorvald Madsen. Salmonella research. 1938-41

Western Reserve University School of Medicine
Joseph T. Wearn. Mechanism of heart failure. 1938-44

Johns Hopkins University School of Medicine
Lawson Wilkins. Endocrines in relation to growth and development. 1938-50

Yale University School of Medicine
Milton C. Winternitz. Study of shock and vascular disease. 1938-48

University of Pennsylvania School of Medicine
Stuart Mudd. Study of the streptococcus. 1938-41

Harvard Medical School
Edwin J. Cohn. Apparatus for protein studies. 1938-39

Western Reserve University School of Medicine
Joseph T. Wearn. Study of leukemia. 1938-46

Western Reserve University School of Medicine
E. E. Ecker. Chemical factors in resistance to disease. 1938-48

Columbia-Presbyterian Medical Center
Dickinson W. Richards, Jr., André Cournand. Cardiorespiratory physiology. 1939-50

Harvard Medical School
J. Howard Mueller. Nutritive requirements of bacteria. 1939-51

New York University College of Medicine
Homer W. Smith. Study of human kidney function. 1939-52

Columbia-Presbyterian Medical Center
Dorothy N. Andersen. Chronic malnutrition in infants and children. 1939-52

Columbia-Presbyterian Medical Center
Frank E. Meleney. Surgical bacteriological study. 1940-43

New York City Department of Hospitals
Research Council of Department Hospitals.
Marijuana study. 1940-44

Columbia-Presbyterian Medical Center
B. P. Watson. Mechanisms of labor. 1940-45

Western Reserve University School of Medicine
Carl J. Wiggers. Peripheral circulation and shock. 1940-46

Memorial Hospital, New York
C. P. Rhoads. Disturbed chemical function in relation to cancer. 1940–48

Columbia–Presbyterian Medical Center
Hattie Alexander. Study of influenza bacillus. 1940–50

Washington University School of Medicine
Harvey L. White, Peter Heinbecker. Endocrine function with reference to kidney. 1940–46

Cornell University Medical College
George N. Papanicolaou. Diagnostic uses of the vaginal smear. 1940–51

University of Chicago School of Medicine
Paul E. Steiner. Cancer-producing substances from human tissue. 1941–44

Columbia–Presbyterian Medical Center
Dana W. Atchley. Clinical review of essential hypertension. 1941

Jackson Memorial Laboratory
C. C. Little, George W. Woolley. Physiological factors in susceptibility to cancer. 1941–50

Harvard Medical School
Alan Butler, Nathan B. Talbot. Endocrine study; pediatric endocrinology. 1941–58

Columbia–Presbyterian Medical Center
A. O. Whipple, Edmund N. Goodman. Diagnostic technique for cancer of the stomach. 1942–44

Washington University School of Medicine
Robert Elman. Shock due to hemorrhage and burns; systemic effects of injury. 1942–51

University of California School of Medicine
I. L. Chaikoff. Studies of the thyroid gland. 1942–46

Columbia–Presbyterian Medical Center
Tracy J. Putnam. Research in neurology. 1942–47

University of California School of Medicine
I. L. Chaikoff. Studies of the thyroid gland. 1942–46

University of Pennsylvania School of Medicine
Max Lurie. Resistance and susceptibility to experimental tuberculosis. 1942–57

Tufts College, Navy Air Service
Leonard Carmichael. Stereoscopic vision at low levels of illumination. 1942–44

Massachusetts General Hospital
Fritz Lipmann. Studies of cellular metabolism. 1942–53

Board for Investigation of Epidemic Disease in the Army, War Department
Francis G. Blake. Study of respiratory disease. 1942–43

Washington University School of Medicine
Robert Moore. Functional studies of autopsy material. 1942–44

Washington University School of Medicine
Sherwood Moore, Louis Hempelman. Radioactive phosphorus in treatment of cancer. 1942–44

New Jersey Agricultural Experiment Station
Selman A. Waksman. Study of antibiotics. 1943–49

Washington University School of Medicine
W. Barry Wood, Jr., Carl G. Harford. Cellular mechanisms in natural resistance to infection. 1943–52

New York University
H. A. Charipper. Means to increase resistance to low atmospheric pressures. 1943–44

Vanderbilt University School of Medicine
John B. Youmans, George M. Meneely. Diagnostic service for chronic chest diseases. 1944–47

University of Pennsylvania, Institute for Gynecologic Research
Douglas P. Murphy. Familial distribution of cancer of the uterus and breast. 1944–51

University of California School of Medicine
Philip A. Cavelti. Pathogenesis of nephritis and rheumatic fever. 1945–47

University of Montreal Faculty of Medicine
Hans Selye. Endocrine factors in cardiovascular disease. 1945–50

University of Alabama Medical School (initiated at Johns Hopkins)
Richard J. Bing. Physiological studies of children with congenital heart defects. 1945–53

New York Botanical Garden
William J. Robbins. Study of antibiotics from fungi. 1946–50

New York University College of Medicine
A. M. Pappenheimer. Study of diphtheria toxin. 1946–51

Washington University School of Medicine
Peter Heinbecker. Physiological controls centering in the pituitary gland. 1946–54

University of Chicago
Heinrich Klüver. Study of porphyrins. 1947–59

State University of New York, Downstate Medical Center
Jean Oliver. Histochemical studies of the nephron. 1947–50

Mt. Sinai Hospital Laboratories
Gregory Schwartzman. Study of a new antibacterial agent. 1947–50

Harvard Medical School
Benjamin Alexander. Study of hemophilia. 1947–50

Massachusetts General Hospital
Paul D. White, Howard B. Sprague. Study of coronary artery disease. 1947–50

University of Pennsylvania School of Medicine
Julius Comroe. New techniques of respiratory physiology. 1947–50

State University of New York, Downstate Medical Center
Janet Watson. Study of sickle cell anemia. 1948–50

Memorial Hospital, New York
Konrad Dobriner. Physiology of steroid compounds in health and disease. 1948–51

University of Wisconsin, Enzyme Institute
David E. Green. Study of integrated enzyme action. 1948–52

University of Washington, Seattle
Alexander H. Bill. Surgical experimentation for relief of mitral stenosis. 1948–50

University of Pennsylvania School of Medicine
T. N. Harris. Mechanisms of antibody formation. 1948–53

Medical College of Virginia (initiated at Harvard Medical School)
David M. Hume. Control of pituitary function. 1949–61

University of Pennsylvania School of Medicine
Seymour Cohen. Chemical study of virus formation. 1949–61

University of California School of Medicine, Los Angeles
Horace W. Magoun. Physiological basis of brain waves; neural correlates of mental activity. 1949–57

Washington University School of Medicine
Harvey L. White. Endocrine influence on kidney function. 1949–51

New York Academy of Medicine
Sam Levine, Howard R. Craig. Study of neonatal mortality. 1950–51

Cornell University Medical College
David P. Barr. Blood fats in relation to arteriosclerosis. 1950–51

Yale University, Child Study Center
Milton J. E. Senn. Emotional development in early childhood. 1950–59

Tulane University School of Medicine
Robert H. Heath. Research on schizophrenia. 1950–61

New York University, Department of Biology
Robert Chambers. Synthesis of studies of the living cell. 1950–53

Swarthmore College
Wolfgang Köhler. Direct electric currents to the brain. 1951–52

Harvard University, Department of Biology
Alexander Weinstein. Genetic studies of the mechanism of crossing-over. 1951–56

New York University College of Medicine
Hans-Lukas Teuber. Studies of cerebral function. 1952–59

University of Chicago School of Medicine
Isidore Gersh. Histochemical studies of submicroscopic organization of cells and extracellular substances. 1952–62

Harvard Medical School
Somers Sturgis. Psychiatric research in gynecology. 1952–59

Columbia University, Institute for Study of Human Variation
Richard H. Osborne. Twin study of hereditary and environmental factors in body build. 1953–58

Harvard Medical School, McLean Hospital
Mark D. Altschule. Physiological studies of the pineal gland. 1953–59

Worcester Foundation for Experimental Biology
Oscar Hechter. Biological role of the steroids. 1953–61

Institute for Muscle Research, New York City
Albert Szent-Gyorgyi. Chemical mechanisms of intracellular energy transmission. 1954–62

Cornell University Medical College
Edward C. Mann. Psychiatric study of habitual abortion. 1955–58

University of Colorado, Department of Physics
Theodore Puck. Studies in biophysics (fluid support). 1955–61

University of Colorado School of Medicine, Child Research Council
Robert W. McCammon. Study of growth and development. 1955–63

University of California School of Medicine, Berkeley
William F. Ganong. Neuroendocrine responses to environmental stimuli. 1956–62

Sloan Kettering Institute for Cancer Research
Leonard D. Hamilton. Structure and function of nucleic acids and nucleoproteins. 1956–62

Washington University School of Medicine
Seymour Reichlin. Neural mechanisms in regulation of pituitary thyrotropic hormone secretion. 1956–58

Henry Ittleson Center for Child Research
William Goldfarb. Study of childhood schizophrenia. 1956–62

California Institute of Technology, Division of Chemistry and Biology.
Linus Pauling, George Beadle. Fluid funds for support of research. 1956–59

Medical College of South Carolina (initiated at University of Illinois)
W. Curtis Worthington, Jr. Vascular studies of pituitary gland. 1956–61

University of Arkansas School of Medicine
Samuel A. Corson, Roscoe A. Dykman. Neural influences on kidney function. 1957–59

Saskatchewan Hospital, Weyburn
Humphrey Osmond. Relation of ward design to patient behavior. 1957

Baylor University College of Medicine.
William T. Lhamon. Fluid support for research in department of psychiatry. 1957

Eye Bank for Sight Restoration
Electron microscope (equipment). 1958

Mary Imogene Bassett Hospital, Cooperstown, New York
Joseph W. Ferrebee, E. Donall Thomas. Study of whole-body radiation (equipment). 1958

Harvard Medical School
Nathan B. Talbot. Management of patients with chronic disabilities. 1959–65

Saskatchewan Hospital, Weyburn
Humphrey Osmond. Application of learning theory techniques to altering behavior in psychiatric patients. 1959–61

Worcester Foundation for Experimental Biology
Hudson Hoagland. Blood studies in reference to the psychoses. 1960–62

Massachusetts Institute of Technology
Hans-Lukas Teuber. Studies of relation between brain and behavior. 1965

Columbia University College of Physicians and Surgeons
Division of Orthopedic Research Laboratories (equipment). 1971

Albert Einstein College of Medicine
Robert D. Terry. Research into the major cause of senile dementia: Alzheimer's disease. 1982–83

Johns Hopkins University School of Medicine
Donald L. Price. Research into the major cause of senile dementia: Alzheimer's disease. 1982–83

Yale University School of Medicine
Elias E. Manuelidis. Research into the major cause of senile dementia: Alzheimer's disease. 1982–83

Mount Sinai School of Medicine
Diane E. Meier. Reducing the burden of osteoporosis. 1984–

Appendix E

Grants to Medical Schools for Programs in Comprehensive Care

University	Year*	Amount
Cornell	1953	$ 36,000
	1954	447,468
	1957	280,000
	1960	200,000
U. Colorado	1951	264,912
	1954	52,482
	1955	293,942
	1957	10,000
Temple U.	1957	298,574
	1960	300,000
U. North Carolina	1953	160,000
	1955	50,000
	1957	28,000
Boston U.	1950	60,000
	1952	68,000
	1954	215,200
	1958	120,000

*End of fiscal year

Appendix F

Planning New Schools and Reorganizing Existing Schools of Medicine

School*	Year (or 1st grant)	Amount	Purpose
U. of Arizona	1965	$ 240,000	Planning for a college of medicine
Brown U.	1960	830,000	Planning and implementing program in medical education
	1963	500,000	Program in medical education
	1967	600,000	Development of program in medical science
	1974	600,000	Transition to an M.D. degree program
Dartmouth Coll. and Med. School	1958	1,000,000	Refounding of medical school
	1965	300,000	Full-time dept. of medicine
	1969	750,000	Development of 4th yr. curriculum
Drew Postgrad. Med. School	1970	100,000	Planning program for school's development as a community-based academic medical center
Duke U.	1965	750,000	New curriculum
Albert Einstein Coll. of Med.	1966	30,000	Evaluation and modification of program of medical education
U. of Florida	1952	96,500	Planning for new medical school
	1955	143,650	Additional planning grant

*Partial list

School*	Year (or 1st grant)	Amount	Purpose
U. of Hawaii	1964	120,000	Study of feasibility of establishing a program of basic medical sciences
	1965	350,000	Planning for 2 yr. medical school
U. of Kentucky	1957	73,400	Planning for new medical school and support for Dept. of Community Medicine
	1965	370,000	
Mayo Clinic	1972	450,000	Establishment of new medical school
Medical College of Pennsylvania	1973	25,000	Completion of long-range planning and organization
Meharry Med. Coll.	1968	700,000	Developmental program in basic sciences
U. of Miami	1966	45,000	Preparation of new curriculum
Michigan State U.	1961	483,000	To develop integrated program for teachers of medicine; educational research and evaluation
Mount Sinai Hosp.	1968	500,000	Development of basic sciences faculty
U. of Nevada	1969	418,078	Establishment of new medical school
	1973	50,000	Establishment of a clinical teaching program in southern Nevada
Oxford College	1967	534,800	Reform of university's medical curriculum
U. of Rochester	1964	396,000	New program of medical education
Stanford U.	1967	500,000	Planning for new University hospital
SUNY–Stony Brook	1969	333,550	Planning study for new medical school and Health Sciences Center
Tulane U.	1966	258,000	Planning a new medical center and curriculum;
	1969	329,000	Basic development of school
	1971	$ 185,500	Basic development of school

Appendix F

School*	Year (or 1st grant)	Amount	Purpose
U. of Utah	1958	60,000	Planning for new medical center
WAMI	1971	996,678	Regional plan for medical education of residents of Washington, Alaska, Montana and Idaho
George Washington U.	1965	150,000	New curriculum
Western Reserve U.	1950	1,635,000	Restructuring of medical curriculum and its later evaluation
Women's College, U. of Pennsylvania	1970	100,000	Program for basic redevelopment of the college

Appendix G

Capital Grants to Medical Schools

Name	Amount	Board Rept.	Placed in Endowmt.	Use
Harvard	$1,000,000	11/55	Yes	Experimental revisions of medical curriculum in basic sciences. Tutorial plan, integrated teaching.
Western Reserve	1,000,000	11/55	Yes	Income: added expenses of revised medical education programs. Principal: saved for projects in medical education, medical care, or related problems; continued development of clerkships.
Cornell	750,000	11/55	$650,000	Principal and income: teaching program. Remainder: new ventures, particularly experiments in medical education. Study of curriculum of Medical College; salary increases and additions to staff in dept. of anatomy; increase in basic budget of dept. of medicine; costs of patient care and teaching in Comprehensive Care and Teaching Program.

Name	Amount	Board Rept.	Placed in Endowmt.	Use
New York University	$ 750,000	11/55	No	Entire amount placed in separate invested account for continuation of educational planning programs underway for past 10 years. Principal and income: continuing study of objectives of medical center; establishment of Honors and Merit Scholarship Program; initiation of pilot programs in medical education.
Columbia	750,000	11/55	Most	Salaries for new personnel; increases in salaries of present staff in basic science depts. Supplements for salaries of technicians and junior staff.
Yale	750,000	11/55	No	Entire grant, plus income accrued to June 1957, budgeted for expenditure over next 15 years, largely for salary increases in clinical depts. (medicine, surgery, pediatrics, pathology).
Tulane	750,000	11/55	No	Matching grant. Used as fluid fund for additional faculty, increase in salary scales (in 1955: depts. of surgery, obstetrics, gynecology, pathology, and biochemistry; planned: depts. of pediatrics and tropical medicine).
Emory*	600,000	11/55	Yes	Income: basic sciences, including salaries of new faculty members, fellowships for graduate students, new equipment for teaching personnel in expanded graduate program. Seed money for pilot projects.
U. of Chicago	500,000	11/55	$400,000	Project in religion and health, summer scholarships in physiology, summer lectures on sociology and medicine, program of student health. New plans: strengthening dept. of psychiatry, study by curriculum committee.

Name	Amount	Board Rept.	Placed in Endowmt.	Use
U. of Southern California	$ 300,000	11/55	No	Three new full-time faculty in depts. of surgery, microbiology, and pathology; increase in salaries of all full-time faculty; faculty travel, educational experiments, planning. Pilot lecture series in humanities for medical students.
Northwestern	300,000 from income	2/56	No	Grant to be expended over 10 years. Supervision of new clinical clerkships in last two years of medical school; development of new plan for comprehensive care in outpatient clinics; planning of better correlation of pre-medical and medical work through joint study of University and Medical School faculties.
Tufts	300,000 from income	2/56	No	Completion of reorganization, based on ambulant care, of dept. of preventive medicine; revision of last two years of clinical teaching; alteration of research labs.; salaries of psychiatrist and experimental pathologist; support of the home care program; partial support of basic science depts., especially bacteriology.
Albany Med. Coll. of Union University	500,000 from income	5/56	No	Grant to be spent over next 10 years for acquisition of faculty, underwriting of projects in educational program. Two full-time chairs established in depts. of surgery and obstetrics.
George Washington	500,000	5/56	No	Eight new full-time positions in basic science depts. and one half-time position in psychiatry. Salary increases for faculty in basic sciences. Planning and partial support for new dept. of preventive and environmental medicine, modernization of teaching equipment.

Name	Amount	Board Rept.	Placed in Endowmt.	Use
Boston U.	600,000	5/56	No	Entire grant applied to construction costs, by matching a federal grant.
Johns Hopkins	1,000,000	5/56	Yes†	Income for 1956–57 added to capital to be used for reorganized educational program in 1959.
U. of Pennsylvania	500,000	5/56	No	Educational survey of school of medicine's program and organization; matched federal government grant for construction of research wing; $225,000 unallocated, but intended for implementation of educational survey.
Stanford	$1,000,000	5/56	Yes‡	Building costs if necessary. Income: basic science and clinical depts. Help in moving medical school to Palo Alto campus, reorganization of medical education.
U. of Rochester	750,000	5/56	No	Income: study of educational practices of School of Medicine and Dentistry. Proposed was establishment and support of dept. of preventive medicine and public health.

*On the basis of this grant, Emory was able to obtain $1,000,000 from the Rockefeller Foundation.
†Deposited in expendable account functioning as endowment, but available for disbursement.
‡Carried in Controller's office as Invested Plant Fund, marked for eventual classification as an Endowment Fund.

Appendix H

Selected Grants Awarded during the Presidency of J. Quigg Newton, Jr.

The Transition

Year	Amount	Program
1963	$250,000	Community Blood Council of Greater New York, Inc.—New York Blood Center
1964	150,000	National Board of Medical Examiners—Program of Evaluation of Medical School Performance
	524,045	University of Puerto Rico School of Medicine—Library
	105,000	Planned Parenthood–World Population—Film for Medical Students and Physicians on Conception Control
	165,387	Cornell University Medical College—Program with University of Bahia School of Medicine, Brazil
1965	150,000	Tufts University School of Medicine—Further Development and Strengthening of the School
	150,000	Western Reserve University School of Medicine—Division of Research on Medical Education
	190,520	University of Kentucky College of Medicine—Program in Community Medicine
	100,000	Population Council—Biomedical Fellowships
	150,000	International Mass Education Movement—Rural Reconstruction in Colombia and Guatemala
	450,000	Johns Hopkins University School of Medicine—Program to Strengthen Selected Foreign Medical Schools

Year	Amount	Program
1965	$ 90,000	University of Rochester School of Medicine and Dentistry—Exchange Program with University of Lagos Medical School, Nigeria
1966	350,000	Boston University School of Medicine—New Instructional Building and Addition to Research Building
	128,700	Columbia University College of Physicians and Surgeons—Project to Strengthen Instruction in Urology
		Harvard Medical School
	110,000	—Studies of Medical Education by Daniel H. Funkenstein, M.D.
	125,000	—Planning for the School's Role in Meeting Future Social Needs
	500,000	Johns Hopkins University School of Medicine—Developmental Program to Strengthen Johns Hopkins as a University Medical Center
	180,000	Michigan State University College of Human Medicine—Office of Medical Education Research and Development
	168,141	University of Toronto Faculty of Medicine—Research in Medical Education
	100,000	University of Utah College of Medicine—Construction and Equipment of Health Sciences Library
	253,998	University of Colorado School of Medicine—Training of Pediatric Public Health Nurse Practitioners
	150,000	Planned Parenthood–World Population—Special Fund to Assist the Work of the International Planned Parenthood Federation
	200,000	Population Council—Implementation of Family Planning in Large Delivery Hospitals
	100,000	Association of Canadian Medical Colleges—Development of Basic Program
	176,475	Columbia University—Institute for the Study of Science in Human Affairs

Appendix I

Selected Grants Awarded during the Presidency of J. Quigg Newton, Jr.

The Vice-Presidency of Colin M. MacLeod

Year	Amount	Program
1967	$ 158,100	Albany Medical College–Rensselaer Polytechnic Institute—Integrated Program of Premedical and Medical Education
	176,475	Columbia University—Institute for the Study of Science in Human Affairs
	158,465	Rensselaer Polytechnic Institute—Integrated Program of Premedical and Medical Education with Albany Medical College
	500,000	Vanderbilt University School of Medicine—Expansion of Facilities of the Department of Medicine and the Clinical Research Center
	300,000	Albert Einstein College of Medicine—Health Careers Program at Lincoln Hospital
	600,000	Harvard Medical School—Research, Education, and Demonstration in Health Care
	375,000	University of Southern California School of Medicine—Development of New Programs in Community Medicine
	165,000	University of Washington—University-wide Program in Health Affairs
	180,000	Cornell University Medical College—Program with University of Bahia School of Medicine, Brazil
	534,800	Oxford University Faculty of Medicine—Reform of the University's Medical Curriculum
	120,000	Pan American Federation of Associations of Medical Schools—Development of Federation's Executive Office

Year	Amount	Program
1968	$ 104,000	Association of American Medical Colleges—Comprehensive Evaluation of Curriculum Reform in United States and Canadian Medical Education
	270,000	Boston University School of Medicine—Development of Accelerated Medical Education as an Integral Feature of the School
	1,500,000	Columbia–Presbyterian Medical Center—Construction of New Research Wing for the Center's Eye Institute
	270,000	Johns Hopkins University School of Hygiene and Public Health—Strengthening the University's Role as a Center of Research and Education in Health Care
	700,000	Meharry Medical College—Developmental Program in the Basic Sciences
	500,000	Duke University School of Medicine—Training Unskilled Women as Home-Care Health Aides—Experiment in the Training and Use of Physicians' Assistants
	500,000	Duke University School of Medicine—Teaching, Research, and Demonstration in the Health-Care Field
	145,700	Planned Parenthood of New York City—Experiment in Sex Education, Counseling, and Related Medical Services for Urban Ghetto Youth
	165,000	Population Council—Planning Program with the International Institute for the Study of Human Reproduction, Columbia University, to Integrate Family Planning into Rural Maternal-Care Services
	600,000	American University of Beirut—Development of the University's Role in Strengthening Medical Education and Health Care in the Middle East
	500,000	National Academy of Sciences—Expansion of Endowment for Unrestricted Operating Income
	150,000	National Academy of Sciences—Development of the Initial Program of the Academy's Newly Established Board on Medicine
	300,000	National Board of Medical Examiners—Research Program in Educational Testing and Measurement
1969	115,000	Boston University Medical Center—Trustee and Faculty Study to Strengthen Policies and Processes for the Center's Advancement
	298,100	Collaborative Program among Five Universities for New Patterns of Residency Training and Continuing Education of Physicians (Clinical Scholars Program)
	126,750	University of Florida College of Medicine—Planning and Evaluation Program for the Integration of Premedical and Medical Studies and Related Student Advisory Systems

Year	Amount	Program
1969	$ 655,000	Massachusetts Institute of Technology—Planning and Initial Development with Harvard University of a Joint Program in the Health Sciences
	136,000	Michigan State University College of Human Medicine—Office of Medical Education Research and Development
	110,062	State University of New York, Upstate Medical Center at Syracuse—Planning Study for a Health Services Research Center
	236,725	University of Colorado—Experimental Curriculum to Train Pediatric Associates
	280,000	Johns Hopkins University School of Medicine—Program to Strengthen Selected Foreign Medical Schools

Appendix I

Appendix J

Selected Grants Awarded during the Presidency of J. Quigg Newton, Jr.

The Vice-Presidency of Robert J. Glaser

Year	Amount	Program
1970	$ 250,000	Johns Hopkins University School of Medicine—University-wide Program in the Development of Systems of Community Health Care
	600,000	Mount Sinai School of Medicine—Development of Health Care Systems in East Harlem and Other Urban Communities
	778,575	National Urban Coalition—Development of a Health Program
	600,000	University of Pennsylvania School of Medicine—Development of New Programs in Community Medicine
	2,000,000	Yale University School of Medicine—Comprehensive Program Addressed to the National Health Problem of Trauma
	285,000	Alderson-Broaddus College—Baccalaureate Program to Train Physicians' Assistants
	300,000	Planned Parenthood / World Population—Center for Family Planning Program Development
	100,000	Population Council—Biomedical Fellowships
	150,000	Pan American Health Organization—Regional Library of Medicine for Latin America
1971	150,000	Associated Medical Schools of Greater New York—Establishment of a Full-Time Executive Office
	117,500	Boston University School of Medicine—Development of Accelerated Medical Education as an Integral Feature of the School

Year	Amount	Program
1971	$ 361,800	National Board of Medical Examiners and the American Board of Internal Medicine—The Development and Validation of a Computer-Based System to Teach and Test Clinical Competency
	230,748	Maternity Center—National Program to Expand the Training and Use of Nurse-Midwives
	242,985	National Commission on Accrediting—Establishment of a Study Committee to Reform the Accreditation Process in the Education of Allied Health Manpower
	150,000	University of Florida College of Medicine—Institution-wide Program of Education, Research, and Experimentation in Community Medical Care
	210,000	Johns Hopkins University School of Hygiene and Public Health—Strengthening the University's Role as a Center of Research and Education in Health Care
	180,000	University of Miami School of Medicine—Basic Study to Improve the Processes of Medical Care for Ethnically Diverse Populations of the Inner City
	278,142	University of Colorado Medical Center—Research and Demonstration in the Treatment and Prevention of Parental Child Abuse
	308,569	University of Pennsylvania—Center for the Study of Sex Education in Medicine
	505,686	Stanford University School of Medicine—Establishment of a University-wide Program on Aggression and Violence in Modern Society
	150,000	Pan American Federation of Associations of Medical Schools—Development of the Federation's Executive Office
	300,000	John F. Kennedy School of Government, Harvard University—Program to Prepare Future Leaders for Public Policy Responsibility in Health Affairs and Other Fields
	361,800	National Board of Medical Examiners and the American Board of Internal Medicine—The Development and Validation of a Computer-based System to Teach and Test Clinical Competency
1972	300,000	University of Minnesota Medical School—Teaching and Research Program in Human Sexuality for Students in Medicine and Other Professions
	750,000	Yale University School of Medicine—Establishment of a Division of Cell Biology as a New Scholarly Resource within the School and the University
	425,000	Cornell University Medical College—Training of Allied Health Personnel to Assist Surgeons in Hospital Care

Year	Amount	Program
1972	$ 236,677	University of Southern California School of Medicine—Establishment of a Division of Allied Health in the Department of Community Medicine and Public Health
	300,000	Beth Israel Hospital, Boston—Training, Research, and Demonstration Program for the Advancement of Ambulatory Health Care
	194,700	Bowman Gray School of Medicine—County-wide Development of Community Health Care Services in the Winston-Salem Area
	750,000	Columbia University College of Physicians and Surgeons—Area-wide Program to Improve Systems of Health Care in New York City and Other Urban Communities
	600,000	Massachusetts Institute of Technology and Harvard University—Joint Program in Health Sciences and Technology
	300,000	Vanderbilt University School of Medicine—University-wide Program on Health Care Problems in the Mid-South
	255,000	University of Vermont College of Medicine—Campus-based Community Medical Practice to Teach Ambulatory Medical Care
	450,000	Drug Abuse Council, Inc.
	174,000	Stanford University School of Medicine—Team Approach to Multifactorial Problems, including Sexual Dysfunction
	400,000	American University of Beirut—Regional Program to Strengthen Medical Education and Health Care Development in the Middle East
	200,000	Johns Hopkins University School of Medicine—Exchange Programs with the American University of Beirut, Lebanon, and the University Cayetano Heredia, Lima, Peru

Appendix K

Selected Grants Awarded during the Presidency of J. Quigg Newton, Jr.

The Vice-Presidency of Carleton B. Chapman

Year	Amount	Program
1973	$ 317,300	The Children's Hospital Medical Center—Training of Pediatricians and Psychiatrists in Leadership in Teaching and Research in Child Development
	312,000	Yale University—Regional Center for Service, Education, and Research in the Problems of Early Childhood Development
	530,625	Yale University Law School—Graduate Education and Research Program in Law, Science, and Medicine
	309,650	University of California, San Francisco—Graduate Program to Train Teachers, Researchers, and Administrators in Medical Information Science
	240,000	Baylor College of Medicine—New Approaches to Comprehensive Health Care for Houston's Mexican-American Community
	300,000	Duke University—Establishment of a Center for Education and Research in Formulation and Analysis of Health Policy
	300,000	Mt. Sinai School of Medicine—Creation of a Center to Study and Advance the Integration of Service, Education, and Research in Prepaid Group Practice
	331,566	University of Pennsylvania School of Medicine—Support for Key Faculty in the Department of Community Medicine
	300,000	Rush–Presbyterian–St. Luke's Medical Center—Network of Teaching Hospitals in Cook County to Improve Health Manpower Distribution and Medical Care

Year	Amount	Program
1973	$ 200,000	Planned Parenthood / World Population—Center for Family Planning Program Development
	100,000	Planned Parenthood of NYC, Inc.—Creation of an International Training Center for Physicians and Allied Health Workers in the Field of Family Planning
1974	189,535	Peter Bent Brigham Hospital / Children's Hospital Medical Center—Shortened Curriculum, for the Preparation of Clinically Oriented Cardiologists Able to Provide Both Adult and Pediatric Care
	5,000,000	Columbia–Presbyterian Medical Center—Construction of a Major "Library–Health Sciences Center" and Other Capital Campaign Projects
	225,000	Harvard University—Support for Postdoctoral Fellowships at the Center for Community Health and Medical Care
	225,000	Mount Zion Hospital and Medical Center—Model Program to Train a New Category of Practitioner in the Field of Mental Health
	100,000	The Community Blood Council of Greater New York, Inc.—Construction or Renovation of Facilities for Service, Research, and Education
	225,000	Harvard University School of Public Health—Center for the Evaluation of Clinical Procedures
	600,000	National Academy of Sciences—Core Support for the Institute of Medicine
	100,000	National Health Council, Inc.—Program to Strengthen Private-Sector Organizations and Agencies Working in Health
	287,379	University of Rochester School of Medicine and Dentistry—Post-Graduate Program to Prepare Pediatricians for Teaching and Research in the Emerging Field of Child Development
	346,628	Roosevelt Hospital of New York—Model for Comprehensive Consumer Health Education in the Community Hospital Setting
	120,000	Tufts–New England Medical Center—Definition of the Role and Educational Requirements of the "Primary Care Physician"
	300,000	Planned Parenthood / World Population—Center for Family Planning Program Development
	78,500	The Population Council—Prepackaged Lecture Series on Population for Use in Medical and Nursing Schools in the Developing World
	319,731	Stanford University School of Medicine—Renewed Support for University-wide Program on Aggression and Violence in Modern Society
1975	250,000	Association of American Medical Colleges—Creation of a "Division of Faculty Development" to Spur Improvement of Medical School Educational Activities

Year	Amount	Program
1975	$ 450,000	Cornell University Medical College / The Rockefeller University—Coordinated M.D.-Ph.D. Program for Preparation of Teachers and Researchers in Biomedical Science
	339,152	Howard University College of Medicine—Associated B.S.-M.D. Program for Exceptional Students
	2,500,000	Yale University—Center for the Study of Human Genetics
	100,000	Spelman College—Support for the College's Division of Natural Sciences in Educating Black Women for the Health Professions
	375,000	Mt. Sinai School of Medicine—Improvement of Service, Teaching, and Research in the Outpatient Department of Elmhurst Hospital Center
	450,000	New York University School of Medicine—Development of Service and Teaching in Community Medicine as an Integrated Effort of the Medical Center
	300,000	Drug Abuse Council, Inc.—Support for the Final Two Years of the Council's Operations

Appendix L

Institutions Receiving $1 Million or More for Medical Education, 1949–1977

School	Amount
Columbia P & S	$15,870,520
Yale U.	12,402,469
Harvard U.	8,352,086
Cornell-Rockefeller U.	5,006,087
Duke U.	4,925,000
Johns Hopkins U.	4,713,115
Rochester U.	4,037,914
Case Western U.	3,598,848
Boston U.	3,500,321
Tulane U.	2,955,559
Stanford U.	2,820,973
U. Pennsylvania	2,808,612
U. Chicago	2,674,736
U. Colorado	2,405,078

School	Amount
Dartmouth	$ 2,100,000
Brown U.	2,030,000
Mt. Sinai (New York)	1,827,140
Vanderbilt U.	1,630,000
New York University	1,571,371
MIT	1,550,000
Albany-Rensselaer	1,434,355
U. Washington (Seattle)	1,433,629
Northwestern U.	1,358,691
U. Southern California	1,329,677
Tufts U.	1,255,000
U. Vermont	1,074,994
George Washington U.	1,050,000
American University of Beirut	1,000,000

Appendix M Commonwealth Fund Grants, 1919–1984

Year	Child Welfare	Mental Health	Community Health	Rural Hospitals	Medical Research
General Director: Max Farrand					
1919	$ 19,000	$ 10,000			
1920	146,000	10,000			
General Director: Barry C. Smith					
1921	216,270	40,000			$ 87,000
1922	527,200		$232,016		10,000
1923	399,075		26,750		10,100
1924	697,437		57,540		
1925	376,994	523,000	20,000	$ 95,000	13,500
1926	436,134	555,900	29,500	20,000	7,500
1927	434,471	697,387	18,000	413,950	30,000
1928	53,500	845,204	424,859	358,438	31,800
1929	34,500	563,398	291,780	305,300	59,200
1930		619,251	555,294	93,389	169,600
1931		616,036	440,586	140,667	328,100
1932		363,057	439,750	143,720	203,987
1933		203,749	423,305	205,414	105,216
1934		213,945	418,919	239,853	308,553
1935		217,650	427,255	357,220	123,147
1936		203,840	420,955	398,870	281,190
1937		219,479	439,043	395,496	308,825
1938		208,563	591,683	477,574	472,748

*Included are grants to Experimental Health Services, which were supported from the late 1940s to the late 1970s (see p. 317).

Medical Education*	Fellow- ships in Health Field	Publications	President's Revolving Fund	Totals
General Director: Max Farrand				
	$15,000			$ 165,500
				1,530,600
General Director: Barry C. Smith				
$300,000				1,776,270
				1,208,966
				949,275
26,500				934,477
37,850				1,339,294
				1,360,303
				1,952,091
2,000		$78,464		2,081,515
2,000		94,000		1,991,723
102,000		81,785		2,095,910
1,500		91,375		2,187,161
1,000		78,105		1,556,119
25,750		86,051		1,656,495
15,500	$25,500	79,829		1,714,602
15,500	17,097	59,150		1,568,558
266,835		55,777		1,961,351
	4,800	67,250		1,827,184
61,500	30,100	73,990		2,260,633

Year	Child Welfare	Mental Health	Community Health	Rural Hospitals	Medical Research
1939		$193,329	$456,519	$491,606	$293,870
1940		148,089	409,518	472,263	441,550
1941		156,820	311,038	122,176	366,712
1942		163,820	354,911	338,598	385,955
1943		163,284	262,340	86,278	324,462
1944		141,305	278,053	49,675	295,586
1945		188,814	356,740	295,380	375,880
1946		294,040	320,544	581,567	447,391
1947		265,020	267,181	242,697	436,022

General Director: Donal Sheehan

Year	Child Welfare	Mental Health	Community Health	Rural Hospitals	Medical Research
1948		241,505	287,657	128,101	554,808

President: Malcolm P. Aldrich

Year	Child Welfare	Mental Health	Community Health	Rural Hospitals	Medical Research
1949			418,160	323,945	487,068
1950		89,500	492,344	58,500	380,002
1951		60,000	679,471		454,768
1952			429,500	3,568	413,569
1953			224,323		517,101
1954			182,280		627,149
1955			137,750		887,926
1956			72,000		717,546
1957			206,070		815,625
1958		7,120	47,500		188,083
1959		64,870			990,959
1960		70,000			466,279
1961		5,000	45,500		22,465
1962					154,255
1963					

President: J. Quigg Newton, Jr.

Year	Child Welfare	Mental Health	Community Health	Rural Hospitals	Medical Research
1964					
1965					108,926
1966					
1967					
1968					
1969					
1970					
1971					
1972					
1973					
1974					
1975					

Medical Education*	Fellow-ships in Health Field	Publications	President's Revolving Fund	Totals
	$ 39,600	$ 75,050		$ 1,913,297
$ 48,160	55,350	74,300		1,992,980
46,800	19,200	71,900		1,399,976
70,600	24,600	64,350		1,733,539
25,800	8,850	61,850		1,486,768
83,150	18,650	66,260		1,245,983
23,000	16,000	62,975		1,613,161
184,000	40,850	62,750		2,109,961
42,900	9,650	82,890		1,597,554

General Director: Donal Sheehan

Medical Education*	Fellow-ships in Health Field	Publications	President's Revolving Fund	Totals
334,200	92,000	89,470		1,954,438

President: Malcolm P. Aldrich

Medical Education*	Fellow-ships in Health Field	Publications	President's Revolving Fund	Totals
241,256	131,800	90,355		2,014,226
593,370	100,000			1,941,523
1,008,242	121,040	50,708		2,779,382
1,057,554	160,000	125,000		2,574,736
602,977	75,000		$ 3,012	1,798,575
1,527,261	100,000		3,158	3,321,737
1,954,071	416,650		3,575	3,469,972
13,159,723	383,310		2,660	15,140,154
1,803,275	564,056	100,000	4,885	3,808,911
2,173,605	747,060	70,000		3,662,293
1,289,123	848,923	85,000	1,300	3,803,325
4,263,808	100,900	125,000	7,686	6,183,672
3,102,300	512,641	150,000	6,289	4,204,195
4,057,980	751,000	100,000	9,820	5,493,235
2,522,936	715,900	100,000	6,528	4,060,364

President: J. Quigg Newton, Jr.

Medical Education*	Fellow-ships in Health Field	Publications	President's Revolving Fund	Totals
3,341,432	574,000	125,000		4,833,432
5,283,022	550,000	125,000	12,500	7,067,448
5,326,770	350,000	180,980	4,165	7,001,915
5,901,190		60,000	30,000	7,059,190
6,209,374	100,000	325,000	87,000	7,633,374
4,582,516		175,000	80,400	5,609,916
6,217,517		211,000	133,872	7,293,389
5,347,990		175,000	136,603	6,393,593
6,799,502		203,000	148,800	8,132,002
5,412,816			225,000	6,495,131
9,710,732		175,000	225,000	10,916,922
5,936,402		320,000	225,000	7,555,236

Year	Child Welfare	Mental Health	Community Health	Rural Hospitals	Medical Research
President: Carleton B. Chapman					
1976					
1977					
1978					
1979					
1980					
President: Margaret E. Mahoney					
1981					
1982					
1983					
1984					
Totals	3,340,581	8,362,975	11,496,634	6,839,245	13,704,423

Medical Education*	Fellow- ships in Health Field	Publications	President's Revolving Fund	Totals
President: Carleton B. Chapman				
5,342,088		75,000	225,000	6,518,344
6,974,621		275,000	225,000	8,480,326
7,411,000		275,000	240,906	9,272,213
3,080,544		475,000	250,000	5,384,219
4,918,000		450,000	275,000	7,783,334
President: Margaret E. Mahoney				
3,953,725		1,130,000	275,000	8,845,096
6,495,490			275,000	7,809,285
6,292,174		484,000	275,000	7,857,696
5,892,896		480,000	350,000	7,668,558
161,518,827	7,704,527	8,272,614	3,748,159	269,033,103

Notes and References

Abbreviations

AR Annual Report of the Commonwealth Fund

GD Quarterly reports of the director of the Commonwealth Fund to its Board of Directors. From 1919 to 1948, these reports were known as "Reports of the General Director to the Directors of the Commonwealth Fund." In 1948, they took the title "Reports of the Staff to the Directors of the Commonwealth Fund," and since 1949, they have been known as "Reports of the General Director and Staff to the Directors of the Commonwealth Fund."

CF Arch Commonwealth Fund Archives, The Rockefeller Archives Center, Hillcrest-Pocantico Hills, North Tarrytown, New York 10591.

Secondary Sources

Arnove, R., ed. *Philanthropy and Cultural Imperialism: The Foundations at Home and Abroad.* Boston: G. K. Hall, 1980.

Bremner, R. *American Philanthropy.* Chicago: University of Chicago Press, 1960.

Brown, E. R. *Rockefeller Medicine Men: Medicine and Capitalism in America.* Berkeley and Los Angeles: University of California Press, 1979.

Cassedy, J. H. *Charles V. Chapin and the Public Health Movement.* Cambridge: Harvard University Press, 1962.

Curti, M. and Nash, R. *Philanthropy in the Shaping of Higher Education.* Rutgers, N. J.: Rutgers University Press, 1965.

Duffy, J. *A History of Public Health in New York City, 1866–1966.* New York: Russell Sage Foundation, 1974.

Ettling, J. *The Germ of Laziness: Rockefeller Philanthropy and Public Health in the New South*. Cambridge: Harvard University Press, 1981.

Flexner, A. *Funds and Foundations*. New York: Harper and Bros., 1952.

Kaufman, M. *American Medical Education: The Formative Years, 1765–1910*. Westport, Conn.: Greenwood Press, 1976.

Ludmerer, K. M. *Learning to Heal: The Development of American Medical Education*. New York: Basic Books, 1985.

Numbers, R. L., ed. *The Education of American Physicians*. Berkeley and Los Angeles: University of California Press, 1980.

Rosen, G. *A History of Public Health*. New York: MD Publications, 1958.

Rosenkrantz, B. *Public Health and the State*. Cambridge: Harvard University Press, 1972.

Shryock, R. *American Medical Research, Past and Present*. New York: Commonwealth Fund, 1947.

Introduction

1. Extensive use has been made of John Z. Bowers's essay Influences on the development of American medicine. In: Bowers, J. Z. and Purcell, E. F., eds. *Advances in American Medicine: Essays at the Bicentennial*. Vol. 1. New York: Josiah Macy, Jr., Foundation, pp. 26–35, 1976.

2. *The Commonwealth Fund: Historical Sketch, 1918–1962*. New York: Commonwealth Fund, 1963; Wooster, J. W., Jr. *Edward Stephen Harkness, 1874–1940*. New York: Commonwealth Fund, 1949.

1. The Harkness Family and the Genesis of the Commonwealth Fund

1. Background material derives largely from Wooster, J. W., Jr. *Edward Stephen Harkness, 1874–1940*. New York: Commonwealth Fund, 1949.

2. Wooster, *Edward Stephen Harkness*, p. 20.

3. Obituary, *New York Times*, June 8, 1957.

4. Billings, J. S. Address at the formal opening of the Johns Hopkins Hospital, May 7, 1889. Cited in Harvey, A. M. *Adventures in Medical Research*. Baltimore: Johns Hopkins University Press, 1976, p. 4.

5. *New York Times*, October 13, 1928. Cited in Wooster, *Edward Stephen Harkness*, pp. 62–66.

6. Wooster, *Edward Stephen Harkness*, p. 66.

2. The Fund Searches for a Focus

1. AR, 1919, p. 12.

2. Farrand became director of the Huntington Library and Art Gallery in 1927, serving until 1941. While professor of history at Yale, he edited the three-volume *Records of the Federal Convention of 1787*, an authoritative account of the drafting

of the Constitution of the United States; in 1935, President Franklin D. Roosevelt placed him on the United States Constitution Sesquicentennial Committee. He was a fellow of the American Academy of Arts and Sciences and of the American Philosophical Society, a member of the Advisory Board of the Guggenheim Fund in 1931, and a trustee of the American Academy in Rome in 1939. The University of Michigan made him a Doctor of Laws in 1931, and Princeton, a Doctor of Literature in 1942. Farrand died on June 18, 1945. (Obituary, *New York Times*, June 18, 1945.)

3. GD, March 4, 1919, pp. 1–3.

4. Nielsen, W. A. *The Big Foundations: A Twentieth Century Fund Study.* New York: Columbia University Press, 1972, p. 5.

5. Ibid., p. 5.

6. Report of the United States Commission on Industrial Relations, pp. 118–19, 125, 1915. Cited in Nielsen, *The Big Foundations*, pp. 5–6.

7. GD, March 4, 1919, pp. 1–3.

8. GD, March 4, 1919, p. 5.

9. GD, June 25, 1920, pp. 1–2.

10. Special Report, "Medical Appeals," December 13, 1919, p. 9. CF Arch.

11. Special Report, "The Blind," April 8, 1920, p. 6. CF Arch.

12. Special Report, "Medical Appeals," December 13, 1919, p. 5.

13. GD, June 19, 1919, n.p.

14. Harkness, E. S. Note, April 23, 1921. CF Arch.

15. Special Report, "Medical Appeals," December 13, 1919, p. 1.

16. GD, May 6, 1919, p. 2.

17. The Fund sponsored an Educational Research Conference in Atlantic City on October 23 and 24, 1920. Members of the Fund's group who attended were: A. Ross Hill, president, the University of Missouri (chairman); Lotus D. Coffman, president, the University of Minnesota; Charles H. Judd, director, School of Education, the University of Chicago; Paul Monroe, director, School of Education, Teacher's College, Columbia University; Leonard P. Ayres, director, Division of Education, the Russell Sage Foundation; Samuel P. Capen, secretary, the American Council on Education; Paul H. Hanus, professor of education, Harvard University; and Max Farrand, general director, the Commonwealth Fund.

18. AR, 1921, pp. 10–12.

19. Its members were: James Parker Hall, dean, the University of Chicago Law School (chairman); Charles C. Burlingham, of the law firm of Burlingham, Veeder, Masten, and Fearey, New York City; Benjamin N. Cardozo, Judge of the Court of Appeals of New York, John G. Milburn, of the law firm of Carter, Ledyard, and Milburn, New York City; Roscoe Pound, dean, the Harvard Law School; and Harlan F. Stone, dean, the Columbia University School of Law.

20. Special Report, "Education," June 25, 1921, p. 5. CF Arch.

21. Harkness, E. S. Note. Special Report, "Education," June 25, 1921.

22. Lester J. Evans, interview with A. McGehee Harvey, 1982.

23. In a report to the Fund's directors dated January 20, 1920, Farrand said, "It is altogether probable that if the Laura Spelman Rockefeller Foundation takes up the work of child welfare it would not, at least for some time to come, go into the field of delinquency and crime, even of juvenile delinquency, and that field accordingly lies open before us."

24. GD, March 4, 1919.
25. Special Report, "Child Welfare," November 30, 1920. CF Arch.
26. Ibid.
27. This conference met from March 11 to 14, 1921, and the following were invited: Augusta F. Bronner, psychologist and director, the Judge Baker Foundation, Boston; Mrs. Martha P. Falconer, director, Department of Protective Social Measures, the American Social Hygiene Association; Bernard Glueck, Department of Mental Hygiene, the New York School of Social Work; William Healy, managing director, the Judge Baker Foundation; Charles W. Hoffman, Judge of the Juvenile Court, Cincinnati; J. P. Murphy, secretary and superintendent, the Children's Bureau, Philadelphia; Thomas W. Salmon, medical director, the National Commitee for Mental Hygiene; Henry W. Thurston, Department of Child Welfare, the New York School of Social Work; and the general director of the Commonwealth Fund, Max Farrand.
28. Lester J. Evans, interview with A. McGehee Harvey, 1982.

3. The Program in Psychiatry and Mental Health

1. Lester J. Evans, interview with A. McGehee Harvey, September 20, 1981.
2. Smith graduated with the B.A. degree in 1899, taught at the Cutler and Browning Schools in New York until 1913, then studied for a year at the New York School of Social Work. From 1915 to 1918, he was financial secretary of the Charity Organization of New York; during his last two years there, he was secretary of the Bureau of Advice and Information, an organization devoted to protecting foundations against fraudulent appeals. (Obituary, *New York Times*, April 1, 1952.)
3. Barbara S. Quin graduated from Smith College in 1911 and spent the next year at the New York School of Social Work at Columbia University. She received the M.A. degree from Columbia in 1912 and then became a staff member of the Charity Organization Society, serving from 1915 to 1918 as a district secretary. In 1918 Quin became assistant director of the National Information Bureau, where she remained until joining the Commonwealth Fund. At the Fund, she took primary responsibility for investigating appeals (grant requests) and was particularly helpful to Barry C. Smith in shaping the Fund's contributions to medical education and research. In recognition of her share in directing the Fund's child health work in Austria from 1923 to 1929, she received the Golden Cross of Honor of the Austrian Republic. She died on June 6, 1945. (Obituary, *New York Times*, June 8, 1945.)
4. Mildred C. Scoville was a graduate of the University of Nebraska and the Smith College School of Social Work. She served for several years with the Red Cross in Minneapolis, became an assistant director of the National Committee for Mental Hygiene in 1921, and in 1923 joined the Fund's staff. Scoville was instrumental in helping with the development of the Group for the Advancement of Psychiatry, and she headed the American Association of Psychiatric Social Workers. In 1949 she was recognized by the National Committee for Mental Hygiene, which recommended that she receive the Lasker Award (*see* JAMA

141: 1179, 1949). She was the first woman to be appointed to the National Advisory Mental Health Council. (Obituary, *New York Times*, April 27, 1969.)

5. Roderick E. Heffron, interview with A. McGehee Harvey, October 6, 1981.

6. Rosenau, M. *Preventive Medicine and Hygiene.* 2nd ed. New York and London: D. Appleton and Co., 1916.

7. Salmon, T. W. Mental hygiene. In: Rosenau, M. *Preventive Medicine and Hygiene.* 2nd ed. New York and London: D. Appleton and Co., 1916, pp. 331–62.

8. Meyer, A.: Foreword. In: Ebaugh, F. G. and Rymer, C. A. *Psychiatry in Medical Education.* New York: Commonwealth Fund, 1942.

9. Ebaugh and Rymer, *Psychiatry in Medical Education*, p. 619.

10. Ridenour, N. *Mental Health in the United States: A Fifty-Year History.* New York: Commonwealth Fund (Cambridge: Harvard University Press), 1961; Beers, C. W. *A Mind That Found Itself.* New York: Longmans, Green and Co., 1908; Ebaugh and Rymer, *Psychiatry in Medical Education.*

11. Extensive use has been made of the address of Adolf Meyer at the Twenty-fifth Anniversary Dinner of the National Commitee for Mental Hygiene, November 14, 1934. (Mental Hygiene 19: 31, 1935.)

12. Ibid.

13. Ebaugh and Rymer, *Psychiatry in Medical Education.*

14. Healy, W. D. *The Individual Delinquent.* Boston: Little Brown and Co., 1920, p. 24.

15. CF Arch. See also "New school dedicated to honor Dr. Healy," Welfare Bulletin 43 (November–December 1952), pp. 3–8, Van Waters Papers, Folder 26. (The Arthur and Elizabeth Schlesinger Library, Radcliffe College.)

16. Baker, H. H. *Upbuilder of the Juvenile Court.* Boston: Judge Baker Foundation, 1920.

17. Meyer, A. Thirty-five years of psychiatry in the United States and our present outlook. Am. J. Psychiatry 8: 1, 1928.

18. Lee, P. R. and Kenworthy, M. E. *Mental Hygiene and Social Work.* New York: Commonwealth Fund, 1929; see also the Commonwealth Fund Program for the Prevention of Delinquency, published by the Joint Committee on Methods of Preventing Delinquency (50 East 42nd Street, New York). (This statement concerning the purposes, methods, and organization of the Commonwealth Fund's program was republished, in revised and updated form, from the Fourth Annual Report of the General Director of the Commonwealth Fund.)

19. AR, 1922, p. 7.

20. Thurston's recommendations were contained in his report to the board of directors on June 25, 1921 ("Special Report Presenting a Child Welfare Program," Henry W. Thurston, director, Children's Department, the New York School of Social Work). CF Arch.

21. Smith, B. C. Notes on "Special Report Presenting a Child Welfare Program," June 25, 1921. CF Arch.

22. AR, 1922, pp. 10–11.

23. Committees Connected with the Program:

Division I, Committee on Fellowships, the New York School of Social Work: Porter R. Lee (chairman), Bernard Glueck, Barry C. Smith.

Division II, Division for the Prevention of Delinquency, the National Committee for Mental Hygiene, Advisory Committee: Thomas W. Salmon (chairman), Charles W. Hoffman, Emma O. Lundberg, Herbert C. Parsons, Barry C. Smith, Walter E. Fernald, Lewellys F. Barker, Charles H. Judd, Arnold Gesell, and J. Prentice Murphy.

Division III, National Committee on Visiting Teachers, affiliated with the Public Education Association of the City of New York: Howard W. Nudd (chairman), Jane Culbert (secretary), V. V. Anderson, J. H. Beveridge, Henry W. Thurston, Barry C. Smith, Emma O. Case, Anna B. Pratt, M. L. Brittain, R. G. Jones, and Arthur W. Towne.

Division IV, Joint Committee on Methods of Preventing Delinquency: Porter R. Lee (chairman), Barry C. Smith (secretary), V. V. Anderson, Howard W. Nudd, Julia Lathrop, Bernard Glueck, Henry C. Morrison, J. Prentice Murphy, and Thomas W. Salmon.

24. AR, 1922, p. 11.
25. AR, 1922, p. 12.
26. AR, 1923, p. 32.
27. AR, 1924, p. 26.
28. Stevenson, G. S. and Smith, G. *Child Guidance Clinics: A Quarter-Century of Development.* New York: Commonwealth Fund, 1934, pp. 20–22.
29. Stevenson and Smith, *Child Guidance Clinics.*
30. Ibid.
31. AR, 1923, pp. 38–39.
32. AR, 1923, pp. 34–36.
33. Lowrey, L. G. and Sloan, V., eds. *Orthopsychiatry, 1923–1948: Retrospect and Prospect.* New York: American Orthopsychiatric Association, 1948, p. 529.
34. Witmer, H. L. *Psychiatric Clinics for Children.* New York: Commonwealth Fund, 1940, p. 56.
35. Ridenour, *Mental Health in the United States*, p. 39.
36. Kanner, L. The origin and growth of child psychiatry. Am. J. Psychiatry 100: 139, 1944.
37. Lester J. Evans, personal communication to A. McGehee Harvey.
38. GD, November 11, 1924, p. 2.
39. AR, 1926, p. 46.
40. AR, 1927, p. 36.
41. AR, 1928, p. 48.
42. Ibid.
43. AR, 1928, p. 50.
44. AR, 1929, p. 70.
45. AR, 1926, p. 12.
46. Barry C. Smith to Adolf Meyer, February 25, 1926. CF Arch.
47. Program in Mental Hygiene and Child Guidance, April 15, 1926, p. 25. CF Arch.
48. Lester J. Evans, interview with A. McGehee Harvey, 1981.
49. AR, 1927, p. 8.
50. AR, 1930, p. 53.
51. AR, 1929, p. 64.
52. AR, 1928, p. 51.
53. AR, 1933, p. 55.

54. Cited in GD, 1932.
55. AR, 1933, pp. 55–56.
56. AR, 1931, p. 40.
57. GD, October 20, 1926, p. 5.
58. Glueck, B. Psychoanalysis and child guidance. Mental Hygiene 14: 825, 1930.
59. AR, 1930, p. 50. See also Report of the American Psychiatric Association Committee chaired by William A. White of St. Elizabeth's Hospital, in Washington, D.C. Report presented at the Annual Meeting of the American Psychiatric Association, 1933.
60. Ebaugh, F. G. Present status of the teaching of psychiatry. J. Assoc. Am. Med. Coll. 8: 214, 1933.
61. AR, 1932, p. 49.
62. AR, 1933, p. 53.
63. AR, 1923, p. 41.
64. Fellowships were administered by J. H. Meeker, dean, the University of Pennsylvania Graduate School of Medicine; T. H. Weisenburg and Edward A. Strecker, faculty members of the Graduate School of Medicine; Mildred C. Scoville, staff member of the Fund; Frankwood E. Williams, medical director, the National Committee for Mental Hygiene; and Ralph P. Truitt, director, Division for the Prevention of Delinquency, the National Committee for Mental Hygiene.
65. Ten other applications for fellowships were rejected; one was received from William C. Menninger, who chose to accept a position elsewhere. The second group of four fellows included William George Ferguson, Alberta Jenkins (who died of tuberculosis not long after completing her fellowship), Norville C. LaMar, and Raymond W. Waggoner. Waggoner later became president of the American Psychiatric Association.
66. Truitt, R. Special Report to the Fund. CF Arch.
67. AR, 1928, pp. 56–57.
68. GD, June 5, 1928.
69. Information about fellows in the Colorado program was obtained at a reunion in 1950 of a group of forty-four former residents at the Colorado Psychopathic Hospital (CF Arch). Additional data from *Who's Who in America, American Men of Science,* and the membership directory of the American Psychiatric Association. See also AR, 1928, p. 86; Romano, J. The teaching of psychiatry to medical students: Past, present, and future. Am. J. Psychiatry 126: 115, 1970.
70. Report of Mildred Scoville after visit to Baltimore, 1938. CF Arch. See also GD, June 10, 1943, p. 17.
71. AR, 1932, pp. 50–51.
72. AR, 1941, p. 35.
73. AR, 1933, pp. 51–52.
74. Ebaugh and Rymer, *Psychiatry in Medical Education.*
75. AR, 1930, p. 51.
76. Ibid.
77. AR, 1932, p. 51.
78. AR, 1937, p. 8.
79. AR, 1938, p. 15.

80. AR, 1938, pp. 14, 34.

81. AR, 1940, p. 21.

82. Commonwealth Fund Memorandum, May 26, 1936. CF Arch.

83. Ibid.

84. GD, October 28, 1937, quoted from an editorial in the *Louisville Courier-Journal*.

85. Report on the Psychiatric and Neurologic Services in the Peter Bent Brigham Hospital. CF Arch., 19 pp. In a series of letters to Mildred C. Scoville dated January 15, 1949, February 4, 1949, and February 20, 1952, Romano discussed in detail how he developed his interest in bringing psychiatry and general medicine together and described the programs in Boston, Cincinnati, and Rochester. CF Arch.

86. Engel, G. L.; Romano, J.; and Blankenhorn, M. A. Report to the Commonwealth Fund. The teaching of psychosomatic concepts to fourth year medical students assigned to the medical ward service of the Cincinnati General Hospital. June 1, 1946, 14 pp. CF Arch.

87. GD, June 14, 1951, p. 29.

88. GD, June 14, 1951, p. 27.

89. The discussion of the program at Cincinnati is based on the author's interview with Morton F. Reiser on December 1, 1982. For a comparison of the programs at the Peter Bent Brigham Hospital and the University of Cincinnati, see GD, June 16, 1949, p. 17, and GD, June 14, 1951, p. 27. See also GD, June 14, 1945, p. 22.

90. GD, June 16, 1949, p. 24; John Romano, interview with A. McGehee Harvey, April 15, 1982; John Romano to Mildred C. Scoville, February 4, 1949, describing the operation of the Department of Psychiatry at the University of Rochester. CF Arch.

91. Fry, C. C. and Rostow, E. G. *Mental Health in College*. New York: Commonwealth Fund, 1942, pp. xi, xii.

92. Reports to the president and fellows by the deans and directors of several schools and departments for the academic year 1924–1925. New Haven: Yale University, 1925, p. 80.

93. Rostow, E. G. History of the mental hygiene division at Yale. Unpublished manuscript, 1976. Files of the Division of Mental Hygiene, pp. 19, 20.

94. This committee consisted of Arthur H. Ruggles (chairman), James Greenway, Milton C. Winternitz, Edward A. Strecker, and Frankwood E. Williams. Williams had been associated with the Child Guidance Program and other Commonwealth Fund interests in mental health.

95. Other physicians who served in the Division of College Psychiatry and Mental Hygiene at Yale were Ernest F. Russell, Val B. Satterfield, Everett S. Rademacher, Carl F. Wagner, Edgar Van Norman Emery, Wilmoth Osborne, Donald H. Linard, and Ellett M. DeBerry.

96. Fry C. C. (in collaboration with Rostow, E. G.). Preface, *Mental Health in College*. New York: Commonwealth Fund, 1942.

97. Report of the Department of Mental Hygiene to the Commonwealth Fund, 1931–1932. CF Arch.

98. Donald H. Linard (see note 95) selected a group of one hundred cases from the files of the mental hygiene department. These were analyzed intensively

by the staff and were the subject of Dr. Linard's report to the Fund in April 1929.

99. We are indebted to Robert L. Arnstein for supplying much of the information on which this chapter is based (letter, January 6, 1983).

100. Stewart G. Wolf, Jr., interview with A. McGehee Harvey, April 1982.

101. AR, 1944, p. 26.

102. AR, 1945, p. 18.

103. AR, 1945, p. 19.

104. GD, June 14, 1945, p. 16.

105. Ibid.

106. *Psychotherapy in General Medicine: Report of an Experimental Postgraduate Course.* New York: Commonwealth Fund, 1946.

107. John Romano, interview with A. McGehee Harvey, April 15, 1982.

108. AR, 1946, p. 6.

109. A report of the proceedings of this conference may be found in the CF Arch.

110. GD, June 20, 1946, p. 20; GD, June 10, 1948, p. 18; GD, October 27, 1949, pp. 17-19; GD, June 8, 1950, pp. 44-48.

111. William C. Menninger (chairman, GAP), letter to Mildred C. Scoville, September 26, 1949. CF Arch.

112. GD, October 27, 1949, p. 7; GD, October 11, 1951, p. 10.

113. Smith, G. *Human Relationships in Public Health; Report of an Institute on Mental Health in Public Health.* New York: Commonwealth Fund, 1949.

114. Among the distinguished participants were Leona Baumgartner, director, Bureau of Child Hygiene, the New York City Health Department; Donald W. Hastings, professor of psychiatry, the University of Minnesota; M. Ralph Kaufman, psychiatrist, the Mount Sinai Hospital, New York City; Paul V. Lemkau, associate professor of public health administration, the Johns Hopkins University; and Milton J. E. Senn, professor of psychiatry, the Cornell University Medical College.

115. Annual Report of the Carnegie Corporation, 1934. In 1936 Carson Ryan, formerly of Swarthmore College, was engaged by the Fund to make a study of mental hygiene and education. Frederick P. Keppel of the Carnegie Corporation also asked him to prepare—with the consent of the Commonwealth Fund—a program in mental hygiene for his organization. For many years, Keppel said, the Commonwealth Fund was "the only one of the major foundations that had done significant work in mental hygiene." (GD, April 21, 1936, p. 24.)

116. Margo Horn, personal communication to A. McGehee Harvey, 1981.

117. Kohler, R. E. A policy for the advancement of science: The Rockefeller Foundation: 1924-1929. Minerva 16: 480, 1978.

4. The Program in Public Health

1. The availability of facilities for all children was a current topic of discussion worldwide: A resolution at the the International Health Conference in Cannes, France (April 1919), was supported by Sir Arthur Newsholme of Great Britain and two eminent American pediatricians, L. Emmett Holt and Samuel M. Hamill.

2. Mustard, H. S. *Rural Health Practice*. New York: Commonwealth Fund, 1936. Mustard was director of the School of Public Health at Columbia University.

3. Mustard, *Rural Health Practice*.

4. Winslow, C.-E. A. The untilled fields of public health. Science 51 (n.s.): 23, 1920.

5. Freeman, A. Rural health organization in the United States: Past, present, and future. South. Med. J. 27: 517, 1934.

6. Emerson, H. and Lugenbuhe, M. *Local Health Units for the Nation*. Report of the chairman, Subcommittee on Local Health Units, Committee on Administrative Practice, American Public Health Association. New York: Commonwealth Fund, 1945, p. 12.

7. Musacchio, F. A. The history of the modern public health movement. New Orleans Med. Surg. J. 95: 1, 1942; U.S.P.H.S., Public Health Bulletin No. 222: History of County Health Organizations in the United States, 1908–1933.

8. Rosen, G. *Preventive Medicine in the United States, 1900–1975: Trends and Interpretations*. New York: Science History Publications, 1975, pp. 23–26.

9. Winslow, C.-E. A. The untilled fields of public health; Winslow, C.-E. A. *The Evolution and Significance of the Modern Public Health Campaign*. New Haven: Yale University Press, 1923.

10. Winslow, *The Evolution and Significance of the Modern Public Health Campaign*.

11. Ibid., p. 59.

12. Biggs, H. Some of the clinical effects of disease of the myocardium. Yale Med. J. 8: 63, Sept. 1901.

13. New York State Department of Health, Annual Report, 1919, Vol. 1, pp. 7–11; see also memorandum reproduced as appendix A, in Terris, M. Hermann Biggs's contribution to the modern concept of the health center. Bull. Hist. Med. 20: 387, 402, 1946.

14. For a full description of Biggs's plan, see Winslow, C.-E. A. The Life of Hermann M. Biggs, M.D., D.Sc., LL.D. *Physician and Statesman of Public Health*. Philadelphia: Lea and Febiger, 1929, pp. 348–50.

15. Additional references: Biggs, H.M. President's address. Trans. Assoc. Am. Phys. 35: 1, 1920; Biggs, H. M. The state board of health. N.Y. State J. Med. 21: 6, 1921.

16. A summary of this speech appears in Health News 17 (n.s.): 74, March 1922.

17. In a letter to his son in March 1923, Biggs said: "The demands from all sorts of outside activities like the Rockefeller Institute, the Rockefeller Foundation, the International Health Board, the Hartley Foundation, the Milbank Foundation, and the Commonwealth Fund . . . and a dozen other things besides a very large practice and some desperately sick patients and the State Health Department have just swamped me." (Cited in Winslow, *Hermann M. Biggs*, pp. 370–71.)

18. Winslow, *Hermann M. Biggs*, p. 368.

19. Rosen, *Preventive Medicine in the United States*, pp. 23–26.

20. Dinwiddie, C. *Child Health and the Community*. New York: Commonwealth Fund, 1931, pp. 1–13.

21. Report of the Committee on Municipal Health Department Practice of the

American Public Health Association in cooperation with the U. S. P. H. S. Public Health Bulletin No. 136, July 1923.

22. Research Division of the American Child Health Association. *A Health Survey of Eighty-six Cities.* New York: American Child Health Association, 1925.

23. Harwood, M. P. *Public Health Survey of Lafayette, Indiana, and Tippecanoe County, Indiana.* Lafayette, Ind.: Tippecanoe Tuberculosis Association, 1921.

24. AR, 1932, p. 13.

25. Dinwiddie, *Child Health and the Community*, p. 12.

26. Ibid. p. 14.

27. Among this group were: Richard A. Bolt of the American Hygiene Association; L. Emmett Holt; Henry W. Thurston; Richard M. Smith of the Massachusetts General Hospital; Haven Emerson, former New York State commissioner of health; Homer Folks of the State Charities Aid Association; and William Darrach, dean, the Columbia University College of Physicians and Surgeons.

28. The committee comprised: L. Emmett Holt; Sally L. Jean, administrator, the American Child Health Association; Philip Van Ingen, a prominent New York pediatrician and a leader in the New York Academy of Medicine; Livingston Farrand, president of Cornell University; Donald B. Armstrong, medical director, the Metropolitan Life Insurance Company; Richard A. Bolt, staff member, the American Child Health Association; Barbara S. Quin; and Barry C. Smith, chairman. Courtenay Dinwiddie of the Child Health Council was the program's executive director.

29. Informational Reports, Special Projects: GD, February 3, 1925, p. 5.

30. Smith's plan was outlined in an article in the December 1924 issue of Child Health magazine.

31. Born in Alexandria, Virginia, on October 9, 1882, Dinwiddie received his B.A. degree from Southwestern University in 1901 and took two years of postgraduate work at the University of Virginia. From 1905 to 1920, he was secretary to the president of the board of trustees of the Department of Bellevue and Allied Hospitals, executive secretary of the New York City Visiting Committee of the State Charities Aid Association, secretary of the Duluth Charities Aid Association, superintendent of the Duluth City Board of Public Welfare, superintendent of the Cincinnati Anti-Tuberculosis League, and an executive of Cincinnati's Public Health Federation. While executive secretary of the National Child Health Council from 1920 to 1923, Dinwiddie conducted courses in community organization at the Johns Hopkins University. For the next eight years, he was consultant on child hygiene for the New York City health department.

32. Each of the child health demonstrations is discussed in a separate volume, all four published by the Commonwealth Fund: *Five Years in Fargo; A Chapter of Child Health* (Athens and Clarke County, Georgia); *Cross-Sections of Rural Health Progress* (Rutherford County, Tennessee), by Harry S. Mustard; and *Children of the Covered Wagon* (Marion County, Oregon), by Estella Ford Warner and Geddes Smith.

33. Mustard, *Rural Health Practice*, p. 3.

34. GD, November 11, 1924, pp. 1–3.

35. For detailed analyses of nurses' programs, see Winslow, E. A. The measurement of nurse power (reprinted from Public Health Nurse, October 1927 and

February 1928); also *Cross-Sections of Rural Health Progress*, p. 190; *A Chapter of Child Health*, p. 18; and *Children of the Covered Wagon*, p. 70.

36. Dinwiddie, *Child Health and The Community*, pp. 14–16.

37. Evans, L. J. *The Commonwealth Fund: A Thirty-six Year Perspective, 1923–1959*, undated personal memoirs, p. 4. CF Arch.

38. AR, 1923, pp. 19–21.

39. AR, 1927, p. 24.

40. AR, 1924, pp. 16–17.

41. Mustard, *Rural Health Practice*; AR, 1928, p. 37.

42. Bishop, E. L. Foreword. In: Mustard, H. S. *Cross-Sections of Rural Health Progress: Report of the Commonwealth Fund Child Health Demonstration in Rutherford County, Tennessee.* New York: Commonwealth Fund, 1930, p. v.

43. Evans, *The Commonwealth Fund*, p. 5.

44. Dinwiddie, *Child Health and The Community*, pp. 2–3.

45. Professional and Executive Staff, Division of Child Health (AR, 1927, pp. 32–33):

Administrative: Courtenay Dinwiddie, Director of Demonstrations; Cornelia Lyne, Assistant to Director; Emma A. Winslow, Ph.D., Research; Geddes Smith, Publications; and Lester J. Evans, M.D., Medical Assistant.

Fargo: William DeKleine, M.D., Director; Edith B. Pierson, R.N., Director of Nursing Service; Maud A. Brown, Director of Health Education; R.C. Leonard, D.D.S., Director of Dental Service; and Elizabeth L. Brezee, Statistician.

Clarke County—Athens: Bernard W. Carey, M.D., Director; E. D. Andrews, M.D., Director of Medical Service; Myra Cloudman, R.N., Director of Nursing Service; Erna E. Proctor, Director of Health Education; Willie Dean Andrews, Physical Educator; and C. Edith Kerby, Statistician.

Rutherford County: Harry S. Mustard, M.D., Director; J. B. Black, M.D., Deputy Health Officer; O. G. Nelson, M.D., Director of Medical Service; Olive E. Meyer, R.N., Director of Nursing Service; and Cara L. Harris, Director of Health Education; and Carolina R. Randolph, Statistician.

Marion County: Walter H. Brown, M.D., Director; Vernon A. Douglas, M.D., Deputy Health Officer; Estella Ford Warner, M.D., Director of Medical Service; Elnora E. Thomson, R.N., Director of Nursing Service; Anne Simpson, Director of Health Education; Estill J. Brunk, D.D.S., Director of Dental Unit; and Mildred Ihrig, Statistician.

46. AR, 1930, p. 15.

47. A graduate of Bowdoin College in 1909, Scamman received a degree from the Medical School of Maine in 1912, and the M.P.H. degree from the Harvard University School of Public Health in 1922. After serving as director of the Fund's Division of Public Health from 1931 to 1948, Scamman became director of the American Cancer Society's Massachusetts Division, and president of the Massachusetts Public Health Association. (Obituary, *New York Times*, June 27, 1965.)

48. The Fund added several new staff members to the Divisions of Public Health and Rural Hospitals in the mid-1930s. John T. Morrison was a graduate of the University of Wisconsin Medical School and a protégé of William S. Middleton. Morrison had been a member of the administrative staff at the University of Wisconsin Hospital. He took over the Rural Hospital Program's day-to-day educational activities, consultant services, fellowships for staff physicians, and

teaching institutes. Morrison's background made him extremely valuable to community hospitals incorporating public health activities into their programs. Robert Jordan came to the Fund from the Yale–New Haven Hospital. His experience in hospital administration enabled him to develop the routine monthly service and financial reports that would allow local administrators to evaluate their hospital's performance. Sarah P. Lawrence, a nurse trained in Great Britain, also joined the staff to work with nursing education programs in rural hospitals.

49. Trained as an engineer, Walker acquired the D.P.H. degree from the University of Michigan in 1922. Early in his career, he served as a sanitary engineer in the Detroit health department and later as deputy commissioner. He was a first lieutenant in the Sanitary Corps, U.S. Army, during the First World War and then returned to Detroit as superintendent of the Municipal Tuberculosis Sanitorium. From 1923 to 1925, he was a research associate of the American Child Health Association, which was surveying health work in eighty-six American cities; in late 1925 the Committee on Administrative Practice of the American Public Health Association chose him as field director.

50. Editorial. Am. J. Publ. Health 31: 1208, November 1941.

51. Randolph was a graduate of Agnes Scott College and held a master's degree in Public Health from the Johns Hopkins University. (Obituary, *New York Herald Tribune*, March 2, 1958.)

52. Vincent, G. E. *The Rockefeller Foundation: A Review for 1927*.

53. Evans, *The Commonwealth Fund*, p. 56.

54. The original members of the committee were: Barry C. Smith, chairman; Donald B. Armstrong, second vice-president in charge of health and welfare, Metropolitan Life Insurance Company; Livingston Farrand, director, the National Tuberculosis Association; W. F. Draper, director, general medical services, the American National Red Cross; W. S. Leathers, dean and professor of preventive medicine, the Vanderbilt University School of Medicine; Sophie C. Nelson, a registered nurse; Philip Van Ingen, a pediatrician practicing in New York City; and W. Frank Walker.

55. Among the members added in 1939 were: A. C. Bachmeyer, director, University of Chicago Clinics; C. C. Bass, dean, the Tulane University School of Medicine; E. L. Bishop, director of health, Tennessee Valley Authority; C. Sidney Burwell, dean, the Harvard Medical School; John F. Bush, executive vice-president, the Presbyterian Hospital; A. Grant Fleming, dean, Faculty of Medicine, McGill University; Ira V. Hiscock, professor of public health, the Yale University College of Medicine; Harry S. Mustard, professor of preventive medicine, the New York University College of Medicine; W. S. Rankin, director, Hospital and Orphan Sections, the Duke Endowment; Lowell J. Reed, professor of biostatistics, School of Hygiene and Public Health, the Johns Hopkins University; John L. Rice, Commissioner of Health, City of New York; Elliott S. Robinson, director, Division of Biological Laboratories, the Massachusetts State Department of Health; and Marion W. Sheahan, director, Division of Public Health Nursing, the New York State Department of Health. Both Robinson and Reed were also consultants to the Fund in scientific research.

56. By 1946, when the committee disbanded, its members included: Walter Bauer, associate professor of medicine, the Harvard Medical School; William W.

Frye, professor of preventive medicine, Vanderbilt University; Walter W. Palmer, professor of medicine and chairman of the Department of Medicine, Columbia University College of Physicians and Surgeons; Samuel H. Proger, medical director, the Joseph H. Pratt Diagnostic Hospital in Boston; Thomas A. C. Rennie, associate professor of psychiatry, the Cornell University Medical College; D. W. Richards, Jr., professor of clinical medicine, Columbia University College of Physicians and Surgeons; Milton J. E. Senn, associate professor of pediatrics (psychiatry), the Cornell University Medical College; and Ernest L. Stebbins, professor of public health administration and director of the School of Hygiene and Public Health, the Johns Hopkins University. (AR, 1930; AR, 1939; AR, 1946; Evans, *The Commonwealth Fund*, pp. 53, 79.)

57. Emerson and Luginbuhe, *Local Health Units*.

58. Sumner County in Tennessee was known as a "Commonwealth County." One of its most successful activities was a training program for administrative personnel that concentrated on medical records and forms. (John C. Hume to A. McGehee Harvey, September 10, 1984.)

59. GD, The Scope of the Commonwealth Fund's Activities in Public Health, 1930–1947, December 11, 1947.

60. Bigelow, G. H. and Knowlton, W. W. A solution of rural health service in Massachusetts. N. Engl. J. Med. 203: 477, 1930. Bigelow was the state health officer, and Knowlton headed the state unit for the development of local health organizations.

61. AR, 1932, p. 18.

62. Bishop, E. L. Foreword. In: Mustard, *Cross-Sections of Rural Health Progress*, pp. v–vi.

63. AR, 1932, pp. 18–20.

64. Mustard, *Rural Health Practice*.

65. AR, 1934, p. 12.

66. GD, 1920–29, personal copies of E. S. Harkness. CF Arch.

67. Special Report, "Medical Appeals," December 13, 1919. CF Arch.

68. GD, April 8, 1920, p. 21.

69. Special Report, "Medical Appeals," December 13, 1919, pp. 1–3.

70. Terris, M. Hermann Biggs's contribution to the modern concept of the health center. Bull. Hist. Med. 20: 387, 1946; Biggs, H. M. The problem of health in the rural districts. Health News 37: 74, 1922; Biggs, H. M. Presidential address. Trans. Assoc. Am. Phys. 35: 1, 1920.

71. GD, June 3, 1925, pp. 8–17; GD, November 4, 1925, pp. 17–18. Consultants included: Homer F. Sanger, American Medical Association; Charles F. Neergaard, hospital consultant; S. S. Goldwater, director, the Mount Sinai Hospital in New York; and N. P. Colwell, secretary, Council on Medical Education, the American Medical Association.

72. GD, January 6, 1926; Wright, H. Special Report, " Rural Hospital Program," January 6, 1926. CF Arch.

73. AR, 1929, p. 46.

74. Public health nurses in Tennessee kept their records in "family folders." These gave them a good picture of the health and socioeconomic situation of the family and its individual members. It also frequently saved unnecessary home

visits, since needed services to all members could be handled at one time. This practice may have had its roots in the Fund's programs in Murfreesboro or Farmville. (John C. Hume to A. McGehee Harvey, September 10, 1984.)

75. AR, 1929, p. 48.
76. AR, 1931, p. 3
77. AR, 1930, p. 40.
78. GD, February 14, 1929.
79. AR, 1932, p. 33.
80. Evans, *The Commonwealth Fund*, pp. 60–63.
81. Southmayd, H. J. and Smith, G. *Small Community Hospitals*. New York: Commonwealth Fund, 1944.
82. Ibid.
83. GD, April 7, 1931, p. 22.
84. Ibid.; Fitz, R. H.; Mawardi, B. H.; and Wilbur, J. Scholarships for rural medicine: The Commonwealth Fund experience with a pre–World War II indenture program. Trans. Am. Clin. Climat. Assoc. 88: 191, 1976.
85. Wright, H. Special Report, "Rural Hospital Program," January 6, 1926, p. 2. CF Arch.
86. AR, 1932, p. 36.
87. AR, 1933, p. 35.
88. Fellows attended the following medical and dental schools for postgraduate study:

From Murfreesboro, Tennessee: Columbia, 1; Harvard, 2; Johns Hopkins, 1; New York Post-Graduate, 9; New York Polyclinic, 2; Tulane, 3.

From Beloit, Kansas: Columbia, 1; New York Post-Graduate, 6; Northwestern, 1; Tulane, 1; Washington (St. Louis), 2.

From Glasgow, Kentucky: Columbia, 1; Harvard, 1; New York Post-Graduate, 2; New York Polyclinic, 4; Tulane, 7; Vanderbilt, 2.

From Farmville, Virginia: Columbia, 2; Cornell, 1; Harvard, 3; Johns Hopkins, 1; New York Post-Graduate, 8; New York Polyclinic, 1; Northwestern, 1; Tulane, 2.

From Farmington, Maine: Albany Medical College, 1; Columbia, 1; Harvard, 2; New York Post-Graduate, 5.

From Wauseon, Ohio: Harvard, 1; New York Post-Graduate, 3; Northwestern, 1; Tulane, 2; Washington (St. Louis), 1. (AR, 1930, p. 43.)

89. GD, February 8, 1927.
90. A number of medical educators were consulted, including G. H. Meeker, dean, the University of Pennsylvania School of Medicine; William Darrach, dean, the Columbia University College of Physicians and Surgeons; A. C. Bachmeyer, dean, the College of Medicine, Cincinnati University; Walter B. Cannon, acting dean, the Harvard Medical School; G. Canby Robinson, dean, the Vanderbilt University School of Medicine; Lewis H. Weed, dean, the Johns Hopkins University School of Medicine; Walter Palmer, the Presbyterian Hospital; and Michael Davis, secretary, the Committee on Dispensary Development (GD, February 8, 1927).
91. AR, 1928, p. 45.
92. AR, 1929, p. 45.

93. The grant to Vanderbilt University in support of public health and preventive medicine yielded satisfying results. "No student graduating during the mid- and late thirties had any doubts that public health could provide a respectable and satisfying career for individuals so inclined." The staff at Vanderbilt included W. S. Leathers, dean and professor of preventive medicine; Henry E. Meleney, the outstanding parasitologist; and William Frye, also a parasitologist, later dean of the medical school and vice-chancellor at Louisiana State University. (John C. Hume to A. McGehee Harvey, September 10, 1984.)

94. GD, April 21, 1938.

95. Fitz, Mawardi, and Wilbur. Scholarships for rural medicine.

96. Evans, L. J. to Carl Malmberg, Acting Staff Director, Subcommittee on Wartime Health and Education, United States Senate, January 30, 1945. CF Arch.

97. AR, 1935, p. 25.

98. GD, December 12, 1933. See also Dean's Office correspondence labeled "Commonwealth Fund" at the Francis Countway Library, Boston.

99. AR, 1936, p. 25.

100. AR, 1936, pp. 26–29.

101. AR, 1936, p. 26.

102. AR, 1942, p. 11.

103. AR, 1944, p. 19.

104. AR, 1946, p. 25.

105. AR, 1932, p. 37.

106. Evans, *The Commonwealth Fund*, pp. 67–69.

107. AR, 1933, p. 38.

108. Southmayd, H. J. Confidential Memorandum: Suggestion for an Experiment in the Regional Organization of Hospitals, September 1943. CF Arch.

109. Evans, L. J. Memorandum to Barry Smith, November 30, 1944, regarding the Regional Hospital Plan; Evans, L. J. Memorandum: Regional Hospital Development—A Comparison of Richmond and Rochester Areas, August 17, 1945; Evans, L. J. Memorandum to Southmayd covering support of a regional hospital plan (essentially disapproval of Rochester in favor of Richmond), August 31, 1945. CF Arch.

110. AR, 1945, pp. 21–23.

111. GD, April 9, 1948, pp. 3–10; GD, October 27, 1949, pp. 15–17; GD, February 20, 1953, pp. 34–38.

112. Consultative Council on Medical and Allied Services, Ministry of Health of Great Britain: Interim Report on the Future Provision of Medical and Allied Services. London: H. M. Stationery Office, 1920.

113. See McCombs, C. F. Business management of the Community Chest participating hospitals of Rochester, New York—June 1938. CF Arch.

114. For further details, see GD, October 11, 1945, p. 15; GD, April 9, 1948, p. 3; GD, October 27, 1949, p. 15; GD, April 20, 1951, p. 33.

115. For an example of the type of studies made in the areas of hospital administration and health care delivery, see Lembcke, P. A. Evolution of the medical audit. J.A.M.A. 199: 543, 1967. (Lembcke was associate director of the Rochester Regional Hospital Council.)

116. Rosenfeld, L. S. and Makover, H. B. *The Rochester Regional Hospital*

Council. New York: Commonwealth Fund (Cambridge: Harvard University Press), 1956.

117. Lester J. Evans, personal communication to A. McGehee Harvey.

118. Robert L. Berg, interview with A. McGehee Harvey, April 15, 1982.

119. Robert L. Berg, personal communication to A. McGehee Harvey.

120. AR, 1939, p. 3.

121. Editorial. The Country Doctor. *New York Times.* Cited in GD, October 29, 1929.

122. Editorial. Am. J. Publ. Health 31: 1208, November 1941.

123. During the 1930s, many hospitals found it difficult to make ends meet. There was little encouragement for new hospital construction, and many existing hospitals were allowed to deteriorate. More than one thousand counties had no hospital facilities of any type. During the war years, a number of small hospitals were built, often of flimsy construction, to deal with the emergency requirements of communities crowded with munitions, shipyard, and other wartime workers.

The Hill–Burton Act of 1946 required each state requesting funds to establish an advisory council with consumer and professional representation. Large states were divided into regions, each with its own advisory body. Before requesting funds, the state had to submit a survey indicating the need for hospitals in specific localities, and particular attention was paid to the needs of rural communities. The federal government provided only a portion of the funds requested for each new hospital, its shared determined by variable matching formulas. The Act expressly forbade government interference in the hospitals' operation.

In 1964, the original Act was amended to provide support for construction of nursing homes, diagnostic and treatment centers, chronic-disease hospitals, and rehabilitation facilities. Grants were also made available for research and demonstrations that would enhance the effective use of hospitals.

124. Starr, P. *The Social Transformation of American Medicine.* New York: Basic Books, 1982, pp. 347–51. See also Mountin, J. W.; Pennell, E. H.; and Hoge, V. M. Health service areas—Requirements for general hospitals and health centers. Public Health Bulletin No. 292. Washington, D.C.: U.S. Government Printing Office, 1950; Mountin, J. W. and Greve, C. J. Public health areas and hospital facilities. Public Health Publication No. 42. Washington, D.C.: U.S. Government Printing Office, 1950; Senate Committee on Education and Labor, 79th Congress, 1st Session, Hearings on Hospital Construction Act, Senate Bill 141. Washington, D.C. U.S. Government Printing Office, 1945; Commission on Hospital Care, Hospital Care in the United States. New York: Commonwealth Fund, 1947; New York State Health Preparedness Commission: Planning for the Care of the Chronically Ill—Regional Aspects, Legislative Document No. 78A, Albany, New York, 1945.

125. GD, April 20, 1939, pp. 4–5.

126. Between 1965 and the end of fiscal 1974, Congress appropriated another $2 billion in matching funds under the Hill–Burton program. Annual appropriations through this program reached a maximum of $270 million in 1967, followed by a sharp drop from 1969 to 1970 from $267 million to $172 million. After 1970 the emphasis shifted from construction of new hospitals and nursing homes to modernization of existing hospitals and construction of facilities for the care of outpatients. The total Hill–Burton appropriation for 1974 was $18 million. (Bordley,

J. III and Harvey, A. M. *Two Hundred Years of American Medicine.* Philadelphia: W. B. Saunders, 1976; see also GD, April 9, 1948, p. 3.)

127. Somers, A. R. Why not try preventing illness as a way of controlling Medicare costs? N. Engl. J. Med. 311: 853, 1984.

128. Ibid.

5. Early Programs in Medical Education and Medical Research

1. AR, 1921, pp. 20–21.
2. Evans, *The Commonwealth Fund*, p. 57.
3. Lester J. Evans, personal communication to A. McGehee Harvey.
4. Heffron, R. *Pneumonia, with Special Reference to the Pneumococcus in Lobar Pneumonia.* New York: Commonwealth Fund (London: Oxford University Press), 1939, 1006 pp.
5. Heffron was born in Chicago, Illinois, on September 28, 1901. He attended the University of Illinois at Champaign–Urbana and began medical school at the University of Illinois College of Medicine in Chicago, transferring to Harvard after his first year. (Roderick E. Heffron, interview with A. McGehee Harvey, October 6, 1981; Obituary, *New York Times*, October 29, 1983.)
6. Warren was a 1926 graduate of Cornell University. He received the M.D. degree from the Cornell University Medical College in 1937, and the Ph.D. from New York University. (Obituary, *New York Times*, July 26, 1963.)
7. Evans, *The Commonwealth Fund*, p. 31.
8. AR, 1937, p. 1.
9. AR, 1939, pp. 22–24.
10. AR, 1940, p. 15.
11. AR, 1938, p. 12.
12. GD, April 10, 1941, pp. 30–31.
13. GD, April 10, 1941, p. 31.
14. GD, June 10, 1943, p. 36.
15. AR, 1939, p. 21.
16. GD, October 23, 1947, p. 18.
17. AR, 1941, pp. 25–27.
18. GD, October, 23, 1947, p. 20.
19. GD, June 16, 1949, pp. 66, 69.
20. GD, May 13, 1954, pp. 56–57.
21. GD, October 27, 1949, pp. 12–15.
22. GD, November 17, 1955, p. 62.
23. GD, November 17, 1955, pp. 63–64.
24. The National Institute of Health, the National Cancer Institute, the Mental Health Institute, and the National Heart Institute together (as units of the United States Public Health Service) offered about $1,150,000 for fellowships in 1949. About one-quarter was targeted for training at the bachelor of science level, and the rest for postdoctoral (M.D. or Ph.D.) training. These fellowships were generally pointed toward research, but those for mental health included graduate study and clinical training among their objectives. The Atomic Energy Commission

awarded the significant part of another $1 million to support medicine and biology. The National Research Council administered for the Rockefeller Foundation, the American Cancer Society, and other agencies graduate medical fellowships amounting to about $375,000. The American Heart Association, the Life Insurance Medical Research Fund, and the Jane Coffin Childs Foundation (for cancer research) had among them some $200,000 for fellowships, and the Markle Foundation offered fellowships aimed specifically at the promotion of medical teaching. In addition, state health officers had the authority, subject to federal approval, to spend any part of annual federal subsidies of $30 million for fellowships in general health services, venereal disease control, and tuberculosis control. The Fund estimated that between $2 million and $3 million was so used in 1948. (GD, June 16, 1949, pp. 70–71.)

25. GD, May 17, 1956, p. 70.
26. GD, May 8, 1958, p. 37.
27. AR, 1963, p. 50; AR, 1964, p. 11.
28. Letters and identification of excerpts on file in CF Archives.
29. GD, May 14, 1964, p. 28.
30. GD, May 13, 1965, p. 24.
31. AR, 1967, p. 45.
32. AR, 1968, p. 58.
33. GD, May 26, 1970, p. 45–47; Recommendations to the Board of Directors of the Commonwealth Fund on Programs for the 1970s, Special Meeting of the Board, April 14, 1971, p. 3.
34. GD, May 11, 1978, p. 17.
35. AR, 1920, p. 13.
36. Lape, E. E. Summary of results of medical research projects. October 1, 1931–September 30, 1936. CF Arch.
37. Heffron, *Pneumonia*. See also Lord, F. T. and Heffron, R. *Pneumonia and Serum Therapy, with Special Reference to the Massachusetts Pneumonia Study*. New York: Commonwealth Fund (London: Oxford University Press), 1936, 91 pp. rev. ed., 1938, 148 pp.
38. Weisenburg, T. and McBride, K. E. *Aphasia: A Clinical and Psychological Study*. New York: Commonwealth Fund (London: Oxford University Press), 1935, 634 pp.
39. Huddleston, I. F. *Brucella Infections in Animals and Man*. New York: Commonwealth Fund (London: Oxford University Press), 1934, 108 pp.
40. New York Academy of Medicine, Committee on Public Relations. *Maternal Mortality in New York City: A Study of All Puerperal Deaths, 1930–1932*. New York: Commonwealth Fund (London: Oxford University Press), 1933, 290 pp.
41. Julianelle, L. A. *The Etiology of Trachoma*. New York: Commonwealth Fund (London: Oxford University Press), 1938, 634 pp.
42. Medical Research Review: 1936–1944. Projects Supported during the Eight-Year Period from October 1, 1936 to September 30, 1944. Dated September 1946. CF Arch.
43. AR, 1942, p. 6.
44. Waksman, S. A. *Microbial Antagonisms and Antibiotic Substances*. New York: Commonwealth Fund (London: Oxford University Press), 1945, 350 pp. 2nd ed., 1947, 411 pp.

45. For further details, see Hardy, J. B. *Tuberculosis in White and Negro Children*. Vol. 1: *The Roentgenographic Aspects of the Harriet Lane Study*. 122 pp.; Brailey, M. E. Vol. 2: *The Epidemiological Aspects of the Harriet Lane Study*. 122 pp. New York: Commonwealth Fund (Cambridge: Harvard University Press), 1958.

46. Wiggers, C. J. *Physiology of Shock*. New York: Commonwealth Fund (London: Oxford University Press), 1950, 459 pp.

47. The Mayor's Committee of the City of New York: *The Marijuana Problem in the City of New York*. Lancaster, Pa.: Jacques Cattell Press, 1944, 220 pp.

48. Third Medical Research Review, October 1, 1944 to December 31, 1951. Dated February 1953, CF Arch.

49. AR, 1946, p. 15.

50. Deignan, S. L. and Miller, E. The support of research in medical and allied fields for the period 1946 through 1951. Science 115: 321, March 28, 1952.

51. GD, October 14, 1948, pp. 41–46; GD, October 11, 1951, pp. 38–41.

52. GD, October 23, 1947, pp. 25–30.

53. GD, April 9, 1948, pp. 26–27.

54. Wilkins, L. *The Diagnosis and Treatment of Endocrine Disorders in Childhood and Adolescence*. Springfield, Ill.: Charles C Thomas, 1950.

55. GD, June 8, 1950, pp. 15–19; GD, November 20, 1952, pp. 28–31.

56. GD, June 8, 1950, pp. 19–22; GD, April 20, 1951, pp. 40–45.

57. GD, October 14, 1948, pp. 22–26.

58. Cournand, A.; Baldwin, J.; and Himmelstein, A. *Cardiac Catheterization in Congenital Heart Disease: A Clinical and Physiological Study in Infants and Children*. New York: Commonwealth Fund (London: Oxford University Press), 1949, 108 pp.

59. GD, December 11, 1947, pp. 30–32.

60. GD, October 23, 1947, pp. 21–25; GD, June 8, 1950, pp. 26–30; GD, October 11, 1951, pp. 41–42.

61. Oliver, J. *Nephrons and Kidneys* (A qualitative study of developmental and evolutionary mammalian renal architectonics). New York: Commonwealth Fund (New York: Hoeber Medical Division, Harper and Row), 1968, 117 pp.

62. GD, June 8, 1950, pp. 30–35; GD, May 9, 1952, pp. 34–40; GD, February 25, 1954, pp. 27–36; GD, February 10, 1957, pp. 58–66.

63. Senn, M. J. E. and Hartford, C. L. *The Firstborn: Experiences of Eight American Families*. New York: Commonwealth Fund (Cambridge: Harvard University Press), 1968, 91 pp.

64. GD, November 20, 1952, pp. 22–28.

65. Medical Research Review No. 4: January 1, 1952–December 31, 1958. CF Arch.

66. GD, April 18, 1947, pp. 47–53; GD, February 20, 1953, pp. 29–34. See also Wilson, M. G. *Rheumatic Fever: Studies of the Epidemiology, Manifestations, Diagnosis, and Treatment of the Disease during the First Three Decades*. New York: Commonwealth Fund (London: Oxford University Press), 1940, 595 pp.; Wilson, M. G. *Advances in Rheumatic Fever: 1940–1961*. New York: Commonwealth Fund (New York: Hoeber Medical Division, Harper and Row), 1962, 249 pp.

67. GD, October 11, 1951, pp. 21–29.

68. Ropes, M. W. and Bauer, W. L. *Synovial Fluid Changes in Joint Diseases.* New York: Commonwealth Fund (Cambridge: Harvard University Press), 1953, 150 pp.

69. Short, C. L.; Bauer, W. L.; and Reynolds, W. *Rheumatic Arthritis: A Definition of the Disease and a Clinical Description Based on a Numerical Study of 293 Patients and Controls.* New York: Commonwealth Fund (Cambridge: Harvard University Press), 1957, 480 pp.

70. GD, June 16, 1949, pp. 45–49.

71. Talbot, N. B. et al. *Functional Endocrinology from Birth through Adolescence.* New York: Commonwealth Fund (Cambridge: Harvard University Press), 1947, 618 pp.; Spanish translation, Buenos Aires, n.d.; Talbot, N. B.; Richie, R. H.; and Crawford, J. D. *Metabolic Homeostasis: A Syllabus for Those Concerned with the Care of Patients.* New York: Commonwealth Fund (Cambridge: Harvard University Press), 1959, 132 pp.

72. GD, June 16, 1949, pp. 40–45; GD, January 11, 1951, pp. 26–27; GD, May 9, 1952, pp. 23–28; GD, February 25, 1954, pp. 21–27.

73. GD, April 20, 1951, pp. 36–40; May 16, 1957, pp. 43–48; GD, May 21, 1959, pp. 32–35.

74. GD, April 1950.

75. Grant to the Western Reserve University School of Medicine—survey of the work of the Child Research Council (University of Colorado School of Medicine). $5000 grant approved by Executive Committee Board on November 20, 1953. Presented at Director's meeting of February 25, 1954. CF Arch; Report to the Rockefeller Foundation and the Commonwealth Fund of a Committee to Review the Activities of the Child Research Council at the University of Colorado (F. Howell Wright, chairman; Robert B. Reed, John H. Dingle). Submitted May 20, 1954, 8 pp. CF Arch. (Appendix by Dr. Reed, 4 pp.)

76. The University of Colorado School of Medicine—Child Research Council. Evans, L. J. Comment on Wright Report, June 10, 1954. 5 pp. CF Arch; Washburn, A. H. Child Research Council, Study of Growth and Development; Heffron, R. E. General Summary, Memorandum and Visit to Project, June 14–18, 1954. Dated July 13, 1954, 29 pp. CF Arch.

77. Roderick E. Heffron to Robert S. Morison, associate director, Division of Medicine and Public Health, the Rockefeller Foundation, August 31, 1954. CF Arch.

78. Interview with Robert W. McCammon, director, and some of his associates, October 19, 1964. Comments by Roderick E. Heffron, November 6, 1964, 8 pp. CF Arch; preparation of a series of volumes on human growth and development, May 3, 1966. Unsigned, 7 pp. CF Arch.

79. Robert W. McCammon to A. McGehee Harvey, October 19, 1982, and November 15, 1982.

80. McCammon, R. W. *Human Growth and Development.* Springfield, Ill.: Charles C Thomas, 1969.

81. X-rays of chest, long bones, back—Fels Research Institute, Antioch, Ohio; anthropometric measurements—Fels Research Institute; dental casts, head x-rays, hand x-rays—University of Oklahoma Health Sciences Center, Orthodontic Department, School of Dentistry; copies of dental cases and cephalometric x-rays—University of Connecticut School of Dentistry and Pedidontic

Division, University of Illinois School of Dentistry; electrocardiographic tracings—Health Care Research Foundation, Denver; microfilm library of all data except x-rays and electrocardiographic tracings—McCammon's office.

82. Boyd, E. *Origins of the Study of Human Growth.* Portland: University of Oregon Health Sciences Center Foundation, 1980.

83. Papanicolaou, G. N. *Atlas of Exfoliative Cytology.* New York: Commonwealth Fund (Cambridge: Harvard University Press), 1954, 220 pp.; Papanicolaou, G. N. and Traut, H. F. *Diagnosis of Uterine Cancer by Vaginal Smear.* New York: Commonwealth Fund (London: Oxford University Press), 1943, 47 pp.; Papanicolaou, G. N.; Traut, H. F.; and Marchetti, A. A. *Epithelia of Woman's Reproductive Organs. A Correlative Study of Cyclic Changes.* New York: Commonwealth Fund (London: Oxford University Press), 1948.

84. George N. Papanicolaou to Roderick E. Heffron, June 4, 1952. CF Arch. See also Carmichael, D. E. *The Pap Smear: Life of George Papanicolaou.* Springfield, Ill.: Charles C Thomas, 1973, pp. 14–15; Berkow, S. C. A visit with Dr. George N. Papanicolaou. Obstet. Gynecol. 16: 243–252, 1960; Papanicolaou, G. N. The evolutionary dynamic and trends of exfoliative cytology. Tex. Rep. Biol. Med. 13: 901, 1955; Cameron, C. S. Dedication of the Papanicolaou Cancer Research Institute. J.A.M.A. 182: 556–559, 1962; Papanicolaou, G. N. A new cancer diagnosis. Proc. Third Race Betterment Conference, Battle Creek, Michigan, January 2–6, 1928.

85. Peabody, F.; Draper, G.; and Dochez, A. R. *A Clinical Study of Acute Poliomyelitis.* Monograph No. 4. New York: Rockefeller Institute of Medical Research, 1912, 187 pp.; Maxcy, K. F., ed. *Papers of Wade Hampton Frost, M.D.* New York: Commonwealth Fund (London: Oxford University Press), 1941. See also Paul, J. R. Wade Hampton Frost and the beginning of statistical epidemiology. In: Paul, J. R. *History of Poliomyelitis.* New Haven: Yale University Press, 1971, p. 137.

86. Report of the Dean, the Johns Hopkins University School of Hygiene and Public Health, to the President of the University, 1937–1938, p. 3.

87. Fee, E. Johns Hopkins Magazine, October 1983, p. 27.

88. Report of the Dean, The Johns Hopkins University School of Hygiene and Public Health, to the President of the University, 1932–1933, pp. 2–3.

89. Brailey, M. E. A study of tuberculous infection and mortality in the children of tuberculous households. Am. J. Hyg. 31, Sec. A: 1, 1940; Frost, W. H. The age selection of mortality from tuberculosis in successive decades. Am. J. Hyg. 30, Sec. A: 91, 1939; Frost, W. H. and Gover, M. The incidence and time distribution of common colds in several groups kept under continuous observation. Publ. Health. Rep. 47: 1815–1841, Sept. 2, 1932; Frost, W. H. Risk of persons in familial contact with pulmonary tuberculosis. Am. J. Publ. Health 23: 426–432, May 1933.

90. Maxcy, *Papers of Wade Hampton Frost,* p. 583.

91. Read, F. E. M.; Ciocco, A.; and Taussig, H. B. The frequency of rheumatic manifestations among the siblings, parents, uncles, aunts and grandparents of rheumatic and control patients. Am. J. Hyg 27: 719, 1938; Gauld, R. L. and Read, F. E. M. Studies in rheumatic disease: V. The age at onset of primary rheumatic attack. J. Clin. Invest. 19: 729, 1940; Gauld, R. L. and Read, F. E.

M. Studies of rheumatic disease: III. Familial association and aggregation in rheumatic disease. J. Clin. Invest. 19: 393, 1940.

92. Maxcy, *Papers of Wade Hampton Frost.*

93. Ebert, R. H. Presidential address. Trans. Assoc. Am. Phys. 86: 1, 1973.

94. Ibid.

95. Ibid.

96. Medical Research Review No. 4, 1952–1958, p. 70.

97. GD, February 16, 1922, pp. 13–22; Report to the Executive Committee, "Special Report on the American Society for the Control of Cancer," February 14, 1929. Smith had conferred with Curtis Lakeman, a former executive of the Society for the Control of Cancer, and with Dean William Darrach and Professor of Medicine W. W. Palmer of the Columbia–Presbyterian Medical Center.

98. Other consultants were Robert E. Greenough of Harvard University; Francis C. Wood of Columbia University; and William Darrach, dean, Columbia University. Dr. C. C. Burlingame of the Presbyterian Hospital made a special independent investigation for the Commonwealth Fund at Smith's request. In all, over thirty experts were consulted, others being: Franklin H. Warton, director general, the American College of Surgeons; James B. Murphy, the Rockefeller Institute; and Joseph C. Bloodgood, oncologist at the Johns Hopkins University School of Medicine.

99. Henry A. Christian to Barry C. Smith, 1929. CF Arch. Cited in GD, December 18, 1929.

100. Henry A. Riley to Barry C. Smith, 1929. CF Arch. Cited in GD, December 18, 1929.

101. GD, April 8, 1924. Smith chose the following consultants to evaluate the proposal: David L. Edsall, Harvard University; Walter L. Niles, Cornell University; William Darrach, Columbia University; Lindley R. Williams, Secretary, the National Tuberculosis Association; W. D. Cutter, dean, the Post-graduate Medical School; and Arthur I. Kendall, dean, Northwestern University. All except Cutter agreed that the board had had a very favorable effect on the standards of medical education.

102. Barry C. Smith to Chairman of Subcommittee on Wartime Health and Education, 1944. CF Arch.

103. Evans, L. J. Memorandum, Post-War Medical Education Activities. May 2, 1945, 45 pp. CF Arch.

104. AR, 1943, pp. 8–10.

105. Smith, B. C. Memorandum to Board of Directors, February 28, 1947. CF Arch.

106. Malcolm P. Aldrich to W. E. Stevenson, January 31, 1949. CF Arch.

6. Support of Comprehensive Medicine

1. After leaving the Fund, Sheehan served as chairman of the Scientific Committee of the New York University—Bellevue Medical Center and dean of the New York University College of Medicine.

2. GD, January 11, 1952, pp. 18–26.

3. Evans, *The Commonwealth Fund*, pp. 91–93.
4. GD, Special Report on General Policy, March 1948.
5. Report of the Presidential Research Board, John R. Steelman, chairman, October 1947. Cited in GD, Special Report on General Policy, March 1948.
6. GD, Special Report on General Policy, March 1948, pp. 27–28.
7. GD, April 9, 1948, p. 4.
8. GD, June 10, 1948, p. 17.
9. GD, October 27, 1949, pp. 7–12; February 20, 1953, pp. 18–24.
10. GD, June 14, 1951, pp. 27–33.
11. GD, June 12, 1947, pp. 13–18; June 16, 1949, pp. 17–30.
12. GD, June 16, 1949, pp. 73–75.
13. Barr received his medical degree from the Cornell University Medical College in 1914 and after internship training at Bellevue began work in the Russell Sage Institute of Pathology at Cornell, studying with Eugene F. DuBois. In 1924 Barr became chairman of the Department of Medicine at the Washington University Medical School in St. Louis. His work included several classic papers, with John P. Peters, on the respiratory mechanism in cardiac dyspnea, and he described the disease produced in a patients with adenoma of the parathyroid gland, coining the term "hyperparathyroidism." Just before World War II, Barr succeeded DuBois as chairman of the Department of Medicine at Cornell.
14. GD, April 9, 1948, p. 14.
15. John Romano, interview with A. McGehee Harvey, April 19, 1982.

7. Programs in Medical Education and Community Service

1. Aldrich maintained strong ties with Yale over the years; in 1957, he was president of the University Council, and in 1973 he received the Yale Medal for service to the university.
2. Eberhart received the B.A. degree in psychology from the University of Oregon in 1929, and the Ph.D. in the same field from Northwestern University in 1934. He remained at Northwestern until 1943; from 1943 to 1946, he served as an air combat intelligence officer in the Navy. He then spent a year as a postdoctoral student with the Social Sciences Research Council, studying the psychology of politics in the House of Representatives. In 1947, Eberhart joined the National Institute of Mental Health (NIMH) as a training specialist in psychology, returning to the NIMH as director of intramural research when he left the Fund. Eberhart remained at the NIMH for twenty years and eventually became senior advisor to the deputy director of science at the National Institutes of Health.
3. Aldrich's consultants included James B. Conant of Harvard University; Devereux C. Josephs, former president of the Carnegie Corporation; Chester I. Barnard, president of the Rockefeller Foundation; Robert M. Hutchins, president of the University of Chicago; Rev. Donald Aldrich, dean, the Princeton Cathedral; and Jackson Reynolds, banker.
4. GD, April 20, 1951, pp. 1–12.
5. John C. Eberhart, interview with A. McGehee Harvey, December 18, 1981.

6. Robert J. Glaser, interview with A. McGehee Harvey, February 1982.

7. A 1925 graduate of the Johns Hopkins University School of Medicine, Berry took his residency training in medicine at the Johns Hopkins Hospital. After three years at the Rockefeller Institute for Medical Research, he was appointed professor and chairman of the Department of Medicine at the University of Rochester School of Medicine and Dentistry. There, his interest turned to medical administration, and in 1941, he became assistant and then associate dean before moving to Harvard in 1949.

8. GD, May 13, 1954, pp. 19–34.

9. Robert J. Glaser, interview with A. McGehee Harvey, February 1982.

10. George P. Berry, interview with A. McGehee Harvey, December 10, 1981.

11. Ibid.

12. The group included John M. Russell of the Markle Foundation; Frank G. Boudreau of the Milbank Fund; Alan Gregg of the Rockefeller Foundation; Leonard Carmichael of the Carnegie Foundation for the Advancement of Teaching; John W. Gardner, vice-president of the Carnegie Corporation; and Evans.

13. Saunders, L. *Cultural Difference and Medical Care.* New York: Russell Sage Foundation, 1954, p. 7. Cited in Evans, L. J. *The Crisis in Medical Education.* Ann Arbor: University of Michigan Press, 1964, p. 8.

14. Evans, *The Crisis in Medical Education*, p. 36.

15. Evans, L. J. Memorandum, Fund Assistance to Medical Education. October 27, 1948, 43 pp. CF Arch; Memorandum to staff. December 15, 1949, 16 pp. CF Arch.

16. Evans, L. J. Memorandum, The Commonwealth Fund and Medical Education. May 10, 1949, 21 pp. CF Arch.

17. Lester J. Evans, personal communication to A. McGehee Harvey.

18. Evans, L. J. Memorandum, 1951. CF Arch.

19. Medical Education Planning Grants, April 7, 1959, 29 pp.; Eberhart, J. C. Memorandum to Lester J. Evans: Fund Support for Medical Education, March 21, 1955, 5 pp.; GD, May 9, 1952, pp. 1–4; GD, February 10, 1955, pp. 1–6; Evans, L. J. Memorandum, Medical Education Planning Grants, April 7, 1959, 29 pp.; Lee, P. V. Review of Commonwealth Fund Experiments in Medical Education, Part II, October 8, 1959, p. 18; GD, February 25, 1954, pp. 1–13; GD, February 10, 1957, pp. 1–13; GD, February 8, 1962, pp. 17–23.

20. Lester J. Evans, interview with A. McGehee Harvey, September 24, 1981.

21. GD, May 13, 1954, pp. 34–45; February 10, 1955, pp. 52–67; GD, May 13, 1954, pp. 34–46.

22. Lee, P. V. Review of Commonwealth Fund Experiments in Medical Education. Part I, April 21, 1959. Pt. 2, October 8, 1959. CF Arch.

23. Information on the individual programs derives largely from the formal applications and yearly progress reports of grant recipients. These sources portray both the information initially available to the staff on receipt of a proposal and the material on which the board of directors based its decisions about funding. In order to display the opinions of the staff that were transmitted to the directors—a crucial step in the decision-making process—particular use has been

made of material in the reports of the president and staff to the directors of the Fund.

24. Reader, G. G. and Soave, R. Comprehensive care revisited. Milbank Memorial Fund Quarterly 54: 391, Fall 1976; Alfort, J. S. and Charney, C. The Education of Physicians for Primary Care. Washington, D.C.:U.S. Department of Health, Education and Welfare; Delbanco, T. C. The teaching hospital and primary care. J. Med. Educ. 50: 29, 1975; Sanazaro, P. J. and Bates, B. A joint study of teaching programs in comprehensive medicine. J. Med. Educ. 43: 777, 1968; Snoke, P. S. and Weinerman, E. R. Comprehensive care programs in university medical centers. J. Med. Educ. 40: 625, 1965.

25. George G. Reader, interview with A. McGehee Harvey, December 1981.

26. AR, 1949, p. 2.

27. Reader, G. G. Comprehensive medical care. J. Med. Educ. 28: 34, July 1953. See also GD, June 14, 1951, p. 11; GD, May 13, 1954, p. 1; GD, May 16, 1957, p. 1.

28. Connie Myers Guion (1882–1971), considered by many to be the "complete general physician," was associated with the Cornell University Medical College for many years. Her impression of the Comprehensive Care Program may be found in her oral history deposition in the Oral History Collection of Columbia University.

29. George G. Reader, interview with A. McGehee Harvey, December 1981.

30. Reader, G. G. and Goss, M. E. W, eds. *Comprehensive Medical Care and Teaching.* Ithaca, N.Y.: Cornell University Press, 1967; Mary Goss, interview with A. McGehee Harvey, December 1981.

31. The background, evolution, and objectives of the program appear in Reader, G. The Cornell Comprehensive Care and Teaching Program. In: Merton, R. K.; Reader, G. G.; and Kendall, P. L., eds., *The Student Physician*, New York: Commonwealth Fund, 1954.

32. Reader, G. G. and Olencki, M. Cost of care to ambulant patients under a comprehensive care program. Am. J. Publ. Health 50: 1114, 1960.

33. Lee, P. V. Review of Commonwealth Fund Experiments in Medical Education. Dated April 21, 1959. CF Arch.

34. Notes on the Conference on Evaluation Studies in Medical Education, held May 7–8, 1954, at Harkness House, New York City. See also Dingle, J. H. et al. An approach to evaluation of medical education at Western Reserve University. J. Med. Educ. 33: 113, 1958; Adams, W. R. The psychiatrist in an ambulatory clerkship for comprehensive medical care in a new curriculum. J. Med. Educ. 33: 211, 1958; Mawardi, B. H. A career study of physicians. J. Med. Educ. 40: 658, 1965.

35. George G. Reader, interview with A. McGehee Harvey, December 1981.

36. Patricia L. Kendall to A. McGehee Harvey, June 18, 1984.

37. Kern, F, Jr. The general medical clinic of the University of Colorado. Am. J. Publ. Health 45: 47, 1955.

38. Hammond, K. and Kern, F., Jr. *Teaching Comprehensive Medical Care.* Cambridge: Harvard University Press, 1959.

39. For further details see Hammond, K. R. et al. *Teaching Comprehensive Medical Care; A Psychological Study of Change in Medical Education.* New York: Commonwealth Fund (Cambridge: Harvard University Press), 1959, 642 pp.;

Lee, P. V. Review of Commonwealth Fund Experiments in Medical Education. Dated April 21, 1959. CF Arch; Lee, P. V. *Medical Schools and the Changing Times.* Evanston, Ill.: Association of American Medical Colleges, 1962.

40. Lee, P. V. Review of Commonwealth Fund Experiments in Medical Education. Dated April 21, 1959. CF Arch.

41. Steiger, W. A. and Hansen, A. V. The teaching of comprehensive medicine at Temple University School of Medicine and Hospital. J. Med. Educ. 32: 580, 1957; English, O. S. and Hoffman, F. H. The goals of undergraduate psychiatric education at Temple University School of Medicine. J. Med. Educ. 35: 1030, 1960; Steiger, W. A. et al. A definition of comprehensive medicine. J. Health Hum. Behav. 1: 83, 1960.

42. Proposal to the Commonwealth Fund for support of certain curricular changes and activities based on the general clinic of the North Carolina Memorial Hospital, April 1, 1957, CF Arch; William L. Fleming, interview with A. McGehee Harvey, October 5, 1982; Fleming, W. L. Teaching of family physician's approach by a department of preventive medicine. J.A.M.A. 161: 711, 1956; White, K. L. and Fleming, W. L. Improving teaching on ambulant patients. J. Med. Educ. 32: 30, 1957.

43. This section represents the view of a participant, T. Franklin Williams, who was an active member of the General Clinic as a major part of his faculty assignment. Williams was interviewed by A. McGehee Harvey on April 15, 1982. Also interviewed (in October 1982) was W. L. Fleming, the director of the clinic.

44. Williams, T. F. et al. The referral process in medical care and the university clinic's role. J. Med. Educ. 36: 899, 1961.

45. Robert Huntley, for example, joined the group after being in family practice. A good researcher and teacher, he eventually became chairman of the Department of Community Medicine at the Georgetown University School of Medicine. Daniel Martin became head of the general ambulatory service and public health section at a clinic in Kentucky, while James Bryan took a position as head of ambulatory services at the University of North Carolina at Chapel Hill.

46. Lee, P. V. Report to the Commonwealth Fund on Experiments in Medical Education. CF Arch.

47. GD, May 9, 1952, pp. 4–11.

48. Lee, P. V. Review of Commonwealth Fund Experiments in Medical Education. Pt. 2, October 8, 1959. CF Arch.

49. Bissonnette, A. Memorandum to Joseph J. Stokes, June 19, 1984.

50. This group included George G. Reader from Cornell University, Henry J. Bakst and Ed Myra from Boston University, Cecil G. Sheps from the Beth Israel Hospital, Frank Furstenberg from the Sinai Hospital in Baltimore, Clifton Himmelbad from the USPHS Hospital, and a few others. A complete list appears in the attendance records of the outpatient department workshops of the University of North Carolina at Chapel Hill.

51. The details of the development of the program, its integrated curriculum, and its revision in 1968 appear in Williams, G. *Western Reserve's Experiment in Medical Education and its Outcome.* New York: Oxford University Press, 1980. Published by the Commonwealth Fund and the Cleveland Foundation. Extensive use has been made of Williams's book in the preparation of this vignette.

52. Commonwealth Fund staff memorandum, November 2, 1945. CF Arch.
53. Commonwealth Fund staff memorandum, February 4, 1948. CF Arch.
54. Joseph T. Wearn to Lester J. Evans, February 20, 1948.
55. Transcript of Commonwealth Fund staff conference, January 6–7, 1949. Staff members present: Lester J. Evans, Roderick E. Heffron, Harry E. Handley, Charles O. Warren, Robert Jordan, Mildred C. Scoville, Geddes Smith, and Henry J. Southmayd. Visitors: Joseph T. Wearn and John L. Caughey, Jr. CF Arch.
56. Commonwealth Fund staff memorandum, April 20, 1949. CF Arch.
57. Ibid.
58. Commonwealth Fund staff memorandum, June 9, 1949. CF Arch.
59. Commonwealth Fund staff memorandum, October 5, 1949. CF Arch.
60. Ibid.
61. Commonwealth Fund staff memorandum, November 14, 1949. CF Arch.
62. GD, January 19, 1950.
63. Ibid.
64. Williams, *Western Reserve's Experiment*, chapter 35.
65. Wearn, J. T. Wandering thoughts and observations on medical education. Trans. Assoc. Am. Phys. 67: 1, 1954.
66. GD, January 19, 1950.
67. Williams, *Western Reserve's Experiment*, p. 332.
68. Commonwealth Fund staff memorandum, November 14, 1951. CF Arch.
69. Wearn, J. T. et al. The evolution of an experimental program of medical education at Western Reserve University. Proceedings of the Annual Congress of Medical Education Licensure. Chicago, February 8–10, 1953.
70. Williams, *Western Reserve's Experiment*, p. 335.
71. Dietrick, J. E. and Berson, R. C. *Medical Schools in the United States at Mid-Century*. New York: McGraw-Hill, 1953, pp. 323–24.
72. Merton, Reader and Kendall, *The Student Physician*, p. 35.
73. Commonwealth Fund staff memorandum, November 23, 1953. CF Arch.
74. Commonwealth Fund staff memorandum, May 25, 1954. CF Arch.
75. Horowitz, M. J. *Educating Tomorrow's Doctors*. New York: Appleton-Century Crofts, 1964; Horowitz, M. J.; Brozgal, J. L.; and Eaton, J. W. Observations of first-year students in preceptoral groups. J. Med. Educ. 33: 118, 1958.
76. Commonwealth Fund staff memorandum, May 25, 1954. CF Arch.
77. Williams, *Western Reserve's Experiment*, p. 340
78. Ibid.
79. Joseph T. Wearn, to Malcolm P. Aldrich, February 21, 1958.
80. Ham, T. H. The student as colleague: Medical education experience at Case Western Reserve. Ann Arbor, Mich.: University Microfilms, International, 1976.
81. Williams, *Western Reserve's Experiment*, chapter 35.
82. Lee, P. V. Medical schools and the changing times: Nine case reports on experimentation in medical education, 1950–1960. J. Med. Educ. 36: 45, Pt. 2, December 1961.
83. Ebert, R. H. Foreword. In: Williams, *Western Reserve's Experiment*.
84. Ibid.
85. The monies given were allocated as follows: teaching program, 1950–59, $1,125,920; construction and equipment, 1951–52, $276,428; evaluation studies

of curriculum, 1953–56, $88,200; capital grant, 1955, $1,000,000; division of research in medical education—program and project support, 1967–78, $610,396; health sciences library, 1963, $500,000.

86. GD, February 13, 1958, pp. 1–6; GD, February 8, 1962, pp. 10–16.

87. Handler, P. and Wyngaarden, J. B. The bio-medical research training program of Duke University. J. Med. Educ. 36: 1587, 1961.

88. GD, November 3, 1966, p. 125.

89. Memorandum: Duke University School of Medicine, site visit December 15, 1964. Notes by Roderick E. Heffron. CF Arch.

90. GD, February 25, 1965, p. 3.

91. Gifford, J. F., Jr., et al., eds. *Undergraduate Medical Education and the Elective System: Experience with the Duke Curriculum, 1966–1975*. Durham, N.C.: Duke University Press, 1978.

92. See also: Davison, W. C. Liberalizing the curriculum. South. Med. J. 21: 983, 1928; Davison, W. C. An M.D. degree five years after high school. J.A.M.A. 90: 1812, 1928; Davison, W. C. The Duke University School of Medicine. Trans. Med. Soc. State North Carolina 74: 35, 1927; Warren, C. O. Memorandum. Duke University School of Medicine, Durham, N.C., September 15, 1955. CF Arch; Philip Handler, to Lester J. Evans, December 26, 1957. CF Arch; James B. Wyngaarden, to Roderick E. Heffron, November 30, 1961. Letter and enclosures in CF Arch; Barnes Woodhall to Philip Handler, December 6, 1961. In: Philip Handler papers; Handler, P. A new curriculum in the Duke University School of Medicine. Undated. In: Philip Handler papers; C. G. Child III, to William G. Anylan, November 13, 1964. Copy in Thomas D. Kinney papers; Robert J. Glaser to J. Quigg Newton, Jr., September 23, 1964; L. T. Coggeshall to Roderick E. Heffron, October 2, 1964; W. B. Wood, Jr. to Roderick E. Heffron, September 30, 1964. CF Arch; Joseph T. Wearn to Roderick E. Heffron, October 17, 1964. CF Arch; Heffron, R. E. Memorandum, Duke University School of Medicine, December 15, 1964. CF Arch; Memorandum, Duke University Medical School, New Curriculum, February 25, 1965. CF Arch; Duke Medical School *Bulletin*, 1966, pp. 4–5.

93. Scoville, M. C. Memorandum, Some Thoughts on College Preprofessional and Professional Education. January 22, 1951, 4 pp., CF Arch.; GD, January 11, 1952, pp. 1–10.

94. GD, January 11, 1952, p. 3.

95. George P. Berry to Lester J. Evans, November 17, 1951. CF Arch.

96. George P. to Malcolm P. Aldrich, December 10, 1951. CF Arch.

97. Emanuel Suter to Charles O. Warren, July 7, 1953. CF Arch.

98. Karnovsky, M. L. A rearrangement of the curriculum in the preclinical years at Harvard. Harvard Medical Alumni Bulletin, April 1957, pp. 7–11.

99. Lee, P. V. Review of the Commonwealth Fund Experiments in Medical Education. Pt. 2, October 8, 1959. CF Arch.

100. Robert H. Ebert, interview with A. McGehee Harvey, April 29, 1982.

101. Asper, S. P. A revised program of medical education at Johns Hopkins. J. Med. Educ. 33: 225, 1958.

102. Keefer, C. S. The training of the physician: Experiment with the medical-school curriculum at Boston University. N. Engl. J. Med. 271: 401, 1964.

103. Cooper, J. A. D. and Prior, M. A. A new program in medical education at Northwestern University. J. Med. Educ. 36: 80, 1961.

104. Golmor, M. E.; Kessler, R. H.; and Eckenhoffer, J. E. *The Honors Program in Medical Education at Northwestern University (1961–1976): A Critical Review.* Chicago: Northwestern University Medical School, August 1977.

105. Lee, P. V. Report to the Commonwealth Fund on Experiments in Medical Education. CF Arch.

106. Soutter, L. et al. *A New Combined Liberal Arts—Medical Program of Medical Education. Report of a Joint Committee.* Boston: Boston University, 1959. See also GD, May 25, 1971, p. 24.

107. Blaustein, E. H. and Kayne, H. L. The accelerated medical program and the liberal arts at Boston University. J.A.M.A. 235: 2618, 1976; Lanzoni, V. and Kayne, H. L. A report on graduates of the Boston University six-year combined liberal-arts–medical program. J. Med. Educ. 51: 283, 1976; Blaustein, E. H. and Kayne, H. L. Boston University and accelerated medical education: The first five cohorts. J. Med. Educ. 55: 202, 1980; Culbert, A. J.; Blaustein, E. H.; and Sandson, J. I. Special report: The modular medical integrated medical curriculum. An innovation in medical education. N. Engl. J. Med. 306: 1502, 1982.

108. Kanter, G. S. The Rennsselaer Polytechnic Institute–Albany Medical College six-year biomedical program. J. Med. Educ. 44: 1139, 1969; GD, May 26, 1970, p. 3.

109. Stowe, L. M. The Stanford plan: An educational continuum for medicine. J. Med. Educ. 34: 1059, 1959.

110. Robert J. Glaser, personal communication to A. McGehee Harvey.

111. Robert J. Glaser to A. McGehee Harvey, August 14, 1984.

112. Chapman, C. B. On experiments in medical education. N. Engl. J. Med. 297: 1347, December 15, 1977. See also A combined liberal-arts and medical curriculum (editorial). N. Engl. J. Med. 261: 405, 1959; Berry, G. P. Medical education in transition. J. Med. Educ. 28: 17, March 1953; Blumberg, M. S. Accelerated programs of medical education. J. Med. Educ. 46: 643, 1971; Cooper, J. A. D. Major factors involved in reconstructing the medical curriculum. J.A.M.A. 170: 452, 1959; Darley, W. Studies and research in medical education, their timeliness and importance. J. Med. Educ. 34: 625, 1959; Petersen, E. S. Evolution of the comprehensive care concept in the medical school clinics. Q. Bull. Northwestern Univ. Med. School 33: 352, 1959; Scott, G. H.; Levitt, M.; and Gardner, E. D. Five years' experience with the 2–4–2 program at Wayne State University. J. Med. Educ. 40: 510, 1965; Thomas, L. Notes of a biology-watcher: How to fix the premedical curriculum. N. Engl. J. Med. 298: 1180, 1978; Wolf, G. A., Jr. Integration of the last year of college and the first year of medical school. J. Med. Educ. 32: 573, 1957; Young, R. H. Medical education in the United States. J. Med. Educ. 34: 802, 1959.

113. Poor, R. S. *Planning Florida's Health Leadership: A Summary.* In: Maloof, L. J., ed. Medical Center Study Series. Vol. 1. Gainesville: University of Florida Press, 1954; J. W. Reitz, president emeritus, University of Florida, personal communication to A. McGehee Harvey.

114. Poor, *Planning Florida's Health Leadership.*

115. J. W. Reitz, personal communication to A. McGehee Harvey.

116. Poor, *Planning Florida's Health Leadership.*
117. Ibid.
118. Ibid. See also MacLachlan, J. M. *Planning Florida's Health Leadership: Florida's Doctors at Mid-Century.* Medical Center Study Series. Vol. 2. Gainesville: University of Florida Press, 1954; *Health and the People in Florida.* Vol. 3, 1954, *Florida's Hospitals and Nurses.* Vol. 4, 1954; *Medical Education in the University.* Vol. 5, 1955.
119. Harrell, G. T., Jr. The university in medicine: Concept of the new program at the University of Florida. J.A.M.A. 161: 700, 1956.
120. George T. Harrell, Jr., interview with A. McGehee Harvey, April 18, 1983.
121. AR, 1971, p. 35.
122. AR, 1963, p. 6.
123. Office of the Dean, Mission Statement, John A. Burns School of Medicine, February 7, 1984.
124. GD, November 12, 1964, pp. 21–29.
125. AR, 1971, pp. 22–23.
126. Terence A. Rogers to A. McGehee Harvey, June 19, 1984.
127. Terence A. Rogers to A. McGehee Harvey, July 16, 1984.
128. AR, 1977, pp. 44–45.
129. Letter from John S. Wellington accompanying the report of the conference. Additional details of the founding of this school and its subsequent development may be found in: Bowers, J. Z. and Purcell, E. F., eds. *New Medical Schools at Home and Abroad: Report of a Macy Conference.* Josiah Macy, Jr., Foundation, 1978; Rogers, T. A. and Jones, G. B. The John A. Burns School of Medicine. Manoa: University of Hawaii, pp. 45–84; Conference on Curriculum, October 12–14, 1979, CF Arch; Report to the Senate of the 10th Legislative Regular Session of 1979, State of Hawaii, March 21, 1979, CF Arch; Chapman, C. D. et al. Medical Education at the University of Hawaii: A Report to the President of the University. CF Arch.
130. Terence A. Rogers to A. McGehee Harvey, July 16, 1984.
131. I. J. Schatz (chairman of the Department of Medicine) to Alvin R. Tarlov, May 4, 1984.
132. Terence A. Rogers to A. McGehee Harvey, June 19, 1984.
133. Lester J. Evans, personal communication to A. McGehee Harvey.
134. Summary of notes, personal files of Lester J. Evans, CF Arch.
135. Miller, G. E.: Bedside teaching for first-year students. J. Med. Educ. 29: 28, 1954; see also Miller, G. E. *Educating Medical Teachers.* New York: Commonwealth Fund (Cambridge: Harvard University Press), 1980.
136. Miller, G. E. Adventure in pedagogy. J.A.M.A. 162: 1448, 1956.
137. Summary of notes, personal files of Lester J. Evans, CF Arch.
138. Eberhart, J. C. Memorandum on site visit to Buffalo, March 1955. CF Arch.
139. Eberhart, J. C. Memorandum on site visit to Buffalo, April 1957. CF Arch.
140. Miller, *Educating Medical Teachers,* p. 60.
141. Becker, D. R. Cover letter, February 1961, Final Report to the Commonwealth Fund, CF Arch.

142. Miller, *Educating Medical Teachers,* p. 83.

143. Ibid., pp. 86-91.

144. Evans, L. J. Memorandum after site visit to University of Illinois, May 1958. CF Arch.

145. Proposal, University of Illinois College of Medicine, 1958. CF Arch.

146. Miller, *Educating Medical Teachers,* p. 133.

147. Berry, G. P. Preface. In: Gee, H. H. and Cowles, J. T., eds. *The Appraisal of Applicants to Medical School.* Evanston, Ill.: Association of American Medical Colleges, 1957.

148. Sanazaro, P. J. The placebo effect in medical education. J. Med. Educ. 35: 416, 1960.

149. Steiner, J. Educational research for decision-making. Proceedings of the Fourth Pan American Conference on Medical Education, multilith. University of Toronto, p. 23, 1973. In: Miller, *Educating Medical Teachers,* p. 205.

150. Miller, *Educating Medical Teachers,* p. 207.

151. Ibid., p. 210.

152. Ibid., p. 210-211.

153. GD, February 14, 1957, pp. 1-12.

154. AR, 1962, p. 2; GD, February 8, 1962, pp. 17-23.

155. Deuschle, K. W. and Fulmer, H. S. Community medicine. A "new" department at the University of Kentucky College of Medicine. J. Med. Educ. 37: 434, 1962.

156. Deuschle, K. W. and Wiggins, W. S. The use of nitrogen mustard in the management of two pregnant lymphoma patients. Blood 8: 576, 1953.

157. McDermott, W.; Deuschle, K. W.; and Barnett, C. R. Health care experiment at Many Farms. Science 175: 23, 1972; Deuschle, K. W. and Adair, J. An interdisciplinary approach to public health on the Navajo Indian Reservation. Medical and anthropological aspects. Ann. N.Y. Acad. Sci. 84: 887, 1960.

158. Willard, W. R. et al. Philosophy of medical education at the University of Kentucky, 1956. Mimeographed report, CF Arch.

159. Tapp, J. W.; Fulmer, H. S.; and Deuschle, K. W. Medical students in Appalachia: A training program in community medicine. Human Organization 25: 225, 1966; Deuschle, K. W. et al. The Kentucky experiment in community medicine. Milbank Memorial Fund Quarterly 44: 9, January 1966 (pt. 1); Deuschle, K. W. and Eberson, F. Community medicine comes of age. J. Med. Educ. 43: 1229, 1968.

160. Kurt W. Deuschle, interview with A. McGehee Harvey, April 1982.

161. Tapp, J. W., Jr. and Deuschle, K. W. The community medicine clerkship: A guide for teachers and students of community medicine. Milbank Memorial Fund Quarterly 47: 411, October 1969.

162. GD, November 12, 1964, pp. 13-20.

163. Burke, W. M. et al. An evaluation of the undergraduate medical curriculum: The Kentucky experiment in community medicine. J.A.M.A. 241: 2726, June 1979.

164. GD, February 19, 1970, pp. 3-7.

165. GD, May 17, 1973, pp. 19-22.

166. See also Bosch, S. J. and Deuschle, K. W. The role of a medical school in the organization of health-care services. Bull. N.Y. Acad. Med. (2nd series)

53: 449, 1977; Merins, R.; Rose, D. N.; and Bosch, S. W. A medical school's involvement in the development of a community-board health center. J. Comm. Health 8: 130, 1982; Bosch, S. J. and Fischer, E. The role and functions assumed by a department of community medicine in planning a group practice. Health Policy and Education 2: 167, 1981.

167. GD, November 21, 1974, pp. 8–13.

168. For additional information on Deuschle's programs see Deuschle, K. W. et al. The community medicine clerkship: A learner-centered program. J. Med. Educ. 47: 931, 1972; Bosch, S. J.; Fischer, E.; and Deuschle, K. W. A framework for participation: The contribution of a medical school to local health planning. Mt. Sinai J. Med. 46: 552, 1979; Deuschle, K. W. and Bosch, S. J. The community medicine–primary care connection. Israel J. Med. Sci. 17: 86, 1981; Deuschle, K. W. Urban health and academic medicine. The Merrimon Lecture, University of North Carolina School of Medicine at Chapel Hill, October 15, 1975; Deuschle, K. W. and Diaz, M. The shortfall in Hispanic health manpower: The national and Mount Sinai–East Harlem picture. Mt. Sinai J. Med. 48: 339, 1981; Deuschle, K. W. Community-oriented primary care: Lessons learned in three decades. In: Connor, E. and Mullan F., eds. Institute of Medicine Conference Proceedings. Washington, D. C.: National Academy Press, 1982, pp. 1–15.

169. Kurt W. Deuschle, interview with A. McGehee Harvey, April 1982.

170. Lee, P. V. Review of Commonwealth Fund Experiments in Medical Education. Pt. 2, October 8, 1959, pp. 41–46. CF Arch.

171. Lester J. Evans and Charles O. Warren, interview with Leon R. Lezer, October 31, 1958. (Notes by Warren.) CF Arch.

172. AR, 1956, p. 21.

173. AR, 1957, p. 9.

174. Leon R. Lezer to A. McGehee Harvey, July 24, 1984.

175. GD, November 10, 1971, p. 22; GD, May 13, 1976, p. 17.

176. Tufo, H. M. Project Report, The University of Vermont Given Health Care Center. March 9, 1979.

177. Ibid., p. 4.

178. Henry M. Tufo to A. McGehee Harvey, July 13, 1984.

179. In an address delivered at the convocation exercises of the University of Chicago on December 17, 1907, William Henry Welch said, "the historical and proper home of the medical school is the university of which it should be an integral part coordinate with the other faculties." (J.A.M.A. 50: 1, 1908.) Professor Everett Hughes had stressed that the education of the medical profession was only a part of medical education, which he defined as "the whole series of processes by which the medical culture is kept alive (which means more than merely imparted) through time and generations, and by which it is extended to new populations of elements of the population, and by which it is added to through new learning and experiment." (Proposal to Study Medical Education in the University of Kansas. Submitted to the Commonwealth Fund by Community Studies, Inc., Kansas City, Missouri.)

180. Thomas, L. *The Youngest Science*. New York: Viking, 1983, pp. 121–22.

181. Vernon W. Lippard, interview with A. McGehee Harvey, December 2, 1982.

182. Smith, G. and Evans, L. J. Preventive medicine: An attempt at a definition. Science 100: 39, July 21, 1944; Evans, L. J. The metamorphosis of preventive medicine. Presented before the Conference of Professors of Preventive Medicine, St. Louis, Missouri, October 30, 1950. Conference of Professors of Preventive Medicine Newsletter 2 (1): 31 March 1951.

183. Robert L. Berg, interview with A. McGehee Harvey, April 15, 1982.

184. A full account of the Hunterdon project was published in Trussel, R. E. *Hunterdon Medical Center: The Story of One Approach to Rural Medical Care.* New York: Commonwealth Fund (Cambridge: Harvard University Press), 1956. See also Wescott, L. B. The rise and fall of a medical Camelot. N. Engl. J. Med. 300: 952, April 26, 1979; Editorial, N. Engl. J. Med. 300: 977, 1979; Letters, N. Engl. J. Med. 301: 504, August 30, 1979; GD January 11, 1951, pp. 1–11; GD, October 11, 1951, pp. 17–21; GD, May 9, 1952, pp. 11–23.

185. Lester J. Evans, interview with A. McGehee Harvey, September 1982.

186. Trussell, *Hunterdon Medical Center,* pp. 17–18.

187. Evans L. J. Memorandum. CF Arch.

188. Aldrich, M. P. Recommendation B, in Report to the Board of Directors, January 5, 1950.

189. Trussell, *Hunterdon Medical Center,* p. 138.

190. Ibid., pp. 154–173.

191. Lloyd B. Wescott, letter to A. McGehee Harvey, June 5, 1984.

192. Pellegrino, E. D. Role of the community hospital in continuing education—The Hunterdon experiment. J.A.M.A. 164: 361, 1957.

193. McKinsey and Co.: Report of Hunterdon project. 1971. CF Arch.

194. Pellegrino, E. D. Two decades before its time. In: Curry, H. B., et al. *Twenty Years of Community Medicine: A Hunterdon Medical Center Symposium.* Columbia Publishing, Frenchtown, N.J.: 1974, p. 43.

195. Lloyd B. Wescott to A. McGehee Harvey, June 5, 1984.

196. GD, February 10, 1977, pp. 27–30.

197. Somers, A. R. Editorial. Hunterdon—"May it never be forgot." N. Engl. J. Med. 300: 977, 1979.

198. Edmund D. Pellegrino to A. McGehee Harvey, June 4, 1984.

199. GD, January 13, 1949.

200. Bluestone, E. M. Some fundamental problems in hospital administration. Modern Hospital 23: 514, 1924.

201. Bluestone, E. M. What is the place of the aged in the medical scheme? Modern Hospital 35: 61, 1930.

202. Bluestone, E. M. The place of the long-term patient in the modern hospital. Bull. Am. Coll. Surg. 31: 104, 1946.

203. Bluestone, E. M. Health services. Jewish Social Service Quarterly 24, September 1947.

204. Montefiore Medical Center: Home Care and Extended Services Department: Program Evaluation and Annual Report, 1982. Submitted by Marilyn P. Rahmond, director, Home Care and Extended Services Department.

205. Liberal use has been made of an article by Dorothy Levenson, The origins of the department of social medicine at Montefiore: Montefiore medicine, which appeared in Montefiore Medicine on the department's thirtieth anniversary, and

of her book *Montefiore: The Hospital as Social Instrument* (New York: Farrar, Straus and Giroux, 1984).

206. Cherkasky, M. The Montefiore Hospital home care program. Am. J. Publ. Health 39: 163, 1949.

207. Levenson, D. The origins of the department of social medicine at Montefiore.

208. Baehr, G. The Peckham experiment. Milbank Memorial Fund Quarterly 22: 352, 1944.

209. Bluestone, E. M. Social medicine arrives in the hospital. Modern Hospital 75: 59, August 1950.

210. Silver, G. A. and Kissick, W. A social medicine residency program. J. Med. Educ. 37: 1217, 1962.

211. Ibid.

212. Levenson, D. The origins of the department of social medicine at Montefiore.

213. Consultants included former president Herbert C. Hoover; Irving Olds; John S. Dickey, president, Dartmouth College; Harold W. Dodds, president, Princeton University; John S. Millis, president, Western Reserve University; and Lee A. DuBridge, president, the California Institute of Technology.

214. Review of four Commonwealth Fund Mental Health Projects by Iago Galdston. January 8, 1959, 20 pp.; GD, November 20, 1952, pp. 16–22. See also Massie, W. A. *Medical Services for Rural Areas: The Tennessee Medical Foundation.* New York: Commonwealth Fund (Cambridge: Harvard University Press), 1957.

215. After Aldrich's retirement, the Commonwealth Fund endowed a research chair in ophthalmology at Columbia University in his name. He received a citation from the American Medical Association for Distinguished Service, as well as honorary degrees from Southern Massachusetts University and Boston University.

8. The University and the Community

1. Newton's career included membership in the National Advisory Mental Health Council (1964–68) and in the Institute of Medicine, National Academy of Sciences (1972–present). He is a fellow of the American Academy of Arts and Sciences and holds honorary degrees from the University of Denver, Adams State College, Colorado College, and the University of Colorado.

2. The other members of the board were Roger M. Blough, chairman of the board, United States Steel Corporation; George P. Berry, dean, the Harvard Medical School; Fredrick M. Eaton, partner in the law firm of Shearman and Sterling; John A. Gifford, partner in the law firm of White and Case; William H. Moore, chairman of the board, Bankers Trust Company; Hulbert S. Aldrich (Malcolm's brother); and Leo D. Welch. Joining the board in 1963 was Calvin H. Plimpton, who had been professor of medicine at the American University in Beirut and was later president of Amherst College.

3. Participants were (in addition to Newton and Glaser): H. Stanley Bennett,

dean, Division of Biological Sciences, the University of Chicago School of Medicine; Francis S. Cheever, dean, University of Pittsburgh School of Medicine; Julius B. Richmond, chairman, Department of Pediatrics, State University of New York Upstate Medical Center; W. Barry Wood, Jr., chairman, Department of Microbiology, the Johns Hopkins University School of Medicine; and Joseph T. Wearn, consultant for medical affairs, Western Reserve University. The extensive notes taken at this meeting are in the Commonwealth Fund Archives.

4. Interviews with John A. Gifford (September 10, 1964), Fredrick M. Eaton (July 11, 1964), and Leo D. Welch (September 24, 1964). CF Arch.

5. Among those interviewed were: Kerr L. White, University of Vermont College of Medicine (September 21, 1964); Victor R. Fuchs, National Bureau of Economic Research (July 23, 1964); Milton Singer, pediatrician, voluntary staff, Columbia–Presbyterian Hospital (July 1966); Charles P. Noyes, former member of the Rockefeller Foundation staff (June 30, 1964); Robert F. Loeb, professor of medicine, the Columbia University College of Physicians and Surgeons (December 17, 1963); Robert K. Merton, professor of sociology, Columbia University (July 9, 1964); Robert S. Morison, director of medical and natural sciences, the Rockefeller Foundation (July 17, 1964); Eleanor B. Sheldon, Russell Sage Foundation (July 6, 1964); George G. Reader, professor of medicine, the Cornell University Medical College (July 7, 1964); W. Homer Turner, vice-president and executive director, United States Steel Foundation (July 21, 1964); and Gordon McLachlan, the American Hospital Association (January 15, 1965). CF Arch.

6. Newton, J. Q., Jr. Position paper, November 12, 1964. CF Arch.

7. Starr, P. *The Social Transformation of American Medicine*. New York: Basic Books, 1982, p. 381.

8. Report of a press conference, *New York Times*, July 11, 1969. Cited in Starr, *The Social Transformation of American Medicine*, p. 381.

9. It's time to operate. Fortune 81: 79, January 1970. Cited in Starr, *The Social Transformation of American Medicine*, p. 381.

10. GD, February 13, 1964, p. 11; GD, November 14, 1963, p. 7; GD, November 12, 1964, p. 49.

11. AR, 1967, p. 19; GD, May 11, 1967, pp. 3–13.

12. AR, 1942, p. 23; AR, 1944, p. 32; AR, 1945, pp. 27, 29; AR, 1947, p. 27; AR, 1924, p. 48; AR, 1926, pp. 69–70; AR, 1928, p. 47; AR, 1936, p. 35; AR, 1931, p. 8; AR, 1938, pp. 30–31.

13. AR, 1937, p. 31.

14. GD, June 16, 1949, p. 73; AR, 1950, p. 24.

15. GD, January 11, 1951, p. 31.

16. GD, January 11, 1951, p. 32.

17. GD, January 11, 1951, pp. 31–34.

18. GD, November 20, 1952, pp. 64–65.

19. GD, February 25, 1954, pp. 43–44.

20. GD, February 10, 1955, pp. 52–53.

21. GD, November 13, 1958, p. 55.

22. GD, May 13, 1954, pp. 34–36.

23. GD, May 13, 1954, p. 44.

24. GD, November 17, 1955, p. 83.

25. GD, May 16, 1957, pp. 90-91; GD, May 21, 1959, pp. 58-60; AR, 1964, p. 43.

26. GD, May 12, 1966, p. 3.

27. Fine, L. L. and Silver, H. K. Comparative diagnostic abilities of child health associate interns and practicing pediatricians. J. Pediatr. 83: 332, 1973; Silver, H. K.; Ford, L. C.; and Day, L. R. The pediatric nurse-practitioner program: Expanding the role of a nurse to provide increased health care for children. J.A.M.A. 204: 298, 1968; Day, L. R.; Egli, R.; and Silver, H. K. Acceptance of pediatric nurse practitioners: Parents' opinion of combined care by pediatrician and a pediatric nurse practitioner in a private practice. Am. J. Dis. Child. 119: 204, 1970; McAtee, P. R. and Silver, H. K. Nurse practitioners for children—Past and future. Pediatrics 54: 578, 1974.

28. Loretta C. Ford, R. N., Ed. D., left Colorado to become dean and director of nursing at the University of Rochester Medical Center. Ford is now one of the country's ranking leaders in academic nursing.

29. Silver, H. K. New health professionals for primary ambulatory care. Hosp. Pract. 9: 91, April 1974. McAtee, P. R. and Silver, H. K. What about a national nurse-practitioner program? RN 38: 22, December 1975; Silver, H. K. and Duncan, B. Time motion study of pediatric nurse practitioners: Comparison with regular office nurses and pediatricians. J. Pediatr. 44: 62, 1969; Schiff, D. W.; Fraser, C. H.; and Walters, H. L. The pediatric nurse practitioner in the office of pediatricians in private practice. Pediatrics 44: 62, 1969.

30. GD, November 14, 1968, p. 13.

31. Silver, H. K. New allied health professionals: Implications of the Colorado child health associate law. N. Engl. J. Med. 284: 304, 1971.

32. Silver, H. K. and Hecker, J. A. The pediatric nurse practitioner and the child health associate: New types of health professionals. J. Med. Educ. 45: 171, 1970; Machotka, P. et al. Competence of child health associates. I. Comparison of their basic science and clinical knowledge with that of medical students and pediatric residents. Am. J. Dis. Child. 125: 199, 1973; Silver, H. K. and Ott, J. E. The child health associate: A new health professional to provide comprehensive health care to children. Pediatrics 55: 1, 1973.

33. GD, May 26, 1970, p. 30.

34. AR, 1970, p. 31.

35. Silver, H. K. and McAtee, P. R. Summary Report to the Commonwealth Fund on the Pediatric Nurse Practitioner and School Nurse Practitioner Programs. February 14, 1977, 13 pp. CF Arch.

36. Silver, H. K. and McAtee, P. R. Summary Report to the Commonwealth Fund on the Pediatric Nurse Practitioner and School Nurse Practitioner Programs. February 14, 1977. CF Arch; Silver, H. K.; Igoe, J. B.; and McAtee, P. R. Draft, The school nurse practitioner: Providing improved health care to children; Silver, H. K.; Igoe, J. B.; and McAtee, P. R. The school nurse practitioner: Providing improved health care to children. Pediatrics 58: 580, 1976; McAtee, P. R. Nurse practitioners in our public schools? An assessment of their expanded role. Clin. Pediatr. 13: 360, 1974; Silver, H. K. The school nurse practitioner program: A new and expanded role for the school nurse. J.A.M.A. 216: 1332, 1971.

37. GD, February 19, 1970, p. 21.

38. Estes, E. H., Jr., and Howard, R. D. Potential for newer classes of personnel: Experiences of the Duke physician's assistant program. J. Med. Educ. 45: 149, 1970; AR, 1970, p. 35.

39. Sadler, A. M., Jr.; Sadler, B. L.; and Bliss, A. A. *The Physician's Assistant—Today and Tomorrow.* 2nd ed. Cambridge, Mass.: Ballinger Publishing, 1975, pp. 1–2.

40. Reisz, W. G.; Cawley, J. F.; and Barry, W. S. The current status of physician assistants. Md. State Med. J. 33: 288, 1984.

41. GD, May 11, 1972, p. 14.

42. Report of the Committee on Sex Education in Medicine. Cited in AR, 1975, p. 73.

43. Lief, H. I. and Ebert, R. K. A survey of sex education in U.S. medical schools. CF Arch. (Paper presented at meeting, Education and Treatment in Human Sexuality. The training of Health Professionals. Geneva, February 6–12, 1974; Summary of Accomplishments of the Center for the Study of Sex Education in Medicine: 1968–1974. 9 pp. CF Arch.)

44. AR, 1974, p. 79, p. 84; AR, 1975, pp. 65–74; GD, November 21, 1974, p. 70; GD, November 9, 1972, pp. 37, 52.

45. GD, May 12, 1966, p. 11.

46. Victor R. Fuchs to J. Quigg Newton, Jr., May 21, 1969. CF Arch.

47. Victor R. Fuchs to J. Quigg Newton, Jr., December 21, 1977. CF Arch.

48. MacLeod, C. M. Notes for board of directors' meeting, May 11, 1967. CF Arch.

49. Terrance Keenan, interview with A. McGehee Harvey, May 28, 1982.

50. GD, November 9, 1967, p. 93; AR, 1968, p. 26.

51. AR, 1962, p. 33.

52. GD, May 26, 1969, p. 69.

53. GD, May 26, 1970, p. 9.

54. AR, 1970, p. 44; AR, 1971, p. 39; GD, May 11, 1972, p. 28.

55. GD, May 17, 1973, p. 34.

56. GD, May 9, 1974, p. 37.

57. Information for prospective participants in the Fellowship Program in Academic Medicine for Minority Students, November and December 1983. CF Arch.

58. Sullivan, L. W. The status of blacks in medicine. Philosophical and ethical dilemmas for the 1980s. N. Engl. J. Med. 309(13): 807, 1983.

59. GD, November 9, 1967, p. 14.

60. Lloyd C. Elam to Reginald H. Fitz, October 9, 1974. CF Arch.

61. GD, February 13, 1969, p. 3.

62. London, I. M. The university, the community and the nation's health. J. Med. Educ. 46: 18, 1971.

63. GD, November 10, 1971, p. 28.

64. J. Quigg Newton to Irving M. London, November 12, 1971.

65. J. Quigg Newton to Hulbert S. Aldrich, chairman of the board of directors, the Commonwealth Fund, February 3, 1976.

66. Irving M. London, interview with A. McGehee Harvey, March 1982.

67. Margaret E. Mahoney, interview with A. McGehee Harvey, June 1, 1982.

68. Material about the Commonwealth Fund's collaboration with the Carnegie

Corporation is based on A. McGehee Harvey's interview with Margaret E. Mahoney, June 1, 1982.

69. The Endicott conference resulted in a monograph, *Medical Education Revisited,* and the Swampscott Study was discussed in Cope's book *Man, Mind and Medicine. The Doctor's Education.* Philadelphia: J. B. Lippincott, 1968, 144 pp.

70. GD, February 10, 1966, p. 23.

71. GD, February 7, 1967, p. 3.

72. Ibid., pp. 3–17.

73. Ibid.

74. Ibid.

75. GD, February 19, 1970, p. 15.

76. Robert H. Ebert, interview with A. McGehee Harvey, April 29, 1982; Robert H. Ebert, to A. McGehee Harvey, May 9, 1983.

77. Yale Trauma Program. A Proposal to the Commonwealth Fund, 1969. CF Arch.

78. Yale Trauma Program, First Progress Report (1969–71); Second Progress Report (1971–73). CF Arch.

79. Robson, M. G. Third Progress Report of the Yale Trauma Program. June, 1974, p. 1. CF Arch.

80. Press release from Thomas J. Meskill, Governor of Connecticut, February 25, 1972.

81. A complete summary of this report appears in the Second Progress Report of the Yale study. Also included in the Second Progress Report is a complete draft of the proposed legislation. CF Arch.

82. Co-principal investigators were William Frazier, Paul Lally, and Joseph F. Cannon.

83. Terrance Keenan (vice-president for special programs, the Robert Wood Johnson Foundation), to A. McGehee Harvey, December 22, 1982. Keenan was executive secretary of the Commonwealth Fund at the time of the grant to the Yale Trauma Project.

84. For a full report of the project, see Regional Emergency Communications Systems. Final Report of the Committee on Regional Emergency Medical Communications Systems. Assembly of Life Sciences, National Academy of Sciences, Washington, D.C. 1978.

85. This project is fully described in the Third Progress Report of the Yale Trauma Program (June 1974).

86. Baker, C. C. et al. The impact of a trauma service on trauma care in a university hospital. Presented at the meeting of the New England Surgical Society, October 1984.

87. Christopher C. Baker, to A. McGehee Harvey, August 31, 1984.

88. Ibid.

89. AR, 1968, p. 1.

90. AR, 1968, pp. 1–2.

91. AR, 1968, pp. 2–3.

92. Two years later, MacLeod accepted an assignment to review the work of the SEATO Cholera Laboratory in Bangladesh for the United States Public Health Service. He died suddenly en route to this assignment, in 1972.

93. Glaser's professional affiliations were numerous: fellow of the American Academy of Arts and Sciences; member of the American Clinical and Climatological Association, the American Society for Clinical Investigation, the Association of American Physicians, and the Institute of Medicine of the National Academy of Sciences; assistant secretary of the Association of American Medical Colleges from 1956 to 1959 (chairman of the Committee on Education and Research from 1958 to 1962, member of the Executive Council from 1959 to 1962, and chairman of the Executive Council and Assembly from 1968 to 1969).

94. Walter Donway was twenty-seven years old when he joined the Fund's staff as Keenan's assistant. Born and educated in the public schools of Worcester, Massachusetts, he attended Brown University from 1962 to 1966, where his major interests were in creative writing, history, and philosophy. After graduation with honors, he spent two and one-half years studying philosophy in the graduate school of Boston University. Deciding that creative writing was his principal interest, Donway joined the staff of the *Worcester Telegraph* as a general reporter, later reporting on business and finance. From there he returned to Brown, where he worked in the development office preparing grant proposals to foundations. Although he had no medical background, Donway knew how medical institutions operated. Keenan was interested at this time in a staff member who could help disseminate information about the Fund, and Donway's responsibilities included preparing press releases on all major grants—a practice that was later discontinued. (Walter Donway, interview with A. McGehee Harvey, December 8, 1982.)

95. Walter Donway, interview with A. McGehee Harvey, December 8, 1982.

96. GD, April 14, 1971.

97. GD, November 12, 1970, p. 15.

98. GD, November 12, 1970, p. 10.

99. GD, November 12, 1970, p. 34.

100. Somers, A. R., ed. The Kaiser–Permanente Medical Care Program. One Valid Solution to the Problem of Health Care Delivery in the United States. Proceedings of a Symposium. New York: Commonwealth Fund, 1971, 238 pp.

101. GD, February 24, 1971, p. 3.

102. C. Henry Kempe, to A. McGehee Harvey, December 29, 1982.

103. GD, February 24, 1971, p. 3.

104. Suter, E. Book review, *Recent Trends in Medical Education.* J. Med. Educ. 52: 950, 1977.

105. GD, November 12, 1970, p. 3.

106. August G. Swanson to A. McGehee Harvey, November 11, 1982; M. R. Schwarz to A. McGehee Harvey, January 25, 1983.

107. The names of all those who contributed to the success of the WAMI program are too numerous to mention. Schwarz has emphasized the following: as WAMI coordinator for each state, Wayne W. Myers and Richard Lyons at the University of Alaska were highly influential, as was Guy R. Anderson at the University of Idaho. Frank Newman and Marshall Cook at Montana State University and Ron Atkins at Washington State University were also, in his opinion, true pathfinders. Among the central support staff at WAMI at the University of Washington were Roger Bennett, who dealt with finances; Charles Thomas Cullen, who performed the evaluation of the program; Marion Johnson, who

prepared the learning resources, the public relations, and the satellite program; Robert Davidson, who covered continuing medical education; and John Boor, who handled the satellite and technical aspects of the program. In addition, Gary Stricker and John Loeser supervised the curriculum development, and Ben Belkamp and Werner Samson, the admission. Dean Robert L. Van Citters provided vital support and encouragement. Governors who endorsed the program included Daniel J. Evans of Washington, Cecil Andrews of Idaho. Thomas Judge of Montana, and Richard Egan of Alaska. Among the university presidents who provided encouragement were Charles E. Odegaard of the University of Washington, Glenn Terrill of Washington State University, William Wood of the University of Alaska, Carl McIntosh of Montana State University, and Ernest Hartung of the University of Idaho. In addition, there were innumerable physicians, both in the practicing community and on the faculty at the University of Washington, who played influential roles. (M. R. Schwarz to A. McGehee Harvey, January 25, 1983.)

108. Schwarz, M. R. The WAMI program: A progress report. West. J. Med. 130: 384, April 1979.

109. See also AR, 1971, p. 5; Carline, J. D. et al. Career preferences of first and second year medical students: The WAMI experience. J. Med. Educ. 55: 682, 1980; Swanson, A. G. WAMI: A proposal for the regionalization of medical education in the Pacific northwest. Undated. CF Arch; Schwarz, M. R. WAMI— An experiment in regional medical education. West. J. Med. 121: 333, 1974.

110. Kingman E. Brewster, to J. Quigg Newton, Jr., June 27, 1966; Draft, Statement of Goals and Objectives of the Yale–New Haven Medical Center, dated March 14, 1969. CF Arch; Report on the Reappraisal of Yale University's Medical Programs during 1966–69, supported by a grant from the Commonwealth Fund, dated February 12, 1969, 20 pp. CF Arch.

111. Leon E. Rosenberg, interview with A. McGehee Harvey, December 3, 1982.

112. GD, May 8, 1975.

113. Leon E. Rosenberg, interview with A. McGehee Harvey, December 3, 1982.

114. GD, November 10, 1971, p. 9.

115. Russell J. Barrnett to A. McGehee Harvey, December 2, 1982.

116. The group included Russell J. Barrnett, Lubert Stryer (professor of molecular biophysics and biochemistry), and Gerhart Geibisch (chairman of the Department of Physiology).

117. GD, February 14, 1974, p. 52.

118. Evans, L. E. Memorandum, The Ambulant Patient as a Focal Point for the Re-Orientation of Medical Education. June 8, 1950. 14 pp. CF Arch.

119. GD, May 11, 1972, p. 3; AR, 1972, p. 11.

120. GD, November 21, 1974, p. 27.

121. Thomas L. Delbanco to A. McGehee Harvey, August 29, 1984. For further information about BIAC, see Delbanco, T. L. and Parker, J. N. Primary care at a teaching hospital: History, problems, and prospects. Mt. Sinai Med. J. 45: 628, 1978; Berarducci, A. A.; Delbanco, T. L.; and Rabkin, M. T. The teaching hospital and primary care: Closing down the clinics. N. Engl. J. Med. 292: 615, 1975; Goodson, J. D., ed. *Primary Care at Harvard: Practice and*

Postgraduate Training. Boston: Harvard Medical School, 1984; Winsten, M. S.; Makadon, H. J.; and Delbanco, T. L. Financing a hospital-sponsored general medical practice: The Beth Israel Ambulatory-Care Program. In: Altman, S.; Lion, J.; and Williams, J., eds. *Ambulatory Care: Problems of Costs and Access.* Lexington, Mass.: Lexington Books, 1983, pp. 111–121; Lawrence, R. S. Evolution: A decade of primary care. Harvard Medical Alumni Bulletin 58: 18, 1984; *Wellbeing at the Beth Israel Hospital.* Boston: Beth Israel Public Relations, October 1980.

122. GD, February 8, 1973, p. 82.

123. Wald, H. J. A hospice for terminally ill patients. Unpublished master's thesis. Columbia University School of Architecture, May 21, 1971.

124. GD, February 13, 1975, p. 3; AR, 1975, p. 42.

125. Lack, S. A. and Buckingham, R. N. III. *The First American Hospice: Three Years of Home Care.* New Haven: Hospice, Inc., 1978.

126. Morris A. Wessel, interview with A. McGehee Harvey, December 1, 1982; Wessel, M. A. To comfort always. Yale Alumni Magazine, June 1975, p. 17; AR, 1973, p. 108.

127. Florence S. Wald to A. McGehee Harvey, March 8, 1983. See also Wald, F. S. A Nurse's Study of Care for Dying Patients. U.S.P.H.S. Grant NU 00352, Principal Investigator, 10/1/69–9/30/71; Wald, F. S. An Interdisciplinary Study of Care for Dying Patients and Their Families. ANF Grant #2–70–023, Principal Investigator, 2/1/70–1/31/71; Wald, F. S. Patients with Terminal Illness: A Nurse's Diary (book in progress). Grant-in-Aid, The Commonwealth Book Fund, 1979–1981.

128. GD, May 25, 1971, p. 3.

129. Ibid., p. 7.

130. Ibid.

131. AR, 1971, p. 44.

132. Renewal application to the Commonwealth Fund, Studies of Stress and Conflict, June 1973, p. 8. CF Arch.

133. Ibid., pp. 4–15.

134. Ibid., p. 17.

135. Ibid., p. 18.

136. Ibid.

137. Ibid., p. 20.

138. Chapman, C. B. Memorandum. August 27, 1973. CF Arch.

139. Ibid.

140. GD, November 8, 1973, pp. 19–24.

141. AR, 1974, p. 74.

142. Report to the Commonwealth Fund from the Stanford Laboratory of Stress and Conflict, 1977, p. 4.

143. Ibid., pp. 4–8.

144. Hamburg, D. A., to Reginald H. Fitz, October 15, 1975. CF Arch. See also Newsweek, June 21, 1975.

145. H. C. Kraemer (associate professor, co-investigator of the Laboratory for Stress and Conflict) to the Commonwealth Fund, November 30, 1976. CF Arch.

146. Memorandum, site visit to the Laboratory of Stress and Conflict, Stanford

University, by Reginald H. Fitz and Walter Donway, November 10–11, 1976 (notes by Fitz), p. 6. CF Arch.

147. Ibid.

148. J. Quigg Newton, Jr. to Jane van L. Goodall and David A. Hamburg, November 15, 1974. CF Arch.

149. Memorandum, site visit to the Laboratory of Stress and Conflict, Stanford University, by Reginald H. Fitz and Walter Donway, November 10–11, 1976 (notes by Fitz).

150. David A. Hamburg to A. McGehee Harvey, April 10, 1984.

151. AR, 1971, p. 40.

152. Don K. Price to Reginald H. Fitz, November 12, 1974. CF Arch.

153. Ibid.

154. Earl P. Steinberg to A. McGehee Harvey, December 19, 1984.

155. Ibid.

156. GD, September 14, 1973.

157. Ibid.

158. GD, February 8, 1973, p. 14.

159. GD, February 10, 1977, p. 15.

160. GD, February 14, 1974, p. 11.

161. Hiatt, H. A. Report to the Commonwealth Fund, September 1975. CF Arch.

162. Center for the Analysis of Health Practices. Report to the Commonwealth Fund, January 20, 1976. CF Arch.

163. Center for the Analysis of Health Practices: Report to the Commonwealth Fund, January 1977. CF Arch.

164. Proposal for a Joint Venture: Research Department, Harvard Community Health Plan and the Center for the Analysis of Health Practices, June 1, 1983. CF Arch.

165. AR, 1980, p. 35.

166. Drew, L. W. Harvard doctors on the fiscal frontier. Harvard Medical Alumni Bulletin 58: 10, Spring 1984.

167. McNeil, B. J. and Komaroff, A. L. Annual Report: Center for Cost-Effective Care. Brigham and Women's Hospital. October 1982–October 1983. CF Arch.

168. Ibid.

169. John G. Simon to Carleton B. Chapman, December 12, 1979.

170. Margaret E. Mahoney, interview with A. McGehee Harvey, June 1, 1983.

171. GD, May 15, 1953; AR, 1962, p. 34; GD, February 25, 1965, p. 49; GD, November 9, 1967, p. 98; GD, May 11, 1972, p. 91.

172. GD, May 21, 1959, p. 64.

173. For a complete list of the topics and speakers as well as the list of distinguished participants, see GD, November 10, 1965.

174. GD, May 11, 1967, p. 100.

175. The advisory committee included such educational leaders as Eugene A. Stead, professor of medicine, Duke University; and Robert J. Glaser, then dean of the Stanford University School of Medicine.

176. See Cope, O. *Man, Mind and Medicine: The Doctor's Education.* Philadelphia: J. B. Lippincott, 1968, 144 pp.

177. R. C. Reynolds to A. McGehee Harvey, June 15, 1983.

178. J. Quigg Newton, Jr., interview with A. McGehee Harvey, February 11, 1982.

9. Integrating Medical Education into the University

1. Chapman, C. B. Review of J. Quigg Newton, Jr.'s April 1971 report to the board of directors of the Commonwealth Fund. June 1974; Chapman, C.B. to the board of directors, July 3, 1974. CF Arch.

2. Carleton B. Chapman, interview with A. McGehee Harvey, December 10, 1982.

3. Ibid.

4. Kennan, E. T. The curriculum period. In: *Disorders in Higher Education.* Englewood Cliffs, N.J.: Prentice-Hall, 1979, pp. 166–181.

5. Chapman, C.B. The Flexner report. Daedalus 103: 105, Winter 1974.

6. Carleton B. Chapman, interview with A. McGehee Harvey, November 7, 1983.

7. Huxley, T. Address at the Johns Hopkins University, September 12, 1876.

8. Survey of Educational Experiments, 1974. CF Arch.

9. Simpson, M. A. A mythology of medical education. Lancet 1: 399, March 9, 1974.

10. Notes on board of directors' meeting, February 13, 1975. CF Arch.

11. AR, 1975, p. 1.

12. The Fund issued a formal statement explaining the Interface Program in June 1976. CF Arch.

13. AR, 1976, p. 12.

14. Irving Spar, interview with A. McGehee Harvey, April 15, 1982.

15. Ibid.

16. GD, May 8, 1980; Neimi, R. and Phillips, J. E. Interim Report of the Evaluation Committee on Phase 1 of the Rochester Plan, June 29, 1979, p. 35. CF Arch.

17. GD, May 8, 1980, p. 6.

18. Irving Spar, interview with A. McGehee Harvey, April 15, 1982.

19. Ibid.

20. Final Report of Rochester Plan, February 8, 1982. CF Arch.

21. GD, May 13, 1976, p. 25; AR, 1976, p. 19.

22. AR, 1979, p. 14.

23. Consultants included Paul R. Gross, president and director, the Marine Biological Laboratory and former dean of graduate studies, the University of Rochester; and James V. Warren, professor of medicine, the Ohio State University School of Medicine.

24. GD, November 18, 1976.

25. Consultants were Gordon Meiklejohn, professor and former chairman, Department of Medicine, the University of Colorado School of Medicine; Paul

R. Gross, professor of biology and dean of the graduate school, the University of Rochester; and Mack Lipkin, professor of psychiatry (medicine) and family practice, University of Oregon Medical School, and a part-time consultant to the Fund.

26. GD, February 14, 1980. Consultants included Paul R. Gross, Mack Lipkin, and James V. Warren.

27. GD, February 10, 1977, p. 3.

28. L.T. Bowles (director, Division of Curriculum and Instruction, Association of American Medical Colleges) to Carleton B. Chapman, April 26, 1973:

> There are currently nine medical schools which accept high school graduates into six year programs which combine baccalaureate and medical education. These schools are as follows:
> 1. Northwestern University
> 2. University of Michigan
> 3. Albany Medical College
> 4. Boston University
> 5. Jefferson Medical College
> 6. Hahnemann Medical College
> 7. Medical College of South Carolina
> 8. Louisiana State University–Shreveport
> 9. University of Missouri–Kansas City
>
> In addition to the above, Brown University has expanded to a degree-granting school and has some experience providing the first two years of medical school in its graduate school of human biology.
>
> Florida State University in Tallahassee provides the first two years of medical school for students accepted into their medical program. These students transfer to Gainesville as third-year students when they complete their studies in Tallahassee.
>
> The University of Illinois utilizes two basic science campuses, one in Champaign–Urbana and the other in Chicago to provide the first year of basic medical science for medical students through the university's graduate departments. Students then transfer to one of three clinical campuses basd in Rockford, Peoria and Chicago.
>
> The University of Indiana uses six campuses for first-year medical students in addition to the main campus in Indianapolis. The graduate school on each campus is responsible for implementing the first basic science year curriculum, and all students then move to Indianapolis for their second year and the remainder of their training.
>
> One other school that might fall into your sphere of interest is Virginia Commonwealth University, which is now parent to the Medical College of Virginia [MCV]. Basic science teaching for MCV students is conducted by the graduate school of the parent university and basic science faculty are responsible to the graduate school dean, not the medical school dean.

29. Special Report: The modular medical integrated curriculum. N. Engl. J. Med. 306: 1502, June 17, 1982.

30. Consultants were Mack Lipkin; Lee D. Peachey, Ph.D., University of Pennsylvania School of Medicine; Peter A. Stewart, M.D., Division of Biological and Medical Sciences, Brown University; and James V. Warren.

31. AR, 1979, p. 17; Pozen, J. T.; Meyers, A. R.; and Scharf, K. Boston University MMEDIC Program, Phase I, Final Evaluation Report, September 1980; Annual Report, Modular Medical Integrated Curriculum, Boston University, July 1, 1981–June 30, 1982. CF Arch. Consultants were Paul R. Gross; Mack Lipkin (by then senior medical consultant to the Fund); and James V. Warren.

32. GD, May 12, 1977.

33. Ibid., p. 10.

34. Ibid, p. 8.

35. Executive Summary, The Program in Liberal Medical Education, Brown University, October 19, 1983. CF Arch.

36. Ibid.; Annual Progress Report to the Commonwealth Fund for the Academic Year 1980–81 from the Interface Program, Brown University; Annual Progress Reports, 1981–82, 1982–83. CF Arch.

37. GD, May 12, 1977, p. 15.

38. Ibid., p. 17.

39. Ibid., p. 20.

40. AR, 1980, p. 24. Consultants included Paul R. Gross and James V. Warren.

41. GD, February 12, 1980, p. 17; GD, February 12, 1980, p. 22.

42. Progress Report, The Interface Program at Dartmouth, July 15, 1982. CF Arch.

43. Ibid.

44. AR, 1978, p. 18; Johns Hopkins Gazette, March 16, 1978; Application to the Commonwealth Fund for Continued Support of Human Biology Program, Johns Hopkins University, December 16, 1980. CF Arch.; GD, May 1978; Progress Report, Human Biology Program, Johns Hopkins University, 1980. CF Arch.

45. AR, 1978, p. 18.

46. Report of the Joint Committee on Human Biology and Medicine, July 1973. See AR, 1978, p. 19. Complete report available in Alan M. Chesney Medical Archives, the Johns Hopkins Medical Institutions.

47. Report of the Biological Sciences Task Force, November 1976. See AR, 1979, p. 20. Complete report available in Alan M. Chesney Medical Archives, the Johns Hopkins Medical Institutions.

48. AR, 1978, p. 30; GD, February 14, 1974, p. 16. See also AR, 1974, p. 14; Gellhorn, A. and Scheuer, R. The experiment in medical education at the City College of New York. J. Med. Educ. 53: 574, 1978.

49. AR, 1978, p. 33.

50. AR, 1978, p. 34.

51. AR, 1980, p. 30.

52. Report: Education for Medicine, A Program of the Commonwealth Fund, June 1976. CF Arch.

53. Ibid.

54. Ibid.

55. Premedical-Preclinical Interface Program, Final Recommendations of the Ebert Committee. CF Arch.

56. Margaret E. Mahoney, letter, September 29, 1980.

57. The two consultants on the evaluation committee were Paul R. Gross and James V. Warren. Reginald H. Fitz, the Fund's vice-president, and Walter Donway, the Fund's executive associate, acted as the committee's staff.

58. A condensed version of Alfred Gellhorn's report appeared in AR, 1980, p. 13.

59. Gellhorn, A. An Evaluative Report of the Interface Programs Supported by the Commonwealth Fund. April 1980, 70 pp. CF Arch.

60. Ibid.

61. This section is based mainly on A. McGehee Harvey's interview with Carleton B. Chapman on December 10, 1982.

62. AR, 1980, p. 1.

63. AR, 1980, pp. 1–11.

64. Report of Yale University for the 1979 Reaccreditation Review, Natural Sciences Section, pp. 125–127. CF Arch.

65. Clouser, K. D. Philosophy in medical education. In: *The Role of the Humanities in Medical Education*. Norfolk: Eastern Virginia Medical School, 1978, p. 28. K. Danner Clouser was philosopher-in-residence at the Pennsylvania State University College of Medicine (Hershey Medical Center).

66. Carleton B. Chapman, interview with A. McGehee Harvey, December 10, 1982.

67. Ibid.

10. Programs for the 1980s

1. Newhouse, J. P. *Medical Care Expenditures: A Cross-National Survey. Policies for the Containment of Health Care Costs and Expenditures*. Washington, D.C.: U.S. Government Printing Office, 1978, pp. 67–79.

2. Data Resources, Inc. *The Data Resources United States Long-Term Review*. Lexington, Mass.: Data Resources, 1980; Wharton Economic Forecasting Associates: *The Pre-Meeting Solutions*. Philadelphia: The Wharton School of Business, University of Pennsylvania, 1980; The Economist Intelligence Unit: *The Major European Economies, 1980–1985*. London: The Economist, 1980.

3. Freeland, M; Calat, G; and Schendler, C. Projections of National Health Expenditures, 1980, 1985, and 1990. Health Care Financing Review 1: 11, 12, 16. Winter 1980.

4. Ibid.

5. Stein, H. How to pay for survival. Commentary 70(2): 28, August 1980.

6. Center for Health Services Research and Development. *Health Care Issues: Physician and Public Attitudes*. Chicago: American Medical Association, 1979.

11. The Book Program

1. AR, 1935, p. 51.
2. Chapman, C. The Commonwealth Fund Book Program, 1973. CF Arch.
3. AR, 1937, p. 44.

4. Chapman, *The Commonwealth Fund Book Program*, pp. 4, 13.
5. AR, 1937, p. 42.
6. AR, 1928, pp. 80–81.
7. AR, 1932, p. 66.
8. AR, 1943, p. 47.
9. GD, October 29, 1929.
10. AR, 1936, pp. 38–39.
11. AR, 1935, p. 52.
12. GD, October 14, 1948, p. 5.
13. Chapman, *The Commonwealth Fund Book Program*, p. 14.
14. AR, 1950, p. 35.
15. GD, June 8, 1950, p. 35.
16. GD, June 14, 1951, p. 69.
17. Chapman, *The Commonwealth Fund Book Program*, p. 17.
18. GD, February 13, 1964, p. 40.
19. Chapman, *The Commonwealth Fund Book Program*, pp. iii, iv, 2.
20. Chapman, C. B. to A. McGehee Harvey, December 8, 1983.
21. *The Frontiers of Science*. Announcement of the Commonwealth Fund Book Program. February 1983.
22. Thomas, L. A statement from the editor. In: *The Frontiers of Science*. Announcement of the Commonwealth Fund Book Program. February 1983.

Epilogue

1. Rich, A. R. Reflections on the relation of the curriculum to certain problems in medical education. Bull. Johns Hopkins Hosp. 49: 121, 1931.
2. Rosen, G. Critical levels in historical process—A theoretical exploration dedicated to Henry Ernest Sigerist. J. Hist. Med. 13: 179, 1958. Cited in Bordley, J. III and Harvey, A. M. *Two Centuries of American Medicine*. Philadelphia: W. B. Saunders, 1976, p. viii.
3. Rich, The curriculum in medical education.
4. *The Commonwealth Fund: A Historical Sketch*. New York: Commonwealth Fund, 1963, p. 40.
5. AR, 1949, pp. 1–3.
6. For example, Loeb, R. L. Values in undergraduate medical education. Trans. Assoc. Am. Phys. 58: 1, 1955.
7. Evans, L. J. Memoranda. 1947. CF Arch.
8. Evans, L. J. *The Crisis in Medical Education*. Ann Arbor: University of Michigan Press, 1964, p. 36.
9. Culliton, B. J. Medical education under fire. Science 226: 419, October 26, 1984.
10. Chapman, C. B. Letter to the editor. Harvard Magazine, pp. 35–37, September–October 1984.
11. *Physicians for the Twenty-first Century*. Report of the Panel on the General Professional Education of the Physicians and College Preparation for Medicine. Association of American Medical Colleges, 1984. Cited in Culliton, Medical education under fire.

12. Ibid.; Bok, D. The President's Report, 1982–1983. Harvard University.
13. Culliton, Medical education under fire.
14. Ibid.
15. Bok, The President's Report.
16. Chapman, Letter to the editor.
17. Bok, The President's Report.
18. Chapman, Letter to the editor; Culliton, Medical education under fire; Culliton, B. J. New curriculum at Harvard Medical School. Science 227: 153, 1985.
19. Bok, The President's Report.
20. Brown will merge premedical and M.D.-degree programs. *New York Times*, September 23, 1984.
21. Arthur, R. J. and Yager, J. Future work conditions for physicians: Implications for medical education. Pharos 47: 12, Summer 1984.
22. Bok, The President's Report; Physicians for the Twenty-first Century.
23. Paul, J. R. President's address. Trans. Assoc. Am. Phys. 69: 4, 1956.
24. Bok, The President's Report.
25. Ibid.
26. See also Institute of Medicine: Medical education and societal needs: A planning report for the health professions. Publication No. ION 83–02, July 1983; Relman, A. S. The new medical-industrial complex. N. Engl. J. Med. 202: 963, 1980.
27. Muller, S. Medicine: A learned profession? Address at the 95th meeting of the Association of American Medical Colleges, Chicago, Illinois.
28. Ibid.
29. Relman, A. S. Who will pay for medical education in our teaching hospitals? Science 226: 20, October 5, 1984.
30. Reynolds, R. C. Editorial. The narrowing gap between practicing and academic physicians. J. Med. Educ. 54: 514, 1979.
31. Pellegrino, E. D. Research in medical education: The views of a friendly Philistine. J. Med. Educ. 46: 750, 1971; see also Miller, G. E. A perspective on research in medical education. J. Med. Educ. 45: 694, 1970.
32. Margaret E. Mahoney to Pierre M. Galetti, vice-president (biology and medicine), Brown University, November 8, 1984.
33. Ibid.

Index of Names

References to illustrations are printed in italic type

Aagaard, George, 77
Abel, John, 164
Abrahamson, Stephen, 293, 295
Abrams, Herbert K., 302
Ackerly, S. Spafford, 65
Adair, John, 299
Adams, Anthony, 302
Adler, Alfred, 35
Albright, Fuller, 156, 157
Aldrich, Hulbert S., 512
Aldrich, Malcolm Pratt (second president of CF), 200, 210, *212*, 341, 452, 454, 512, 557, 648nn. 1, 3, 659n.215; administration of, 211–37; as chairman of the board, 338–39, 406; and Harkness, 15, 211; retirement of, 337, 659n.215
Aldrich, Robert, A., 455
Alexander, Benjamin, 175
Allen, Willard, 187
Alpers, Bernard J., 57
Anderson, Donald G., 296
Anderson, Forrest N., 57
Andrews, Samuel, 10
Angell, Rose Z., 318–19
Anylan, William G., 258, 482, 483–84
Appel, Kenneth E., 527
Arluke, Arnold, 444
Avery, O. T., 365

Bacon, Francis, 541
Baehr, George, 195, 333
Baker, Christopher C., 400
Bakst, Henry J., 240, 241
Ball, Eric, 261, 262
Bannard, Otto T., 19, *20*
Barnett, Thomas B., 238
Barr, David Prestwick, 74, 75, 209, 216, 226, 227, 648n.13
Barrnett, Russell J., 421–22, 423
Bauer, Walter, 77, 146, 174, 179, 180
Baumgartner, Leona, 388
Beck, John C., 383
Becker, Donald R., 291
Beers, Clifford W., 35, 36, 557
Belin, Harriet Bundy, 512
Benjamin, John, *58*
Bennett, Granville, 293, 294
Berg, Robert L., 139, 317
Berry, George P., 216–17, 220, 230, 261–63, 265, 338, 341, 387–88, 649n.7
Berson, Robert, 250
Bert, Robert A., 444, 445
Bidder, T. George, 249
Bigelow, George H., 147
Biggs, Hermann M., 30, *32*, 87, 88, 89, 90, 94, 115, 539, 634n.17
Bilbo, Robert L., 391

675

Billings, Edward G., *58*
Binet, Alfred, 34
Bing, Richard J., 177, 179
Bishop, E. L., 105, 112, 113
Blackfan, Kenneth, 65, 530
Blalock, Alfred, 177
Blankenhorn, Marion A., 68, 69
Blendon, Robert, 386
Bliss, Ann, 392
Bloodgood, Joseph C., 120, 195
Bloom, Benjamin, 288
Bluestone, Ephraim Michael, 328–29, 330, 331, 332, 333, 334
Blumenthal, David, 439
Boas, Ernst P., 332
Bodian, David, 530
Bok, Derek C., 381, 549–50
Bond, Douglas D., 77, 253
Bond, Earl D., 527
Boole, Mary Everest, 38
Bosch, Samuel J., 305
Bowers, John Z., 369
Bowman, John G., 115
Bowman, Karl M., 65
Brailey, Miriam, 169, 191
Branscomb, Lewis M., 469
Brask, Thomas, 398
Braunwald, Eugene, 450
Brewster, Kingman, 418–19, 420, 428
Bridge, Edward W., 286, 287
Brooks, Barney, 120
Brosin, Henry W., 77, 79
Brozgal, Joseph L., 251, 252
Bruce, Alexander, 59
Buck, Carl E., 141
Burch, George E., 75
Butler, Alan, 170

Cadbury, William E., 369, 370, 371
Calderone, Mary S., 359
Calkins, David, 439
Campbell, Charles Macfie, 59
Campbell, Willis, 120
Cantor, Nathaniel, 288
Capen, Samuel P., 25
Carnegie, Andrew, 2
Carstens, C. C., 26
Caughey, John L., Jr., 243, 244, 245, 247, 249, 253
Chalmers, Thomas C., 306
Chan, Lo-Yi, 429
Chapman, Carleton Burke (fourth president of CF), 275–77, 284, 434–35, *462*, 557; administration of, 461–514; as vice-president of CF, 339, 440–43, 533
Cherkasky, Martin, 329, 330, 332, 333, 334
Childgren, Richard A., 360
Christian, Henry A., 196
Clark, Mary A., 527
Cleaveland, Frederic N., 484
Cluff, Leighton E., 455, 456, 457–58
Cobb, Stanley, 147
Cohen, Seymour, 174, 182
Cohn, Edwin J., 163, 166, 168
Cole, Jack W., 392, 399
Collins, William, 399
Comroe, Julius, 177
Cooper, John A. D., 270
Cope, Oliver, 384
Corwin, E. H. L., 195, 319, 321, 530
Cournand, André, 176, 177, 179, 319
Crane, Robert A., 530, 533
Crawford, Albert B., 71
Crede, Robert H., 67
Crothers, Bronson, 62
Cullen, Thomas S., 195
Cumming, Hugh S., 96
Cummings, Martin, 533
Cunningham, Nicholas, 305

Dana, Bessie S., 306
Dargassies, Sainte-Anne, 157
Darley, Ward, 230, 232
Darrach, William, 22, 195
Davis, Terrell, *58*
Davison, Wilburt C., 257, 278
deForest, Robert W., 15
de la Chapelle, Clarence, 319
Delbanco, Thomas L., 425
Delgado, Richard, 444
Denson, Paul, 390
Deuschle, Kurt W., 299–301, 303, 304–5, 306
Dewey, John, 37
Dickes, Robert, Jr., 151
Diers, Donna, 429
Dietrick, John E., 250
Dingle, John H., 249
Dinwiddie, Courtenay, 93, 94, 96, 635n.31
Dixon, James P., 232
Dobihal, Edward F., Jr., 427, 428
Dochez, A. R., 151
Dollard, Charles, 221
Dollard, John, 71
Donway, Walter, 405–6, 407, 436, 664n.94
Dorsey, Joseph L., 390

Dorsh, Joseph, 391
Douglas, William O., 338
Dummer, Mrs. W. F., 38
Dunn, Mary K., 429
Durfee, Marion, *58*

Eaton, Joseph W., 251
Ebaugh, Franklin G., *57*, 60
Eberhart, John C., 212, 216, 250, 251, 289–91, 292, 648n.2
Ebert, Paul A., 358
Ebert, Richard V., 441
Ebert, Robert H., 193, 265, 378, 388, 389–90, 391, 507
Ecker, E. E., 168
Edwards, Lydia, 169
Eisenhower, Dwight D., 140
Elam, Lloyd, 368, 377
Elman, Robert, 171
Elsas, Louis J., 420
Embree, Edwin R., 115
Endicott, Kenneth, 415
Engel, George L., 67
English, O. Spurgeon, 236
Erickson, Gregory, 504
Estes, Harvey, Jr., 356
Evans, Herbert McLean, 157
Evans, John, *58*
Evans, Lester J., 4, 77, 97–100, *98*, 106, 107, 110, 163, 183, 203, 212, 337, 453; characteristics of, 220–22, 230, 459, 511, 512–13, 536; and comprehensive medicine, 224, 225, 227, 229, 231, 242, 544; and grants, 160, 188, 313, 317, 464; and health care, 323, 423; and Hunterdon project, 319, 320, 321; and medical education, 197, 206, 220–23, 242, 243, 244–45, 246, 248, 249, 287, 288–89, 292, 293, 295, 543, 546, 548, 550; retirement of, 337, 339, 557; and rural hospitals, 123–24, 128, 133
Ewalt, Jack, *58*
Ewing, James, 195

Farrand, Livingston, 88
Farrand, Max (first general director of CF), 19–26, 537, 557, 626n.2, 627nn. 17, 23, 628n.27
Fein, Rashi, 284, 390
Feinberg, Harvey, 439
Fell, Honor, 157
Ferris, Eugene B., 67
Findlay, Edgar, *58*

Fineman, Robert, 421
Fisher, Lawrence, 294
Fisher, Samuel H., 15, 19, *20*, 211
Fitz, Reginald H., 404–5, 436, 533, 534
Flagler, Henry M., 10, 11
Fleming, William L., 238
Flexner, Abraham, 2, 22, 24, 218, 276, 277, 373, 466, 467, 505, 543, 549
Folks, Homer, 26, 88
Folsom, Marion B., 140
Ford, Loretta C., 350, 661n.28
Forssmann, Werner, 177
Franklin, Philip, *58*
Frazier, Howard, 391, 447
Frazier, William, 399
French, William J., 94, 107–8
Freud, Sigmund, 35, 37
Frost, Wade Hampton, 169, 183, 188–90, *189*, 191, 192
Frothingham, Channing, 404
Fry, Clements, 71, 73
Fuchs, Victor R., 364
Fulmer, Hugh Scott, 302
Furnas, Clifford C., 289, 290

Galletti, Pierre M., 491
Gardner, John, 455
Gates, Frederick T., 2
Gellhorn, Alfred, 500, 507–8
Gellis, Sydney S., 155
Gertler, Menard M., 531
Gesell, Arnold L., 71
Gifford, John A., 339
Glaser, Robert Joy, 216, 340–41, *404*, 407, 457, 470, 514, 664n.93; on conflict of interest, 217; as vice-president of CF, 339, 403–40, 441, 442
Glock, Charles, 228
Glueck, Bernard, 41, 96
Goldenberg, Ira, 427, 428
Goldwater, S. S., 115
Goodall, Jane, 432, 433, 436
Grace, William J., 75
Graef, Irving, 369, 371
Green, David E., 176
Guion, Connie Myers, 226, 650n.28

Hall, Granville Stanley, 35
Ham, Thomas Hale, 244, 249, 252, 253, 296
Hamburg, Betty, 436, 437
Hamburg, David A., 431, 432, 434–35, 436, 437
Hamilton, Jefferson M., 278, 279

Handler, Philip, 257
Handley, Harry E., 212
Hansen, A. Victor, Jr., 236, 237
Hardy, Janet, 174
Harkness, Anna (wife of Stephen Vanderberg), 1, 9, 11, 13, *14*, 17, 19
Harkness, Charles, 10–11, 13, 15
Harkness, Daniel, 9
Harkness, David, 9
Harkness, Edward Stephen (first president of CF), *12*, *20*, 23, 344, 452, 454; administration of, 2, 4, 13–19, 520–21, 536, 557; and Aldrich, 211, 216, 339; family of, 9–11; on government Department of Education, 25; on hospitals, 114–15; 1937 gift of, 146, 148, 163, 165, 167, 207, 541
Harkness, Lamon, 9
Harkness, Martha Cook (mother of Stephen Vanderberg), 9
Harkness, Mary, 10
Harkness, Stephen Vanderberg, 9
Harkness, William, 9
Harkness, William (grandson of William), 9
Harrell, George T., 278, 279, 280, 281
Harris, Jerome S., 257
Harris, T. N., 175
Hart, Deryl, 257
Harvey, A. McGehee, 455–58
Hastings, Donald W., 77
Heald, Henry T., 340
Healy, William, 26, 38, 46, 537
Heath, Robert G., 216
Heffron, Roderick E., 146–47, 152, 158, 160, 162, 185, 188, 243, 300, 302, 529, 642n.5
Helmholz, Henry F., 96
Hertwig, Richard, 186
Hevesy, Georg, 156
Heyman, David, 333
Hiatt, Howard H., 429, 446, 447
Hillman, Richard, 421
Hinkle, Lawrence E., 75
Hinsey, Joseph C., 230
Hiscock, Ira V., 143
Holder, Angela, 444
Hollingshead, August B., 308
Holman, Halsted R., 383
Hoover, Herbert C., 93, 96
Horowitz, Milton J., 251, 252
Howe, Howard A., 530
Howell, William H., 190
Howlett, K. S., 120
Hume, David M., 178

Hume, Edward, 122
Hume, Michael, 532
Hunt, Andrew, 295, 320, 321
Hutchins, Robert, 549
Huxley, Thomas H., 466–67, 549

James, George, 303–4
James, Walter B., 22
Jason, Hilliard, 295
Jobling, J. W., 163
Johnson, Howard W., 378
Johnson, Mrs. J. Seward., 325
Jordan, Robert, 337
Julianelle, Louis A., 165
Jung, Carl Gustav, 35

Kaiser, Albert D., 135, 140
Kanner, Leo, 46
Karnovsky, Manfred, 264
Kaufman, Moe, 77
Keenan, Terrance, 339–40, 386, 391, 405–6, 407, 415, 456, 663n.83
Keggi, Kristaps J., 392
Kemeny, John G., 494
Kempe, C. Henry, 412
Kennan, Elizabeth, 464
Kern, Frederick, Jr., 228, 232
Kerns, Harry, 71
Kerr, Clark, 282
Keys, Ancel, 441
Kimball, Stockton, 289
Kinney, Thomas D., 254
Kirstein, George, 333
Kissick, William L., 334
Klüver, Heinrich, 174
Komaroff, Anthony L., 451
Kraepelin, Emil, 34, 37, 59
Krebs, Hans, 176
Krevans, Julius R., 383
Kriedler, Robert N., 369
Krizek, Thomas J., 399
Krogh, August, 156
Kubitschek, Paul E., 57

Labate, John S., 151
Lack, Sylvia A., 429
La Guardia, Fiorello, 333
Lakeman, Curtis E., 527
Langford, W. S., 62
Lape, Esther Everett, 163
Leathers, W. S., 120
Lee, Peter V., 225, 239, 240, 253, 254, 264, 308–9

Lee, Porter R., 25, 41, 96
Lee, Porter R., Jr., 530
Lee, Sidney S., 388, 391
Leicester, Mrs. William F., 318, 319, 320
Leiderman, Herbert, 360
Lein, Allen, 505
Lein, John N., 414
Leutner, Winfred G., 243
Levine, Maurice, 67
Levine, Seymour, 436
Levy, David M., 49–50
Lewis, Jerry, 371
Lezer, Leon R., 307, 308
Lief, Harold I., 360, 532
Lipmann, Fritz A., 146, 175, 176, 179
Lippard, Vernon W., 278, 317
Little, C. C., 170
Lock, Frank R., 358, 359
Lockwood, Richard A., 282, 283
London, Irving M., 378–80, 381–82
Loosli, Clayton, 155
Lord, Frederick T., 529
Lowrey, Lawson G., 49
Ludwig, Alfred O., 532
Lumsden, L. L., 86
Lurie, Max, 174

McAtee, Patricia R., 351
McBride, Katherine E., 529
McCann, William S., 238
McCammon, Robert W., 185
McDermott, Walsh, 227, 284, 285, 299, 494
McIntosh, Rustin, 65
MacLachlan, John M., 278
MacLean, Basil C., 132, 134, 278
MacLean, Franklin Chambers, 367–68, 369
MacLeod, Colin M., 303, 316, 339, 340, 365, 366, *366*, 367, 378, 382, 403, 456, 663n.92
McNamara, M. J., 302
McNeil, Barbara J., 451
Magoun, Horace W., 174, 179, 181
Mahoney, Margaret Ellerbe (fifth president of CF), 4, 194, 391, 507, 514, *518*, 557, 558; administration of, 517–21; and Carnegie Corporation, 382, 383, 386, 424, 457, 462
Mahoney, Morris, 420–21
Maloney, William, 292
Manly, Basil, 21
Margolis, Simeon, 499
Marie, Pierre, 59
Marriott, W. McKim, 99, 100

Meadow, Henry, 388
Mee, Mrs. Robert G., 195
Meiklejohn, Gordon, 404
Menninger, William C., 79
Merton, Robert K., 228, 250
Meskill, Thomas J., 396, 397
Meyer, Adolf, 30, *32*, 33, 35–36, 46; and child psychiatry, 37, 39, 50, 62; and psychiatric training, 58, 59, 60, 538
Michels, Robert, 361
Miles, Catherine C., 71
Miles, Walter R., 71
Miller, George E., 288, 293, 294, 297
Miller, James Alexander, 319
Miller, J. Hillis, 278
Miller, Neal, 71
Miller, Roscoe, 269
Milstone, Jacob Haskell, 151
Monroe, Russell R., 532
Moore, F. L., 114
Moore, Gordon, 391
Morgan, Thomas E., 414
Morgan, Thomas Hunt, 186
Morrison, Robert S., 284
Moses, Henry, 333
Mulholland, John, 150
Muller, Steven, 499, 552
Mulley, Al, 439
Murray, George W., 19, *20*
Murray, John, 77
Murrow, Edward R., 200
Muschenheim, Carl, 299
Musser, John H., 75
Mustard, Harry S., 113

Nesson, H. Richard, 390
Newman, Howard H., 450
Newton, James Quigg, Jr. (third president of CF), 232, 242, 258, 312, *339*, 464, 520, 557, 659n.1; administration of, 338–460; 1971 report of, 461, 462, 463
Nissl, Franz, 59
Nixon, Richard M., 341, 357, 369, 469
Noe, William L., Jr., 120
Noguchi, Hideyo, 165
Northrop, John H., 151
Nudd, Howard W., 41

O'Connor, John F., 361
Odegaard, Charles E., 415
Oliver, Jean, 177
Oswald, John, 302

Packman, Seymour, 421
Palade, George E., 421, 422–23
Palmer, George T., 94
Palmer, W. W., 195
Papanicolaou, George N., 170, 179, 183, 186, *187*, 188, 531
Park, Edwards A., 191
Park, William H., 84, 87
Parry, Herbert, *58*
Paton, Stewart, 71
Paul, John R., 550–51
Pearl, Raymond, 190
Pearson, G. H. J., 57
Pellegrino, Edmund D., 320, 321, 324, 326–28, 556
Penrose, Lionel, 158
Perkins, James A., 28
Petersdorf, Robert G., 449, 451
Pifer, Alan, 382
Plimpton, Calvin H., 469
Pollack, Jerome, 388, 390–91
Poor, Russell S., 278
Powdermaker, Florence, 155
Powers, Charles A., 195
Price, Don K., 439
Prince, Morton, 35
Pritchett, Henry S., 2, 22
Putnam, Tracy J., 170
Pyle, Thomas O., 391

Quin, Barbara S., 30, *31*, 47, 100, 211, 628n.3

Rakic, Pashko, 423
Randolph, Carolina R., 108, 114
Rappleye, Willard C., 320
Reader, George G., 74, 75, 209, 226, 227, 228, 229–30, 231, 300, 303
Redlich, Frederick C., 422
Reed, Lowell J., 169, 183, 190, 191, *192*
Reichlin, Seymour, 181
Reiser, Morton F., 67, 69
Reitz, J. Wayne, 281
Relman, Arnold S., 553
Rennie, Tom, 77
Reznikoff, Paul, 74
Rhead, William, 421
Rich, Arnold R., 535
Richards, A. Newton, 171
Richards, Dickinson W., Jr., 146, 171, 176, 177, 179, 319
Riley, Henry Alsop, 196
Ripley, Herbert, 74

Roberts, Stewart B., 120
Robson, Martin, 399
Rock, Miriam, 476
Rockefeller, John D., 10, 11, 87
Rockefeller, Winthrop, 320
Rogers, David E., 284, 386
Rogers, James Gamble, 116
Rogers, Terence A., 285
Romano, John, 33, *58*, 66–67, 69, 77, 209, 455
Roosevelt, Franklin D., 143, 332, 627n.2
Rose, Wickliffe, 87
Rosen, George, 535
Rosenau, Milton J., 31, 40
Rosenbaum, Milton, 67
Rosenberg, Leon E., 419, 420, 421
Rosenberg, Mark, 439
Rosinski, Edwin F., 292–93
Ross, Richard S., 499
Rubin, Harry, 305
Rudhe, Ulf, 157
Ruggles, Arthur H., 70, 71–72, 73
Rutstein, David D., 378, 388, 389
Rymer, Charles A., *58*

Sabin, Florence R., 141, 232
Sadler, Alfred M., Jr., 392, 398
Sadler, Blair L., 392, 397, 398
Sage, Dean, 17
Salmon, Thomas W., 26, 31, 32, 34, *36*, 36–37, 55, 537
Sanazaro, Paul J., 296
Sandson, John I., 486
Sanford, Terry, 482
Saunders, Cicely, 427
Saunders, Lyle, 221
Sayles, Mary B., 527, 528
Scammon, Clarence L., 108, 636n.47
Schwarz, M. Roy, 414, 415–16
Scoville, Mildred C., 30, *31*, 47, 100, 212, 511, 628n.4; and mental health programs, 33, 57–58, 61, 70, 77, 79, 80, 82
Seashore, Margretta R., 421
Sedgwick, W. T., 86
Senn, Milton J. E., 151, 173, 178, 216
Shannon, James A., 374, 378
Sharp, Sally, 444
Sheehan, Donal (third general director of CF), 203–10, *204*, 214, 225, 341, 557, 647n.1
Sieker, Herbert O., 258
Silver, George, 334

Silver, Henry K., 349, 350, 351, 352, 353, 355
Simmons, Henry E., 325
Simon, Théodore, 34
Simpson, Frank F., 195
Simpson, Michael, 467–68
Smith, Alfred E., 90
Smith, Barry Conger (second general director of CF), 29–30, *30*, 628n.2; administration of, 2, 26, 29–200, 341, 344, 452, 511; and Book Program, 525, 536, 539, 557; on CF's first twenty-five years, 199–200; on government aid, 196; and juvenile deliquency program, 40–41, 46, 47, 50; and medical education, 145, 146, 148; and public health programs, 84, 90, 92–93, 94, 100, 107, 109, 110; retirement of, 200, 203, 209, 211; and rural hospital programs, 115, 116, 122, 125, 143–44; and training of psychiatrists, 33, 55, 57–58, 61, 82
Smith, Geddes, 77, 194, *212*, 215, 225, 227, 246, 247, 527
Smith, Homer W., 169, 179
Smith, Rufus, 370
Smith, Winford H., 115
Solnit, Albert J., 430
Somers, A. R., 326, 412
Southmayd, Henry J., 116, 133, 144, 212
Spar, Irving, 473–77
Spiro, Howard M., 445
Starr, Paul, 444
Stead, Eugene A., Jr., 257, 259, 355, 407
Steinberg, Earl P., 439–40
Stepto, Robert C., 369
Stewart, Michael M., 305
Stockard, Charles, 186
Strecker, Edward A., 72
Strickler, James C., 494
Studdiford, W. C., 170
Sturgis, Somers H., 532
Suter, Emanuel, 456
Swank, Roy L., 66
Swanson, August G., 414, 415
Sydenstricker, Edgar, 190

Tabor, Ben Z., 360
Talbot, Nathan B., 174, 179, 180
Tapp, Jesse W., Jr., 302
Taussig, Helen B., 177, 530
Taylor, Charles H., 422
Taylor, Graham Romeyn, 42, 526, 530

Taylor, H. C., 170, 195, 419
Thayer, William S., 24
Thomas, Lewis, 193, 316, 402, 520, 534
Thompson, Lloyd J., 71, 72
Thurston, Henry W., 40
Tibbles, Lance, 444
Tilney, Frederic, 165
Tosteson, Daniel C., 257, 477, 479
Touloukian, Robert, 399
Towler, Martin, *58*
Towne, Arthur H., 42
Traut, Herbert F., 186, 187
Treuting, Theodore, 75
Trussell, Ray E., 320, 321
Tschirgi, Robert D., 282, 283
Turner, Joseph C., 151
Turner, Thomas B., 459
Tyler, Ralph, 294

Uretz, Robert B., 480

Van Citters, Robert L., 418
Vandervoort, Herbert E., 361
van Lawick-Goodall, Jane. *See* Goodall, Jane
Vincent, George E., 109

Waitzkin, Michael, 444
Waksman, Selman, 146, 168–69
Wald, Florence S., 427, 428, 430
Wald, Henry J., 429
Wald, Lillian, 88
Walker, W. Frank, 108, 114, 143, 144, 637n.49
Waring, James, 404
Warner, A. R., 115
Warren, Charles O., 147, 212, 229, 244, 245, 250–52, 289, 292, 642n.6
Washburn, Alfred H., 173, 179, 182, 183–84, *184*, 185, 186
Wasson, W. Walter, 183
Watson, Robert F., 227
Wearn, Joseph T., 242, 243, 244, 245, 248, 249, 250, 253, 258–59, 423, 425, 546; on medical students, 246–47
Webster, Bruce P., 227
Weed, Lawrence L., 309
Weinstein, Alexander, 174
Weisberger, Austin S., 383, 385
Weisenburg, Theodore H., 164, 529
Weiss, Edward, 236, 237
Weiss, Robert, 390
Weiss, Soma, 66

Welch, William Henry, 88, 115, 190, 555, 657n.179
Wellington, John S., 286
Wescott, Lloyd B., 319, 320, 321, 324–25
Wessel, Morris A., 427, 428
White, Kerr L., 239, 242
White, Paul D., 531
White, William A., 46
Whitehorn, John C., 59, 497
Whittam, Ronald, 156
Wickman, E. K., 337
Wiesner, Jerome R., 378, 381
Wiggers, Carl J., 171, 179
Wilkins, Lawson, 175
Willard, William R., 253, 279, 299, 302
Williams, Frankwood E., 72
Williams, T. Franklin, 238, 239, 242
Wilson, May G., 167, 174, 179
Winslow, C.-E. A., 30, 88, 89
Winslow, Emma, 526
Witmer, Lightner, 38
Wolf, Barry, 421
Wolf, George A., Jr., 307
Wolf, Stewart G., Jr., 73, 74
Wolff, Harold G., 73, 74, 77, 209, 226
Wood, Francis Carter, 195
Wood, Harland G., 244, 249, 253
Wood, W. Barry, 403
Woodhall, Barnes, 257
Worlin, George, 183
Wright, Henry C., 116, 126
Wyngaarden, James B., 256, 383

Zacharias, Jerrold, 384
Zeckhauser, Richard, 440
Zimmerman, Kent A., 151
Zinsser, Hans, 195

Index of Subjects

AAMC. *See* Association of American Medical Colleges
Affiliated Hospitals Center, Inc. (AHC), 365, 403, 448–52; Center for Cost-Effective Care (CCC) at, 449–52
Albany Medical College, 265, 273, 320, 322, 345
Albany-RPI Program, 273–75. *See also* Rensselaer Polytechnic Institute
Albert Einstein College of Medicine, 345, 378, 379
Alcoholism, 306, 324, 410, 427, 442
Alderson-Broaddus College, 402
Alzheimer's disease, support of research on, 194
Ambulatory Pediatric Association, 353
American Academy of Pediatrics, 352
American Academy of Physicians' Assistants, 357
American Association for the Advancement of Science, 182
American Association of Planned Parenthood Physicians, 532
American Association of Psychiatric Social Workers, 53
American Board of Internal Medicine, 409, 411
American Board of Neurology and Psychiatry, 539
American Cancer Society, 157, 195, 643n.24
American Child Health Association, 40, 91, 93, 95, 108
American Child Hygiene Association, 93
American College of Hospital Administrators, 132
American College of Physicians, Richard and Hilda J. Rosenthal Award of, 418
American College of Surgeons, 115, 117, 119, 144, 195, 399
American Federation for Clinical Research, 239, 651n.45
American Heart Association, 157, 643n.24
American Hospital Association, 115, 132, 143, 195, 328
American Journal of Psychiatry, 526
American Journal of Public Health, 530
American Lung Association, 371
American Medical Association (AMA), 110, 117, 130, 143, 195, 313, 332, 358; Council of Medical Education of, 127
American Nurses Foundation, 427
American Orthopsychiatric Association, 53
American Psychiatric Association (APA), 53, 56, 61, 79, 539; Mental Hospital Institute service of, 80
American Public Health Association (APHA), 88, 95, 104, 113, 143, 539; Committee on Administrative Practice of, 100, 101, 108, 141, 142
American Social Hygiene Association, 23

683

American Society for the Control of Cancer (ASCC), 23, 90, 195. *See also* American Cancer Society
American Society of Parenteral and Enteral Nutrition, 440
Annual Conference on Research in Medical Education, 296
Anthropology, and medicine, 248, 299, 301, 504
APHA. *See* American Public Health Association
Arthritis, 172, 174, 180
Associated Jewish Charities of Baltimore, 329
Association of American Medical Colleges (AAMC), 217, 313, 359, 402, 412, 441, 537; and comprehensive medicine, 230; and minorities, 369, 373, 374; teaching institutes of, 296
Association of American Physicians, 246
Association for the Prevention and Relief of Heart Disease, 90
Atlas of Exfoliative Cytology (Papanicolaou), 531
Atomic Bomb Casualty Commission (Japan), 156

Babies' Hospital (New York), 62, 63, 65. *See also* Columbia-Presbyterian Medical Center
Bacteriology, 17, 86, 87, 218, 264, 535
Bellevue Hospital, 171, 195, 458
Beth Israel Hospital (Boston), 175, 388, 439, 446; Ambulatory Care Center at, 386–87, 413, 423–27, 447
Binet and Simon measuring scale, 34
Bingham Associates Fund, 134
Biochemistry, 162, 218, 263, 264, 265, 276, 277, 336, 375, 436, 482, 493–94, 495, 498, 542
Biology, 181–82, 205, 255, 263, 272, 276, 376, 421–22; as educational theme, 280, 281; and health professionals, 356; human, 380, 381, 470, 477, 478, 479, 480, 497, 498, 503, 504; and Interface Program, 474, 475, 484; molecular, 224, 482, 504; and premedical education, 503, 510
Biophysics, 218, 255
Blood banks, 136, 137
Bloomingdale Hospital (New York), 57
Blue Cross/Blue Shield, 311, 429
Blue Cross/Massachusetts, Hospital Association Fund for Cooperative Innovation, 451
Book Program (CF), 405, 512, 520, 525–34
Boston City Hospital, 147, 240, 241; Thorndike Laboratory at, 244
Boston Hospital for Women, 449
Boston Psychopathic Hospital, 33, 39, 58, 59–60
Boston University, 225, 402, 550; Home Medical Service of, 226, 240, 241; Human Ecology Program of, 240–41; Interface Program at, 485–89, 505, 506, 507; Liberal Arts-Medical Education Program, 485–86; Modular Medical Integrated Curriculum (MMEDIC), 265, 266, 272, 276, 343, 485, 486, 487–88, 489, 670n.30; School of Medicine of, 155, 240–42, 271–72, 302, 402, 487, 488, 489
Bowman Gray Medical College, 345, 358, 359
Brain, research on, 165, 181
British Medical Journal, 529
Brookings Institution, 336, 402
Brown University, 345, 467, 549; Interface Program at, 489–92, 505, 507, 508
Bruner Foundation, 355
Bureau of Children's Guidance (NYC), 41, 42, 46, 49
Bureau of Health Manpower Education, 349, 357, 397. *See also* National Institutes of Health
Butler Hospital (Providence, R.I.), 72

California Institute of Technology, 408
California State Department of Health, 81, 633n.114
Cambridge (Mass.) City Hospital, 390
Cancer: control of, 89, 195; fellowships for study of, 151; and home care, 330, 427, 429, 430; research on, 163, 170, 183, 186–88, 195; tests for, 301; X-ray therapy for, 195, 647n.98. *See also* Hospice in New Haven
Cardiology, 177, 242. *See also* Research
Carnegie Corporation, 1, 355, 356, 517; and collaboration with Commonwealth Fund, 281, 411, 453, 454, 455, 457, 462; and health care, 386, 387, 424; and medical education, 221, 296, 375, 382, 383, 384–85, 402, 403, 425, 467; and mental hygiene, 82, 633n.115

Carnegie Foundation for the Advancement of Teaching, 1, 22, 367
Carnegie Institution of Washington, 1
Case Western Reserve University, 220, 258, 293, 309, 334, 652n.85; and comprehensive medicine, 214, 229, 243; curriculum reform at, 225, 242–54, 276, 287, 290, 292, 297, 342, 405, 423, 464, 510, 546, 550; medical research at, 168, 171
Center for the Analysis of Health Practices, 391, 445–48, 450
Center for Health Research. See Center for the Analysis of Health Practices
Centers for Disease Control, 439, 447
CF. See Commonwealth Fund
Chicago Commission on Race Relations, 527
Chicago Juvenile Psychopathic Institute, 38, 39
Child abuse, 306, 398, 409, 412–13, 432, 453
Child Abuse Advisory Committee, 398
Child development, 182–86. See also Child Research Council of Denver
Child guidance clinics, 3, 31, 34, 42, 43–46, 47, 520; and child welfare, 45, 198, 537, 538; increase in, 50; and juvenile deliquency, 39, 41–46, 197; and psychiatrists, 52, 56–57, 60, 62, 64, 198. See also Institute for Child Guidance
Child Health Council, 26
Child Health Demonstration Program (CF), 31, 91, 92–103, 109, 538, 539; in Athens, Georgia, 101–2; committee for, 93–95, 107, 635n.28; and dental hygiene, 101–2; in Fargo, North Dakota, 97–101, 106, 108, 110; in Marion County, Oregon, 103, 107; publications of, 635n.32; results of, 103–7, 114, 142; in Rutherford County, Tennessee, 102, 104, 105, 108, 110, 113
Child Health Organization, 89, 93–94. See also American Child Health Association
Child hygiene, 54–55. See also Child welfare; Mental health
Child Hygiene Association, 23
Child Labor Committee, 38
Child psychiatry, origins and growth of, 37–40, 41, 43, 44, 45–46, 48. See also Child guidance clinics; Psychiatry
Children's Bureau, 349
Children's Hospital (Boston), 62, 63, 65
Child Research Council of Denver, 163, 183–86, 206, 231–32
Child welfare, 3, 25–26, 31, 40, 91–97, 194, 537–39, 627n.23; and demonstrations, 26, 43–46, 91–101; and well-baby clinics, 99
Child Welfare League of America, 26
Cincinnati General Hospital, psychosomatic ward in, 67
City University of New York (CUNY), 304, 406; City College of, 499; courses in community health at, 500–501; Interface Program at, 499–502, 508; Program in Biomedical Education at, 500–501
Clinical Scholars Program, 383–86, 462
Clinic for Comprehensive Care (Cornell University), 227–29
College of Physicians of Philadelphia, 402
College of Physicians and Surgeons (Columbia University), 15, 17, 162, 165, 176, 320, 331, 361, 404. See also Columbia University
Colorado General Hospital, 233
Colorado Psychopathic Hospital, 33, 58, 60–61
Columbia-Presbyterian Medical Center, 62, 151, 170, 171, 216, 334, 344, 345, 458; Library-Health Sciences Center at, 442; Vanderbilt Clinic at, 442. See also Columbia University; Presbyterian Hospital
Columbia University, 22, 290, 345, 458, 467; Bureau of Applied Social Research at, 228, 250; and health studies, 362; Institute of Administrative Medicine at, 138; Medical Center of, 17; Medical School of, 15, 17; Neurological Institute of, 162; research at, 228, 250; School of Dental and Oral Surgery at, 163
Commission on Hospital Care, 143, 328
Committee on Economic Security, 143
Committee on Social Medicine, 333
Commonwealth Fund (CF): administrative structures of, 47, 96–97, 209, 411, 512, 537; appeals to, 19, 22, 215; board of directors of, 4, 19, 209, 215, 339, 512, 521, 659n.2; Committee on Public Health of, 109, 637nn. 54, 55, 56; concern for community welfare of, 539–41; consultants to, 638n.71, 639n.90, 647n.98, 648n.3, 659n.213, 668nn. 23, 25, 669n.26, 670n.30; decision making in, 4–5, 23, 24, 25, 47, 199, 209–10, 214–24, 313–14, 405–7, 507, 536, 546, 649n.23; directors of, 4, 5, 13, 19–26, 29–31, 200, 211; Division of Community Clinics of, 46, 48; Division of Publications of, 4, 46, 214,

Commonwealth Fund (CF) (*continued*)
337, 412, 461, 520, 526–34, 538; Educational Research Committee of, 25, 26; and Educational Research Conference (1920), 627n.17; Experimental Health Services of, 212, 318, 335, 452, 556; first half-century of, 401; first twenty-five years of, 197; founding of (1918), 1, 2, 13, 15, 536; and health professionals, 345–58; health studies of, 107, 108–9; history of, 3, 4; investment policy of, 520; and juvenile delinquency, 40–56, 82, 96, 197, 222, 525, 526; Legal Research Committee of, 25; and medical records, 118, 137; and New York City programs, 511, 519; and personal giving, 17, 23; President's Discretionary Fund of, 454–58, 511, 667n.175; programs of, in 1950s, 214; programs of, in 1980s, 519–21; and sex education, 359–62; and "socialized medicine," 333; and social programs, 387; staff of, 511, 513–14, 636nn. 45, 48; traditions of, 4, 458–60, 511–13, 521, 536; and universities, 463, 467–546; during World War II, 196–97; writers in, 4, 215, 526, 527. *See also* Child welfare; Education, medical; Fellowships; Grants; *individual programs*; Mental health; Public Health; Health; Research

Commonwealth Fund Books, 532. *See also* Book Program

Community Blood Council (New York), 452

Community Mental Health Centers Act: of 1963, 383; of 1965, 383

Community Service Society, 334

Comprehensive Health Manpower Training Act, 357, 371

Comprehensive medicine, 173, 184, 203–10, 218, 224, 225–42. *See also* Clinic for Comprehensive Care

Computers, grants for, 411–12, 550, 553

Congress, U.S., 192–93, 196, 315; Office of Technology Assessment, 517

Connecticut Commission on Hospitals and Health Care, 429

Connecticut Committee on Emergency Medical Services (EMS), 393, 396, 400

Connecticut Committee on Public Health and Safety, 396

Connecticut Council on Hospitals and Health Care, 396

Connecticut Medical Service, 429

Connecticut Regional Medical Program, 392, 429

Connecticut Society for Mental Hygiene, 36

Connecticut State Act Concerning the Correction of Child Abuse, 398

Cornell University, 250, 290, 299

Cornell University Medical College, 53, 147, 151, 209, 344, 357; and comprehensive medicine, 225, 226–31, 544; Pilot Clinic for a Broader Medical Service at, 33, 73–75; research at, 170, 183, 186; training of surgical assistants at, 357–58

Cytology, 186–88, 301, 423

Danforth Foundation, 373

Dartmouth-Hitchcock Medical Center, 450

Dartmouth University: medical school at, 403, 441, 464, 492; Interface Program at, 492–97, 506, 507

Demonstrations, 26, 41, 141, 197, 520; of child guidance clinics, 43–45, 47, 49, 53, 57; of child health program, 31, 91–103, 526; in health care, 389, 390, 520. *See also* Child Health Demonstration Program

Denver General Hospital, 232, 233, 234–35, 404

Department of Education, U.S., 25

Department of Health, Education and Welfare (HEW), U.S., 165, 196, 364, 424–25, 426, 517

Department of State, U.S., 282

Diagnostic Related Groups (DRG), 440

Diphtheria, 84, 88, 89, 103, 112, 119, 190

Disease, 2, 3, 34, 145, 150, 168, 176; bacteriology and, 535; chronic, 169, 174, 191, 330, 332, 427; classification systems for, 195–96; communicable, 87–88, 89, 92, 95, 102, 103, 104, 112, 119, 143, 190, 191, 264, 538; prevention of, 16, 84–85, 86, 87, 144, 145, 222; research on, 162–72, 193; and study of normal growth, 535; venereal, 89, 190, 191. *See also* Epidemics; Epidemiology; Immunization; Preventive medicine

Drug abuse, 397, 409–10, 431, 433, 453; in schools, 353–54; and study of marijuana, 171–72; and violence, 434, 435

Drug Abuse Council, 387

Duke University, 402, 467, 480, 481, 482; Biomedical Research Program Training Program at, 255–57; and clinical scholars, 385; curriculum revision at, 254–60;

and health care, 386; and Interface Program, 480–85, 506, 507, 668n.25; Trinity College of, 481, 482, 483, 484, 485

Education, 24–25, 288–89, 526, 548; health, 102, 104, 198, 389, 426; and health care, 408; liberal, 466–68, 472, 483, 503, 504, 506, 509, 510; and mental health, 32, 45; public, 45, 79, 185
Education, medical, 3–4, 15–16, 29, 131–32, 145, 194, 197, 198–99, 212, 411; aid to programs in, 218–312, 335, 336, 344, 442, 537, 538, 541–43, 545; combined with science and engineering, 378–82; and the community, 214, 298–312, 553; conferences on, 384, 663n.69; continuing, 205–6, 311, 323, 409, 463, 539, 553, 554, 555; and creative scholarship, 153–62; and curriculum reform, 242–77, 342, 408, 409, 442, 463–68; directions for 1980s in, 553–57; financing, 312–17, 343, 553, 555; and health care, 222, 226, 366, 382; interdisciplinary, 148–49; international, 410, 462; and liberal arts, 466–68, 472, 483, 497, 502, 506; for minorities, 367–82; problems of, 219, 402, 509, 548, 549–53; and psychiatry, 79; and public health, 106, 109, 144; redefinition of, 469; regionalization of, 413–18; and research, 148, 162, 174, 193; specialization in, 218–19, 223, 554; technology in, 411–12, 417–18; and universities, 657n.179. *See also* Fellowships; Grants
Electronmicroscopy, 421, 423
Emergency medical technicians (EMTs), 396–97
Emory University, 120, 348, 454
Endocrinology, 170, 173, 174, 175, 178, 180–81, 188, 545
Epidemics, 89, 189
Epidemiology, 183, 188–92, 300, 306, 499, 501
Epilepsy, 162, 170
Exploratory Conference on Medical Services and Medical Education (1966), 384

Family practice, 224, 243, 280, 323, 351, 386
Federal Trade Commission, 526

Fellowships, 146–61; advanced medical, 148–53, 154, 156, 192, 198, 410, 442; for creative scholarship, 153–60, 532, 642n.24; increase in, 49, 53, 146; individual, 55, 160–62, 410, 463, 541; for nurses, 347; in psychiatry, 57, 58, 59, 60, 61, 63, 64, 148, 212; for rural physicians, 120, 126–32, 198, 639nn. 88, 90, training, 33, 34, 42, 198; traveling, 49; to visiting teachers, 53. *See also* National Medical Fellowships, Inc.
Field Foundations, 368
Finger Lakes Health Systems Agency, 140
Fisk University, 375, 376
Flexner Report (1910), 129, 277, 466, 467, 468, 510, 541
Ford Foundation, 82, 185, 315, 336, 338, 340, 373, 375, 387, 391
Fort Lauderdale Conference of 1966, 455
Foundations, 4, 21, 340, 514; capabilities of, 557–58; collaboration of, 367, 375, 382–87, 411; function of, 197, 207, 312, 335, 462, 535; hostility to, 21, 24, 84; and research, 162, 193
Franklin C. MacLean Fund for Blacks in Medicine, 368. *See also* National Medical Fellowships, Inc.
Fund for the Advancement of Medical Education, 288

General Education Board, 1, 467. *See also* Rockefeller Foundation
Genetics, 223, 255, 264, 282, 336, 366, 418–21, 474, 496
Geriatrics, 308, 351, 411, 551
Gombe Stream Reserve (Tanzania), 432, 436. *See also* Stanford University, Laboratory of Stress and Conflict of
Government: and aid to community programs, 426; and aid to medical education, 369, 371, 541; vs. foundations, 462; and health care, 438, 518–19; influence of comprehensive medicine on, 242; and medical programs, 469; and nurse-practitioners, 349, 355; spending of, on public health, 318, 336; support of, for medical research, 196, 207, 209, 214, 218, 335. *See also* United States Public Health Service
Grants: and capital funds, 312–17; CF's attitude to, 513; classification of, 173; for comprehensive care, 227, 232; and conflict-

Grants (*continued*)
  of-interest, 217; for construction, 337, 343, 377; evaluation of, 228, 249–52; ideas for, 165–66; 313–14; and medical institutions, 344; planning, 223, 227, 244, 379, 388, 424, 513, 520; post–World War II, 172–78; timing of, 535; unrestricted, 314–17. *See also* Medical schools; Research
Greater New York Fund, 329
Group for the Advancement of Psychiatry (GAP), 33, 79–80, 455, 539
Group practice, 243, 333, 343, 390, 412, 424

Harkness fortune, 10–13
Harper and Row, Hoeber Medical Division of, 531, 532
Harriet Lane Home (Johns Hopkins University), 175, 191
Hartford Foundation, 288
Harvard Community Health Plan, 387–92, 402, 424, 448, 545
Harvard Medical School, 33, 59, 146, 216, 244, 450, 480; and community health, 387, 387–92, 426; grants to, 66, 163, 170, 175, 178, 180. *See also* Children's Hospital; Harvard Community Health Plan; Peter Bent Brigham Hospital
Harvard-MIT Division of Health Sciences and Technology, 378–82
Harvard University, 344, 345, 459; Center for Community Health and Medical Care at, 425; Center for the Evaluation of Clinical Procedures, 446; collaboration with MIT, 378–82; Department of Pediatrics at, 387; Department of Social Relations at, 153; Harvard Planning Group at, 551; health-care delivery programs at, 345; and health studies, 362; integrated curriculum at, 260–65; Medical Center of, 217, 387; medical research at, 166, 168, 170, 175, 178, 180; Oliver Wendell Holmes Society at, 549; and rural physicians, 127, 128, 129; School of Public Health at, 346, 379, 389, 439, 443, 446. *See also* Harvard Community Health Plan; Harvard Medical School; John F. Kennedy School of Government
Harvard University Press, 531, 532, 534
Hastings Center (New York), 452
Haverford College, 369
Hawaii Medical Association, 282
Health, 3, 4; community, 208, 241, 500, 538; economics of, 362, 379; environmental, 86, 87, 332, 411, 453, 496, 501; maintenance of, 205; as social responsibility, 197
Health care, 2, 3, 199, 407, 411, 517–19, 536; ambulatory, 224, 448, 457, 532; community, 208, 241, 300–303, 306, 387–92, 501; costs of, 144, 306, 309, 326, 343, 351, 362, 382, 443, 519, 549, 556, 557; crisis in, 341–42, 382, 389, 408, 547; international, 410, 459, 462; national, 306, 310, 311, 323; primary, 253, 281, 285, 299, 326, 350, 355, 426, 540, 553; research in, 162, 239, 651n.50; rural, 89–90; in Scandinavia, 159; and universities, 312, 344–45, 389, 402, 420, 496–97, 504, 547, 549. *See also* Home care
Health centers: community-based, 208, 241, 299, 456, 546; university-based, 243, 245, 556. *See also* Health; Health care
Health insurance, 23, 305, 311, 323, 326, 332, 343; of New York City employees, 333, 391
Health Insurance Plan of Greater New York, 333, 334
Health professionals: and physicians, 543; training of, 345–58; 377, 463, 465, 469, 478, 504, 547; and university advisors, 483–84
Health Training Improvement Act, 357
Henry Phipps Psychiatric Clinic (Baltimore), 33, 39, 58–59
Hershey conference (Hershey, Pa.), 76, 77, 78, 79
Hill-Burton Hospital Survey and Construction Act (1946), 143, 144, 196, 207, 214, 242, 318, 325, 641nn. 123, 126
Home care, 328–34, 337, 425; and medical education, 224, 226, 228, 229, 231, 240, 241; for terminally ill, 429, 430. *See also* Montefiore Hospital
Hospice in New Haven, 413, 427–31, 556
Hospital Construction Act, 137
Hospital of Saint Raphael, 378
Hospitals, 3, 23, 34, 198, 199, 427; and blacks, 115; building of, 520, 540, 641nn. 123, 126; cost of, 328; and medical schools, 15–17; outpatient departments of, 120; regional, 132–41, 540; rural, 31, 107, 110, 114–26, 198, 214, 367, 539, 540; teaching, 552
House of the Good Samaritan (Boston), 163
Howard University, 368, 373, 374

Hunterdon Medical Center (N.J.), 318–28, 540–41, 658n.184; financing medical care at, 323–28; medical care at, 321–22; teaching programs at, 322–23
Hyams Trust, 426
Hygiene: dental, 101–2; teaching of, 88, 89, 109
Hypertension, 165, 169, 184, 448
Hypertension: A Policy Perspective (Center for the Analysis of Health Practices), 448

Illinois Board of Higher Education, 345
Immunization, 84, 85, 87, 193, 223, 538; diphtheria, 84, 88, 103
Industrial District Nursing Association, 88
Influenza, 119, 189, 190
Institute for Child Guidance (CF), 46, 48–56. *See also* Bureau of Children's Guidance
Institute of Juvenile Research, 57
Institute of Medicine, 386
Institute for Policy Studies, 455
Inter-Agency Task Force on Medical Education of Minority Students, 370
Interface Program (CF), 463–511, 548, 669n.28; Board of Director's response to, 469–70; and curriculum reform, 550; development of, 463–69; diversity of, 505–6, final recommendations of, 507–9; ground rules of, 512–13; retrospective look at, 509–11
International Conference on Mental Hygiene, 53
International Council for Educational Development, 284
International Institute for the Study of Human Reproduction, 361
Ittleson Family Fund, 429, 430

Jane Coffin Childs Foundation, 643n.24
Jefferson Medical College, 322
John F. Kennedy School of Government (Harvard University), 413, 438–40; Public Policy Program of, 438–40
Johns Hopkins Hospital (Baltimore), 58–59, 115, 190, 191
Johns Hopkins University, 335, 385, 386, 458, 552; experiment in medical education, 225, 342, 402; first joint medical school-hospital at, 17; integrated curriculum at, 265, 266, 267–68, 276; Interface Program at, 497–99, 505, 506, 507; medical research at, 164, 165, 169, 175;
School of Hygiene and Public Health of, 188, 190, 191; School of Medicine of, 23, 24, 120, 164, 169, 198, 287, 439, 440, 459, 497
Joint Commission on Accreditation of Hospitals, 137
Joint Committee on Methods of Preventing Delinquency, 42, 525, 526
Josiah Macy, Jr., Foundation, 2, 217, 333, 355, 367, 369, 375, 376, 382
Journal of the American Medical Association, 143, 364, 530
Journal of Medical Education, 252
Judge Baker Foundation (Boston), 39, 57, 63, 387
Julius Rosenwald Fund, 1, 367, 368, 373
Juvenile courts, 38, 39, 40, 43, 46, 59, 537. *See also* Judge Baker Foundation
Juvenile delinquency, 23, 25, 26, 40–48, 537, 627n.23. *See also* Juvenile courts; Program for the Prevention of Juvenile Delinquency
Juvenile Protective Association, 38, 39
Juvenile Psychopathic Institute, 39

Kaiser Family Foundation, 311, 365, 386, 387, 403, 440
Kaiser Health Plan, 324
Kaiser-Permanente Medical Care Program, 324, 412
Kankakee Hospital (Ill.), 35
Kellogg Foundation, 284, 288, 367, 375, 376
Kresge Foundation, 419

Laboratory of Zoophysiology (Copenhagen), 156
Lafayette County Health Center (Fla.), 456–57
Lakewood conference (N.J.; 1921), 26, 40, 628n.27
Lenox Hill Hospital (New York), 322
Life Insurance Medical Research Fund, 643n.24
Lincoln Hospital (New York), 458
London School of Hygiene and Tropical Medicine, 346
Long Island College of Medicine, 151, 177. *See also* State University of New York
Lord Dawson Report (Great Britain), 134
Lucille P. Markey Charitable Trust, 217

McGill University, 385
McKinsey and Company, 323

Macy Conferences, 2. *See also* Josiah Macy, Jr., Foundation
Malpractice insurance, 324
Marijuana, 171–72. *See also* Drug abuse
Markle Foundation, 2, 185, 255, 375, 643n.24
Marriage Council of Philadelphia, 360
Mary Imogene Bassett Hospital, 454–55
Massachusetts Department of Public Health, 164
Massachusetts Department of Public Welfare, 241
Massachusetts Eye and Ear Infirmary, 447
Massachusetts General Hospital, 146, 156, 175, 195, 332, 439, 447
Massachusetts Institute of Technology (MIT), 86, 345, 378, 408; College of Health Sciences, Technology, and Management (Whitaker College) at, 381; Lincoln Laboratory of, 424
Massachusetts Medical Society, 128
Massachusetts State Department of Public Health, 147
Maurice Falk Medical Fund, 375
Medicaid, 241, 306, 310, 323, 326, 374, 448, 517, 555, 557
Medical Care Prices (federal report), 455
Medical College of Virginia, 292–93
Medical schools: admissions policies of, 265–66; CF support of, 208, 341; and comprehensive medicine, 208; curriculum in, 219–20; founding of new, 277–86, 403; growth of, 342, 554; and health care, 342, 389–90, 408, 545, 552; and hospitals, 15–17; improvement in, 204, 222–23, 544; postgraduate teaching in, 131, 146; and preventive medicine, 106–7; and psychiatry, 56, 61, 336; and public health, 106–7; research in, 552; revitalization of departments of, 418–40; sex education in, 358–62, 409, 442, 453, 459; and six-year programs, 669n.28; specialization in, 218, 260; state, 242; and universities, 312, 657n.179. *See also* Fellowships; *individual universities*; Teachers
Medicare, 242, 306, 310, 323, 326, 331, 341, 374, 383, 440, 517, 555, 557
Medicine: and anthropology, 248, 299, 301, 504; basic sciences of, 218; community, 281, 299–307, 311–12, 417, 424, 545; comprehensive, 173, 184, 203–10, 218, 224, 225–42, 303, 307, 311, 335, 336, 539, 542–48, 556; definition of, 221; ethics of, 411, 549, 550, 557; Harkness's interest in, 15–18; holistic, 67, 68, 197, 204–5, 224, 332, 544; and law, 443–45; "scientific," 218–19, 224, 542; social, 243, 334, 388, 542; sociology of, 336; specialization in, 218, 222, 382, 423, 542; and technology, 219, 223, 450, 553, 554, 557. *See also* Preventive medicine; Psychosomatic medicine; Research
Meharry Medical College, 367, 368, 373–77, 402; George W. Hubbard Hospital of, 373, 374
Mental health, 3, 30, 31–32, 34–37, 41; and child health, 38, 45, 184; and comprehensive medicine, 335–36; legacy of program in, 81–83; measurement of, 34–35. *See also* Child guidance clinics; National Institute of Mental Health; Psychiatry
Mental Health Materials Center, Inc., 359
Mental Hygiene Bulletin, 54
Michigan State College, 164
Michigan State University, 448; College of Human Medicine, 295
Midwifery, 452, 459
Milbank Memorial Fund, 2, 334, 375, 386
Millis Report, 253
Model Cities Program, 304
Montefiore Hospital: Division of Social Medicine of, 332–34; Family Health Maintenance Demonstration of, 333, 334; Home Care Program of, 328–34, 541; Medical Group of, 333
Mount Sinai Hospital (New York), 115, 195; hospitals affiliated with, 304, 305; School of Medicine of, 303–7, 311, 333, 364, 402, 406

National Academy of Sciences, 398, 402, 436, 537
National Association for the Advancement of Colored People (NAACP), 370
National Association for Public Health Nursing, 96
National Board of Medical Examiners, 249, 252, 302, 368, 409, 502; and certification standards, 196, 647n.101; grants to, 402, 411–12
National Bureau of Economic Research (NBER), 362–65
National Cancer Institute, 429, 642n.24. *See also* United States Public Health Service
National Center for Health Services Research, 242, 365
National Child Health Council, 39

Index of Subjects

National Child Labor Committee, 25
National Commission on Certification of Physicians' Assistants, 357
National Committee for Health Manpower, 340
National Committee for the Improvement of Nursing Services, 346
National Committee for Mental Hygiene, 23, 25, 26, 36; and CF, 26, 30, 47, 526; and child guidance clinics, 34, 47, 51, 52; and child psychiatry, 60; Division of Community Clinics of, 63; Division of Psychiatric Education of, 57; Division of Rehabilitation of, 76–77
National Committee on Visiting Teachers, 41, 42, 53
National Conference on Medical Costs, 455
National Conference on the Nomenclature of Disease, 195
National Conference on Social Work, 53
National Education Laboratory for the Blind, 23
National Foundation for Infantile Paralysis, 368
National Fund for Medical Education, 313
National Heart Institute, 642n.24. *See also* United States Public Health Service
National Information Bureau, 29
National Institute for Child and Maternal Health, 185
National Institute of Mental Health (NIMH), 59, 82, 336, 343, 433, 435, 447, 642n.24. *See also* United States Public Health Service
National Institutes of Health (NIH), 165, 196, 292, 374, 546; budget of, 469; decision making at, 214–15; fellowships of, 157, 642n.24; grants from, 255, 400, 532; and hospices, 429; and medical education, 378, 382, 384, 419, 420, 422; and medical research, 179, 192–93, 342, 399, 554. *See also* Bureau of Health Manpower Education; United States Public Health Service
National League for Nursing, Inc., 346–47, 348
National Library of Medicine, 450, 533
National Medical Fellowships, Inc. (NMF), 367–73
National Mental Health Act, 207
National Mental Health Association, 537
National Research Council, 643n.24
National Science Foundation, 469

National Sex Forum, 361
National Tuberculosis Association, 26
Neurological Institute (New York), 23, 165
Neurology, 147, 165, 170, 174, 181
Neurophysiology, 255
Neuropsychiatry, 33, 37, 57, 61–62
Neurosciences, 495–96
New England Medical Center (Boston), 134
New Haven Health Care, Inc., 397
New Haven Visiting Nurse Association, 429
New Jersey College of Medicine and Dentistry, 322
New School for Social Research, 53
New York Academy of Medicine, 164, 171, 319, 320, 455
New York Academy of Sciences, 454
New York Arbitration Society, 453
New York Child Labor Committee, 25
New York City Cancer Committee, 329
New York City Commitee for Mental Hygiene, 53, 75
New York City Health Department, 406; Division of Child Hygiene in, 39
New York City Mission, Woman's Board of, 88
New York Committee on Aftercare of Infantile Paralysis Cases, 25
New York Foundation, 333
New York Hospital, 63, 76, 163, 167, 179, 186; Children's Clinic of, 64; Payne Whitney Psychiatric Clinic at, 61. *See also* Cornell University Medical College
New York Nursery and Child's Hospital, 25
New York Postgraduate School, 127
New York School of Social Work, 25, 26, 29, 40, 41, 42, 47, 49, 51–52, 53, 530. *See also* Institute for Child Guidance
New York State Charities Aid Association, Mental Hygiene Committee of, 51
New York State Health Department, Division of Child Hygiene in, 39
New York State Hospitals, Pathological Institute of, 35
New York State Joint Hospital Survey and Planning Commission, 137–38
New York State League of Women Voters, 90
New York University, 319, 320; College of Medicine of, 150–51, 203, 209, 290, 320, 365, 366, 402; Honors Program at, 316; and preventive medicine, 128; research at, 164, 169, 170–71. *See also* New York University-Bellevue Medical Center

Index of Subjects

New York University-Bellevue Medical Center, 320, 322
NMF. *See* National Medical Fellowships, Inc.
Nomenclature, unified medical, 537
North Carolina Memorial Hospital, 238
Northeastern University, 402; nursing school of, 348
Northwestern University, 225, 265, 266, 268–71, 276, 315, 343
Nurse practitioners, 160, 349–51, 357, 547; pediatric, 349–50; school, 353–55
Nurses: education of, 136; fellowships for, 136, 345–49; public health, 88, 89, 142, 229, 233, 345, 349, 638n.74
Nurse Training Act, 357
Nursing, 136, 224, 307; new concepts of, 349–50; schools of, 346–48, 383. *See also* Nurses

Obstetrics, 24, 148, 151, 264; and comprehensive care, 233, 425; and nurse practitioners, 351; research in, 164–65, 170–71
Office of Economic Opportunity, 349, 458; Health Centers Program of, 383
Old Dominion Foundation, 73
Organism-environment interaction, 179–80, 207, 218
Outpatient clinics, 224, 227, 231, 232–35, 236–38, 254, 423, 555
Oxford University, 345

Paramedical personnel, 393, 399, 400, 401, 409, 457, 463, 547
Partnership for Health Act of 1966, 383
Pathological Institute (Ward's Island, N.Y.), 59
Patient Care Planning Council, 140
Peckham Experiment (London), 333
Pediatrics, 24, 51, 163, 175; and child health associates, 351–53; and comprehensive medicine, 233, 264; fellowships for, 148, 151, 153, 208–9; and nurse practitioners, 349–51, 353–55; preventive, 99, 198; and psychiatry, 33, 60, 61–65, 69, 73, 78, 81, 538
Peter Bent Brigham Hospital (Boston), 66, 178, 404, 448
Pharmacology, 218, 264, 375
Philadelphia General Hospital, 120
Philanthropy, early twentieth-century, 1–3, 13, 15
Physicians, 4, 205, 246–47, 256, 261, 469, 544; assistants to, 355–57, 547; and comprehensive medicine, 224, 231; family, 253, 280, 307, 543; and hospice idea, 430; income of, 552, 555; and liberal education, 466–67; and medical schools, 554; and nurse practitioners, 349, 350; and patients, 205, 224, 233, 237, 280, 306, 310, 543; postgraduate education for rural, 126–32; and psychiatry, 33, 36, 39, 49; and public health, 90, 106–7, 110, 300, 540; ratio of black, to black population, 373; and rural hospitals, 121–23; school, 89; shortage of, 277, 345, 349, 357, 383, 414; in society, 558; as teachers, 16, 257. *See also* Education, medical; Family practice; Group practice
Physicians' Forum, 332
"Physicians for the Twenty-First Century" (AAMC), 549, 550, 552
Physiology, 156, 169, 172–73, 199, 218, 263, 367, 375, 441; cardio-respiratory, 176–77, 179
Planning Act of 1966, 140
Presbyterian Hospital (New York), 15–16, 17, 22, 23, 195
President's Office of Science and Technology, 378
Preventive medicine, 4, 16, 22–23, 31, 300, 343, 537, 542, 548; and child development, 184; and comprehensive medicine, 230, 232, 233, 240; and environment, 37; experiments in, 333–34, and hospitals, 115, 140; and medical training, 205, 225–26, 240, 243, 298, 308, 501; and public health, 86–89, 93, 100, 109, 144, 198, 232, 539; and research, 309
Princeton University, 217, 324; Institute for Advanced Study at, 336
Proceedings of the American Sociological Society, 526
Program in Mental Hygiene (CF). *See* Program for the Prevention of Juvenile Delinquency
Program in Mental Hygiene and Child Guidance (CF), 46. *See also* Joint Committee on Methods of Preventing Delinquency
Program for the Prevention of Juvenile Delinquency (CF), 40–46, 49, 96, 197, 538; committees connected with, 629n.23
Provident Medical Associates, 367–68. *See also* National Medical Fellowships, Inc.
Psychiatrists: and child guidance, 50–51, 52; and comprehensive care clinics, 236,

248, 424, 501; and Cornell pilot clinic, 74; demand for, 79, 82; and juvenile delinquency, 38, 41, 43, 44, 198; salaries of, 55; training of, 31, 33, 44, 49, 50, 51, 52, 54, 56–62, 72, 79, 538; and Yale experiment, 55

Psychiatry, 29–33, 34, 35, 38; and child guidance, 38, 55–56, 198, 222; and comprehensive medical care, 208, 214, 228, 232, 233, 236, 240; fellowships for study of, 57, 58, 59, 60, 61, 63, 64, 148, 198, 208; government funding of, 207; and juvenile deliquency program, 82, 198; and medicine, 65–66, 69, 73–78, 83, 206; and pediatrics, 60, 61–65, 148, 198, 222, 537; psychoanalytic school of, 35, 67, 216; and public health, 80–81; and violence, 431; and Yale experiment, 72, 73. *See also* Psychiatrists

Psychologists, 37, 73, 250, 550; and child guidance, 38, 41, 43, 44, 50–51, 52, 53, 185; training of, 49, 50, 52, 54, 538

Psychosomatic medicine, 71, 74, 243; and comprehensive care, 226, 233, 236, 551; John Romano's programs in, 33, 66–69

Psychometric testing, 38, 52, 53

Public Education Association of the City of New York, 41, 42

Public health, 2, 22, 23, 26, 30, 31, 84–144, 194, 536; ancillary programs in, 141–42; and bacteriology, 84, 86, 87; and child welfare, 84, 633n.1; and comprehensive medicine, 230, 307, 311, 539; and education, 89, 106; federal funds for, 130, 214; and first diagnostic laboratory, 539; and government, 85, 86–87, 90, 318; and health centers, 89–90, 198, 214; and medical service, 89, 222, 320; and mental health, 81; and nursing, 89; and personal hygiene, 88; and physicians, 90, 106–7, 110, 300; and prevention of disease, 88, 89, 198, 550; and psychiatry, 33; public attitude toward, 84, 86, 92, 105; and rural services, 3, 106, 109–13, 539, 540, 638nn. 58, 60

Public Health Council of New York, 89

Race Betterment Conference (Battle Creek, Mich.), 187

Rensselaer Polytechnic Institute (RPI), 265, 273, 345

Research: biomedical, 2, 3, 259–60, 343, 554; cancer, 23; and child guidance, 51, 182–86; educational, 31, 537; grants for; 165–66, 172–78; health-services, 385, 389, 390, 520; legal, 25, 31, 537; longitudinal, 173–74, 178, 182–86, 207; medical, 3, 24, 29, 83, 109, 145–47, 148, 161–94, 196, 199, 214, 218, 335, 342, 537, 541–43, 544; and pharmaceutical companies, 174; psychiatric, 69, 74, 216; public understanding of scientific, 520; and regional hospitals, 136; reports of, 527; in social hygiene, 26; surgical, 17; and teaching, 296–97, 342; war-related, 167–68

Resident Physician's Handbook, The (CF), 120

Rheumatic fever, 163, 167, 174, 179–80, 190, 191, 320

Richard King Mellon Foundation, 384

Rip Van Winkle Foundation (Hudson, N.Y.), 318

Robert B. Brigham Hospital (Boston), 449

Robert Wood Johnson Foundation, 2, 284, 355, 365, 372, 386, 405, 494; and Center for the Analysis of Health Practices, 447; and community service, 426, 457; and emergency medical service, 398; and health-care delivery, 462, 517, 547; and home care, 241; and medical education of minorities, 371, 377

Rochester Regional Hospital Association. *See* Rochester (N.Y.) Regional Hospital Council

Rochester (N.Y.) Regional Hospital Council, 135, 138, 139–41

Rochester (N.Y.) Regional Hospital Plan, 133, 134–41

Rockefeller Foundation, 1, 115, 185, 190, 336, 355; and health care, 386, 387, 391; and medical education, 271, 288, 367, 373, 375, 467; and medical fellowships, 146, 203, 643n.24; and psychiatry, 82, 83; and public health, 98, 109, 110, 113

Rockefeller Institute for Medical Research, 1, 36, 151, 232, 365

Rockefeller Sanitary Commission, 2, 87

Rockefeller University, 423

Roscoe B. Jackson Memorial Laboratory (Bar Harbor, Maine), 170

Rosenwald Fund, 113

Russell Sage Foundation, 336

Rutgers University Medical School, 344

Rutherford Hospital (Murfreesboro, Tenn.), 118–19, 120

Index of Subjects 693

Salomon Winter Foundation, 183
St. Vincent's Hospital (New York), 322
Science: and humanities, 464, 465–66, 471–72; and law, 443–45; and medicine, 3, 15, 255–57, 261, 263, 281, 378, 464, 466, 510, 535, 544; and philanthropy, 2; public support for, 520, 534; teaching of basic, 245, 255–58, 260–65, 375, 377, 379, 509–10, 548, 551; writing on, 526, 534. *See also individual sciences*
Senate Subcommittee on Wartime Health and Education, 196
Sex Information and Education Council of the United States (SIECUS), 359
Sheppard and Enoch Pratt Hospital (Baltimore), 57
Sheppard-Towner Act, 39
Sloan Foundation, 368, 369, 375
Smith College School of Social Work, 42, 49, 50, 52, 53
Social sciences, 153, 204, 336, 379, 401, 520, 534, 544
Social Science Research Council, 336
Social workers: and child guidance, 50, 51, 52; and comprehensive care, 229, 231, 233, 248, 424; psychiatric, 43, 49, 50, 51, 53, 54, 63, 538; training of, 41, 44, 50, 54; and Yale experiment, 72, 73
Sociologists, 228–29, 250, 251, 307, 308, 344, 444
Southern Regional Education Board, 346, 347, 348, 374
Stanford University, 223, 265, 295, 335; Alcohol and Violence Clinic at, 433, 434; Human Biology Program at, 433; Laboratory of Stress and Conflict of, 413, 431–40; Outdoor Primate Facility at, 435; School of Medicine of, 274–75, 293, 360, 385, 403, 550
Stanford University Hospital, Child Psychiatry Clinic at, 61, 63; classification system at, 195; program in health-care delivery at, 345
State University of New York, 53; College of Medicine of, 177; at Stony Brook, 550
Strangeways Laboratory (Cambridge, Eng.), 157
Strong Memorial Hospital (Rochester, N.Y.), 69, 132, 133, 136, 139, 278
Subcommittee on Public Health, 143
Surdna Foundation, 391
Surgery, 24, 327, 445–46, 554
Surgical assistants, 357–58

Swampscott Study on Behavioral Science in Medicine (1966), 384

Teachers: fellowships for young, 148; training of, 3, 24, 41, 49, 102, 286–92, 296–98; visiting, 41, 42, 45, 49, 52, 53, 96
Technology, 2, 193, 326, 378, 553, 554, 557
Temple University, 225, 226; Comprehensive Medicine Program at, 235–38
Temple University Hospital, 237
Texas University, nursing school at, 348
Tuberculosis Preventorium for Children, 25
Tufts University, 127, 128, 315
Tulane University, Department of Medicine at, 75, 127, 128, 216, 402, 458, 532

United Nations Educational, Scientific, and Cultural Organization (UNESCO), 434
United States Children's Bureau, 113, 144
United States Commission on Industrial Relations, 21
United States Public Health Service (USPHS), 80, 96, 113, 141, 143, 334; budget of, 207; and CF, 114, 144, 209, 214; classification system of, 195; Department of Nursing Resources of, 427; fellowships of, 642n.24; and health economics, 364; and medical research, 174, 185, 191, 214; and medical school facilities, 279; Mental Health Council of, 80; and sanitation, 86
University of Alabama, 177, 348
University of Alaska, 415, 416
University of Buffalo School of Medicine, 286–95, 550
University of California Hospital, 64
University of California at San Diego, 467, 502–5; Health Professions Honors Program (HPHP) at, 504–5; Interface Program at, 502–5, 508; Warren College at, 502, 503, 504, 505
University of California at San Francisco, 361, 467
University of California School of Medicine, 64–65, 181, 208, 282
University of Chicago, 155, 362, 448, 467, 549; Graduate School of Social Service Administration at, 49; Interface Program at, 470, 471, 477–80, 505, 507; Liberal Arts of Biology and Medicine Department (LABM) at, 478–79; Pritzker School of

Medicine at, 477, 478, 479; Program for Education in the Arts and Sciences Basic to Human Biology and Medicine (ASHUM) at, 479–80, 668n.25

University of Cincinnati, 33, 66, 69

University of Colorado, 60, 173, 206, 214, 221, 290, 338, 340, 405; child-abuse program at, 412; and Child Health Associates Program, 351–53; comprehensive medicine experiment at, 225, 226, 228, 229, 231–35, 544; health-care delivery program at, 345; nurse-practitioner programs at, 349–51, 353–55. *See also* Child Research Council of Denver

University of Florida, medical school of, 223, 225, 277–81, 335, 455–58

University of Hawaii, 281–86; East-West Center of, 282; John A. Burns School of Medicine at, 284; Pacific Biomedical Research Center of, 282

University of Illinois, 293–94; Office of Research in Medical Education (ORME) at, 294

University of Kentucky, 223, 279; School of Medicine at, 298–303, 306, 311, 550

University of Long Island, 208

University of Louisville School of Medicine, 65, 80–81, 208, 300

University of Maryland, 348

University of Massachusetts, 448

University of Michigan, 292, 362; School of Public Health of, 346

University of Minnesota, 44, 441; program in human sexuality at, 360; teaching of psychotherapeutic medicine at, 77–78, 79, 80

University of Minnesota Hospital, 63, 78

University of New Mexico, 405

University of North Carolina, 225, 238–40, 242, 348

University of Pennsylvania: Center for the Study of Sex Education in Medicine, 359–60; fellowships at, 49, 57, 631nn. 64, 65; Leonard Davis Institute of Health Economics at, 323; medical research at, 164, 165, 171, 175, 177, 181–82; psychological clinic at, 38; school of dentistry at, 500; school of medicine of, 322, 323, 359, 402

University of Pennsylvania Hospital, 57, 527

University of Rochester, 290, 317, 455, 458–59; Department of Psychiatry at, 33, 69–70; Genesee Regional Educational Alliance for Health Personnel of, 412; Interface Program at, 470, 471–77, 505, 506; School of Medicine of, 69, 133, 139, 140, 353–54, 412, 471, 472, 473, 474

University of Southern California (USC), 295, 311, 345

University of Tennessee, 102, 120

University of Texas, 441

University of Toronto, 455

University of Vermont School of Medicine, 307–11, 348

University of Washington, 345, 414–17, 455

University of Wisconsin, 176

Urban Coalition, 403

Van Ameringen Foundation, 429, 430

Vanderbilt University: School of Medicine at, 64, 120, 127, 128, 129, 130, 345, 640n.93; School of Nursing at, 345, 348

Veterans Administration, 76, 80, 241, 435, 457

Violence, studies of, 409, 413, 431–40, 442

Violence and the Struggle for Existence (Stanford University), 431

Visiting Nurse Service of New York, 329

WAMI (Washington, Alaska, Montana, and Idaho) program, 413–18, 664n.107

Washington University (St. Louis), 467; medical research at, 165, 171, 181; Well Baby Clinic at, 99

Western Reserve University. *See* Case Western Reserve University

Whitaker College. *See* Massachusetts Institute of Technology

White House Conference on Child Health and Protection, 53

Willard Report, 253

Worcester Hospital (Mass.), 35

World Health Organization (WHO), 434

World War I, 146, 537, 538

World War II, 59, 130, 150, 167, 196, 518

Yale Law School Program in Law, Science, and Medicine, 443–45

Yale-New Haven Hospital, 398, 399, 400

Yale-New Haven Medical Center, 419, 427

Yale Physicians' Associate Program, 397

Yale Trauma Program, 387, 392–401, 402, 556

Yale University, 29, 345, 458; Child Study Center at, 177–78, 430; Department of Anatomy at, 413, 421–23, 665n.116; Department of Mental Hygiene and Psychiatry at, 33, 70–71, 632nn. 94, 95; and Harkness family, 10, 11, 13, 15, 116, 216; Program on Non-Profit Organizations of, 452; research at, 173, 178; School of Medicine of, 67, 70, 317, 445; School of Nursing at, 348, 419, 427; science teaching at, 509; student health service at, 70–73

Young Men's Christian Association of New Haven, 15

A. McGehee Harvey, M.D., who spent three years researching and writing this book, is Distinguished Service Professor of Medicine at the Johns Hopkins University School of Medicine and Physician-in-Chief, Emeritus, at the Johns Hopkins Hospital. Among his other books are *Research and Discovery in Medicine: Contributions from Johns Hopkins* and *Science at the Bedside: Clinical Research in American Medicine,* both available from Johns Hopkins. Susan L. Abrams is an editor at the Johns Hopkins University School of Medicine.

The Johns Hopkins University Press

"For the Welfare of Mankind"

This book was set in Century Old Style text and Franklin Gothic Condensed display type by EPS Group, from a design by Chris L. Smith. It was printed on 50-lb. Eggshell Cream Offset paper and bound in Roxite A by the Maple Press Company.